THE ROUTLEDGE COMPANION TO PERFORMANCE AND MEDICINE

The Routledge Companion to Performance and Medicine addresses the proliferation of practices that bridge performance and medicine in the contemporary moment.

The scope of this book's broad range of chapters includes medicine and illness as the subject of drama and plays; the performativity of illness and the medical encounter; the roles and choreographies of the clinic; the use of theatrical techniques, such as simulation and role-play, in medical training; and modes of performance engaged in public health campaigns, health education projects and health-related activism. The book encompasses some of these diverse practices and discourses that emerge at the interface between medicine and performance, with a particular emphasis on practices of performance.

This collection is a vital reference resource for scholars of contemporary performance; medical humanities; and the variety of interdisciplinary fields and debates around performance, medicine, health and their overlapping collaborations.

Gianna Bouchard is Head of the Department of Drama and Theatre Arts at the University of Birmingham, UK.

Alex Mermikides is D'Oyly Carte Senior Lecturer in Arts and Health at King's College London, UK.

ROUTLEDGE THEATRE AND PERFORMANCE COMPANIONS

For more information about this series, please visit: www.routledge.com/handbooks/products/SCAR30

THE ROUTLEDGE COMPANION TO PERFORMANCE AND MEDICINE

Edited by Gianna Bouchard and Alex Mermikides

Routledge
Taylor & Francis Group

LONDON AND NEW YORK

Designed cover image: *Habitation* (2021) Helen Pynor. Photograph by Helen Pynor. © Helen Pynor. Image courtesy of the artist.

First published 2024
by Routledge
4 Park Square, Milton Park, Abingdon, Oxon OX14 4RN

and by Routledge
605 Third Avenue, New York, NY 10158

Routledge is an imprint of the Taylor & Francis Group, an informa business

© 2024 selection and editorial matter, Gianna Bouchard and Alex Mermikides; individual chapters, the contributors

The right of Gianna Bouchard and Alex Mermikides to be identified as the authors of the editorial material, and of the authors for their individual chapters, has been asserted in accordance with sections 77 and 78 of the Copyright, Designs and Patents Act 1988.

British Library Cataloguing-in-Publication Data
A catalogue record for this book is available from the British Library

ISBN: 978-0-367-47773-8 (hbk)
ISBN: 978-0-367-47776-9 (pbk)
ISBN: 978-1-003-03650-0 (ebk)

DOI: 10.4324/9781003036500

Typeset in Times New Roman
by Apex CoVantage, LLC

CONTENTS

Contents

ILLUSTRATIONS

CONTRIBUTORS

Addie, Yewande O., RTI International, College of Journalism and Communications, University of Florida, United States. Yewande O. Addie is a narrative researcher at RTI International. She received her PhD in mass communications in 2022 and her MPH in 2019 from the University of Florida. Her research interests revolve around identity and culture in health messaging, arts and health edutainment and narrative storytelling interventions.

Aung, April Thant, Medical Humanities Research Cluster, Nanyang Technological University, Singapore. April Thant Aung is a PhD candidate working on theatre-based pedagogical intervention in medical education in Singapore. Her research interests are in the intersection of medicine, theatre, literature and medical education. She is a recipient of the NTU Research Scholarship, and her scholarly work has been published in *The Journal of Medical Humanities*.

Baldauf, Uta, Independent artist, United Kingdom. Uta Baldauf is a German-born British artist. She studied at Dartington College of Arts, which led to a wide range of projects in theatre, performance, video, music, curation and creative writing. Language and human vulnerability are recurring themes which are relevant to her current work as a registered nurse.

Barrett, Andy, De Montfort University and Artistic Director, Excavate Theatre Company, United Kingdom. Dr Andy Barrett is a community playwright and researcher whose company, Excavate, has created shows across the East Midlands since 2000, working with thousands of people in largely place-based communities. He has been involved in several international and interdisciplinary health-based projects, including producing audio stories for the End-of-Life Care for All NHS training programme.

Başar, Deniz, Atatürk Institute for Modern Turkish History, Boğaziçi University, Turkey. Deniz Başar is a theatre researcher, puppet maker and two-time national award-winning playwright from Turkey. In 2021, she finished her PhD at Concordia University with her work on contemporary Turkish theatre, entitled *A Dismissed Heritage: Contemporary Performance in Turkey Defined through Karagöz*. Her work has been published in numerous anthologies and peer-reviewed journals since 2019.

Beniston, Judith, University College London, United Kingdom. Judith Beniston is Professor of Austrian Literature and Cultural History at University College London and has published widely in that field. She co-edited the yearbook *Austrian Studies* from 2003 to 2011 and is one of the editors of *Arthur Schnitzler digital. Digitale historisch-kritische Edition (Werke 1905–1931)*.

Bichuetti, Jorge Antônio Nunes, Gregório Franklin Baremblitt Foundation, Félix Guatarri Institute and Psychosocial Care Center Maria Boneca, Brazil, Dreamer, poet, life artist, a potent creator and a star listener. Jorge was a physician, psychotherapist, schizodramatist, institutional analyst and schizoanalyst. For many years he was the Clinical Director of the Gregório Franklin Baremblitt Foundation. He was also a professor at the Félix Guatarri Institute in Belo Horizonte state of Minas Gerais in Brazil. Jorge passed away on a cloudy Wednesday on 5 October 2022.

Bleakley, Alan, Plymouth Peninsula School of Medicine, University of Plymouth, United Kingdom. In heading a department of medical education research at Peninsula Medical School UK, Emeritus Professor Alan Bleakley introduced an innovative core, compulsory and assessed medical humanities programme. He developed an international reputation in medical education and medical humanities, publishing widely, including twenty books. He is also a poet, with six collections.

Bogaert, Brenda, Institute of Humanities in Medicine, Lausanne Switzerland, France and Switzerland. Brenda Bogaert is a researcher in medical ethics at the Institute of Humanities in Medicine (CHUV/UNIL) in Lausanne, Switzerland. She has a PhD in philosophy, an important part of which involved developing a forum theatre play with epilepsy patients. Her research focuses primarily on patient participation.

Bouchard, Gianna, University of Birmingham, United Kingdom. Dr Gianna Bouchard is Head of the Department of Drama and Theatre Studies at the University of Birmingham. Her research focuses on medical discourse and practices in relation to contemporary performance, with a particular focus on identity politics and the ethics of display.

Bouchet, Pauline, Université Grenoble-Alpes, France, Lecturer in Theatre Studies. Pauline Bouchet has taught in France and Quebec. Specialist in contemporary dramaturgy, she is in charge of an 'Arts-Santé' research programme within Litt&Arts laboratory. She is interested in the links between the care environment and the theatre environment in 'shared dramaturgy' projects between carers and playwrights and is also involved in training doctors in the patient–carer relationship.

Burke, Katherine, Cleveland Clinic Lerner College of Medicine of Case Western Reserve University, United States. Katherine Burke is the Director of the Program in Medical Humanities at Cleveland Clinic Lerner College of Medicine. She lives in Ohio with her amazing daughter Vivian. Burke is pursuing a PhD in bioethics and medical humanities at Case Western Reserve University, focusing on the use of Theatre of the Oppressed for health justice.

Case, Gretchen A., University of Utah, United States. Dr Gretchen A. Case is the Director of the Center for Health Ethics, Arts, and Humanities at the University of Utah, where she is a faculty member in the Department of Theatre and the Department of Internal Medicine. She has taught arts and humanities at six universities and four medical schools.

Chandradasan, Artistic Director, Lokadharmi Theatre, Kochi, India. Dr Chandradasan is a designer, director, dramaturg, actor, playwright, writer, editor and translator. He is a recipient of the Fulbright–Nehru Fellowship for professional and academic excellence. He has visited the US, Finland, Lithuania, Bangladesh and Greece to direct plays, conduct workshops, participate in seminars, carry out research and perform in theatre festivals.

Coleman, Lucinda, Edith Cowan University, Australia. Dr Lucinda Coleman is a choreographer, writer, director, researcher and educator. She delights in teaching, making and performing and was founding Dance Maker of the performing arts collective *Remnant Dance*, 2010–2020. Her research interests include dance-making as a site for social justice arts engagement, collaboration, collective practices, site-specific dance-making and cross-cultural performance.

Dalton, James, University of Sydney, Australia. James Dalton is a director, dramaturg and PhD candidate based in Sydney, Australia, and a sessional academic for the BFA and MFA programs at the National Institute of Dramatic Arts, Australia.

Das, Shilpa, National Institute of Design, Ahmedabad, India. Shilpa Das teaches at the National Institute of Design, Ahmedabad, and has cumulative work experience of three decades in the education, publishing and voluntary sectors. She is on the advisory boards of the Missing Billion Initiative & Philips Inclusive Health Facility Co-Design Project, London, and the Centre for Disability Research and Training, KMC, Delhi University.

Day, Giskin, School of Medicine, Imperial College London, United Kingdom. Giskin Day is a principal teaching fellow at Imperial College London, where she leads an intercalated BSc in medical humanities. Her doctoral research, conducted at King's College London, consisted of an interdisciplinary inquiry into the role of gratitude in health care.

Dean, Bec, Independent curator and producer, Australia. Bec Dean is a curator, writer and educator and has worked for multi-disciplinary contemporary arts organisations in Australia as curator and producer since 1996. Since 2020 she has held the role of Senior Manager of Policy and Partnerships at Create NSW, the New South Wales state arts funding agency.

Dennis, Sarah-Mace, Independent Artist/Scholar, Ravensbourne University, United Kingdom and Australia. Sarah-Mace Dennis is an artist/filmmaker working at the intersections of critical writing, performance, spatial practice and the moving image. She has been commissioned to create public projection works in the UK and Australia. Her writing and films on consciousness, dance and brain plasticity have been exhibited and published internationally.

Fakhrkonandeh, Alireza, University of Southampton, United Kingdom. Alireza Fakhrkonandeh is an assistant professor in modern and contemporary drama and literary theory at the University of Southampton, UK. He completed his PhD at Warwick University in 2015. He is the author of two books, entitled *Body and Event in Howard Barker's Theatre of Catastrophe* (2019) and *Oil and Modern World Dramas* (2023). Fakhrkonandeh's works have featured in various journals, including *Symploke*, *Textual Practice*, *TDR*, *Angelaki*, *Comparative Drama*, *English Studies* and *JCDE*.

Fakunle, David O., Morgan State University, United States. David O. Fakunle, PhD, is a 'mercenary for change' primarily serving as Assistant Professor at Morgan State University in Baltimore.

Fakunle's interests include stressors within the built environment; manifestations of systemic oppression; and the utilisation of arts and culture to cultivate holistic health through humanity, justice, equity and ultimately liberation.

Fortuna, Cinira Magali, University of São Paulo at Ribeirão Preto College of Nursing, Brazil. Dr Cinira Magali Fortuna is a nurse and associate professor at University of São Paulo at Ribeirão Preto College of Nursing. She is also one of the Coordinators of the Center for Studies and Research in Collective Health (NUPESCO) Profa. Dra. Maria Cecília Puntel de Almeida. She is a former violin student and also a former choir singer. She is an admirer of the simple things in life. She is the grandmother of one baby girl called Ana Liz.

Garner Jr., Stanton B., University of Tennessee, United States. Stanton B. Garner Jr. is James Douglas Bruce Professor of English and Theatre at the University of Tennessee. His books include *The Absent Voice: Narrative Comprehension in the Theatre* (1989), *Bodied Spaces: Phenomenology and Performance in Contemporary Drama* (1994), *Trevor Griffiths: Politics, Drama, and History* (1999), *Kinesthetic Spectatorship in the Theatre: Phenomenology, Cognition, Movement* (2018) and *Theatre & Medicine* (2023).

Gotman, Kélina, King's College London, United Kingdom. Kélina Gotman is Professor of Performance and the Humanities at King's College London. She is author among others of *Choreomania: Dance and Disorder*, editor of *Theories of Performance: Critical and Primary Sources*, and co-editor among others of *Foucault's Theatres*. She writes widely on the history and philosophy of science and medicine, disciplines and institutions, language, performance and dance.

Hooker, Claire, Sydney Health Ethics, Sydney School of Public Health, University of Sydney, Australia. Dr Claire Hooker is Associate Professor in Health and Medical Humanities at Sydney Health Ethics and President of the Arts Health Network NSW/ACT.

Kelly, Traci, Independent artist and researcher, United Kingdom and Denmark. Traci Kelly is Honorary International Associate Research Fellow at the Institute of Drama, Dance & Performance Studies of De Montfort University. In 2023, the university acquired her solo archives and also those of the collaborative project, *hancock & kelly*, where they form part of the teaching and research ecology.

Lammer, Christina, Academy of Fine Arts Vienna, Austria. Christina Lammer is a research sociologist, filmmaker and bodywork practitioner based in Vienna. Her work combines sensory ethnography with analog film, video and body art. Lammer holds a PhD in sociology from the University of Vienna.

Lobel, Brian, Rose Bruford College, United Kingdom. Brian Lobel is a performer, teacher and curator whose work has shown work internationally from Harvard Medical School to Lagos Theatre Festival. Books include *Theatre & Cancer*, *BALL & Other Stories About Cancer* and *Purge*, and performances include *24 Italian Songs & Arias*, *BINGE* and *Sex with Cancer*. Brian is Professor of Theatre & Performance at Rose Bruford College.

Low, Katharine E., King's College London, United Kingdom. Dr Katharine E. Low is a practitioner-researcher with over twenty years' experience in socially engaged theatre and health, working in the fields of sexual health, gender equity and violence, in the UK and internationally.

Her collaborative research practice is embedded in collaborations with arts and cultural organisations, medical practitioners and NGOs to co-facilitate participatory theatre and arts-based projects.

Marshall, Robert, University of Exeter College of Medicine and Health, United Kingdom. Robert Marshall is an honorary associate professor at the University of Exeter Medical School, where he was involved in the medical humanities aspect of the curriculum. His research and publications have concentrated on the relevance of Homer's *Iliad* and *Odyssey* to medical education, culminating in the book *Rejuvenating Medical Education*.

Matumoto, Silvia, University of São Paulo at Ribeirão Preto College of Nursing, Brazil. Dr Silvia Matumoto is a nurse and an associate professor at University of São Paulo at Ribeirão Preto College of Nursing. She is also one of the Coordinators of the Center for Studies and Research in Collective Health (NUPESCO) Profa. Dra. Maria Cecília Puntel de Almeida. She is also a crochet and sewing lover.

Mermikides, Alex, King's College London, United Kingdom. Alex Mermikides is D'Oyly Carte Senior Lecturer in Arts and Health at King's College London. Her research into the interface between performance and medicine bridges scholarly publication (most recently *Performance, Medicine and the Human* [2020]); practice research with her company, Chimera; and curriculum development within the School of Medical Education.

Neumann, Annja, Cambridge Digital Humanities, University of Cambridge, United Kingdom. Annja Neumann is a cross-disciplinary artist-researcher with a background in digital humanities and medical humanities. Her recent work explores the staging of medical spaces in relation to questions of digital change and agency. Research performances she has produced include the hospital drama *Professor Bernhardi* and the online performance *Dr Tulp and the Theatre of Zoom*.

Numanoglu, Alp, Division of Paediatric Surgery, Faculty of Health Sciences, University of Cape Town, South Africa. Alp Numanoglu is a paediatric surgeon with an interest in the Minimally Invasive Surgery and Surgical Skills Training Centre. He has established the Surgical Skills Training Centre in Cape Town, where state-of-the-art training in a safe environment is provided for the surgeons in training.

Oliveira, Maria de Fátima, Gregório Franklin Baremblitt Foundation and Psychosocial Care Center Maria Boneca, Brazil. Maria de Fátima is a psychologist, schizodramatist and specialist in mental health and public health. She is also one of the founders of the Gregório Franklin Baremblitt Foundation and the Psychosocial Care Center Maria Boneca, Uberaba, Minas Gerais, Brazil. She is a dancer. A body with no tethers. A free body in a universe of feelings.

Ong, Adelina, Independent Researcher, Singapore/United Kingdom. Dr Adelina Ong is an independent applied performance researcher. Her synthetic (AI) applied performance practice is inspired by urban arts, placemaking practices and Death Cafes. She has published in *Theatre Research International* and *Research in Drama Education (RiDE)*. She is currently co-editing *Performing Homescapes* with Prof. Sally Mackey.

Orton, Liz, Independent artist, United Kingdom. Liz Orton is an artist working with archival practices, both real and imagined, to explore the tensions between personal and scientific forms of knowledge. Before taking time out of work in 2021 due to chronic illness, she was a lecturer in photography at London College of Communication and Associate Artist with Performing Medicine.

Parry, Simon, University of Manchester, United Kingdom. Simon Parry is Senior Lecturer in Drama and Arts Management at University of Manchester. His research explores the politics and aesthetics of creative practice at the intersection of health, science and the arts. His publications include *Science in Performance: Theatre and the Politics of Engagement* (Manchester: MUP, 2020).

Paterson, Katie, Guildhall School of Music & Drama, United Kingdom. Katie Paterson is Senior Creative Practice Tutor at Mountview and a PhD candidate at the Guildhall School of Music & Drama, where she also lectures in contextual studies. Paterson's practice research looks at the potential of queer feminist performance to illuminate lived experience and validate embodied knowledge(s).

Plastow, Jane, University of Leeds, United Kingdom. Jane Plastow is Professor of African Theatre at the University of Leeds. She has spent some forty years making, researching, training and writing about African theatre, having lived and worked in a number of countries across the continent. She is the author of the two-volume *A History of East African Theatre* (2020/2021, Palgrave Macmillan).

Pufahl, Jeffrey, University of Florida and Rutgers University, United States. Jeffrey Pufahl is a publicly engaged applied theatre scholar exploring the intersections of theatre and wellness. His research focuses on how participating in theatre and the arts improves wellness and how theatre can catalyse public engagement and critical dialogue around social justice and health issues.

Purcell-Gates, Laura, Bath Spa University, United Kingdom. Laura Purcell-Gates is Reader in Drama at Bath Spa University and co-artistic director of UK-based puppetry company Wattle and Daub, through which she conducts practice-based research on puppetry, object performance and non-normative bodies.

Pynor, Helen, Independent Artist, Australia/United Kingdom. Dr Helen Pynor is an artist and researcher whose work explores philosophically and experientially ambiguous zones, such as the life-death boundary. Pynor's work has been exhibited widely nationally and internationally, most recently at ZKM Center for Art and Media | Karlsruhe, and she has been awarded an Honorary Mention at Prix Ars Electronica, Austria.

Rauch, HG Laurie, Faculty of Health Sciences, University of Cape Town, South Africa. Dr HG Laurie Rauch is an adjunct senior lecturer in neurobiology of exercise. He supervises PhD and masters students and presents at international scientific conferences. Rauch's research explores the neurobiological underpinnings of mastering bodily stress reactivity and performing under pressure, whether it be in the sporting, corporate, artistic, academic or wellbeing arena.

Redling, Ellen, University of Birmingham, United Kingdom. Dr Ellen Redling is a lecturer in drama and theatre arts at University of Birmingham, UK. She has written numerous articles on contemporary theatre and co-edited a volume on *Non-Standard Forms of Contemporary Drama and Theatre*.

She is currently working on a new monograph project, *Theatres of Disruption in 21st-Century Britain* (forthcoming with Bloomsbury).

Reid, Steve, University of Cape Town, South Africa, As Chair of Primary Health Care at the University of Cape Town. Steve is a family physician with a background in rural medicine and an advocate for rural health. As a musician, he is also interested in the medical humanities and the role of the arts in health.

Rodríguez, Verónica, University of Alicante, Spain. Verónica Rodríguez is Lecturer in the Department of English Studies at University of Alicante, Spain and co-researcher at Contemporary British Theatre Barcelona (see www.ub.edu/cbtbarcelona/) and currently focuses on the intersection of theatre and performance practice and women's health. She is also a commissioned playwright, poet and certified women's health coach.

Russell, Emily, Rollins College, United States. Emily Russell is the Kenneth Curry Professor of Literature at Rollins College, US. She is the author of *Transplant Fictions: A Cultural Study of Organ Exchange* (2019) and *Reading Embodied Citizenship: Disability, Narrative, and the Body Politic* (2011).

Santos, Felipe Lima dos, University of São Paulo at Ribeirão Preto College of Nursing and CY Cergy Paris Université, Brazil. Felipe Lima dos Santos is a nurse and a PhD candidate in a double degree at the University of São Paulo at Ribeirão Preto College of Nursing and at CY Cergy Paris Université. He is also a member of the Center for Studies and Research in Collective Health (NUPESCO) Profa. Dra. Maria Cecília Puntel de Almeida. He was born and raised in the city of Manaus, in the state of Amazonas in Brazil.

Sidi, Leah, University College London, United Kingdom. Dr Leah Sidi is a lecturer in health humanities at University College London. Her research examines representations of mental distress and care in contemporary theatre, with a focus on feminist theatre and theory. Her monograph *Sarah Kane's Theatre of Psychic Life* was published by Methuen Drama in 2023.

Souraya, Sally, Clown Me In, United Kingdom/Lebanon. Sally Souraya is a multi-disciplinary artist, using activism and performance to promote social change. As a performer and trainer with Clown Me In, Souraya aims to empower communities and advocate for justices through arts, laughter and play. Souraya is also a mental health expert working on improving health systems and integrating art to promote wellbeing.

Sümbül, Yiğit, Ankara Hacı Bayram Veli University, Turkey. Yiğit Sümbül is an assistant professor at the Department of English Language and Literature at Ankara Hacı Bayram Veli University, Turkey. He completed his PhD at Ankara University, Turkey, in 2018 with a dissertation on a selection of Howard Barker's plays and published journal articles and book chapters on contemporary British drama, comparative literature and contemporary continental philosophy.

Summerskill, Clare, Freelance academic, United Kingdom. Clare Summerskill is a freelance academic, a playwright and a stand-up comedienne. Her publications include *Creating Verbatim Theatre from Oral Histories* (Routledge, 2021) and *Gateway to Heaven: Fifty Years of Lesbian and Gay Oral History* (Tollington, 2012), and she co-edited *New Directions in Queer Oral History. Archives of Disruption* (Routledge, 2022).

Tembeck, Tamar, Artist-run centre OBORO, Montreal, Canada. Tamar Tembeck, PhD, is an art historian, cultural worker, curator and writer with a background in the performing arts. Her research interests include visual cultures of illness and medicine, as well as performance and media studies. She is artistic director of the artist-run centre OBORO in Montreal, Canada.

Thompson, James, University of Manchester, United Kingdom. James Thompson is Professor of Applied Theatre at the University of Manchester. He has run theatre projects internationally and has written widely on applied theatre and socially engaged arts. His books include *Performance Affects* (2009); *Humanitarian Performance* (2014); and, edited with Amanda Stuart Fisher, (2020) *Performing Care*. His new book, *Care Aesthetics*, was published in summer 2022.

Underwood-Lee, Emily, University of South Wales, United Kingdom. Emily Underwood-Lee is Professor of Performance Studies at the University of South Wales. Her work focuses on contemporary performance and first-person narratives. She has a particular interest in stories of the maternal, gender, health/illness and heritage and the differences that sharing these stories can make for both teller and listener.

Verlander, Freya, University of Warwick, United Kingdom. Freya Verlander works at the University of Warwick in the Theatre and Performance Studies department. Her research interests are, broadly, in the field of skin studies. Recent publications include *(Skin)Aesthetics (The First Manifesto)* and an article in *Performance Research* exploring the role of touch in pandemic theatre. Her wider research interests include exploring the interfaces between science, the senses and different modes of performance.

Whalley, Joanne 'Bob', University of the Arts London, United Kingdom. Joanne 'Bob' Whalley is an artist, dramaturg and acupuncturist who focuses on radical kinship and politics of care. She is Director of Doctoral Training and Development at University of the Arts London, UK. Her book *Between Us: Audiences, Affect and the In-Between* (Palgrave Macmillan, 2017) celebrates spaces which cause an affecting and bodies affected.

Willson, Suzy, Clod Ensemble, United Kingdom. Suzy Willson creates original performance rooted in movement and music. She is Co-Artistic Director of Clod Ensemble and has directed all of their productions to date. She also leads the company's Performing Medicine initiative and is Professor of Movement, Arts & Medicine at Queen Mary University of London.

Wilson, Michael, Loughborough University, United Kingdom. Michael Wilson is Professor of Drama at Loughborough University, where he is also Director of the Storytelling Academy, a research centre focused on applied storytelling for social change, with projects across the globe relating to health, environment and education. His research interests lie broadly within the field of popular and vernacular performance.

Wisser, Wilfried, Medical University Vienna, Austria. Wilfried Wisser is Associate Professor of Surgery at the Department of Cardiac Surgery of the Medical University in Vienna, Austria. In his research he focuses on minimally invasive cardiac surgery. He has collaborated with sociologist and filmmaker Christina Lammer since 2015.

ACKNOWLEDGEMENTS

Our first thanks go to all authors who have contributed to this volume. It has been a long time in the making, especially because its development and initial stages coincided with the global pandemic. Working with authors from around the world meant that the waves of infections and intensities of the illness affected everyone differently, and we are, therefore, very grateful for our contributors' efforts, that they found time to read and think and write in the midst of other pressures. We are grateful, too, for everyone's patience and understanding as we worked with each contributor to best accommodate their own timescales and pressures. It has been an exciting and stimulating dialogue, and we have very much enjoyed collaborating with such a diverse range of scholars and practitioners. We hope that you enjoy the volume and that it allows further opportunities for exchange and collaboration among an excitingly eclectic field of enquiry and creativity.

Thanks also go to our colleagues in our respective institutions. To Gianna's colleagues at the University of Birmingham, whose continued support and friendship is so important for her work and thinking. For Alex, the development of this project straddled her move from Guildhall School of Music & Drama to the School of Medical Education at King's College London, that is, from one specialist institution dedicated to nurturing the next generation of performing artists to one cultivating tomorrow's doctors. Her appreciation goes to colleagues in each of these environments, whose openness and encouragement helped sustain her curiosity about the interface between performance and medicine. Throughout, our students continue to be vital to our thinking, too, so thanks for their energy and insights. Special thanks, too, to Katie Paterson and Michał Kawecki, for your patient and painstaking assistance with the editorial process. We would also like to thank Routledge for supporting this project and helping to bring it to publication.

Finally, but by no means least, our deepest thanks go to our families and loved ones, who keep us going with their love and encouragement. Living with an academic is not always easy, especially when they are working on a book of this scale. Alex gives a special thanks to her partner, Matt, for his steadfast support; for keeping the home fires burning during writing retreats and conference trips; for giving the children love, attention and bubble tea; and for providing comic relief at times of stress. Special thanks also from Gianna to her partner Paul for his constant support, for being an inspiration and guide and for sharing a love for a cup of tea!

And our thanks go to each other – the journey is so much more interesting when you are travelling with a friend!

INTRODUCTION

Gianna Bouchard and Alex Mermikides

This edited collection addresses the proliferation of practices that bridge performance and medicine in the contemporary moment and which come from different perspectives – epistemological, philosophical, professional, disciplinary and artistic. As such, the scope of the volume includes but is not limited to medicine and illness as the subject of theatre and performance, the performativity of illness and the medical encounter, the roles and choreographies of the clinic; the use of theatrical techniques, such as simulation and role-play, in medical training; and modes of performance engaged in public health campaigns, health education projects and health-related activism. With a particular emphasis on performance practices, the chapters reveal the diverse approaches and discourses that emerge at the interface between medicine and performance. In other words, the contributors consider how medicine is experienced in and through performance, on the stage and in the everyday, and how performance is made in response to medicine, as exploration, resistance and critique. Throughout the book, medicine and performance are understood as equally valid epistemologies and sets of practices that intersect and overlap in different ways: medicine can be a form of performance, and performance can operate as a sort of medicine. This conjunction of medicine and performance is a particularly rich ground for interdisciplinarity, enabling debate and dialogue around prescient issues such as subjectivity, identity, embodiment, health and illness, often in the face of complex and troubling bio-ethical dilemmas, which appear as much in the current moment as in the past. The unequal relations between medics and patients, between medical knowledge and lay expertise, underpinned by professional practices, languages and technologies, can all contribute to exploitative, coercive, manipulative and prejudicial attitudes and behaviours that are also explored in some of the book's content.

The sub-discipline of performance and medicine is relatively new, but it is a vibrant field, with more publications emerging in relation to an increased proliferation of artistic outputs relevant to this interface and a growing interest in health and wellbeing more widely.[1] At the same time, the medical humanities is strengthening and consolidating, but it often overlooks performance or focuses on only a few of its facets, such as narrative and empathy or performance as a mode of therapy.[2] There is also less attention given to more performative modes of practice related to medicine, health care and health, such as lived and performed experiences of illness or health care in the everyday. We hope that this volume redresses some of that imbalance, introducing new voices and creative approaches that demonstrate the vitality of the field and the significance of the

DOI: 10.4324/9781003036500-1

imbrication of performance and medicine across a range of locales, actors and topics. The book takes stock of current thinking and practices whilst also identifying key shifts in the field over the last two decades or so and new work.

Focusing mainly on the contemporary period, given the richness of the present time in relation to the subject, the book still gives due attention to the complexity of the histories of this interface, particularly in order to contextualise the current state of play. It is organised thematically to loosely follow a medical journey, from a patient's symptoms and their lived experience or the performativity of illness, to diagnosis and the performance of medicine as the patient is medicalised, through to treatment and recuperation, the ethics and effects of these encounters and practices, and finally to various medical futures, in terms of experiments, limit cases and new horizons. Performance is broadly understood as including the 'everyday', for example, the performance of professional and social identities in the consulting room, as well as incorporating various forms of practice, such as plays, dance, ritual and puppetry. Medicine is examined mainly from a Western perspective because of its place as the current dominant paradigm and because the ambivalent position it holds in the public imagination merits discussion. Western medicine pervades contemporary subjectivity and not only in the so-called Western world. The book, therefore, understands medicine as a historically and culturally contingent set of practices and acknowledges alternative ideas about how the body functions and how best to keep it well and healthy.

As editors, we are both performance scholars, and Mermikides is also a theatre-maker, so the book champions performance practice as well as performance scholarship. Such work takes diverse approaches to its objects of study, which are not confined to what happens on stage or in the pages of a play text. A global spread of such scholarship and performance-making is represented through contributors who are expert in practices in their own local, regional and/or national contexts. We have also included important perspectives and contributors from beyond the field of theatre and performance studies, for example, from medical sociology and ethnography, medical history, from health care professionals and medical educators. Contributions are either in the form of academic essays or 'snapshots' of practice that focus more exclusively on artistic responses to medicine from a performance perspective.

Given the scope and depth of the interface between medicine and performance, this introduction begins by explaining and defining these two key fields and their relationship to each other, making connections with the interdisciplinary aims of the volume and as explored by our contributors. They are not exhaustive accounts but set out the key facets of each to contextualise them and provide insight into the fundamental terms, practices and ideas that have informed their development and which we believe to be significant in understanding the intersections between performance and medicine. This leads into a discussion of critical thinking that has influenced the recent academic and artistic development of the imbrication of performance and medicine, and we then take the opportunity to identify the main shifts in thinking and practice that we have witnessed in the last decade or so in this area. These epistemological and practical transformations are present in the work of our authors as they respond to the cultural, social, political, medical and technological shifts that they have witnessed and which impact their research and creativity. The final section of this introduction provides an overview of the book's structure. We begin, then, with medicine, considering its ubiquity, reach and epistemological development and examining some of its ethical difficulties.

A definition of medicine

For the purposes of this volume, we define 'medicine' quite broadly to encompass biomedical research, where the biomedical 'features the increasingly biological scientific aspects of the practices of clinical medicine', the development and regulation of novel treatments, the provision of health care services by professional workers and their education and the design and dissemination of public health policy (Clarke *et al.*, 2003, p. 162). Western medicine, thus conceived, merits our attention because it is a domain of immense scale and power, with far-reaching, often life-or-death, consequences on individuals, communities, nations and beyond. For this reason, it is practised by those whose expertise and authority have been validated by formal qualifications, within systems and designated institutions of national scale, often sustained through substantial investment from the state, commercial and philanthropic sectors, and subject to close governmental oversight and public accountability (even if these are not consistently achieved across all national contexts). Indeed, its importance often exceeds national boundaries, for example, in research collaborations between nations (the Human Genome Project, 1990–2003, brought together research centres across United States, Europe and East Asia in order to map the entire human genome), the international adoption of regulatory standards for drug development and approval, consensus statements about professional frameworks and education for health care workers and policy responses to large-scale health crises and priorities (as seen with the inclusion of 'Health and Wellbeing' as one of the United Nations' seventeen Sustainable Development Goals).[3]

In putting biomedical research first in our list of practices encompassed by medicine, we are in effect conceiving medicine as an epistemological paradigm as well as a set of institutional practices. Medicine deals with knowledge (of the human body and of the behaviours, environmental substances and factors that might impact its efficient functioning): discovering new insights, translating it into therapies and health guidelines and forming professional categories, career paths and identities based on its demonstration through various academic qualifications and research publications. It often prioritises specific forms of knowledge – empirical and rationalist modes – at least in the context of the laboratory and, especially, the clinical trial where objectivity, reproducibility and predictability of results and generalisability are of paramount importance. The generation and dissemination of such knowledge requires the formation of specialised spaces, where interactions with patients and research materials can be highly specialised: laboratories, hospital wards, operating theatres and a close affiliation or merging with academic institutions. Within these various formal institutional settings, medicine is categorised into multiple disciplines and specialisms, for example, those relating to specific bodily systems or parts (for example, immunotherapy, neurology), diseases (such as cancer, depression, HIV/AIDs) or health threats (for example, addiction or obesity).

In conceiving of the scientific investigation of the body and of pathology as definitive of Western medicine, we are following Michel Foucault, whose *Birth of the Clinic* (published in English in 1973) viewed medicine as a practice rooted in the practices of dissection and anatomy. For him, the move from domestic to hospital-based health care in eighteenth-century Paris gave doctors unprecedented access to the cadavers that could be studied to ascertain the causes and location of disease (an effect of which was the specialisation and spatialisation of medicine noted previously). This in turn instituted new ways of understanding what we are and how we might address our bodily frailty and established a particular way of looking at the bodies of the living – the 'medical gaze'. These offered complex mechanisms through which various signs and symptoms of the body might reveal dysfunction rather than viewing the suffering individual as the object of care and charity. For Foucault, this also led to a stark power differential between the medical professional as an expert and the patient as the object of their investigation. This objectification of both patient and doctor is but one of the many critiques directed at Western medicine by followers of Foucault and by others. Ivan Illich's *Limits to Medicine*, for example, famously declared the medical establishment 'a major threat to health' (1975, p. 3), because of what he saw as its hubristic failure to counter disease (he attributed historically decreasing mortality rates to the development of sanitation, improved housing and better nutrition) and the ineffectiveness or harm caused by its interventions. Biopolitical philosophers such as Roberto Esposito (2008) and Giorgio Agamben (1998) point to the collusion of the medical profession in horrific genocidal and eugenic programmes, such as those of the Nazi regime. Feminist scholars such as Haraway (1991), Grosz (1994) and Shildrick (1997) describe the patriarchal paradigms inherent in medicine's conceptualisations of the body (for example, its tendency to demarcate it from the mind and to take the male body as its norm) and in health care practices that sequester authority to men, privileging masculine forms of knowledge and erasing female experience.

Although we have dedicated one of the five parts of this volume to these and other negative 'side effects' of medicine, we have otherwise attempted to find a balance between chapters that criticise and those that celebrate various aspects of medicine (though rarely to the extent that historian Roy Porter went to in declaring medicine 'the greatest benefit to mankind' [1997]) – the majority taking a more neutral stance to this vast and contradictory phenomenon. We have, however, also decided to broaden the scope beyond this conceptualisation of Western medicine as a scientific enterprise. We have included, for example, in Part 1, a set of chapters focussed on experiences, representations and metaphors of illness. As well as developing the means to appropriately remediate ill health and trauma, medicine has also provided a language to name, describe and understand experiences and states in relation to health, illness, disability, impairment and so on. Medical terminology and its imaginary have entered common parlance, most obviously perhaps in television advertisements that use 'the science bit' to sell even shampoos and skin care. Our experiences of health and illness, however, exist beyond Western medicine and can be understood through different paradigms (spiritual, philosophical and so on), even if it is difficult, in the contemporary era and in the global north, to extricate the biomedical view.

This volume therefore encompasses a wide range of practices and activities directed at understanding and conceptualising the working of the human body and mind and at alleviating suffering associated with ill health or trauma. This includes practices and activities undertaken by people whose understandings and conceptualisations of the human condition are founded in their own experiences of ill health rather than formal medical qualifications or whose approaches to remediating suffering take place outside clinical spaces and biomedical paradigms. Many of these practices have historic roots in domestic (often female), 'folk', indigenous and spiritual healing crafts that predate the emergence of Western medicine in the early modern period – and that have been, at different historical moments, co-opted by it or excluded from it.[4] Think, for example, of the way the male-dominated medical discipline of obstetrics was established in the eighteenth century, at the expense of women's expertise in home-based birthing and midwifery.[5] We also give attention to another human enterprise that sits alongside medicine's pursuit of knowledge: the prosocial drive to help when we are faced with human suffering, to care for others. Again, this predates and operates beyond the institution of medicine, as well as within it. And it is not the exclusive domain of those with medical qualifications. In Part 3 we give attention to performance practitioners attempting, in a similar vein and alongside their medical counterparts, to counter the ravages of illness and associated ills and to promote health with specific communities.

Our broad scope is bolstered by the widening characterisation of health, crystallised in the much-quoted definition by the World Health Organization as 'a state of complete physical, mental and social well-being and not merely the absence of disease and infirmity', which implicitly broadens the remit of health care providers to include support of the 'mental' and 'social' dimensions of human existence.[6] Inflected by shifts in terms of the health conditions of specific patient populations, one key example is the increase in diseases associated with more affluent lifestyles and longer lives (for example, obesity, cancer, dementia) in the global north. An even more radical expansion of the notion of health and its social determinants is a stronger commitment to environmental and planetary health. This goes beyond our recognition of how factors such as air pollution impact our health to more fundamentally rethinking the relations and relative importance of humans to other inhabitants of our planet.

As all this reveals, the scope of our book is expansive, resting on a wide definition of health (and, by implication, ill health) and health *care*. This merits a few clarifying notes about terminology and definitions. In our title and this introduction, we used the term 'medicine' to encompass, among other things, health care. This is contrary to more common usage, which would see medicine as subsection of health care, the former constituting the aspects of health care more directly involved in treating illness (sometimes only physical illness), the latter also encompassing specialities and roles identified more generally with the maintenance of health. An example of this is the way, in some contexts, that nurses, nursing associates, hospital porters and receptionists at a general practice surgery would be considered health care professionals but not necessarily medical ones. In some settings, the term 'medical' is reserved only for those who can boast specific professional qualifications. In a collection of this scope, involving contributors from different geographic domains, such specificity would not be possible, and those terms – 'medicine' and 'health care' – may sometimes be used interchangeably or differently in each chapter. Likewise, there will also be some terminological inconsistency between chapters, especially in relation to health care roles: our contributors may refer to physicians, medics, doctors and more, as appropriate to the locale in which they are writing. Our policy has been to stay true to the native context of the contributor. Please note, too, that we have not attempted a comprehensive engagement with all the professional roles, specialisms or conditions that are encompassed by medical and health care practice: it would not be possible to cover anywhere near the vast array of disciplines. In collating the chapters for this volume, we chose not to decide in advance what medical disciplines to prioritise, for example, by singling out those identified in public health and health care policy (these vary considerably across the global north and south) nor specific branches of biomedical scientific discovery. Rather, we allowed our contributors to inform us, through their choice of theme, what aspects of medicine are currently attracting the interests of performance scholars, practitioners and their audiences.

Speaking of which, our next section introduces performance, tackling its definition and development as a discipline, its critical approach to its objects of study and how it connects to medicine more broadly and within the context of this volume.

A definition of performance

In focusing on *performance* and medicine, this volume understands the term performance in the broadest sense, following scholarship derived from drama and theatre studies, which led into the formation in the 1980s of the field of 'performance studies' in the academy. Theatre practitioner and scholar Richard Schechner was the first to start expanding the idea of performance in the mid-1960s, proposing that ritual, play, games and sport are closely related to theatre as forms of performance (1966, pp. 26–27). Emerging from an engagement with anthropology, Schechner identified some shared 'qualities' across these activities that involve some kind of special ordering or adaption of time (for example, the structuring of time in a play or the duration of a consultation with a doctor), the attachment of value to objects within the context of the activity (such as a prop on stage or the stethoscope hanging round a doctor's neck), a separation from work-based productivity (for instance the community parade or the process of 'scrubbing in' before an operation) and the incorporation of specific rules because of an activity's separation from everyday life (think here of the theatrical convention of sitting in a darkened auditorium or cross-infection protocols in clinical environments) (ibid, p. 28).

The work of anthropologist Victor Turner also bolstered this expansion of the term performance in the latter decades of the twentieth century. He studied ritual practices, focusing on their intensity as liminal, or transitional, events and that as such they were detached from ordinary life in ways that resonated with Schechner's thinking. Turner identified the theatrical nature of ritualised actions, calling them 'social dramas' that incorporated conflict and resolution (Turner, 1957). Analysing social relationships and roles, sociologist Erving Goffman's ideas about 'the enactment of rights and duties attached to a given status' which 'may be presented by the performer on a series of occasions' to an audience have also been seminal in enhancing performance as a conceptual tool (1959, p. 9). In other words, performance is involved in professional and social roles where certain behaviours and actions are expected or required of an individual to maintain their position. This might include the performance of a patient, expected to be compliant and obliging, or the role of the junior doctor in medical hierarchies.

Following this scholarship, the work in this book approaches performance as part of a spectrum or continuum

> ranging from ritual, play, sports, popular entertainments, the performing arts (theatre, dance, music), and everyday life performances to the enactment of social, professional, gender, race, and class roles, and on to healing (from shamanism to surgery), the media and the internet.
>
> (Schechner, 2013, p. 2)

Schechner firmly established performance as action, and its study therefore focuses on the 'doing' of an activity, on behaviours, practices and events. As performance scholar Diana Taylor elaborates, 'doing captures the *now* of performance', and so it can be understood as process but also as product, as a 'thing done' (2016, pp. 7–9, emphasis in original). This neatly encapsulates some of the ways that the chapters in this book engage with performance, as both social and aesthetic practice, concerned with doing, thinking and making. Instances of performance might be a fully staged production, rehearsals in a community setting, choreographies of surgical labour or moments of quiet activism in an AIDS support group, for example.

The work of these scholars suggests that there is no fixed definition of performance, and instead it remains mobile, responsive and malleable as a term, rather than stable and unitary. Schechner states that 'any action that is framed, enacted, presented, highlighted, or displayed is a performance', highlighting its openness as a category and utility as an expanded term (which also has its concomitant drawbacks and challenges, of course, when there seems no limit to its reach) (2013, p. 2). This flexibility and desire to consider performance in a vast range of contexts has meant that performance studies has always had a strong ethical imperative that favours acting 'on or . . . against settled hierarchies of ideas, organizations, and people' (ibid, p. 4). It is likely to challenge the status quo and favour the marginalised and the subversive. We hope that this sense of breadth, ethical concern and inclusivity is evident in the book, where performance is used in a variety of ways and not least as its own epistemology, equivalent to medicine, and capable of revealing important insights about the interface between the two fields.

This is not to say that more conventional theatre practices are omitted from the volume, as they constitute an important part of how performance is made in response to medicine. Medicine and illness are regular subjects of dramas and plays, dealing as they do with matters of life and death, power and knowledge, identity and the human. As theatre scholar Kirsten Shepherd-Barr notes, 'the stage [is] a natural site of speculation about the responsibility and motives of scientists in their acquisition and use of knowledge, and of the delicate tension between knowledge and power' (2006, p. 7). Doctors are therefore frequent players in these scenes, appearing as central protagonists given their social status and level of responsibility and intervention in complex personal situations. Their prevalence is underlined by a quick glance at the London theatre listings of 2022–23, where both *The Doctor*, created by Robert Icke, and *Dr Simmelweiss*, by Stephen Brown, played in the West End. Patients too have been memorably staged, from plays about people with AIDS to those with mental health conditions. Theatre performances have also included more unusual and abstract encounters with and depictions of medical conditions, such as the musical *The Pacifists Guide to the War on Cancer* (2106–17) by Brian Lobel, Byrony Kimmings and Tom Parkinson, which explored the impact of living with a cancer diagnosis and included performers dressed as cancer cells.

Returning to Schechner's ideas about performance, the critical edge that he perceives as being part of the academic study of the discipline is visible too in plenty of theatrical examples. Challenges to the medical status quo come from playwrights interested in the authority conferred on medical practitioners and the sense that this power over patients can be subverted and manipulated for nefarious ends, even when that can be comedic or eroticised. As Harriet A. Washington's book, *Medical Apartheid*, reminds us, medicine has a troubling past in terms of exploiting certain bodies for its own gains, for example, '[d]angerous, involuntary, and nontherapeutic experimentation upon African Americans has been practiced widely and documented extensively at least since the eighteenth century' (2006, p. 7). People subjugated and abused by medical practitioners are increasingly being given visibility and their own voices in contemporary performance, offering important historical correctives for women, people with disabilities and people of colour, amongst others.

The theatrical scope of this book is broader than this, though, moving beyond the stage to include the use of theatrical techniques in medical training and modes of performance being engaged in public health campaigns, health education projects and health-related activism. In medical education, role playing and simulation are valuable pedagogical approaches in training students to be effective communicators and efficient health care professionals.[7] So too are the bedside tutorials where medical students present real case histories to their senior colleagues, all the while performing certain attitudes and embodied know-how meant to convey confidence, understanding and status. Theatre strategies are also used widely in community settings, where public health messages need to be conveyed in informative and enjoyable ways, through public performances, participatory events or smaller-scale, more intimate and supportive peer workshops.

These examples, stretching from staged works performed in front of audiences to 'everyday' performances on wards and in medical consulting rooms, reinforce Schechner's idea of a spectrum of performance. Such a wide-ranging paradigm includes 'performativity', which is both a metaphor and an analytical tool, according to Marvin Carlson, which provides 'new sources of stimulation, inspiration and insight' (2004, p. 6). As a concept, performativity is derived from linguistic analysis, in the work of J.L. Austin. Austin used the term 'performative' to describe particular utterances, such as promises, bets and curses, which not only describe something, but they have an effect in the world: they are 'speech acts' that bring something into being (Austin, 1962). For example, when a judge in a court of law pronounces the accused as 'guilty', it not only describes the altered status of that individual but brings into being a new identity and change in circumstance, possibly resulting in immediate imprisonment, as an example. Speech acts therefore rely upon specific social relations and structures to become intelligible, credible and accepted. To shift the context, for example, to a play set in a courtroom where an actor is found guilty within a fictional world, the speech act would lose its force and meaning, mimicking its logic rather than effecting authentic change.

This idea of the performative has been taken up by performance studies through its 'focus on action', neatly tying into ideas about performance as an act or an embodied doing (Allain and Harvie, 2014, p. 222). It has also been utilised by philosopher Judith Butler to argue that gender identity is a socially constructed performance. The body is socially and medically marked at birth, as female, for example, and then that individual learns how to be feminine (within what Butler calls the heterosexual matrix) through the constant repetition of their gender performance through their lives. In Butler's post-structuralist terms, '[g]ender reality is performative, which means, quite simply, that it is real only to the extent that it is performed' (1988, p. 527). For Butler and other scholars, these ideas have led to a consideration of the body as a material entity shaped, constrained and regulated by certain social, political and cultural practices that are historically and geographically contingent. An understanding of the performativity of everyday life has thus provided further scope for the analysis of roles, identities and behaviours in every aspect of contemporary existence, including those in medical practice. For instance, addressing the performativity of an operating theatre can shed light on the somatic (bodily) practices to be found there. Medical skills are often embedded within complex choreographies in these spaces, where efficiency, teamwork and control are crucial to the success of a medical procedure and its surrounding institutional structures. Effective communication works together with disciplined movement, gestural efficiency and shared understandings of the task, the technologies, the patient's body and each other in the operating theatre. Thinking about this context through performance encourages the close study of these rooms and practices in terms of their scenography, costumes, props, technologies, roles, hierarchies, movement, action and processes in ways that can illuminate the interplay of skills, status, roles and interpersonal relations in a dynamic and multifaceted environment.

In the previous descriptions relating to the operating theatre, there are also parallels that can be drawn with more conventional theatre scenarios, such as the inclusion of rehearsal and improvisation within any surgical procedure; the spatial distinctions between the operating 'theatre' and its backstage areas, such as the scrub and anaesthetic rooms; and in the costumes and roles (Kneebone, 2016). Doing this kind of comparative work suggests that performance can 'transcend disciplinary boundaries', and in doing so it can ask new and vital questions about medical practices (ibid, p. 80). This volume is interested in those questions and some potential answers, through its engagement with the many ways in which performance and medicine interact. Of course, this is not a one-way analysis, and the arguments presented here also reflect on performance, causing us to re-think its meanings, possibilities and parameters. The crucial thing is the status of both disciplines as equals, with each recognised as having epistemological value, rather than old-fashioned, hierarchical and limiting ideas of theatre and performance being 'handmaidens' to medicine. Thinking about this work as 'interdisciplinary' can help to avoid such pitfalls, where 'critical interdisciplinarity, especially from humanistic and creative perspectives, encourages [a] critique of what we know and how we know it' (Condee, 2016, p. 25).

The chapters in the book demonstrate a growing and rich interface between performance and medicine, and we have attempted to capture some of this expansion through a range of examples of practice. Because we have defined both medicine and performance broadly, the field is noticeably eclectic, as indicated previously, from main stage theatre works, to more experimental outputs, to applied practices and to everyday performance in relation to professional health care workers, medical students and patients and incorporating performance within medical settings, as part of public health campaigns and as a mode of patient advocacy. This Companion is an opportunity to experience this global breadth of interdisciplinary and cross-sectoral work, whether conceptual or practical.

Thinking about performance and medicine

Bringing together performance and medicine in this interdisciplinary and cross-sectoral way sets into motion strikingly different, often incompatible, epistemological conceptions of reality and truth. It may be tempting to characterise such epistemological disjuncture in terms of medicine's 'scientific' empiricism and objectivity versus the subjective, interpretative, experiential – and often capricious – notions of reality inherent in performance (and the arts and humanities more generally). Doing so, however, would be an over-simplification. For there is uncertainty and subjectivity in the practices and underpinning conceptual paradigms of medicine and objectivity and empiricism in performance and its study. Performers, for example, understand their bodies in anatomical as well as aesthetic terms, conscious of the muscular-skeletal structures activated when they train and move across the stage; considerations of how the form and colour of an artefact may impact a viewer come into play in medical illustration, modelling and imaging, as well as in scenographic design; lived experience, individual thoughts, feelings and perceptions, are as relevant to the dramaturgy of a real medical encounter as they are to a staged scene.

This is a foundational principle of the volume: to value personal, local, lived, embodied perspectives alongside the supposedly objective and empirical and to explore the overlap between the different epistemological positions attributed to the represented disciplines, be they medical, performance or neither. At the heart of this project is a commitment to give equal credence to objectivist approaches to understanding our lived reality and empirical approaches to knowledge and knowing, with more subjective, inter-subjective, irrational approaches. Recognising the epistemological diversity *within* performance and *within* medicine (as well as *between* performance and medicine) can be destabilising. Comfort comes from a worldview, rooted in the postmodern turn of the mid-twentieth century, that distrusts 'grand narratives' and their claims for universal truth without denying the applicability of specific epistemological paradigms within specific locales. Postmodernist philosophy is characterised by this scepticism towards epistemic certainty and universal meaning, which, for many of its proponents, also involves questioning conventionalised power structures, social roles and identities. The postmodern perspective allows different constructs and values to pertain to different settings, cultures and disciplines – what is important, true and verifiable in a clinical trial is not the same as what is important, true and verifiable in a rehearsal studio. And that is fine.

As this suggests, the late twentieth and early twenty-first century have generated radical shifts in critical thinking that have special relevance to the remit of this volume. These emerging lines of thought are rooted in disciplines (such as philosophy and gender studies) and interdisciplines (for example, the medical humanities and science and technology studies) that lie outside of performance studies per se. Nevertheless, they pertain to phenomena that come into focus at the conjunction between performance and medicine. Additionally, they can help us conceptualise the interrelationship of performance (the arts, humanities) and medicine (science, health care) itself, not least by triangulating different disciplinary perspectives on a topic of mutual concern. An example of this is the topic of the body. Approaching this topic from the dual perspective of performance and medicine reveals a multiplicity of ways the taken-for-granted nature of the human body might be unpacked: the body is at once a complex biological entity; the passive object of anatomical investigation; the site of our experiential and sensory encounter with the world; the vehicle for and expression of our individual selves; and, as an aesthetic medium, staged, manipulated and represented so as to elicit effects in others.

We will further probe the ontological complexity of the body in the following, in the course of outlining some of the other theoretical traditions, which stem from the legacy of postmodernism and that provide scaffolding for our project of bringing performance and medicine into relation with one another. We structure this overview under three themes, which have emerged from our experiences of reading and watching and making and thinking and writing in response to this inter-face. These are: entanglement and intercorporeality, social justice and the distribution of power and lived experience. We view these as significant shifts in the sub-discipline of performance and medicine.

Entanglement and intercorporeality

In addition to postmodernism, what can also be helpful in making sense of a field in which fun-damentally different worldviews co-exist is a recourse to the related field of post-structuralist philosophy. Poststructuralism has an antipathy towards binary ways of thinking, challenging the assumption that reality can be understood through opposition between opposing pairs – male/female, nature/culture, rationalism/emotionality and so on. It can therefore equip us to challenge binary assumptions about the materials of both performance and medicine (bodies, minds, technol-ogy) and about the interrelation between two fields of practice that might otherwise be considered to be defined in contradistinction from one another. Post-structuralism has had a profound impact on performance scholarship and work in the medical humanities. Its ideas have been used, for example, to question language, power structures and knowledge formation through thinkers such as Jacques Derrida and Michel Foucault. For a volume focused on the interface between perfor-mance and medicine, some of the most significant aspects of poststructuralism can be found in its thinking about the body. Understood as a socially and culturally constructed entity, rather than just a biological one, this recognition has had serious implications for issues such as consent, bodily autonomy and the medicalisation of certain conditions, such as hyperactivity, menopause and post-traumatic stress disorder (Conrad, 2007, p. 9). Scholars, such as Judith Butler, have interrogated the complex relationship between the body, gender and identity, highlighting the performative nature of gendered bodies, which has implications for both performance studies (as examined previously) and health care practice. Much of this work has led to explorations of the ethical dimensions of medical and performance practices, considering the representation of bodies in both arenas, with an emphasis on subjectivity and identity that has informed the study of social inequi-ties and intersectionality in both disciplines.

Over the last few decades, and notable in this volume, has been a developing interest in the idea of 'entanglement', initiated from the work of French philosophers and poststructuralists Gilles Deleuze and Félix Guattari. Their concept of the 'rhizome' challenges traditional models of thought that rely on hierarchical and linear structures in favour of a 'rhizomatic' way of conceptualising knowledge and connections (1980). In such a system, elements are interconnected in a web-like manner or network that is fluid and dynamic because it is decentralised and non-hierarchical. Thinking rhizomatically avoids dualisms such as mind/body and subject/object that have been so foundational in academic disciplines, including medicine and performance. 'Entanglement' is then an extension of this model, proposing that bodies and ideas are intricately entwined with each other rather than being separate and autonomous. In other words, entanglement suggests that everything and everybody is connected, interacting and in a constant state of flux. Within the medical humanities, the concept of entanglement has been used to challenge received ideas about how medicine and the humanities interrelate. Notably, Des Fitzgerald and Felicity Callard argue in their contribution to the *Edinburgh Companion to the Critical Medical Humanitie*s, that entanglement follows:

> an intuition that some set of things, commonly held to be separate from one another (indeed, that define themselves precisely with reference to their separability) – science and justice, humans and non-humans, settlers and natives – not only might have something in common, but also, in fact, may be quite *inseparable* from one another.
>
> (2016, p. 40)

This is reflected in our own conceptualisation, outlined previously, of the interrelation between medicine and performance. The concept of entanglement is also closely connected to the idea of 'intercorporeality' developed by philosopher Gail Weiss (1999), which focuses on embodiment and similarly emphasises the idea of bodies as being interconnected and relational:

> As used by Weiss, 'intercorporeality' implies that no form of human embodiment is discrete and self-identical. Rather, each person's experience of being embodied emerges from a field of embodied relationships and continues to refer to, and be modified by, such a field throughout life.
>
> (Waldby, 2002, p. 241)

Where bodies and medicine are concerned, ideas of entanglement and intercorporeality have shifted thinking in transplant studies, for instance. The relationship between donor and recipient bodies has been complicated by anthropological studies of the lived experience of post-transplant patients and donor kin, whose narratives often signal a profound shift in understandings of identity and the self after transplantation. Transplant recipients are aware of their implanted organ(s) coming from another body, which prolongs their life, whilst donor kin often forge intimate blood ties with them, understanding that part of their deceased kin 'lives on' in this other body and person (Sharp, 2006). These narratives run counter to medical protocols and practices that try to establish distance between donor and recipient, actively discouraging the recipient from identifying with the donor and deterring both from seeking contact with each other. But there is a biological entanglement at stake in transplantations that seemingly promotes the 'idiom of fictive kinship' and which

> generates new sentimental ties of sociality, enabled by the sharing of donor flesh. As such, this process minimises the strangeness of the hybrid body – one composed of parts of disparate human origins – replacing it with the shared sense of intimacy.
>
> (ibid, p. 162)

Such bodies are entangled in complex ways that draw attention to ideas of intercorporeality and how all bodies are permeable, affected by their relationality and interactions with others.

Already a deeply entangled medium, these ideas resonate strongly with performance thinkers and makers who have long been interested in the connections between audiences and 'actors', whether they are performers, health care workers or any other individual engaged in 'doing' something. Thinking of (all) bodies as porous, interdependent and materially connected to many others, including the animal, the fungal, the vegetal and the bacterial, offers important new ways of thinking ecologically, ethically and empathically. Extending our thinking beyond the human seems crucial at this time of environmental catastrophe and the extraordinary extraction of resources under late capitalism, whether that pillage is from the human or non-human. This might seem in conflict with medicine, which is surely all about the human, but there is much to be gained from this turn to the body as a permeable and co-dependent form, both theoretically and scientifically.

Social justice and the distribution of power

While we made an important point previously about the limits of binary thinking, we must not ignore long-standing critical and activist efforts that focus on the more oppositional interactions between medicine and various aspects of personal, social and political experience. These efforts often centre on the limits of the 'biomedical model'. There are well-founded critiques from within feminist, LBGTQ+, disability and race studies, for example, of the way this can serve to pathologise and alienate those whose identity, embodiment, behaviour or ability does not comply with narrow (assumed male, white, cis-gendered, able-bodied, middle-class) ideas of normalcy and health. Black British doctor and author Annabel Sowemimo articulates this as 'the problem . . . at the root of medical knowledge', based upon an 'archetypal patient' that 'excludes the symptoms and behaviours of marginalised groups' (2023, pp. 86–87). Such critiques also point to the ways in which the biomedical model disavows individual experiences of embodiment and illness. For feminist scholars of the body, such as Grosz, the concern is with the way the biomedical model ignores the 'leakiness' of the female body, how it perpetuates a Cartesian model that overlooks the interconnectedness of body and mind (1994). Disability activists oppose the biomedical with the social model of disability, the argument being that by situating dysfunction and pathology in the individual, medicine overlooks the fact that people are disabled not by their biomedical idiosyncrasies but by the failure of society to accommodate their needs.

These stark power differentials reflect how medicine operates as a discursive practice. The idea of discursive practices was developed by Michel Foucault in thinking about how language and practices combine to define and produce objects of knowledge (Hall, 1997, p. 44). As a discursive practice, medicine is 'always inextricably enmeshed in relations of power because it [is] always being applied to the regulation of social conduct in practice' (ibid, p. 47). In other words, the language, technologies, institutions and practices of medicine directly affect individuals at both the level of population (through public health initiatives, for example) and as singular subjects (undergoing diagnosis and treatment for specific ailments). Bodies, social relations and lived experiences are all impacted by the ubiquitous force of western medicine, particularly in the global north, and it is this understanding that is generating new insights into the distribution of power in medical training, in clinical encounters, in health care and its outcomes, in medical research and in the history of medicine. To consider medicine as a discursive practice is to examine the ways in which people and bodies can be treated differently depending on things like race, impairments, sexuality, class, gender, ethnicity and age.[8] This thinking has also crucially been extended by the social and political movements of the last two decades, including #MeToo, which since 2006 has focused on empowering survivors of sexual violence to speak about their experiences, and Black Lives Matter, initiated in 2013 when a white Neighbourhood Watch co-ordinator was acquitted of the shooting of black student Trayvon Martin in Florida, US.

There is now an overdue and shameful reckoning with the patriarchal and racist roots of medicine and its complicity with the exploitation, abuse and eugenicide of marginalised communities and individuals. This includes recognition of how the privilege, paternalism, self-interest and hubris of the medical professional has had direct impact on how potentially life-saving treatments were developed and trialled (for instance, the controversies surrounding the HeLa cell line or the Tuskegee syphilis experiment) and who had access to them (the commercialisation of the AIDS

Reagent Program in the early 1980s, for example, which denied treatment for HIV/AIDS to thousands).[9] And there is increased recognition of continuing inequalities within health care, both in terms of patient care and staffing. In the UK, there have been numerous media headlines and investigations into the pay and conditions of immigrant health care workers whom the National Health Service is dependent upon and yet often fails to treat equitably. This has been exacerbated by the coronavirus pandemic, which revealed very poor health outcomes for minority ethnic patients and frontline staff, who were likely to be from the same communities.[10]

Meanwhile, performance and its accompanying scholarship have responded to these social imperatives in multiple ways, from the content of productions addressing histories of racist medical abuse, for example, in the work of playwright Mojisola Adebayo, to undertaking interrogations of performative pandemic responses, such as the 'Clap-for-Carers' phenomenon in this volume. There has been an identifiable shift at the performance and medicine interface to address the colonial, patriarchal and racial histories that are surfacing in wider culture and to examine the precarious and exploitative use of bodies more fully in medical practice, both historical and current. Such works challenge the idea of medical objectivity and point towards its socially and historically contingent nature, whereby it is as much a culturally informed practice as scientific endeavour. This has meant the inclusion of more work from feminist, black studies, queer and disability studies scholars in analysing the emerging practices, and we anticipate this only increasing.

Some of this work is also starting to be focused through an eco-critical lens, producing provocative intersections between medical inequalities and the climate crisis. The work of Marya and Patel, for example, connects modern medicine with colonialism, arguing that

> [d]ecolonizing medicine begins with the project of rehumanizing and reconnection, linking scans to people's faces; patients to their families, their cosmologies, communities, and histories; peoples to their lands and mountains and waters; and relatives to one another across the cast web of life.
>
> (2021, p. 23)

Their idea of 'deep medicine' aims to relocate people in profound relationality with each other and with their local landscapes and ecologies to overcome current environmental and social inequalities which have been and continue to be exacerbated by modern medical practices. More generally, the intersection of performance and medicine may be usefully approached through new materialist perspectives that serve to rethink the interactions and ethical responsibilities among human, animal and material matter (Jane Bennett's concept of 'vibrant matter' [2010] is an especially productive framework in relation to this). Ultimately, as Mermikides points out, there is a 'shared preoccupation, across theatre and medicine, with the human' that highlights the political potential of this interface and its richness and significance in terms of exploring issues of social justice and power (2020, p. 165).

Experience

As the previous outline suggests, there is an expanding and powerful set of standpoint theories that have much to contribute to our understanding of medicine. By this we mean theories which value the knowledge, experience and perspectives of those who occupy specific, marginalised, stigmatised social positions, often aligned with activist movements. It should be noted that standpoint theorists do not always or inevitably critique medicine. A number of scholars within these fields champion the emancipatory possibilities of medical science and technology. For example,

Donna Haraway famously pointed to the way scientific, technological and medical incursion into daily life has fundamentally overthrown unhelpful demarcations between nature and culture in the figure of the cyborg (1991).

Either way, in keeping with their belief in the validity of culturally specific and individual forms of knowledge, poststructuralist and standpoint theorists (who often overlap, notably in the established and powerful field of poststructuralist feminism) sometimes utilise methodologies that pay close attention to lived experience and that are open to forms of knowledge that might be considered nebulous or subjective within more empirical and rationalist paradigms. An important example of this is in Minna Salami's concept of sensuous knowledge, which robustly challenges the notion that 'calculable reasoning is the only worthy way to explain reality', offering instead 'an approach to knowledge that synthetizes the imagination and the rational, the quantifiable and immeasurable, the intellectual and the emotional' (2020, pp. 13–14).

An interest in lived experience is not entirely alien to the medical domain. Indeed, health care providers actively seek out 'patient and public perspectives', and professional and pedagogic frameworks require medical personnel to consider individual experiences, of illness in particular, that go beyond any biomedical definition of disease. This appreciation of patient perspectives plays a key role in the move from so-called 'paternalistic' medicine (the principle that doctor knows best) to patient- or person-centred care and shared decision-making. It also feeds into concerns and debates about doctors' 'empathy' within medical education and professionalism, with frameworks and standards increasingly referring to the capacity to appreciate, acknowledge and understand how patients feel about their diagnoses and treatment. A complementary impetus also seeks to take account of the feelings and experiences of health care professionals, as reflected in recent publications about doctors' feelings.[11]

Within the medical humanities and education, experience has often been packaged in narrative formats, for example, in teaching involving patient educators who tell their own stories about ill health or treatment or through the use of pathographic literary works and self-reflective creative writing activities. This reflects the vast influence of narrative medicine, an approach developed by Rita Charon and widely disseminated within medical education, which employs literary theory to explore the stories inherent in medical experience (2008). Other fields of critical study give credence to the embodied, sensory, affective, emotional and aesthetic aspects of lived experience that may not always be accessed in literary and narrative forms, reflecting a general shift in interest from text to embodied and experiential forms of knowledge.

One of these fields of study is the 'somatic' or 'corporeal turn' of the late twentieth century, characterised by Fraser and Grecos as 'a veritable explosion of interest' in the body, precipitated by Bryan Turner's 'agenda-setting' *The Body and Society* (1984) (Fraser and Grecos, 2005, p. 1). Theorists including Shildrick (1997), Judith Butler (1993), Elizabeth Grosz (1994), Drew Leder (1990) and Elaine Scarry (1985) remind us that bodies matter, that they can be leaky, volatile, absent and in pain. In other words, they argue that the body can be understood as both a material and discursively constructed entity and that our embodiment constructs our social, psychic and political experience and vice versa. Many of these theorists point to the way medicine, science and technology shape experiences and the material composition of the human body. Some also discuss its expressive, creative and aesthetic dimensions. A similarly interdisciplinary approach permeates the field of sensory studies, which since the early 2000s has been investigating perceptual and sensory experience from a cultural and sociological, as well as scientific, perspective. In the introduction to a recent 'manifesto' to the field, David Howes explains the constructed nature of the human sensorium (for example, the eurocentric assumption that there are only five senses) and notes how the field has generated studies of specific senses, such as visuality, sound and touch (2022). Studies of the senses have special relevance to the practice of medicine. The concept of the 'medical gaze', for example, speaks to the way contemporary medical culture prioritises visuality over the other senses, a point developed further by Abraham Verghese in his argument for the significance of the doctor's touch (explicated, for example in his 2013 TED talk). The arts, of course, are concerned with generating sensory experiences, with performance scholars offering analyses of, for example, visuality and aurality in relation to theatre and performance.[12]

Another theoretical field that values experiential dimension is the 'affective turn'. Precipitated by the work of Brian Massumi (2015), this turn concerns itself with affects, that is, our non-conscious responses to sensory and cognitive phenomena. In *Touching Feeling: Affect, Pedagogy, Performativity*, Sedgwick explains how:

> Affects can be, and are, attached to things, people, ideas, sensations, relations, activities, ambitions, institutions, and any number of other things, including other affects. Thus, one can be excited by anger, disgusted by shame, or surprised by joy.
>
> (2003, p. 19)

Both Massumi and Sedgwick investigate the interface between affect, social and political agency and wider institutional structures. While Massumi's stricter definition distinguishes affect from feeling and emotion, we might also consider theorists who explore the latter. Sara Ahmed's *Cultural Politics of Emotion* is an important work in relation to this, interrogating the interconnectedness of the embodied, felt world and the political sphere. In asking what emotions do, Ahmed argues that,

> emotions shape the very surfaces of bodies which take shape through the repetition of actions over time, as well as through orientation towards and away from others. Indeed, attending to emotions might show us how all actions are reactions, in the sense that what we do is shaped by the contact we have with others.
>
> (2014, p. 4)

Ahmed explicates the capacity of emotions – hate, disgust, shame – to orient us towards and away from each other, leading to real-world, sometimes devastating, consequences, for example, in racist and xenophobic behaviours, media discourses and government policies.

Emotion and affect are the main currency within theatre and performance, which often involve both the display of emotions on the part of the performer (which may be simulated, induced, symbolised or otherwise brought into play, according to the specific performance tradition being employed) and the elicitation of emotion in the spectator, including through affects afforded by, among other things, sound, lighting, spatial organisation of the stage and the affective contagion among those who occupy the auditorium. Indeed, theatre and performance have long been fascinated with the drama inherent in medicine and with the emotional lives of patients and health care professionals. Medicine is replete with complex emotion, for we seek it out at times when our health is, at least potentially, compromised and often in the course of significant life events – birth, the onset of serious illness, the shock of injury, the reframing of self that might accompany the onset or diagnosis of disability, death – that elicit strong emotional responses. As noted, the shift towards a more person-centred health care practice also acknowledges the emotionality of the student and practitioners: Bleakley's attention to the 'sensibility' in his work on medical education (2016) illustrates how the emotional lives of future medical practitioner is not only acknowledged, at least within the medical humanities, but also increasingly expected, and scripted, as a component of medical professional identity.

Another theoretical field that may perform a similar bridging function in interdisciplinary endeavours such as ours is care ethics. Developed in the 1980s as a branch of moral philosophy by feminist scholars such as Gilligan (1982) and Noddings (1984), care ethics argues for the 'moral saliency' (Held, 2006, p. 10) inherent in care – that is, activities of nurture, caregiving and maintenance often sequestered to the domestic sphere and devalued as 'female' concerns under patriarchal culture. Care, Held continues, involves 'persons in caring relations' who are 'acting for self-and-other together . . . neither egotistic nor altruistic', and this offers an ethical framework that challenges the normative models that underpin, for example, judicial and penal practices (ibid, pp. 12–13). Thinking around care has revived in recent years, prompted by scholars and activists agitating for a more caring politics, for example, in the work of The Care Collective (see The Care Manifesto, 2020) and in relation to the planet – Maria Puig de la Bellacasa's 'speculative ethics', for example, argues for the extension of care to 'more than human worlds' (2017).

The relevance of care ethics to health care is self-evident, especially for those professional roles associated with care such as nursing. The popular success of author and journalist Madeline Bunting's *Labours of Love: The Crisis of Care* (2020) also speaks to revived interest in philosophies of care in relation to health and social care. Perhaps more surprisingly, however, the topic of care has been given extensive consideration within the field of theatre and performance research, with Thompson and Stuart-Fisher's edited collection *Performing Care* (2020), a land-mark study. Thompson's work illustrates how thinking about care through the lens of performance has enabled a further critical development towards an aesthetics of care, including but not limited to health care.

This move towards the aesthetic of health care activities is especially significant for our study because it evidences the contribution that performance (and creative and imaginative practices more generally) can make towards these theoretical turns. In fact, performance, or at least performativity, already threads through several of the theoretical traditions we outline here, for example, in the work of both Sedgwick and Ahmed. And this in turn lays a path for critical thinking that takes performance not only as the object of study or as conceptual framework but also as research methodology. One entry point for this is the method of sensory ethnography, born at the interface between social science research and sensory studies. Sarah Pink's introduction to this approach advocates for research that takes the sensory experience of both research participant and researcher into account but also for the use of creative methods, including performance, for example, in the dissemination of research findings (2015). This might be seen as an extension of the long-standing association between performance and the social sciences, for example, in the theatrical metaphors used by sociologists studying medical culture (Sinclair's *Making Doctors* [1997] is a key example) or Schechner's engagement with the work of Turner and Goffman noted previously. A parallel methodological paradigm, one more central within performance studies, is practice research (also known as artistic research) defined by one of its earliest proponents, Robin Nelson, as

a research project in which practice is a key method of enquiry and where . . . a practice (creative writing, dance, musical score/performance, theatre/performance, visual exhibition, film or other cultural practice) is submitted as substantial evidence of a research inquiry.

(2013, pp. 8–9)

As will be evident in the chapters that follow, our volume recognises performance-making as a valid epistemological method, capable of generating insights and new theorisations, not least in relation to topics of shared concern across performance and medicine.

These emergent critical approaches to thinking about performance and medicine have impacted the depth of the field, adding crucial attention to inequalities; abusive practices; and the construction of more ethical, healthy and caring relationships. Their imbrication with ecology is starting to be examined, a vital means of extending that care to the wider environment, to indigenous knowledges and to the earth itself. This volume suggests that vital work is happening across the world that is mutually beneficial for both disciplines as they intertwine with each other – collaboratively, respectfully and creatively.

The structure of the volume

We have organised the chapters in this volume to loosely follow the journey and experience of a patient from the development of symptoms to diagnosis, to ideas of care and cure, to possible side effects and then to experimentation and future scanning. These are flexible categories, with much crossover between them and the chapters that reside in each part. The chapters are, therefore, thematically linked but they can also be read as stand-alone pieces. Each part is prefaced by an introduction that provides a summary of the chapters within it, offering a rationale for their positioning and brief insights into their content and connections. In brief, the parts are as follows:

Part 1: Symptoms focuses on representations of ill health and disease on the stage, with many of the case studies exploring the lived experience of illness as depicted in the theatre, including its cultural meanings and social impact. Chapters examine how theatre has represented pain, illness, trauma and disability, as well as how performative techniques can be used by individuals to creatively express and help to process trauma, discrimination and loss. The section ends with a consideration of the entanglements between representations of death and real-life, medicalised practices at the end of life. **Part 2: Diagnosis** explores how medicine is performed on stage and in institutional settings, particularly through an examination of professional medical roles, such as the surgeon, general practitioner, junior doctor, nurse and midwife. The contributions travel from doctors on stage, their power and status dramatised for comedic and political effect, to the construction of medical identity in the hospital through bedside and simulation-based training, props, costume and storytelling, and on to the interconnections between surgery, performance and art. Finally, the interface between performance and medicine is analysed through the 'clap-for-carers' phenomenon, born of the global COVID-19 pandemic and resonating with theatrical applause. Throughout, performance is examined as either a constitutive part of medical identity formation or as a means of critiquing it. **Part 3: Care and Cure** considers performance as a means of caring for people, for example, through arts-in-health, applied performance and activist practices. Our contributors focus on using performance in different contexts, including the personal, in intimate moments of care, and the public, in the form of public health campaigns. The practices as they are described are caring and careful, attentive to inequalities and the specificities of place that require tailored responses that work with and alongside communities. **Part 4: Side Effects** addresses the ambivalent, uncertain and negative impacts of medicine through theatricalised and performed examples, covering recent plays, both mainstream and fringe, and performance art. Much of this section details inequalities and exploitative practices in medicine that are confronted in different ways on the stage and through creative outputs. The importance of thinking through the notion of the biopolitical is foregrounded, even in the case of governmental guidance on opening the performing arts again after a national pandemic lockdown. **Part 5: Experiments** deals with emergent medical knowledge and biotechnologies that raise questions about subjectivity, autonomy, embodiment and our relations with others. Here the laboratory refers to the more experimental and innovative aspects of medicine and performance as a means of testing and exploring ourselves, drawing out the positives, the silences and difficulties, as well as the potentiality of the relationship between the two fields.

Notes

1 See, for example, Garner *Theatre & Medicine* (2023); Bouchard (2020) on the performance of specimens and specimenhood; Mermikides (2020) on the interrelationships of performance, medicine and the human; Conti (2019) on nineteenth-century theatrical representations of specific illnesses; Dakari and Rogers' special issue of *Critical Stages Theatre and/as Medicine* (2018); Bouchard and O'Brien's special issue of *Performance Research On Medicine* (2014); Baxter and Low's *Performing Health and Wellbeing* (2017); Mermikides and Bouchard's *Performance and the Medical Body* (2016); Brodzinski's *Theatre in Health and Care* (2010); and Kuppers' *Scar of Visibility* (2007).
2 The work of Alan Bleakley *et al.* (2017) is unusual in this regard in terms of including experimental performance and live art as part of his medical humanities projects.
3 The United Nations' 17 Sustainable Development Goals can be viewed at: https://sdgs.un.org/goals (Accessed: 20 July 2023).
4 See Marya and Patel for an examination of the imbrication of health, medicine and social injustice.
5 See Park (2021) for a historical overview of the female body in relation to the development of human dissection in the Middle Ages and Cleghorn (2021) for a history of the treatment of women by and through medicine in the west.
6 This is expressed as part of the preamble to the World Health Organization's constitution. Available at: www.who.int/about/governance/constitution (Accessed: 29 July 2023).
7 See Mermikides (2020) *Performance, Medicine and the Human*. London: Bloomsbury Methuen Drama Publishing, pp. 56–85.
8 See, for example, the work of Cleghorn (2021) and Washington (2006).
9 For example, see the work of Reverby (2009) on the Tuskegee study; Sowemimo (2023) on racism and medicine; and Washington (2006) on medical experiments on Black Americans.
10 See, for example, the UK's Local Government Hub on Health Inequalities for further details. Available at: www.local.gov.uk/perfect-storm-health-inequalities-and-impact-covid-19 (Accessed: 29 July 2023).
11 See, for example, Ofri (2014) *How Doctors Feel*.
12 On visuality, see Dominic Johnson (2012) and Maaike Bleeker (2011), and on aurality, see Kendrick (2017).

Reference list

Agamben, G. (1998) *Homo sacer: sovereign power and bare life*. Translated by D. Heller-Roazen. Redwood City, CA: Stanford University Press.
Ahmed, S. (2004/2014) *The cultural politics of emotion*. Edinburgh: University of Edinburgh Press.
Allain, P. and Harvie, J. (eds.) (2014) *The Routledge companion to theatre and performance*. London and New York: Routledge.
Austin, J.L. (1962) *How to do things with words*. London: Oxford University Press.
Baxter, V. and Low, K.E. (eds.) (2017) *Applied theatre: performing health and wellbeing*. London: Bloomsbury Methuen Drama Publishing.
Bennett, J. (2010) *Vibrant matter: a political economy of things*. Durham and London: Duke University Press.
Bleakley, A. (2016) *Medical humanities and medical education: how the medical humanities can shape better doctors*. London and New York: Routledge.
Bleakley, A., Lynch, L. and Whelan, G. (eds.) (2017) *Risk and regulation at the interface of medicine and the arts*. Cambridge: Cambridge Scholars Publishing.
Bleeker, M. (2011) *Visuality in the theatre: the locus of looking*. Hampshire: Palgrave Macmillan.

Bouchard, G. (2020) *Performing specimens: contemporary performance and biomedical display.* London: Bloomsbury Methuen Drama Publishing.

Bouchard, G. and O'Brien, M. (eds.) (2014) 'On medicine', *Performance Research*, 19(4). [special issue].

Brodzinski, E. (2010) *Theatre in health and care.* Hampshire: Palgrave Macmillan.

Bunting, M. (2020) *Labours of love: the crisis of care.* London: Granta.

Butler, J. (1988) 'Performative acts and gender constitution', *Theatre Journal*, 40(4), pp. 524–528.

Butler, J. (1993) *Bodies that matter: on the discursive limits of sex.* London and New York: Routledge.

The Care Collective (2020) *The care manifesto: the politics of interdependence.* London and New York: Verso.

Carlson, M. (2004) *Performance: a critical introduction.* London and New York: Routledge.

Charon, R. (2008) *Narrative medicine: honouring the stories of illness.* Oxford: University of Oxford Press.

Clarke, A.E. *et al.* (2003, April) 'Biomedicalization: technoscientific transformations of health, illness and US biomedicine', *American Sociological Review*, 68(2), pp. 161–194.

Cleghorn, E. (2021) *Unwell women: a journey through medicine and myth in a man-made world.* London: Weidenfeld and Nicholson.

Condee, W. (2016) 'The interdisciplinary turn in the arts and humanities', *Issues in Interdisciplinary Studies*, (34), pp. 12–29.

Conrad, P. (2007) *The medicalization of society: on the transformation of human conditions into treatable disorders.* Baltimore: John Hopkins University Press.

Conti, M. (2019) *Playing sick: performances of illness in the age of Victorian medicine.* London and New York: Routledge.

Dakari, V. and Rogers, C. (eds.) (2018) 'Medicine and/in theatre', *Critical Stages*, 17. [special issue].

Deleuze, G. and Guattari, F. (1980) *A thousand plateaus: capitalism and schizophrenia.* London and New York: Bloomsbury Methuen Drama Publishing.

Esposito, R. (2008) *Bios: biopolitics and philosophy.* Translated by T. Campbell. Minneapolis: University of Minnesota Press.

Fitzgerald, D. and Callard, F. (2016) 'Entangling the medical humanities', in Whitehead, A. *et al.* (eds.) *The Edinburgh companion to the critical medical humanities.* Edinburgh: Edinburgh University Press, pp. 35–49.

Foucault, M. (1973) *The birth of the clinic: an archaeology of medical perception.* London and New York: Routledge.

Fraser, M. and Greco, M. (2005) *The body: a reader.* London and New York: Routledge.

Garner, Jr, S.B. (2023) *Theatre and medicine.* London: Bloomsbury Methuen Drama Publishing.

Gilligan, C. (1982) *In a different voice: psychological theory and women's development.* Cambridge, MA and London, England: Harvard University Press.

Goffman, E. (1959) *The presentation of the self in everyday life.* Edinburgh: University of Edinburgh, Social Sciences Research Centre.

Grosz, E. (1994) *Volatile bodies: toward a corporeal feminism.* Bloomington: Indiana University Press.

Hall, S. (ed.) (1997) *Representation: cultural representations and signifying practices.* London: Sage Publications.

Haraway, D.J. (1991) *Simians, cyborgs and women: the reinvention of nature.* London and New York: Routledge.

Held, V. (2006) *The ethics of care: personal, political, and global.* Oxford: Oxford University Press.

Howes, D. (2022) *The sensory manifesto: tracking the sensorial revolution in the arts and human sciences.* Toronto: University of Toronto Press.

Illich, I. (1975) *Limits to medicine: medical nemesis – the expropriation of health.* London and New York: Marion Boyars.

Johnson, D. (2012) *Theatre and the visual.* London and New York: Palgrave Macmillan.

Kendrick, L. (2017) *Theatre aurality.* London: Palgrave Macmillan.

Kneebone, R. (2016) 'Performing surgery', in Mermikides, A. and Bouchard, G. (eds.) *Performance and the medical body.* London and New York: Bloomsbury Methuen Drama Publishing.

Kuppers, P. (2007) *Scar of visibility: medical performances and contemporary art.* Minneapolis: University of Minnesota Press.

Leder, D. (1990) *The absent body.* Chicago and London: University of Chicago Press.

Marya, R. and Patel, R. (2021) *Inflamed: deep medicine and the anatomy of injustice.* Dublin: Allen Lane.

Massumi, B. (2015) *The politics of affect*. Cambridge and Malden: Polity Press.

Mermikides, A. (2020) *Performance, medicine and the human*. London: Bloomsbury Methuen Drama Publishing.

Mermikides, A. and Bouchard, G. (eds.) (2016) *Performance and the medical body*. London and New York: Bloomsbury Methuen Drama Publishing.

Nelson, R. (2013) *Practice as research in the arts: principles, protocols, pedagogies, resistances*. Houndsmill: Palgrave Macmillan.

Noddings, N. (1984) *Caring: a feminine approach to ethics and moral education*. Berkeley, Los Angeles and London: University of California Press.

Ofri, D. (2014) *What doctors feel: how emotions affect the practice of medicine*. Boston: Beacon Press.

Pink, S. (2015) *Doing sensory ethnography*. London: Sage Publications.

Porter, R. (1997) *The greatest benefit to mankind: a medical history of humanity from antiquity to the present*. London and New York: Fontana Press.

Puig de la Bellacasa, M. (2017) *Matters of care: speculative ethics in more than human worlds*. Minneapolis: University of Minnesota.

Reverby, S.M. (2009) *Examining Tuskegee: the infamous syphilis study and its legacy*. Chapel Hill: University of North Carolina Press.

Salami, M. (2020) *Sensuous knowledge: a black feminist approach for everyone*. London and New York: Zed Books.

Scarry, E. (1985) *The body in pain: the making and unmaking of the world*. New York and Oxford: Oxford University Press.

Schechner, R. (1966, Summer) 'Approaches to theory/criticism', *The Tulane Drama Review*, 10(4), pp. 20–53.

Schechner, R. (2013) *Performance studies: an introduction*. London and New York: Routledge.

Sedgwick, E. (2003) *Touching feeling: affect, pedagogy, performativity*. Durham and London: Duke University Press.

Sharp, L.A. (2006) *Strange harvest: organ transplants, denatured bodies, and the transformed self*. Los Angeles and London: University of California Press.

Shepherd-Barr, K. (2006) *Science on stage: from doctor Faustus to Copenhagen*. Princeton and Oxford: Princeton University Press.

Shildrick, M. (1997) *Leaky bodies and boundaries: feminism, postmodernism and (bio)ethics*. London and New York: Routledge.

Sinclair, S. (1997) *Making doctors: an institutional apprenticeship*. Oxford and New York: Berg.

Sowemimo, A. (2023) *Divided: racism, medicine and why we need to decolonise healthcare*. London: Profile Books and Wellcome Collection.

Stuart Fisher, A. and Thompson, J. (2020) *Performing care: new perspectives on socially engaged performance*. Manchester: Manchester University Press.

Taylor, D. (2016) *Performance*. Durham and London: Duke University Press.

Turner, B. (1984) *The body and society*. London: Basil Blackwell.

Turner, V. (1957) *Schism and continuity*. Manchester: Manchester University Press.

Waldby, C. (2002) 'Biomedicine, tissue transfer and intercorporeality', *Feminist Theory*, 3(3), pp. 239–524.

Washington, H. (2006) *Medical apartheid: the dark history of medical experimentation on black Americans from colonial times to the present*. New York: Anchor Books.

Weiss, G. (1999) *Body images: embodiment as intercorporeality*. London and New York: Routledge.

PART 1

Symptoms

Introduction

Our first part focuses on illness, disease, and other deviations from health; how they are experienced by individuals; and how these experiences may align or clash with both biomedical and cultural conceptions and representations of those conditions. The part is founded upon Susan Sontag's seminal work on illness as a metaphor: the idea that diseases such as cancer or HIV/AIDS accrue specific metaphors in different social and historical contexts and that their meanings cannot necessarily be contained within any strict biomedical definition, which is, in any case, itself ideologically inflected and culturally constructed. Thus, a cancer diagnosis might be understood as celestially ordained fate or random genetic mutation or a manifestation of psychological trauma, depending on whose body is affected, who diagnoses or attempts to treat it, when and where. For example, from the mid-twentieth century, Sontag explains, discourses on the 'war on cancer' in the US were replete with allusions to military action and espionage against a devious enemy, echoing the xenophobic foreign defence policies at play at the time. As this suggests, such meanings and metaphors might reflect or even serve political or ideological ends, as when the earliest waves of what would become known as HIV/AIDS were problematically represented as a 'gay plague' in the worldwide media, further marginalising those discriminated against for their sexual identity and behaviours. The metaphors circling around certain diseases, argue Sontag and several of the contributors in this section, have real-world consequences upon those living with – or dying from – illnesses that are stigmatised or otherwise misunderstood, resulting in deficiencies in medical treatment, public health policy, social support and care.

Analysing representations of ill health on stage and through performance can reveal some of the metaphors that circulate around specific diseases and illnesses and their potentially stigmatising effects. Our first chapter, by April Thant Aung, details how the earliest media reports of the HIV/AIDS epidemic in Singapore in the 1980s were framed through homophobic fears and the perceived threat to Asian values of Western 'immorality'. These prejudices are reflected in two of the plays analysed by Aung – Eleanor Wong's *Jackson on a Jaunt* and Chay Yew's *As if He Hears* – both staged, following state censorship of homosexual and sexually promiscuous characters, in 1989. A decade later, the same theatre staged the production of *Completely With/Out Character*, an autobiographical performance by the first Singaporean to publicly reveal his HIV-positive status, Paddy Chew. Chew 'refuses to conform to a passive and invisible position as demanded by society', and the performance ends with him stripping before the audience: 'the revelation of his frail corporeal form', argues Aung, impels the audience to view people living with HIV/AIDS 'as individuals rather than abstract "deviants" or "degenerates" who are deserving of the disease'.

Chew's performance is an example of pathography, a term describing literary (or, in this case, performed) accounts of illness, often autobiographical ones, that have the potential to counter or complicate medical or other cultural metaphors of illness. In the next chapter, Ellen Redling introduces us to the related genre of allopathography, that is, accounts of *other* people's illness. Staying with the topic of HIV/AIDS, her main examples of allopathographic performances are *Untitled (Portrait of Ross in L.A.)* by Felix Gonzales-Torres (1991) and Karen Finley's *Written in Sand* (1992–ongoing), both by artists who have lost loved ones to this disease. Narrating other people's illness and suffering carries the risk of unethical appropriation or misrepresentation, as revealed and satirised, Redling explains, in the play *pool (no water)* by Mark Ravenhill, written while the playwright was grieving his partner, who had also passed away with HIV/AIDS. In the play, a group of artists turn the artefacts of their friends' illnesses and injuries into artworks, gaining acclaim through installations featuring the catheters and condoms of a person with AIDS or photographs of wounds sustained by the central character after diving into an empty pool. Unlike the callous artists in Ravenhill's play, whose works appeal through sensationalising displays of suffering, Redling argues that Gonzales-Torres and Karen Finley have made 'ethically complex' artworks that use 'the power of the live encounter in performance . . . activating and implicating the spectators' and encouraging 'the viewers to engage with their artworks and the experiences behind them more deeply'.

We confront another fearsome and metaphorically resonant disease in the next chapter, as Verónica Rodríguez examines two plays about cancer: *Family Tree* by Mojisola Adebayo (2021) and *In the Body of the World* by Eve Ensler (2016). Both plays deal with the topic of uterine cancer, drawing on the experiences of real women diagnosed with this disease. The central character in Adebayo's play is based on Henrietta Lacks, a patient at the John Hopkins Hospital in Baltimore, US, whose cancerous cells, taken without her knowledge in the 1950s, seeded the HeLa cell line still used in medical research today. *In the Body of the World* details Ensler's own diagnosis and treatment with uterine cancer while working at the City of Joy rape centre in the Congo. The plays develop an illness metaphor of their own, each, in different ways, associating cancer's uncontrollable proliferation of mutated cells with the trauma inflicted on women's bodies and on the earth through patriarchal, racist and capitalist abuse and exploitation – Adebayo also features versions of three real slave women who had been subjected to horrifying experimental gynaecological surgery by J. Marion Sims in the nineteenth century and a trio of fictional health care workers who had died after contracting COVID-19 at work. The 'diseased, complex and traumatised' wombs represent the trauma of these and other women, but are 'upheld and celebrated rather than punished, disbelieved and disciplined'. In a striking turn, their '(cellular) reproduction' is depicted not only as malignant but also as 'potentially healing'.

We stay with women's bodily experience for the next chapter. Joanne 'Bob' Whalley offers an intensely personal and philosophical 'snapshot' of her practice of performance drawing, a practice developed in response to seven years of recurrent miscarriages. Whereas works such as those of Chew and Ensler are pathographies, Whalley describes her own approach as a form of 'corpography' that is, writing that engages with its creator's experience of their body, their embodiment. Whalley conveys how the miscarrying body, the 'diffracted-self' that emerges in recovery suites while waiting for a clinical intervention or for drugs to take effect, is 'no longer my own' but rather something 'to be handled, dealt with, cleaned-up and sorted out'. Sketching 'crude representations of medical ephemera' (we would contest the term 'crude'), objects that intervene between the body and the world, becomes a way for her to make sense of her corporeal experience. This allows an understanding of miscarriage to emerge that, like the 'uber-performing' wombs in the previous chapter, sees the traumatised female body as 'nonetheless generative', in this case 'of experience, of cellular material, of changes in my body, of grief, of unlimited potential'.

The following chapter is also a creative response to ill health, this time taking the form of a film script that combines 'autobiography, neuroscience, theatrical writing and speculative philosophy', medical records and imagined scenarios, reflecting its author's efforts to recall and reconstitute an identity shattered by the traumatic brain injury sustained in a road accident. Using the script format enables Sarah-Mace Dennis to grasp at flashes of memory that arise out of narrative order and the diffraction of the self, reflected, for example, in the way Dennis variously names herself HER/I, I/ SHE and THEM/US/ME. An especially striking moment is the author's observation that 'the clinical languages used by medicine to rehabilitate damaged brains' – including the 'dances' involved in rehabilitating speech and movement – 'rebuild a patient's identity according to socially acceptable behavioural norms'. Yet, she argues, 'another sort of dance *is* possible when we embrace the new forms of experiential plasticity that emerge from sudden neurological change'.

Another insight into performance practice reveals the potential for forum theatre to expose and challenge the stigma and misunderstandings associated with epilepsy. Brenda Bogaert describes how an independent patient group living with epilepsy in Lyon, France, turned to this methodology, originally developed by Brazilian activist and educator Augusto Boal, in order to share their experiences of workplace discrimination. Members of the group had found their employment prospects and their working lives impacted by prospective employers' and colleagues' surprising misconceptions about epilepsy, including the erroneous beliefs that this neurological condition has a psychological or psychiatric basis, that it is a contagious disease or that any reasonable adjustments made in the workplace were unnecessary or unjust. Forum theatre engages its audiences in actively seeking out solutions in conflictual situations, and in this case, spectators stepping into the group's representations of discriminatory behaviour were able to offer hope for 'creative change to entrenched problems' through empathy and education.

Next, Leah Sidi offers a sharp analysis of three plays, staged in London main houses between 2016 and 2017 at the height of the UK's mental health crisis: Alice Birch's *Anatomy of a Suicide*, Duncan Macmillan's *People, Places, Things* and the revival of Joe Penhall's *Blue/Orange*. The chapter explores how the 'mechanics of theatrical productions – especially its spatial organisation – contribute specific understandings of the construction and experience of mental health and illness to a wider cultural field'. An especially insightful observation is that each play is structured around a 'medical-domestic binary, which seeks to explain mental pathology through the exposure of domestic space'. This sits uncomfortably against the backdrop of the crisis, as pressures on mental health services were pushing care into the community and when the inadequacies in social services were exacerbating mental ill health in people prone to precarious and inadequate housing. It also reveals how the plays are haunted by long-standing discourses around bourgeois female domesticity and mental ill health (for example, hysteria) which peaked in the Victorian age and the Naturalistic theatre. Thus, argues Sidi,

> the spatial politics of theatre . . . keeps alive in the mainstream a version of the experience of mental distress which is not only limited, but potentially actively obscures the real conditions that most mental health service users exist in today.

We end, rather fittingly, with death. Emily Russell reveals how even this most intimate and personal of life events is scripted and performed, arguing that 'the performance of death on stage and in medical settings mutually construct a new shared understanding of the proper way to die'. She examines the rituals and scripts that encircle death in hospital settings, for example, the way the heart-rate monitor, its 'beeping peaks, valleys, and the dreaded flat green line' comes to symbolise death and how the breaking of bad news, even the stages of grieving, are deemed to follow preconceived patterns. She then analyses three examples of staged death: Margaret Edson's *Wit* (1995), Michael Cristofer's *Shadow Box* (1977) and Tony Kushner's *Angels in America* (1993), which, in various ways, complicate the 'consensus vision of the good death'. Taken together, though, both staged and real-life scenarios of life's ending 'confirm and create the dominant scripts for the contemporary enactment of death'.

1

HIV/AIDS ON STAGE IN SINGAPORE

Mass media and stigmatising discourses

April Thant Aung

During the 1980s and 1990s, the human immunodeficiency viruses and acquired immunodeficiency syndrome (HIV/AIDS) epidemic constituted a phenomenon in which a pathology became a global sociocultural event. The initial enigma surrounding the science of the virus and its transmission path, the contested origins of the disease, its high mortality rate and the initially higher infection rate in gay men and Haitians gave rise to various socially, culturally and politically constructed discourses that were saturated with misconceptions, stereotypes, stigma, homophobia and racism. Depictions of HIV/AIDS in theatrical performances in this period highlight how these intersecting and overlapping discourses impinged on people living with the disease. To date, studies on HIV/AIDS and theatre have focused primarily on the United States. These studies analyse plays such as *Rent* (1996) by Jonathan Larson, *Angels in America* (1992) by Tony Kushner and *The Normal Heart* (1985) by Larry Kramer. Whilst these plays are valuable works, they are limited to describing HIV/AIDS illness as experienced by characters who are American, gay, white and mostly male. It is vitally important, therefore, that we examine the illness experience of persons with HIV/AIDS (PWHAs) in other global contexts, such as Southeast Asia, for a broader understanding of local perspectives on the disease across culturally specific contexts. This chapter analyses three approaches to thinking about the HIV/AIDS epidemic in Southeast Asia: 1) the ways in which the authorities' response to HIV/AIDS was shaped by its desire to instil 'Asian' values in Singaporeans to curtail undesirable Western influences even as they were aggressively assimilating modernity for economic gains, 2) the coverage of HIV/AIDS in local media and its influence in shaping the Singaporean cultural understanding of HIV/AIDS and 3) the censorship of positive theatrical representations of homosexual HIV-positive characters in state-run events. The chapter examines three Singaporean HIV/AIDS plays, two of which were written during the years when HIV/AIDS became a full-blown epidemic in the nation between 1985 and 1998 (Cutter *et al.*, 2005, p. 10) and one written in the aftermath of the epidemic. The plays are Eleanor Wong's *Jackson on a Jaunt, or, Mistaken Identities* (1989), Chay Yew's *As if He Hears* (1989) and Paddy Chew's autobiographical play *Completely With/Out Character* (1999). While the plays from the United States are politically subversive and provocative and prominently feature HIV-positive queer male protagonists, the Singaporean plays, with the notable exception of Paddy Chew's, are ambivalent in their critique of media discourses on HIV/AIDS. Nonetheless, they provide insight into the Singaporean cultural and political responses to the epidemic that denied PWHAs discursive control and highlight the

DOI: 10.4324/9781003036500-3

ways in which pathology can be over-determined by the nexus of discourses surrounding HIV/AIDS. Through a close reading of the plays within the unique socio-cultural and political context of 1980s and 1990s Singapore, I argue that these theatrical performances offer alternative imagining of PWHAs in Singapore who were consigned to live in secrecy, shame and fear.

'Asian' values and undesirable 'western' mores

Singapore possesses a significant presence on the global stage. The nation, once a colony of the British empire, has transformed rapidly since its independence in 1965 into one of the wealthiest cosmopolitan smart cities and a global financial and shipping hub. Singapore is an ethnically diverse country with indigenous Malays, diasporic Chinese and Indians forming the three primary ethnic groups of the nation. As the country pursues foreign investment and workforce in its pursuit of meteoric economic development, this diversity has further increased, with Singapore becoming a melting pot of heterogeneous cultures. Despite the government's assimilation of Western science, technology and finance systems to achieve a high standard of living, Singapore has made few strides in freedom of expression and is reluctant to repeal colonial-era laws concerning social and human rights issues, such as the criminalisation of sex between consenting male adults under the British penal code section 377A that was abolished only in January 2023. This contradiction between selective modernisation for economic gains and traditional 'Asian' values undergirded the state's initial response to HIV/AIDS and has had a lasting influence in shaping public perceptions of PWHAs to this day.[1] The cultural representation of HIV/AIDS in Singapore during the 1980s and 1990s was fraught with misinformation, myths, fear and homophobia, primarily due to the ways in which the disease was framed by the local media. News outlets such as *The Straits Times* and the now-defunct *Singapore Monitor* were largely regulated by local press laws and mainly re-reported news about HIV/AIDS from the US media from 1983 onwards.[2]

NBC Nightly News' first story on AIDS in 1982 fashioned a rhetoric that pathologised gay men's sexuality and emphatically propagated them as agents of the virus, announcing on 17 June 1982 that: 'Scientists at the National Centers for Disease Control in Atlanta today released the results of a study that shows that the lifestyle of some male homosexuals triggered an epidemic of a rare form of cancer'. This rhetoric, Larry Gross suggests, 'remained constant throughout much subsequent coverage' in the US mainstream media (2001, p. 97), with *Singaporean* newspapers re-reporting that HIV/AIDS was a disease that was 'first identified among homosexual males' (*The Straits Times*, 1983a) and 'associated with homosexuality' overseas (*The Straits Times*, 1983b). While local news coverage steadily increased as cases rose in the United States, Singaporeans remained unconcerned at first because it was largely viewed as a 'foreign disease' (Lim, 2004, p. 46). In a news article entitled 'Understanding AIDS', a doctor reassured readers that 'the average Singaporean is not likely a victim' since it is only 'male homosexuals, particularly those who have a promiscuous sexual pattern', intravenous drug users, haemophiliacs and 'Haitian immigrants to New York and Miami' who were susceptible to the disease (*The Straits Times*, 1983c). Consequently, the 'average Singaporean' (read heterosexual) was deemed safe, and HIV/AIDS remained a 'foreign disease' for nearly two years, until the first three local cases in 1985. The designation of a virus as a 'foreigner' or 'alien' invader, a common trope of outbreak narratives, is chiefly motivated by political agendas.

Singapore, an 'always-already Westernized' nation by virtue of its Western parentage, was, during the 1980s, self-consciously constructing a national identity distinct from its colonial past (Ang and Stratton, 2018, p. S63).[3] As the sociologist Beng Huat Chua observes, 'the battle [is] always one of the moral East fighting hard to slow down the penetration of the moral decay of the West', and the media played an integral role in the state's fight against the supposed moral decadence (1990, p. 17). The then-editor of *The Straits Times*, Leslie Fong, echoed the government by writing in the newspaper that the press must 'help . . . to prevent the erosion or eclipse of those values that underpin Singapore's success', one of the values being 'the sanctity of the family' (1991, p. 13). Against this backdrop of the exigent need to protect the moral fibre of society and 'Asian' values from the threats of homosexuality and glorification of sex, I would argue that the discursive demarcation of HIV/AIDS as a 'foreign disease' was an attempt to keep what was viewed as a consequence of 'undesirable' Western mores and 'deviant' lifestyles and behaviour, such as homosexuality and sexual promiscuity, at bay. Given that 93% of the respondents of a 1987 nationwide survey cited newspapers as their primary source of information on HIV/AIDS, the characterisation of male sex workers and homosexuals as a particularly potent pool of HIV infection in the media became an increasingly sedimented misconception among the general public, which in turn led to greater prejudice towards gay men, sex workers and PWHAs (Emmanuel, 1991, p. 124).

Censoring HIV-positive homosexual characters

Singaporean discourses on HIV/AIDS that linked it to homosexuality encroached on the local arts community, whose positive theatrical representations of homosexual characters with or without HIV/AIDS were censored from state-run events in Singapore. Eleanor Wong's *Jackson on a Jaunt, or, Mistaken Identities* (*Jackson on a Jaunt* from here on) and Chay Yew's *As if He Hears* were scheduled to be jointly presented by the Ministry of Community Development (MCD) with the drama company TheatreWorks as a double bill under the title 'Safe Sex' in 1988. Wong's script originally included a 'gay yuppie' character in a small role who was 'given false-positive for the AIDS virus in a hospital "mixup" [*sic*]', while Yew's initial script featured two protagonists, one of whom was 'a gay AIDS' volunteer from the local non-governmental organisation, Action for AIDS (AfA), and the other was a 'straight male client' of the volunteer (Chong, 1988, p. 15). AfA was formed in December 1988 by 'a group of concerned physicians and citizens' to 'educate the public on AIDS and to advocate the welfare' of PWHAs, and they pressed for changes in public policy (Leong, 2008, p. 21).

Upon discovering that Wong's and Yew's plays featured a minor and major homosexual character, respectively, the MCD publicly objected to the positive depiction of homosexuality in both plays and withdrew support in a statement by the then–cultural affairs director to *The Straits Times*:

> Homosexuality is portrayed as a natural and acceptable form of sexuality in the play. My ministry will not want to be a joint presenter of the play in its present form. This is in line with the Government's campaign against Aids [*sic*] and homosexuality is one of its main causes. Homosexuality in Singapore is objectionable.
>
> (Chong, 1988, p. 15)

In their responses to the news outlet regarding the censorship, Wong revealed that MCD 'doesn't want him portrayed as a sympathetic gay. It wants the gay character straightened', while Yew disclosed that the ministry wanted him 'to change the character of the gay to that of a woman' (Chong, 1988, p. 15). This is an example of the censorship faced by theatre companies in Singapore since the enactment of Public Entertainments Act 1958. Under this act, the police force's Public Entertainment License Unit officers were tasked with evaluating scripts for theatrical performances. Terence Chong explains that since these police officers were not trained in the arts, they would simply 'respond in a straightforward and didactic manner when confronted with offensive material' instead of contextualising it (2010, p. 239). Wong's and Yew's plays were deemed to contain offensive materials because of the presentation of homosexual characters with HIV/AIDS as normative and in a positive light was perceived as categorically contravening efforts to discourage sexual activities between men who were deemed sources of infection and a threat to the nuclear family. Both plays consequently did not receive a performance license to be staged. As reported by the *New Paper*, it was only six months later, after the playwrights rewrote the scripts, that 'censors g[a]ve Aids play[s] the nod' to be staged (1988, p. 23). The homosexual character in Wong's original play was written out, as 'it was just a minor character who was gay' (Ng, 2020, p. 126). Meanwhile, Yew decided to hint instead at the AIDS volunteer's sexuality through his mannerisms and gait. While the portrayal of heterosexual HIV/AIDS-positive characters helped dispel the misconception of the illness as a 'gay disease', the censorship faced by Wong and Yew signalled an attempt to systematically erase representations of HIV-positive gay men's lived experience.

Giving voices to PWHAs in Singapore plays

Rewritten versions of Wong's *Jackson on a Jaunt* and Yew's *As if He Hears* were eventually staged together in 1989 under the title 'Safe Sex: A Double Bill' at The Drama Centre, a significant venue in the local theatre scene, as it was not only located in Fort Canning Park, a historical landmark, but it was also 'the key platform for local companies starting out in the early 1980s' (Arts House Limited, Drama Centre, n.d.). This chapter uses the recordings of the 1989 productions of both plays as well as the script of *Jackson on A Jaunt* for close analysis (Wong, 2016). The protagonist of Wong's rewritten version, Jackson Ong, is a successful young man who sleeps with multiple women (including Mimi, a sex worker) even though he is about to get married. While visiting a doctor regarding a skin infection, Ong runs into Mimi who coincidentally is at the same hospital undergoing her regular screening for HIV. They are mistakenly given the same patient identification number and their blood samples are subsequently sent to the lab. Mimi tests positive for HIV, but the duplicated identification number means Jackson is also informed of the positive result. It is only in the penultimate scene that Jackson is told of the testing blunder and that he had been misdiagnosed with AIDS. Jackson's moment of euphoria and relief is short-lived, however, as he realises it is Mimi, with whom he has sexual relations, who has tested positive. This tragic farce mocks the media discourses that firmly omitted heterosexuals from the list of groups susceptible to the disease.

Meanwhile, Yew's play depicts the illness experience of an HIV-positive character, Hans, from diagnosis to his death in a non-linear dramatic structure. The play begins with the frail-looking Hans living alone in his apartment six months after testing positive. During a flashback scene to the moment of his diagnosis, he confesses to engaging in extramarital sex – the cause of his HIV infection. His wife leaves him in the aftermath of the diagnosis, taking their young daughter with her. Peter, the volunteer from AfA, becomes his regular companion. The play ends with Hans' death.

The two plays are well meaning in their attempt to provide alternative spaces for PWHAs to be heard and seen through the depiction of loneliness and ostracisation faced by HIV-positive characters and the detrimental impact of the diagnosis on their lives and families at a time when the disease is censured by the media. However, these portrayals of PWHAs are to some extent problematic. For instance, the rewritten versions foregrounded promiscuous characters, Hans, Jackson and Mimi, in place of homosexual characters in the original versions. This approach unfortunately promotes the concept of 'risk group' categorisation, first introduced by health experts and fervently echoed by the media. The play's emphasis on Jackson's and Mimi's promiscuities creates the implication that his infection is a corollary of sexual contact with a sex worker, when it was likely caused by their failures to practice safe sex rather than promiscuity *per se*. Such an association is fallacious, as the transmission risk is dependent on a variety of factors such as the viral load, the type of sex, the presence of sexually transmitted infections and acute and late-stage HIV infection, as evidenced by medical studies (Patel *et al.*, 2014; Shaw and Hunter, 2012). The plays' assumption that promiscuity leads to HIV infection is not altogether surprising considering that the Ministry of Health launched a campaign that focused on 'the risks of promiscuity' in 1985 instead of informative educational campaigns to reduce the transmission of the virus (Kong, 1985, p. 13). The playwright Russell Heng recounted in an interview that 'there wasn't a public campaign to get tested. So none of us did' (Ng, 2020, p. 120).

The profound influence that the media had in shaping discourses on HIV/AIDS is reified in the production of *Jackson on a Jaunt* through its set design. The performance unfolds on a circular platform that is covered with newspaper print and enlarged headlines about the illness. The most prominent headline states: 'AIDS: A time-bomb many ignore'. Two stacks of broadsheet newspapers – tall enough to function as both table and two-seater sofa – are placed on the platform adjacent to each other, three feet apart, and they are the only props present on stage at all times. The unfolding of the play within the newspaper-covered stage and the tall stacks of newspapers connote the media coverage of the disease during the outbreak. Despite falling prey to the fallacy that a 'risk group' rather than risky behaviour is primarily responsible for the spread of the virus as propagated by the media however, both plays subvert the 'homosexual disease' discourse since Jackson and Hans – the 'average' Singaporeans who are deemed safe – are infected. Upon receiving their respective diagnoses, Jackson is caught off guard, while Hans is in complete disbelief and denial.

When the doctor instructs Hans to test for HIV at the Communicable Disease Centre, Hans scoffs with incredulity and coarsely states, 'Isn't that . . . Isn't that AIDS? That's a faggot's disease! How can I get it?!' (Yew, 1989). Their incredulous reactions are evidence of the extent to which the newspapers' disproportionate coverage of HIV/AIDS cases in the gay community has insidiously solidified in lay understandings of the disease.

The voices of PWHAs remained conspicuously absent from cultural products and the media even as HIV/AIDS became a full-blown epidemic. On the rare occasion that a PWHA gave an interview to the press, their voices were distorted and their faces were blurred or omitted to maintain their anonymity. This was due to the stigmatising macro-level discourses that treated an HIV-positive diagnosis as immoral and inflicted shame and stigma on PWHAs, thereby discouraging them from speaking out about their illness experience. Despite this atmosphere, Wong's play provides insight into the ways in which HIV-positive diagnosis and its negative significations impact one's sense of identity. Jackson receives his test result midway through the play from his doctor:

Doctor: You have acquired immune deficiency syndrome.
Jackson: Oh. Is that all? (*To audience*) I wasn't too smart then. (*To doctor*) What's the problem? It's the medicine is it? Very expensive is it?
Doctor: Mr. Ong. I don't think you understand.
　　　　[. . .]
Doctor: Mr. Ong you have AIDS.
Jackson: Ay, ay, wait a minute. You never said anything about AIDS, OK? This, what you call it, syndrome is fine but AIDS as well?
Doctor: Mr. Ong, it's just AIDS

Jackson: Just AIDS? It's really very simple in the final analysis, isn't it? Just AIDS . . . And all this time none of us knew that Jackson was defined 'Just AIDS'.

(Wong, 1989, pp. 194–195)

Jackson's aside to the audience illustrates that HIV/AIDS is an identity-implicating illness where the stigmatised disease becomes the patient's identity. In his self-introduction to the audience in the early part of the play, Jackson defines himself as 'a success', and his mother refers to him as 'the perfect son' prior to his appearance on stage (Wong, 1989, pp. 2–3). Yet the attributes and achievements that define him are stripped away at the very instance of diagnosis and Jackson becomes 'Just AIDS' – the list of negative significations that the abbreviated name stands for becomes his identity. The loss of identity is foreshadowed in a preceding scene before Jackson is informed of the result. The doctor, Mei, addresses the audience directly to draw attention to the same identification number that was given to Jackson and Mimi. As she explains the mix-up, both characters join her on stage:

Doctor: Mr. Ong would appear to be a typical successful man. In the prime of his life, outgoing, not too goodlooking [*sic*].

(Wong, 1989, p. 11)

Jackson is undressed in this scene except for a pair of boxers and socks. Stripped of his long-sleeved formal white shirt, grey formal trousers and black boots that defined him from his first appearance on stage, his vivid semi-naked body is one that is vulnerable to the disease, and the scene is also an instantiation of AIDS shredding a person's identity. Yet, even as the play appears to be making this suggestion, it is not the disease *per se* that takes away his identity. Rather, it is the abbreviated name 'AIDS' imbued with culturally constructed prejudicial meanings that overwrite his identity. The circular stage is shrouded in darkness except for a single harsh spotlight shining on Jackson as he says: 'and all this time, none of us knew Jackson was defined just [as] AIDS' after receiving his test result (Wong, 1989). Left to stand alone by himself with the darkness around him, the visual image alludes to the ostracisation that AIDS brings to the patient, while the surrounding darkness suggests the sepulchral atmosphere that AIDS signifies for PWHAs.

The alienating illness experience that PWHAs undergo is given concrete representation through a carefully orchestrated *mise en scene* in *As if He Hears*. The play opens with Hans sitting alone in the centre of the stage on an off-white sofa in a black bathrobe with clothes strewn across the furniture. A mess of papers and rubbish are at his feet. Opening the play with this scene is at once powerful and revealing – Hans' sloppy and unkempt costume, while he sits alone amidst the surrounding darkness, suggests that he is already alienated from society. When Peter arrives at his apartment with groceries, Hans refuses to turn around to face him. As Peter inches closer to the back of the sofa, Hans moves to the adjacent chair, placing distance between himself and Peter. Hans' body eclipses the whiteness of the chair when he sits on it as his black robe camouflages against the darkness of the stage. Hans' posture exhibits what Eve Sedgwick describes as the '[b]lazons of shame' as he sits with his chin down, eyes lowered, shoulders tense, hands clasped and pulled in towards his body (Sedgwick, 2003). The play's representation of the effects of stigmatising discourses on PWHAs in this manner directs attention to those who were most affected by the virus and whose voices had been suppressed.

Subversive acts: reclaiming autonomy and identity

In 1999, when Chew's play was performed, PWHAs were still compelled to conceal their illness like Jackson and Hans due to the rhetorical strategies employed by the local media in their construction of discourses surrounding the disease. Despite this, Paddy Chew bravely performed Singapore's first autobiographical HIV/AIDS play *Completely With/Out Character* despite not being a performance artist. It was written jointly with the playwright Haresh Sharma and staged from 9 May to 16 May 1999, also at The Drama Centre. Chew was an ordinary citizen who decided to publicly declare that he was HIV positive during the First National AIDS Conference in Singapore on 12 December 1998. In his subsequent interviews with various media outlets after coming out, Chew stated that he was 'fed up of waiting for someone to come out' and wanted to 'do something worthwhile for myself and for the cause' (Lim, 1998, p. 23). The enormity of the stigma towards PWHAs was indicated by the fact that Chew was the first – and only – person with AIDS to disclose his condition to the public, thirteen years after the first case of HIV infection in the country. He passed away, aged thirty-nine, on 21 August 1999, three months after the production of his play. He refused to be treated as merely another statistic by staging a public performance that allowed him to assert his autonomy and individuality and reclaim control over his own body, identity and narrative in the face of stigmatising discourses. Chew's solo performance is a conversational direct address piece that re-enacts and narrates anecdotes from his lived experience as a PWHA. This was a bold intervention that opened Singaporean minds to greater understanding of the condition. In the decade following the stringent censorships that hindered Wong's and Yew's scripts, there were some minor changes in the censorship policies. In 1992, the Censorship Review Committee (CRC) published a report stating that 'theatre groups should be given more room for creativity' provided that they take necessary measures to deny entry to minors if the plays 'contain themes or language unsuitable for children' (Ministry of Information and the Arts, 1992, p. 5). At the same time, however, the CRC also stated that 'materials encouraging homosexuality should continue to be disallowed' (ibid, p. 13). If there was any suspicion that Chew's play encouraged homosexuality or hampered the state's campaigns against AIDS, it was almost certainly dispelled by his expression of remorse for his conduct. In one of the scenes, he expresses regret at choosing a 'gay holiday' and 'having a good time' in Europe instead of fulfilling his late mother's wish to visit the Vatican. He tells the audience, 'I always knew in the back of my head that God was going to punish me' (Chew and Sharma, 1999) even though Chew 'eschew[ed] any institutionalised religion', as observed by C.J.W-L. Wee in his review of the play (1999, p. 12). Chew's apologetic position and the moralistic undertone of the play allayed any anxiety about promoting homosexuality.

Nonetheless, Chew refused to conform to a passive and invisible position as demanded by society. The play opens with him dressed as the character of Pierrot, the sad clown, standing in the centre of the stage with his back to the audience while holding two red balloons.[4] His face is painted with a white base make-up, and he dons an oversized white top with ruffled hems at the end of his sleeves and the bottom edge of the top, a pair of loose-fitting pants and flippers. An unoccupied hospital bed is placed on the left side of the stage, while an unoccupied wheelchair is parked on the right side of the stage beside a table that has a cup and a jug of water placed on top of it. Chew waves at the hospital bed as if there is a patient on it and then waddles towards the bedside to deliver the balloons. He cares for the invisible patient by emptying the bedpan. He then touches his chest with both hands and gestures towards the patient, expressing his love. The character of Pierrot embodies at once Chew's status as an outcast in society due to his HIV-positive status as well as his desire and hope for love, companionship and acceptance for PWHAs. After this opening scene, he shares an anecdote about taking his friends on a shopping trip for his coffin, even climbing into it to test it out and taking his obituary picture afterwards at a photo studio. What is apparent amidst the dark comedy is his desire to assert his autonomy; while he would eventually succumb to the uncontrollable infection, he exerts full command over his impending death by managing minute details of his funeral to preserve his vivacious, extravagant and flamboyant personality. The shopping trip is re-enacted on stage as he delivers the anecdote, including the conversations with his friends, in the form of a monologue. He recalls taking his friends on a surprise 'shopping trip' to the casket shop. He then informs them: 'we are going to buy a coffin for me' (Chew and Sharma, 1999). After asking to see the shopkeeper's 'selection of coffins', he finds one that he likes: 'And there it was. I think that one – the one with the X factor'. He then walks to the hospital bed on the left side of the stage, points at the metaphorical coffin and says, 'mahogany' (ibid, 1999). He waves his hand over the bed gracefully, as if showcasing an exquisite display item, and adds, 'Isn't it beautiful? And look at the green', referring to the colour of the inner lining of the coffin (ibid, 1999). It is a subversive act from Chew to make his impending death visible considering that AIDS-related deaths in the country were being buried quietly out of stigma and shame even after more than a decade since the advent of the epidemic.

By law, the bodies of people with AIDS were placed inside black zipper bags, sealed coffins and cremated within twenty-four hours; this burial method was criticised by AfA for 'encourag[ing] discrimination against people with AIDS' (*The Daily Gazette*, 4 December 2000). The burial rules were lifted only on 4 December 2000 after AfA fought for the changes for four years. Alan John, a journalist who witnessed his friend's body undergo the process, remarked that the 'mad dash' to cremate or bury the body conveyed the message that 'Aids [*sic*] is something to fear mightily and stay away from' (1998, p. 13). While Chew's body will eventually be concealed inside the black cadaver bag when he passes, the vibrant colours of his selected coffin are the antithesis to association with the disease and its patients with decay, decline and disgrace, and they symbolise his refusal to make a muted exit as most HIV/AIDS patients were impelled to do by the stigma surrounding the disease.

In the moments before the climax of the play where Chew disrobes to reveal his emaciated body, he makes an impassioned plea to the audience to accept, love and view PWHAs as 'normal, loving human beings' who deserve 'a full and normal life' (Chew and Sharma, 1999). As mentioned earlier, he had stated in his interviews with the media that he 'wanted to do something worthwhile for the cause', and his sentiments to atone for his 'wayward ways' had surfaced earlier in the play (Lim, 1998, p. 23). Read within this context, the act of disrobing can be interpreted as not only a transgression of the social and cultural boundaries that have marginalised PWHAs, but it is also Chew's construction of the self as a martyr. The scene begins with Chew rolling his wheelchair from the right side of the stage to the centre. As the lights on stage dim and a soft beam of light falls on him, he gets up from the wheelchair and walks to the edge of the stage. He unfastens the drawstrings of his loose-fitting white trousers and drops them to reveal his atrophied legs. He then unbuttons his billowy white shirt and takes it off, unveiling his cachexic body. His gaze unflinchingly traverses across the audience during this provocative act as he takes the time to undress bit by bit, heightening the sense of transgression. Wearing only his underwear and a look of serenity on his face, Chew raises his arms to shoulder level – the movement causes his rib cage to visibly strain against his wasted skeletal muscles. He then slowly turns around twice, pausing each time he faces the audience and again when his back faces them. Although this scene risks creating a spectacle, the baring of his painfully thin HIV-positive body – one that society has deemed an abject or non-compliant body – to the public articulates his refusal to be silenced. HIV/AIDS has hitherto been sensationalised in the media by fixating on the controversial facets of the disease that consequently dehumanise PWHAs. The revelation of his frail corporeal form impels the audience to view PWHAs as individuals rather than abstract 'deviants' or 'degenerates' who are deserving of the disease. With his arms raised and his body unclothed except for his underwear, he is a martyr, baring his soul and bearing at once the devastations suffered by PWHAs, demanding for their voices to be heard and for them to be seen and accepted with compassion.

Conclusion

While PWHAs in Singapore were compelled to live in secrecy and shame in the 1980s and 1990s, the three theatrical performances offer alternative imagining that subverts misconceptions, transgress social conventions and underscore the dialectical relationship between the stigmatising discourses and their tangible effects on the lives of PWHAs. *Jackson on a Jaunt, or, Mistaken Identities* and *As if He Hears* – while problematic in their depictions of promiscuous characters as sources of infection and their presentations of the trope of inexorable decline, and death in the latter – are reflective of the cultural understanding of the disease and the social attitudes towards PWHAs in Singapore during the 1980s. Meanwhile, *Completely With/Out Character* revives the patient's voice that was conspicuously absent due to the stigma that quashed any attempts at self-representation for majority of the PWHAs, except Paddy Chew.

Notes

1 'In 1988, the then Deputy Prime Minister Goh Chok Tong mooted the idea of a set of shared values to buttress Singapore's "Asian values" system against over-Westernization and de-culturation. One of the values, "family as a basic unit of society", was partly intended to discourage Singaporeans from engaging in the "alternative lifestyles" seen in many developed (read Western) countries, such as casual sex and single parenthood' (Lim, 2004, p. 61).
2 The press in Singapore is policed by a number of laws including: Newspaper and Printing Presses Act 1974 to prohibit foreign influence through ownership or funding; Undesirable Publications Act 1967 that prohibits importation, distribution or reproduction of undesirable publications that are 'politically offensive, morally offensive, religiously offensive, and ethnically offensive' (Tan and Soh, 1994, p. 43).
3 Sir Stamford Raffles is officially recognized as the founder of modern Singapore. The country's colonial past, its adoption of the English language as the official language and a parliament and legal system modelled on and derived from the British makes Singapore 'always-already Westernized'.
4 I am grateful to Sophia Hyder for this observation.

Reference list

Ang, I. and Stratton, J. (2018) 'The Singapore way of multiculturalism: western concepts/Asian cultures', *Sojourn: Journal of Social Issues in Southeast Asia*, 33(S), pp. S61–S86, 692196. https://doi.org/10.1355/sj33-Sd

Chew, P. and Sharma, H. (1999, 9 May) *Completely with/out character*. Directed by A. Tan. Singapore: The Necessary Stage. First performance.

Chong, T. (2010) '"Back regions" and "dark secrets" in Singapore: the politics of censorship and liberalisation', *Space and Polity*, 14(3), pp. 235–250. https://doi.org10.1080/13562576.2010.532952

Chong, Y.Y. (1988) 'Ministry says "no" to play on AIDS', *The Straits Times*, Singapore, 16 March. Available at: https://eresources.nlb.gov.sg/newspapers/digitised/article/straitstimes19880316-1.2.28.11 (Accessed: 15 June 2021).

Chua, B.H. (1990) 'Confucianization in modernizing Singapore', paper presented at Beyond the Culture? Conference, Loccum, West Germany.

Cutter, J.L. *et al.* (2005) 'HIV in Singapore – past, present, and future', *AIDS Education and Prevention*, 16, pp. 110–118. https://doi.org/10.1521/aeap.16.3.5.110.35528

The Daily Gazette (2000) 'Singapore lifts burial rules for AIDS victims', 4 December, C12. https://news.google.com/newspapers?nid=OtrppQHxQ5wC&dat=20001204&printsec=frontpage&hl=en (Accessed: 15 June 2021).

Drama Centre (n.d.) *Art house limited.* Available at: https://artshouselimited.sg/venues/dramacentre (Accessed: 15 January 2022).

Emmanuel, S.C. (1991) 'Public awareness of AIDS in Singapore', *Singapore Medical Journal*, 32, pp. 123–126. PMID: 2042073

Gross, L. (2001) *Up from invisibility: lesbians, gay men, and the media in America.* New York: Columbia University Press.

John, A. (1998) 'Let's start facing aids and stop fearing its victims', *The Straits Times*, Overseas education, 19 December. Available at: NewspaperSG Reel no. NL21358 (Accessed: 15 June 2021).

Kong, S.C. (1985) 'Aids: 20,000 cleared', *The Straits Times*, Singapore, 29 November. Available at: https://eresources.nlb.gov.sg/newspapers/digitised/article/straitstimes19851129-1.2.29.12 (Accessed: 15 June 2021).

Kramer, L. (1985) *The normal heart.* New York: Samuel French Inc.

Kushner, T. (1992) *Angels in America: a gay fantasia on national themes.* London: Nick Hern Books.

Larson, J. (1996) *Rent.* New York: Rob Weisbach Books.

Leong, L. (2008) 'Walking the tightrope: the role of action for AIDS in the provision of social services in Singapore', *Journal of Gay & Lesbian Social Services*, 3(3), pp. 11–30. https://doi.org/10.1300/J041v03n03_02

Lim, A. (1998) 'I'm still not sure if it's right thing to do', *The Sunday Times*, 13 December.

Lim, K.G.F. (2004) 'Life goes on: living with HIV and AIDS in Singapore', *Asian Journal of Social Science*, 32(1), pp. 42–65.

Ministry of Information and the Arts (1992) *Censorship review committee report 1992.* Singapore: Ministry of Information and the Arts.

NBC Nightly News (1982) 'Nightly news', 17 June.

The New Paper (1988) 'Censors give aids play the nod', 14 September. Available at: NewspaperSG Reel no. NL16636 (Accessed: 15 January 2022).

Ng, Y.-S. (2020) 'Blooms: the dawn of queer Singapore theatre', in *Black waters, pink sands.* Singapore: Math Paper Press, pp. 102–210.

Patel, P., Borkowf, C.B., Brooks, J.T., Lasry, A., Lansky, A. and Mermin, J. (2014) 'Estimating per-act HIV transmission risk: a systematic review', *AIDS*, 28(10), pp. 1509–1519. https://doi.org/10.1097/QAD.0000000000000298

Sedgwick, E. (2003) *Touching feeling: affect, pedagogy, performativity.* Durham: Duke University Press.

Shaw, G.M. and Hunter, E. (2012) 'HIV transmission', *Cold Spring Harbor Perspectives in Medicine*, 2(11), pp. 1–24, a006965. https://doi.org/10.1101/cshperspect.a006965

The Straits Times (1983a) 'No answer to killer disease', Singapore, 6 January. Available at: NewspaperSG Reel no. NL13884 (Accessed: 15 June 2021).

The Straits Times (1983b) 'Mystery illness that strikes fear in many hearts', Singapore, 17 June. Available at: NewspaperSG Reel no. NL14059 (Accessed: 15 June 2021).

The Straits Times (1983c) 'Understanding AIDS', Singapore, 7 September. Available at: NewspaperSG Reel no. NL14163 (Accessed: 15 June 2021).

Tan, Y.S. and Soh, Y.P. (1994) *The development of Singapore's modern media industry.* Singapore: Times Academic Press.

Wee, C.J.W.-L. (1999) 'Performing performance: paddy chew, sincerity and (re-)staging AIDS', *Substance*, pp. 11–12. Available at: https://tnsarchives.com/index.php/essays-and-writings/2153/performing-performance (Accessed: 26 July 2023).

Wong, E. (1989, 23 November) *Jackson on a jaunt, or, mistaken identities.* Directed by O. Keng Sen. Singapore: TheatreWorks. First performance.

Wong, E. (2016) 'Jackson on a jaunt or mistaken identities', in Ng, K.C. (ed.) *Earlier.* Singapore: Firstfruits, pp. 173–214.

Yew, C. (1989, 23 November) *As if he hears.* Directed by O. Keng Sen. Singapore: TheatreWorks. First performance.

2

THE AIDS CRISIS, BEREAVEMENT AND ALLOPATHOGRAPHIC PERFORMANCE

Ellen Redling

As we emerged from the coronavirus (COVID-19) pandemic in 2021, the medical classification of AIDS had its 40-year anniversary. While the two pandemics shared some common characteristics, the AIDS crisis was associated with more complex moral stigma, meaning that people initially avoided speaking about it (Arthur, 2021, p. 20). American philosopher and activist Susan Sontag was among the first to describe a particular type of stigmatisation and judgement faced by people living with AIDS:

> The unsafe behavior that produces AIDS is judged to be more than just a weakness. It is indulgence, delinquency – addictions to chemicals that are illegal and to sex regarded as deviant. The sexual transmission of this illness, considered by most people as a calamity one brings on oneself, is judged more harshly than other means.
>
> (Sontag, 2002, pp. 74–75)

Sontag also argues that there is a potential danger of increasing the suffering and further stigmatising those confronted with diseases due to the way illnesses are talked about by others. She states that the 'very reputation of [an] illness' can 'add . . . to the suffering of those who have it' (2002, p. 66). In line with Sontag's concern, this chapter concentrates on the AIDS crisis and on performances created by people bereaved by the disease. While the artworks under consideration are also about the performance makers' own mourning processes, they foreground the real lives, illness and death of the artists' friends/lovers, who died of AIDS. The examples chosen for this chapter are Mark Ravenhill's *pool (no water)* (2006), Felix Gonzales-Torres' *Untitled (Portrait of Ross in L.A.)* (1991) and Karen Finley's *Written in Sand* (1992-ongoing). These were selected as they were all created by an artist bereaved by AIDS and explore or illustrate the ethical responsibilities that arise when making art in the aftermath of death from a stigmatised disease. Ravenhill's play is a fictional treatment of the ethical problems that can emerge in this context. Although it is an exaggerated portrayal that satirises the exploitation of trauma and taboo associated with the British art scene of the 1990s, it is at the same time also inspired by personal loss and thus can be used as a lens to help read the other two works from an ethical perspective.

DOI: 10.4324/9781003036500-4

AIDS and art-making

The fact that all of these three pieces are by people bereaved by AIDS exemplifies an interesting practice within the wider field of AIDS-related art-making. The works sit between different categories by being, on the one hand, expressions of the makers' grief and forms of activism and memorialisation. On the other hand, they are examples of allopathography, the portrayal/telling of another person's illness, which is an underexplored inflection of the practice of pathography, i.e. narratives of disease. Whilst these works can be seen as calls to action, they are dissimilar from more confrontational activism, e.g. 'street activism such as, in the US, the "die-ins" or "kiss-ins" staged by ACT UP' (Campbell and Gindt, 2018, p. 7). They are also different from artworks about the fear of contagion – such as Kevin Elyot's *My Night with Reg* (1994) and Russell T. Davies's 2021 series *It's a Sin*. Additionally, they diverge from works that explore the realities of dying from or caring for someone with AIDS – such as the Prior/Louis narrative in Tony Kushner's *Angels in America* (1991–1992) and Peter Friedman and Tom Joslin's 1993 documentary film *Silverlake Life*. The specific focus of the pieces under consideration in this chapter perhaps puts them closer to works of memorialisation, such as the AIDS Memorial Quilt project, in which human rights activist Cleve Jones and a group of people created a giant quilt made out of panels dedicated to friends and loved ones who had died of AIDS (Gambardella, 2001; Krouse, 1994; Stull, 2001). For further discussion of performances made in response to HIV/AIDS see chapters by April Thant Aung and Katharine E. Low in this volume.

Allopathography forms part of the practice of pathography, that is, narratives of illness. However, the more commonly analysed form of pathography is 'autopathography', i.e. the telling or performing of one's *own* experiences of illness and treatment. Autopathography is often seen as an empowering act (Hunsaker Hawkins, 1999), as it can even be about 'establishing a new personal identity' in the face of illness (Fulford *et al.*, 2013). It can work against a potentially limiting and harmful, doctor-oriented 'medical gaze' (Foucault, 1973) and thus against an imbalance in power between a physician and a patient. Unlike the medical history written by a doctor, an autopathographic account is 'subjective' and 'experiential' (Hunsaker Hawkins, 1999, p. 12). By making patients' voices heard, autopathography can also raise awareness of specific conditions and often also demonstrate systematic failures or highlight cases of stigmatisation (Fulford *et al.*, 2013). While this is a significant response to HIV/AIDS, the question that will be explored in this chapter, however, is what happens when artists do not seek to convey their own experiences of illness and treatment, but those of other people. In that case one can speak about 'allopathography', rather than 'autopathography'.

To some extent, I am drawing on the work of Katharina Fürholzer, who in her recent German monograph *Das Ethos des Pathographen* (2019) included a sub-chapter about allopathography in relation to literature. For instance, she talks about why friends or relatives might engage in writing about the illness of their loved ones in the first place, stating that it is often because they feel the need to value the lives of the ones they have lost, rather than allowing these lives to be reduced to statistics like the years of their birth and death (Fürholzer, 2019, p. 136). Allopathography thus has a re-humanising effect (ibid, p. 141). She notes that friends and relatives might turn to writing in order to regain some control in a situation where they, like their ill loved ones, feel out of control (ibid, p. 137). However, as she cautions, if the private accounts about friends/relatives become literature, they then go out to the public, which can create ethical problems (ibid, p. 137). Similarly to G. Thomas Couser (2004, 2005), Fürholzer highlights concerns related to representing ill subjects in literature, which are mainly linked to potentially increasing the vulnerable status of the ill or dying person (2019, p. 152). This seems to be in line with what Susan Sontag maintained in terms of the danger of potentially increasing the suffering of those who are already vulnerable.

Ethics in allopathography

Fürholzer argues that the friends/relatives who write about their loved ones might confuse their own observations with those of the ill person (ibid, p. 138, 140). While she does not elaborate on potential effects of such a confusion, I would like to demonstrate that such a misapplication could lead to harmful assumptions about, or impositions upon, the ill person. I will explore such effects further in my analysis of Ravenhill's *pool (no water)*. Fürholzer goes on to say that friends/ relatives also might misappropriate very intimate and personal material that belongs to the ill and vulnerable person for the purpose of their 'story' (ibid, p. 143, 149), which can raise issues surrounding consent (ibid, p. 147). As I will show in the section about *pool (no water)*, such a lack of consent raises even more ethically complex issues, as it does not only take away the ill person's agency and will, but can also – through misappropriation – override this person's ability to 'establish . . . a new personal identity' in the face of disease, which Fulford *et al.* describe as one of the advantages of autopathography (2013). While allopathography could add a further perspective to the ill person's story, for instance that of the bereaved person, it should not go against the ill person's agency and will. In other words, allopathography should not cancel out what would have been the main benefits if the ill person had told their story themselves.

Similarly to Susan Sontag, who points out that the wider 'reputation of [an] illness' (2002, p. 66) is a crucial point to consider in regard to stigmatisation and the AIDS crisis, Fürholzer states that authors have a responsibility not only towards the ill person but also towards society as a whole. This is because every portrayal of illness can have an effect on the way this disease is perceived by society (for example, negatively, balanced, or positively) (ibid, p. 151). Fürholzer only very briefly hints at what friends/relatives could do to act in an ethically responsible way when creating allopathographic literature. She says they could critically reflect on what they are doing and use distancing methods – for instance, by transforming the subject's 'story' into a poem or by anonymising the names of their ill loved ones (ibid, pp. 147–148). A more in-depth exploration of such ethical allopathographic strategies is missing in her volume.

I will therefore take the analysis of such strategies further and examine them in greater detail. In addition to that, I will move the focus from allopathographic *literature* towards allopathographic *performance*, in which the live encounter between performer(s) and spectators arguably adds another layer of complexity to these ethical issues. Thus, I will discuss how Gonzales-Torres' and Finley's works avoid taking advantage of the illness of others and instead create pieces of memorialisation, contemplation and calls to action that are aimed towards achieving greater empathy and socio-political change. Before doing so, I will analyse Ravenhill's depiction of less ethical artistic responses to bereavement in *pool (no water)* (2006). The play explores some of the ethical dangers that have been highlighted previously.

When I saw a performance of Ravenhill's *pool (no water)* in Munich in 2007, directed by Florian Boesch, I heard the audience gasp audibly upon watching a group of artists exploit the serious injuries of their artist-friend, who had jumped into an empty pool, for the purposes of their art-making and for profit. This happened when the group – instead of showing empathy – took pictures of the bloodied body and commented on the aesthetic value of the different shades and nuances of the colours of the wounds. Their behaviour, as they maintain throughout, is one of justified revenge – as their friend had allegedly acted in the same way, when she created art in the wake of her friends Sally and Ray dying of AIDS. The group, who had been unsuccessful artists so far, note that their famous friend became successful because of her own ruthlessness and because of a lack of care on the part of the public. As the group of friends depict it, the famous artist took items such as Ray's 'blood and bandages and catheter and condoms' (Ravenhill, 2006, p. 3) for her installation piece without his consent after he was dead, and it caused a sensation.

The play can be seen as shocking, but also as actively encouraging reflection on that shock. It is both affect-oriented and (self-)reflective – and takes place both in the moment and on the meta-level. Ravenhill's work is typically linked to the often drastic and violent 'in-yer-face' theatre and its legacy, but for him, sensational scenes are never just gratuitous. Thus, *pool (no water)* addresses questions of exploitative art that arose, for instance, in the context of the notorious *Sensation* exhibition by the so-called Young British Artists in London in 1997. Among other alleg-edly sensationalist installations, this exhibition included Marcus Harvey's painting of the child-murderess Myra Hindley (*Myra*, 1995), which is a large-scale reproduction of her police 'mug-shot' composed entirely out of children's handprints.

In 1990, Ravenhill himself was diagnosed as HIV-positive, and he sadly lost his partner due to AIDS-related complications in 1993. However, he does not portray his own illness in this play and generally seems to avoid autobiographical pieces. Caridad Svich writes: 'Illness and death are frequent subjects in his work, and although his work is rarely directly autobiographical, the spectre of disease haunts his writing' (2011, p. 403). This 'spectre of disease' can be seen in the fact that he was partly inspired to write his new version of Voltaire's *Candide* (Ravenhill, 2013) by reading Barbara Ehrenreich's *Smile or Die* (2009), which criticises the cult of 'positive thinking' surround-ing serious illnesses such as breast cancer, from which the author suffered herself. Ravenhill seems to want to highlight larger perspectives that are perhaps inspired by, but not solely connected to, his personal life.

Such larger perspectives are also signalled by the playtext of *pool (no water)*, which contains no specific character names and therefore leaves it to the director to assign which lines of dialogue are allocated to which characters. However, the artist that has become famous is referred to as 'she', which makes her stand out as a more individualised character from the group of friends. While 'she' is hospitalised and in an induced coma following her traumatic injuries, the friends plot their revenge. They decide to document her wounds by taking pictures of them with the aim of exhibit-ing them (Ravenhill, 2006, p. 13). This raises the issue of consent, as she is unconscious while they are taking the pictures and has not agreed to them doing so. The friends' feeling of excitement about their new project fades completely when the famous artist starts to regain consciousness, finds out about their art project, suddenly takes charge of it and thereby regains her agency. The ethical issue of consent thus becomes resolved, as she re-appropriates the work. Seeing the project slip away from them, the group of friends destroy the photos. At the end of the play, she seems to reveal both her anger and her underlying arrogance:

> I have talent. I have vision. I am blessed. You are not . . . And Sally and Ray died because they were too weak to live, to live and make art. I am the only one of you strong enough ever to really live and nothing you can do will ever destroy me. Because I will always be the stronger.
>
> (Ravenhill, 2006, p. 29)

The play leaves it open to interpretation whether or not this final confrontation takes place or is imagined by the group to project their own lack of ethical considerations onto her and thereby alle-viate their sense of guilt. If this is true, they would have misguidedly assumed that she was never truly concerned about her friends Sally and Ray, who had AIDS, and that she exploited them to achieve success in the art world. As the group of friends continue to claim throughout the play, this (supposed) exploitation is similar to them using her injury in order to avenge themselves, acquire fame and make profit. Ravenhill's play thus not only highlights problems connected to friendship and jealousy, it also shows where the ethical dilemmas of creating a performance about the illness and death of friends might lie. In contrast, Felix Gonzales-Torres and Karen Finley each take a different approach to making art in response to death by AIDS.

Holding and creating space

The most moving moments in Cuban artist Felix Gonzalez-Torres' *Untitled (Portrait of Ross in L.A.)* arguably occur when visitors to his installation take hold of one of the shiny sweets that make up the piece, feel the smooth surface in the palm of their hands, unwrap it and then ingest it. This is because they thereby inadvertently become complicit in the consumption and disappearance of an artwork that stands for the body of someone who has died of AIDS. Much like a child or a lover, they have been given candy, but this sweet then attains also serious, and bitter, connotations. I argue that in this sequence of moments, the visitors are both holding space and creating space in regard to this artwork and what it stands for. They are holding space when the sweet is in their hand and therefore the body, represented by the pile, is in transition between presence and absence. They are then creating space when they are ingesting the sweet. These become ethical moments, if the visitors do not treat these scenes as mere acts of removal and consumption, but rather as prompts towards having compassion with – and reflecting on – the disappearing body.

'Holding space' has become a term that is typically used in the field of mental health and therapy today. It essentially means being present for someone, and open to them, rather than coming to their place of suffering from the position of one's own ego and preconceptions. It can also mean being there for someone in the liminal and transitional space between presence and absence, life and death (Plett, 2020, pp. 16–17). I argue that this is what Gonzales-Torres invited visitors to do with his artworks that were based on his partner Ross Laycock's death from AIDS-related complications in 1991. *Untitled (Portrait of Ross in L.A.)* consisted of a pile of 175lbs (about 80kg) of sweets, individually wrapped in red, silver and blue cellophane, and piled into a corner of the gallery. The sweets were 'commercially available, shiny wrapped confections' (Art Institute of Chicago, 1991: online), and the artwork was interactive: 'as visitors choose to take candy from the work, the volume and weight of the work decrease' (ibid). This candy was then later replenished.

While some critics, such as Anthony Iannacci, have linked the taking and eating of the candy to the ritual of communion, the consumption of the body of Christ and to 'the Christian belief in the circularity of Christ's existence and resurrection' (Watney, 2016, p. 347), Simon Watney argues that the act of taking and ingesting the candy is not narrowly defined, but rather has 'many levels' and does not 'retreat into didacticism' (ibid, pp. 344–345). In this context it is important to note that whilst the candy pile is often regarded as representing Ross Laycock's body (Keats, 2012: online), it was not shaped like Ross's body. It often took on a triangular shape, but 'the physical form of the work changes depending on the way it is installed' (Art Institute of Chicago, 1991: online). Furthermore, it is not necessarily Ross's weight that is represented by the pile, but the 'average body weight of an adult male' (ibid), which arguably leaves room for one's own perspective on it.

I think this openness also creates space – space not only for interpretation but also for empathy with Ross and anyone suffering from AIDS, as the depletion of candy could, for instance, be seen as standing for the 'loss of appetite, which is so often painfully experienced by people with AIDS' (Watney, 2016, p. 344). Despite being named after Ross, the artwork is still also 'Untitled', therefore retaining a certain flexibility and openness. This correlates to a certain extent with what Fürholzer writes in regard to how one can create an ethically responsible allopathographic piece, for example by using certain distancing mechanisms (2019, pp. 147–148). Gonzales-Torres' work thus invites interpretation by association, rather than fixed meaning. Candy – rather than other types of food – was perhaps chosen because it can represent something positive amidst the tragedy of loss, namely, for instance, a gift of love and friendship. But if one links Gonzales-Torres' art to that of Andy Warhol (Watney, 2016, p. 347), one might also connect the 'commercially available', shiny colourful sweets to consumerism and regard the spectator as consuming the work of art.

The live encounter that Gonzales-Torres creates between the work and the spectators, however, goes beyond the distancing mechanisms described by Fürholzer. I argue that Gonzales-Torres employs techniques of *both* distance and closeness. Holding space is an intimate act of engaging with another person and another body – even if the other body is (increasingly) absent. Gonzales-Torres established an ethically responsible piece about his partner's illness through the specific interaction with the spectator and through a blend of lighter elements and tragic ones: sweets and death, presence and absence, thoughts and emotions, fantasy and reality. Whilst, interestingly, the sweets can be – and indeed were – replaced every day, the real suffering body of Ross Laycock cannot be. So, whereas the artwork can live on, despite the daily depletion, Laycock cannot. It becomes an act of memorialisation, but at the same time one of holding space for the absent body in the live encounter with the vanishing pile. The viewers can become aware of presence and absence at the same time. The candy in their hand means it is no longer part of the pile. 'Sweetness' and sorrow become part of the same experience, two sides of the coin. The spectators are not merely consuming the pile, and thereby in a sense 'profiting' from the piece of art; they are shown what the price of that consumption is; and this transparency and meta level, which brings sweetness and tragedy together, is where the ethical dimension of the artwork lies. The daily replenishment also indicates a reach beyond one particular body and shows how the same process is happening to many bodies.

In Gonzales-Torres' work the act of taking something away does not become one of exploitation. It becomes an act of holding and creating space – space for those suffering from HIV/AIDS and for the interpretation itself, which remains open. Participants are enticed to not only be part of the fleeting 'sweetness' but to have lingering thoughts – perhaps beyond the performance – about this process, and to experience their own emotions in connection to this. As Jonathon Keats formulates it, '*Untitled (Portrait of Ross in LA)*' is one of the rare artworks to perfectly balance ideas and emotions' (2012: online). Establishing their own connection with the artwork can enable the viewers to have a meaningful encounter – and empathy with those suffering from HIV/AIDS – rather than just coldly consuming the spectacle.

'Infectious' rage

While Felix-Gonzales' piece might lean more towards quiet contemplation, American performance artist Karen Finley's *Written in Sand* (1992-ongoing), which is about the loss of as many as 60 of her friends during the AIDS crisis, shows the rawness of her grief and rage almost as if she had only just heard of their passing before the start of the show. In this anthology of spoken-word pieces, she expresses her sorrow 'in wails and howls that grab at the viscera of anyone within hearing distance' (Brantley, 2014: online). An especially searing moment for me in the performance happens when Finley enacts emergency calls that go unanswered, as no one seems to listen and no one seems to care about those dying of AIDS, not even close family members. Using an often tense and angry voice, with words that cut 'like knives' (Prior, 2015: online), Finley presents a scene entitled 'Hello mother', in which she tells a mother repeatedly that her son is dying, but also mentions that the mother already knows that, indicating her criticism that the mother has chosen to ignore her son's critical situation due to a fear of stigma:

> Hello mother, hello mother, hello mother. Your son is dying. No, don't hang up. You already knew your son, your son is dying. Hello mother! [louder] Hello mother! Your son is dying! No, don't hang up! You already knew your son, your son is dying! [shrill] . . .
>
> (Finley, 2015: online)

Finley then addresses the 'Soho gallery bullshit', the 'art magazine cover crap' and the 'trendy East Villagers with rich parents', telling them that '[their] friend, [their] artist is dying' (ibid). She is wondering where they are now. She also calls out the paramedics who did not 'realise one of [their] clients' IV came out and he was bleeding all over the place and [they] couldn't give a shit' (ibid). She draws attention to a hospital who did not admit a person with HIV. Then she in turn accuses society, Britain, the World, America, and society again of not answering. The constant and increasingly anguished repetition, which towards the end of this scene moves from shrillness to a lower, but still loud and angry, voice is often reminiscent of an evangelical bellowing and has imprinted itself in my gut and mind.

Finley's performance work about the AIDS crisis is an act of mourning and memorialisation through her visceral expression of grief and rage. She lived through the beginnings of the AIDS pandemic in New York and lost many friends to the disease. *Written in Sand* started in 1992 (then called *Memento Mori*) as an interactive installation piece. It is still ongoing, thus strongly emphasising the continued mourning caused by the losses due to AIDS. As Marc Arthur points out, Finley 'reveals how her experiences of the early AIDS crisis remain chronically present' (2021, p. 25). Joe Turnbull similarly states that Finley shows that mourning someone does not necessarily suddenly end. He describes *Written in Sand* as a 'hugely important show. Lest we forget. Lest we get complacent. Lest we fool ourselves into thinking that the battles over attitudes and for acceptance have already been won' (2015: online).

In this loud and furious performance piece, Finley quotes from a collection of texts, letters, and poetry from 1983–1994 that stem from her experiences living through the AIDS crisis in New York. The performance also includes music played by jazz artist Paul Nebenzahl. In the previously mentioned scene 'Hello Mother', Nebenzahl plays an increasingly shrill sounding flute arrangement. As Turnbull writes, *Written in Sand* 'acts like a musical accompaniment to [her] book [*Shock Treatment*]' (2015: online), and her 'lamenting elegies set to music are interspersed with renditions of songs made by musicians who have since lost their lives to AIDS including Freddy Mercury and the B-52's Ricky Wilson' (ibid: online). Finley uses the intensity of her voice to convey her raw sorrow. It aims to infect the audience with her rage so that they spring into action and call for change themselves.

When Finley started this piece, it was a travelling installation that had the title *Memento Mori* (1992) involving several 'grieving rituals' (Finley, 2000, p. 154). Her idea was to 'take public sculpture further. This sculpture would be created by the public, as they interacted with the installation' (ibid). The first ritual was called 'Ribbon Gate'. Visitors coming to the installation were met by a guide standing at an iron gate. They were then asked to choose a ribbon from a basket and to 'tie the ribbon to gate in memory of someone who had died of AIDS' (ibid). The gate subsequently became fuller and fuller of ribbons. When the installation travelled to Los Angeles, its scale became larger. 'In L.A. there were 12 to 15,000 ribbons tied to the gate' (ibid, p. 157). And for the Los Angeles version of *Memento Mori*, Finley also included an antique chest filled with sand and the ritual of the visitors writing 'the name of someone who had died of AIDS in the sand. They were asked to erase the name back into the sand. Parents, lovers, friends, families, and children of those who had died came to participate' (ibid, p. 158). Similarly to Gonzales-Torres, her piece is thus to some extent also about holding space, and about presence and absence – or remembrance and ephemerality. This is also emphasised by a companion installation called the 'Vacant Chair', which Finley included in Toronto. The main idea behind it was that visitors could sit with the 'vacant chair' which stood for 'the presence of the deceased person' (ibid, p. 160). As Finley notes, '[w]hen a person dies, we feel their presence in their absence – the vacant place at the table, the vacant space in the bed, the empty space in the closet, the vacant chair' (ibid).

Her show *Written in Sand*, which was based on her installation, however, moves away from such quiet contemplation, while still asking audience members to leave 'some seats for those who have departed this life' (Brantley, 2014: online). Turnbull describes it as a 'litany of fury and mourning through the medium of spoken word' (2015: online). This rage can be seen as infectious. As Arthur notes, *Written in Sand* can be regarded as employing 'viral dramaturgy' (2021, p. 26), a term coined by Alyson Campbell and Dirk Gindt which means that such a 'performance works like a virus as it moves initially into the individual body's system, producing change at the physiological level' (Campbell and Gindt, 2018, pp. 8–9). Lyn Gardner draws attention to the potential danger that Finley's own grief takes centre stage (2015: online). However, while Finley's work adds her own perspective of a bereaved and mourning friend, she in no way takes away from the ill people's agency and will. There are parts in the performance which are more about her own experience – such as when she says family members told her '"it must get easier when you've lost so many". This said whilst complaining about their fad-diets or boring marriages; "sometimes," she screams, "I pretend to have their problems"' (in Turnbull, 2015: online).

And there are passages which refer more to her friends' experiences, such as in the 'emergency/ wake-up call' scene detailed previously, or when she revisits, with great intensity, a conversation with her friend Ethyl Eichelberger, an experimental theatre artist and drag performer who contemplated taking his own life rather than die of AIDS:

My friend says he's going to take his own life because he wants me to remember him well, not sick. He says he's had a good life. He says, Karen, if I have it my way, I'm going to be coming back in a more evolved state'.

(Arthur, 2021, p. 26)

To go back, in part, to Fürholzer's notes on ethical allopathographic techniques (2019, pp. 147–148), one can make the following observations: First of all, Finley does not confuse her own observations with those of the ill person. She also critically reflects on what she is doing – at one point in the performance saying: 'Creating this work, one of the challenges was thinking about how can you create a work or express in a theatrical way and with the artifice, a human, real experience' (2015: online). Furthermore, Finley employs distancing mechanisms. She transforms her friends' experiences into a performance that reaches beyond the individual details and becomes a wider-reaching outcry. As Mel Gussow argues, '[t]hough [Finley] often draws her material straight from her life, it is transmogrified into something generic and metaphorical' (2000, p. xiii). However, Finley also goes beyond such distancing mechanisms indicated by Fürholzer, by foregrounding the immediacy of the visceral experience in the live encounter with the audience. Like Gonzales-Torres, she brings distance and closeness together, albeit in a different way.

Employing the lens of affect theory, I argue that Finley aims to establish a deep – and arguably ethical – connection with the audience through the searingly intense experience she creates for the audience. As Melissa Gregg and Gregory J. Seigworth write, 'affect is found in those intensities that pass body to body . . . in those resonances that circulate about, between, and sometimes stick to bodies and worlds' (2010, p. 1). Such an intensity emerging from one body can result in a visceral reaction – and a 'drive . . . toward movement' and 'thought' (ibid) – in another body, for instance in the bodies of the spectators. Finley's fury can thus reverberate in the audience and act as a wake-up call or reminder that the grief over the losses of lives and the rage against a society which seems to have forgotten has not abated. As Turnbull notes, '[h]er ire for the contemporary attitudes towards AIDS was fierce' (2015: online). Whilst affect is not ethical in and of itself, it can become a way of ethically moving someone through a body-to-body transmission of anger at injustice, which can be seen in Finley's performance and which can be interpreted as an urgent call to action.

What Finley seems to conjure up during this performance is the idea that her dead friends are speaking *through* her, rather than that she is speaking *for* them. Aptly, Arthur (2021) notes that Finley resembles a medium during the show. She is thus not really concentrating on her own sense of compassion, but rather saying that a friend who was ill, unlike society more in general, had empathy with others even before contracting AIDS: he 'transform[ed] . . . [his] pain into compassion' throughout his entire life (Finley, 2015: online). Through her performance of fierce outrage, her friends' personal experiences quickly become linked to wider socio-political issues. She is making accusations against a society that has ignored, and continues to neglect, those that die from AIDS-related diseases.

To conclude, both Gonzales-Torres and Finley have created ethically complex works about their partner's or friends' illnesses and death. Unlike the group of friends depicted in Ravenhill's fictional play, they have not exploited the experiences of their loved ones. Rather, through making use of the power of the live encounter in performance and through activating and implicating the spectators, they have encouraged the viewers to engage with their artworks and the experiences behind them more deeply. Both reach out beyond their respective personal context and use distance and closeness, but do so in different ways. Whilst Gonzales-Torres encourages a quieter, reflective holding and creating of space for those who are ill and for the overall interpretation of his artwork, Finley has developed an affect-oriented and vulnerable show, a performance that arguably is able to connect us to those who are suffering and those who died from AIDS. It can 'infect' us with her rage in order to work against forgetting and to incite us to call for change.

Reference list

Art Institute of Chicago (1991) *Untitled (portrait of Ross in L.A.)*, Available at: www.artic.edu/artworks/152961/untitled-portrait-of-ross-in-l-a (Accessed: 25 August 2022).

Arthur, M. (2021) 'Nostalgia and chronicity: two temporalities in the restaging of AIDS', *Theatre Journal*, 73(1), pp. 13–36.

Brantley, B. (2014) 'A raging grief, adamantly undiminished', *The New York Times*, 14 October. Available at: www.nytimes.com/2014/10/16/theater/karen-finley-relives-the-aids-epidemic-in-written-in-sand.html (Accessed: 27 May 2023).

Campbell, A. and Gindt, D. (2018) 'Viral dramaturgies: HIV and AIDS in performance in the twenty-first century', in Campbell, A. and Gindt, D. (eds.) *Viral dramaturgies: HIV and AIDS in performances in the twenty-first century*. Basingstoke: Palgrave Macmillan, pp. 3–46.

Couser, G.T. (2004) *Vulnerable subjects: ethics and life writing*. Cornell: Cornell University Press.

Couser, G.T. (2005) '"Paradigms" cost: representing vulnerable subjects', *Literature and Medicine*, 24(1), pp. 19–30.

Ehrenreich, B. (2009) *Smile or die: how positive thinking fooled America and the world*. London: Granta.

Finley, K. (2000) *A different kind of intimacy: the collected writings of Karen Finley*. New York: Thunder's Mouth Press.

Finley, K. (2015) *Written in sand.* Available at: https://vimeo.com/144354236 (Accessed: 7 May 2022).

Foucault, M. (1973) *The birth of the clinic: an archaeology of medical perception.* Translated by A.M. Sheridan. London: Tavistock.

Fulford, K.W.M. *et al.* (eds.) (2013) *The Oxford handbook of philosophy and psychiatry.* Oxford: Oxford University Press.

Fürholzer, K. (2019) *Das Ethos des Pathographen: Literatur- und medizinethische Dimensionen von Krankenbiographien.* Heidelberg: Winter.

Gambardella, S.J. (2001) 'Absent bodies: the AIDS memorial quilt as social melancholia', *Journal of American Studies*, 45, pp. 213–226.

Gardner, L. (2015) '*Written in Sand* review – reflection on AIDS shot through with rage and grief', *The Guardian*, 29 October. Available at: www.theguardian.com/stage/2015/oct/29/written-in-the-sand-review-karen-finley-the-pit-barbican (Accessed: 7 June 2022).

Gregg, M. and Seigworth, G.J. (2010) 'An inventory of shimmers', in Gregg, M. and Seigworth, G.J. (eds.) *The affect theory reader.* Durham: Duke University Press, pp. 1–26.

Gussow, M. (2000) 'Introduction', in Finley, K. (ed.) *A different kind of intimacy: the collected writings of Karen Finley.* New York: Thunder's Mouth Press, pp. xiii–xv.

Hunsaker Hawkins, A. (1999) *Reconstructing illness: studies in pathography.* West Lafayette: Perdue Research Foundation.

Keats, J. (2012) 'How Felix Gonzalez-Torres continues making art 16 years after his death', *Forbes*, 30 August. Available at: www.forbes.com/sites/jonathonkeats/2012/08/30/how-felix-gonzalez-torres-continues-making-art-16-years-after-his-death/?sh=7eb611c716c0 (Accessed: 7 June 2022).

Krouse, M.B. (1994) 'The AIDS memorial quilt as cultural resistance for gay communities', *Critical Sociology*, 20(3), pp. 65–80.

Plett, H. (2020) *The art of holding space: a practice of love, liberation, and leadership.* Vancouver: Page Two.

Prior, D.M. (2015) 'Karen Finley: ribbon gate | Written in Sand', *Total Theatre*, 3 November. Available at: http://totaltheatre.org.uk/karen-finley-ribbon-gate-written-in-sand/ (Accessed: 27 May 2023).

Ravenhill, M. (2006) *'Pool (no water)' and 'citizenship'.* London: Methuen.

Ravenhill, M. (2013) *Candide: inspired by Voltaire.* London: Bloomsbury Methuen.

Sontag, S. (2002) *Illness as metaphor; AIDS and its metaphors.* London: Penguin.

Stull, G. (2001) 'The AIDS memorial quilt: performing memory, piecing action', *American Art*, 15(2), pp. 84–89.

Svich, C. (2011) 'Mark Ravenhill', in Middeke, M., Schnierer, P.P. and Sierz, A. (eds.) *The Methuen drama guide to contemporary British playwrights.* London: Methuen, pp. 403–424.

Turnbull, J. (2015) *Karen Finley relives the AIDS crisis in 'Written in Sand'.* Available at: https://disabilityarts.online/magazine/opinion/karen-finley-relives-the-aids-crisis-in-written-in-sand/ (Accessed: 7 June 2022).

Watney, S. (2016) 'In purgatory: the work of Felix Gonzales-Torres', in Ault, J. (ed.) *Felix Gonzales-Torres.* Göttingen: Steidl, pp. 333–347.

3

THE UBER-PERFORMING UTERUS OF HENRIETTA LACKS AND EVE ENSLER

Ecologies of the womb in Mojisola Adebayo's *Family Tree* and Eve Ensler's *In the Body of the World*

Verónica Rodríguez

I am lying in a hospital bed at the Admissions Department in an East London hospital. Curtains separate patients. We are all going to have surgery today in different parts of our bodies. My surgery is for endometriosis, a chronic inflammatory illness of the womb that occurs when tissue resembling the lining of the uterus appears elsewhere in the body, a tissue that periodically bleeds whilst having no exit. As I lie in bed, a woman consultant comes to me and, by mistake, says: 'So, today we are operating on your throat, isn't that right?' The anecdote is relevant, as the uterus and the throat are related parts of the body when it comes to early accounts of hysteria. Although hysteria, called today 'conversion disorder', is considered a mental pathology and 'not dependent upon any known organic or structural pathology' (Encyclopaedia Britannica, 2022), two pivotal moments in the history of the concept reveal a strong physical connotation.

Hysteria is etymologically derived from the word uterus in Greek (ὑστέρα/hystera) and was used in Ancient Greece to denote a disease of the uterus. The 'wandering uterus' theory (defended by Plato, among others) stated that the uteruses of women who did not bear children would start to wander in their bodies, reaching such distant places as the throat, creating a sense of choking and breathlessness in the hysteric patient. Anna Furse's play *Augustine (Big Hysteria)* (1991) illustrates another moment in hysteria's history, the nineteenth century, when the uterus and the throat were connected: 'AUGUSTINE is experiencing the typical first experience of an [sic] hysterical attack where the throat constricted' (Furse, 2020, p. 36). Recent medical research has even suggested that hysteria was actually a misdiagnosis for endometriosis, where the uterus can be argued to actually 'travel' and where thoracic endometriosis, for instance, can indeed disrupt breathing (see Nezhat et al., 2012).

Departing from the idea of uteruses that migrate and that affect the health of other parts of the body, following the concept of uteruses that do not necessarily conform to their 'assigned' role of reproduction and opening up to the notion of uteruses characterised by excess, I suggest the phrase uber-performing uterus. The German prefix über- means over, above and/or across. It is cognate with the British word over. Uber (I use the English version) can also mean extreme, or extremely

DOI: 10.4324/9781003036500-5

good (or successful). An uber-performing uterus 'acts' extremely or excessively, works above its function and performs across matter and beyond itself (it may transgress specific locations). An uber-performing uterus is a super-productive or hyper-proliferative uterus. Whatever the uber-performing uterus generates, it is a manifestation of something that is already in the world or that has been prompted in response to the world, hence the use of the phrase 'ecologies of the womb' in this chapter.

In particular, I use the idea of the uber-performing uterus to discuss the hyper-productive wombs of real women Henrietta Lacks (1920–1951) and Eve Ensler (1953–) through intersectional and ecological lenses in the uterine cancer plays *Family Tree* by Mojisola Adebayo (2021) and *In the Body of the World* by Eve Ensler (2016). Adebayo brings to the fore an imagined Lacks who shares her thoughts on her life, case and afterlife (a culture of Lacks's uterine cancerous cells became the fastest self-reproducing cell line in history, giving way to highly successful medical achievements). Ensler's play (originally a memoir) offers her own experience with diagnosis and treatment of uterine cancer. Through short snapshots of her cancer experience, the spectator is embedded within the body of the world – due to the interwoven body politics of the work.

The wombs discussed are both pathologised and pathological (uterine cancer, also known as womb or endometrial cancer), but, as the plays' womb ecologies reveal, they are nevertheless capable of engaging with healing practices. Exploited, traumatised and/or sick in various ways (through rape, medical abuse, undignified or unnecessary surgeries, psychological or other trauma, exposure to the consequences of environmental degradation and various toxicities, genetics and so on), uteruses generate matter and material (cells, illness, tissue, knowledge and so on). While the uber-performing womb-owner suffers or dies as a result, they can leave a legacy of healing positive effects (for instance, HeLa cells in the case of Henrietta Lacks or a cancer memoir regarding Eve Ensler). Indeed, uteruses are revealed both as sites of vulnerability and power, excess and extension, metastasis and ecstasy, walls and holes, death and life.

Contextualising *Family Tree* and *In the Body of the World*

As stated, *Family Tree* (2021) is a play by Mojisola Adebayo, 'a Black British born, Nigerian/ Danish performer, playwright, director, producer, workshop leader and teacher' (2021) and an advocate of the LGBTQIA+ community. *Family Tree* premiered at the Greenwich+Docklands International Festival (GDIF) in 2021, UK, and was performed in the gardens of a former hospital (see Adebayo, 2021).[1] In Adebayo's words, the play deals with 'extractions from Black women's bodies and how this relates to environmental racism, the relationship between gynaecology and gardening, soil and cells and many layers more' (2021).

There are two notorious incidents of medical abuse of Black women directly explored in *Family Tree*. The first is the case of Anarcha, Betsey and Lucy, three Black slave women who lived in Alabama in the nineteenth century and who were victims of surgical experimentation. Characters representing Anarcha, Betsey and Lucy (with the same names) appear in Adebayo's play. Inspired by these three historical figures, Adebayo also reimagines the abuse of three Black women in a contemporary medical setting during COVID-19 times with the three dead nurses in the context of the pandemic Ain, Bibi and Lyn – their names' first letters coincide with the historical triad's initials: A, B and L. The second is the case of the aforementioned uterine cancer sufferer Henrietta Lacks, whose cells have been used since her death in 1951 to find cures to and treatments for many diseases.

The racist and sexist history of gynaecology (see Kapsalis, 1997, pp. 31–32) is directly related to the so-called [sic] J. Marion Sims (ibid, p. 31). Following childbirth, Anarcha, Betsey and Lucy developed vesico-vaginal fistulas that provoked involuntary emptying of the bladder and the bowel. Sims 'surgically experiment[ed] on [these] unanesthetized slave women in his backyard hospital in Montgomery, Alabama, between 1845 and 1849' (ibid, p. 6). The women were watched by Sims and other doctors whilst the operations took place and, unsurprisingly, all operations were a failure. Since the three women could no longer work in the fields, they remained under Sim's control, who continued operating on them and who taught them nursing in order to continue his experiments on them and other women. By 1849, Anarcha had undergone thirty procedures. The thirtieth worked, and Sims closed his clinic and moved. Anarcha, Betsey and Lucy then had to return to their enslavers (see Conrad, 2021).

To delve into Lacks's life, she is mainly known for her uterine immortal cells, which double every 24 hours, the so-called HeLa cells. Given their fast reproducibility, HeLa cells have aided medical research for decades, including for HIV, leukaemia, haemophilia, Parkinson's disease treatment, the polio vaccine, cancer treatments including chemotherapy, gene-mapping, cloning and in vitro fertilisation (IVF). The cells were taken from a tumour biopsy (as part of her diagnosis and treatment) while Lacks was still alive. Despite no consent being required at the time to culture those cells, '[h]er family remained ignorant of her contribution to medical history for almost 20 years after her death' (University of Bristol, 2014). Moreover, if the medical/pharmaceutical corporations have benefited so vastly from the experimental use of HeLa cells, it is only fair that the family also receive financial compensation, which has started materialising only recently (see Witze, 2020).

In the Body of the World (2016) is a uterine cancer memoir adapted for the stage with the same name by Ensler, also known as V. It was performed by Ensler, and it premiered at the American Repertory Theater, Cambridge, Massachusetts, US, in 2016. Ensler is an award-winning American playwright, an internationally best-selling author, performer, feminist and activist. She is perhaps best known as the author of *The Vagina Monologues* (1996). Besides, 'Ensler is the founder of V-Day, the global movement to end violence against women and girls, which has raised over $90 million for local groups and activists and inspired the global action "One Billion Rising"' (Ensler, 2016, p. 160).[2] Raped numerous times by her father, unpopular at school, a former alcoholic and addict (to drugs and sex mainly), abused by her now ex-husband, a war zone traveller and arduous feminist activist, Ensler has widely experienced and witnessed violence in her personal and professional life. These areas become blurred in *In the Body of the World*.

While working with rape victims in the Republic of the Congo in the creation of a centre called City of Joy in 2010 (founded by Christine Schuler Deshryver, Dr. Denis Mukwege and Eve Ensler), which is now a 'sanctuary for healing' with the aim to turn local women's 'trauma and pain into power' (Ensler, 2016, p. 6), she received a severe uterine cancer diagnosis. Ensler reflects: 'Cancer threw me into the center of my body's crisis. The Congo threw me into the crisis of the world, and these two experiences merged' (ibid, p. 6). This reiterated idea of intertwining the personal and the political can be said to exemplify the thesis of the work as a whole. What happens to uteruses is reflected in the work's conception and forms, so the very physical idea of the uber-performing uterus is malleable and can become intricately abstract. This is the case when it is used to describe some of the play's aesthetic mechanisms.

Raw and unapologetic, *In the Body of the World* is an extremely hard-hitting work, where we encounter an eight-year-old girl with a fistula created by gang rape and the cooking and eating of a baby, to mention two of the most gruesome atrocities narrated. As claimed, *In the Body of the World* is divided into what Ensler calls 'scans', brief accounts (1–4 pages long) that chronicle her cancer experience. The rationale is that this is precisely the snapshot-way in which she experienced her cancer journey. It approximately spans her seven-month cancer treatment journey and a final 'scan' narrating the opening of City of Joy, which took place eighteen months after she was cancer free – City of Joy crucially appears at the beginning and the end, remaining a structural element of the work. Ensler has stated that, in fact, seeing City of Joy open was one of her motivations to be cancer free (see 2018).

Being *in* and being *the* body of the world means bodies are political and politics affect bodies. It may also mean that what happens to bodies is connected to the world in many ways; that the violence done to women and the environment are entwined and they both show in women's bodies; that other women's pain and the world's pain infiltrates women's bodies and that life traumas surface biochemically. Ensler suggests that 'we cannot separate trauma from illness' (2018), which she summarises with the idea of cancer trauma, adding that she didn't live in her body because 'The *landscape* was too painful' (Ensler, 2018; emphasis added).

Ecofeminism, environmental narratives and the uber-performing uterus

The theoretical framework this chapter uses to address such a set of intertwined complexities and ecologies of the womb is ecofeminism (see also Fernández-Morales, 2020, p. 245), which is 'about the complex web of interrelations between organisms and the environment' (Daly, 1978, p. 9). Mary Daly's *Gyn/Ecology: The Metaethics of Radical Feminism* (1978), has been critiqued for the lack of extra-European divinity references – notoriously by Audre Lorde (1984) – and its essentialism, as Daly was interested in 'the complex web of living/loving relationships of our own kind' (1978, p. 12), which in a nutshell 'fantasizes an actual transcendent ontology in which self and world are no longer differentiated' (Monagle, 2019, p. 337). However, Daly's ecofeminism (and even a sense of spiritualist ecofeminism, as we will see later) is a productive framework to approach both Adebayo and Ensler's works and the playwrights' ecological understanding of women, women's health, the environment and ultimately the world (women and women's health are understood as open-ended concepts). Chris Cuomo connects ecofeminism, women's health and cancer:

> let me give an example of the kinds of connections that concern ecofeminists. One month last year, I felt bombarded by bad news: six women in my circle of friends and family were found to have cancer – all of the cervix, uterus, or breast. In the midst of my fear, I pondered histories of inadequate health care for women and the poor, the ways in which women's and non-white bodies are devalued, the fact that the meaning of women's lives is so often reduced to their reproductive functions, and the character of a profit-driven, increasingly toxic world.
> (1998, p. 1)

Indeed, both *Family Tree* and *In the Body of the World* fall under the category of environmental narratives whose aim is to 'scrutinise connections between rising incidences of cancer in the industrialised world and degradation of the environment' (DeShazer, 2005, p. 220), whether they establish this explicitly or not. There are books that unequivocally connect cancer to environmental abuse, including Sandra Steingraber's *Living Downstream: An Ecologist's Personal Investigation of Cancer and the Environment* (1998). In addition, within *Family Tree*'s Notes, there is one entitled "Sustainability" that reads: 'the production should be low waste with as light carbon footprint as possible in all aspects including props, set, printing, travel, etc., otherwise the staging will contradict the content' (2023, n.p.). In these environmental narratives, 'each writer weaves her own experience [or the imagined experience of a real person] with cancer into her narrative, creating an ecological and autobiographical tapestry' (DeShazer, 2005, p. 242). An added component is that they adamantly want to eliminate racism and violence towards women. Both works also think about hyper-productive wombs in terms of proliferating cells. Words usually connected to damage done to the environment are used to speak about poor women's health like 'extraction' (of cells) or 'holes/drilling' (fistulas). On a more positive note, both plays emphasise permaculture, a type of agricultural design that supports sustainable and self-sufficient ecosystem functioning.

In response to the world and as part of the world, uteruses may become over-productive. A uterus is a hollow, muscular, pear-shaped organ located in the pelvis, whose two main biological functions are collecting and shedding menstrual blood and child growing and carrying (and eventually delivering) when menstruation does not occur. In this chapter, several overlapping meanings of performance meet: a continuum of everyday practices, the work of tissue in response to stimuli, the performance of cells and the performance of the narratives analysed (which includes the merging of women's bodies and the environment and the intersection of medicine and aesthetic/formal choices). Any uterus can be said to be a performing uterus. The dance of processes that occur in this organ merits at the very least the label 'performance'. Menstruation, for instance, is a big 'show': it is an orchestrated self-injury in order to get rid of no-longer-needed tissue. The microorganisms present in the area and their composition (uterine microbiota) perform in particular processes and ways determining womb health.

The uber-performing uterus is a uterus that has developed out of performing extremely or excessively in response to genetics, life experiences and/or environmental exposures, among other phenomena. The uber-performing uterus may or may not develop uterine disorders, is nonconforming, excessive, inhospitable, ambivalently fertile, perhaps out of place, leaking, 'formed' differently, presented otherwise, protruding, inflamed, rich, transgressing, and so as a result, it may be operated on, removed, dissected, classified, shown, exhibited, objectified, accessed, extracted, stolen, 'cut open, catheterized, chemofied, drugged, pricked, punctured, probed, and ported' (Ensler, 2016, p. 15). The uber-performing uterus performs dangerously, most of the time unknowingly. The person with an uber-performing uterus may want more or feel deprived; seek perfection; care mostly about others; worry too much; react against its reproductive nature; desire to produce too much; have problems with letting go of dead projects, unnecessary people, unmanaged emotions and past traumas; and feel unsafe, unwelcome and/or alone and so on. However, a more positive reading of the uber-performing uterus is that, ecologically interdependent, it may stage protest, take forms that bring knowledge about uteruses and scream for life and health to exist.

As the concept encapsulates theatre and gynaecology, it is pertinent to point out that connections between gynaecology and theatre pre-exist this chapter. For instance, apart from having operated with audiences present (see Kapsalis, 1997, p. 33), Sims is also credited with having invented the speculum, the instrument that permits the separating of the vagina walls and allows seeing inside the vagina and cervix – yet a new theatre. Others have discussed specific concepts at the intersection of gynaecology and theatre, for example, 'the performing pelvis' during vaginal examinations.[3] Although Terri Kapsalis warns that the staging of the performing pelvis may point to the idea of 'a vagina disassociated from a person' (1997, p. 12), it is true that to a certain extent the disconnection between the person and the vagina is dramaturgically conducted to ensure the comfort of the patient. A complete reversal to this dissociation is Annie Sprinkle's *A Public Cervix Announcement* (1991), a performance art piece in which Sprinkle shows her cervix (which connects uterus and vagina) with a speculum to audience members, a process gently guided by herself, resulting in the education of spectators and the de-mystification of these organs and their cells' (mis-)behaviour.

Mojisola Adebayo's *Family Tree*

Set in a garden/cemetery and featuring a DNA model in the shape of a tree, *Family Tree* imagines Henrietta Lacks's reflections and ideas about her cancerous cells' afterlives if she had been able to communicate with us. Although the play's central character is Lacks, Adebayo weaves a complex political narrative that addresses the historical and ongoing abuse of Black people in health care contexts and beyond, and women in particular.[4] Characters include the three afore-mentioned NHS Black dead nurses/nineteenth century victims of gynaecological experimentation (Ain/Anarcha, Bibi/Betsey, Lyn/Lucy) and a mysterious Smoking Man, who traverses the stage space in silence at certain moments throughout the play, symbolising, among other phenomena, slavery, colonialism, patriarchy, capitalism, the smoking (cancerous) industry, racism and white supremacy.

Analogies between the material (capitalism) and matter (cancer) proliferation are highlighted in the Prologue: cells, selling cells (Adebayo, 2023, p. 5). The hyper-expansive nature of capitalism and colonialism and their legacies is reflected in cancer and the uber-performing uterus:

Henrietta: Fuck cancer! Fuck the banks, the bankrupt billionaires, landowners, slave owners, border controllers. Fuck columbus, crusaders and colonisers, occupiers, cowboy debt collectors, company directors, capitalist commanders of all their empires. Fuck the big c, the little c, fuck all of your cells!

(Adebayo, 2023, p. 24)

Beyond this clear critique, an interconnected, intersectional, ecological, transhistorical and political understanding of cancer is highlighted.

The play is also careful not to bio-medicalise the real person or equate 'cells' with the human Lacks was. For instance, *Family Tree* includes puns that speak tenderly about the figure of Lacks in a way that critically re-reads the name given to her cells: ' "HeLa"; Healer?' (Adebayo, 2023, p. 11). Other ways in which this respect to the real Lacks is achieved is by establishing parallels with other historical figures (Anarcha, Betsey and Lucy, as explored previously) relevant to the history of medicine and its related activism. Lacks watches the scenes which she is not in, denoting a sense of justice and knowledge with her ongoing presence. The illustration of the idea of performing medicine, performing cancer and the uber-performing uterus is suggested in this stage direction:

Henrietta: She laughs and dances exuberantly celebrating her miraculous existence. During the dance, another Black woman, dressed exactly like Henrietta, runs and joins in dancing, then another Black woman and another – as many as possible – the Community Chorus are like cells multiplying.

(ibid, p. 22)

Another metaphor for this plural existence, multiplication and omnipresence is the fact that the scenes where Lacks appears occur evenly across the play, perhaps like the uniform presence of her uber-performing uterus in research medical centres internationally.

Black women have been crucial to the history of the National Health Service and hold many of the nursing and health care job roles in the UK. However, the play sadly still needs to insist on the persistence of racism towards Black health care professionals today (whether in their roles as nurses or patients):

Lyn: he starts coughing and shouting. "I wanna English nurse! Get this fucking coon offa me!"

(Adebayo, 2023, p. 30)

And:

Bibi: I had the surgery during my lunch break. That bitch is pulling at my polyp for *ten minutes*. And I'm breathing through it, going on about gynaecology, how it all started during slavery, experiments of Black women and she's just pretending not to hear.

(ibid, p. 31, italics in original)

As noted, the genealogy of medical testing and dubious treatments on Black women's bodies for commercial purposes is not something of the past only, which the play summarises:

Ain: And when they wanna cure an STD the first people they wanna try the drugs out on is us. Or pretend to be curing us from syphilis when they're really just watching how we die.

(ibid, p. 32)

Bibi replies to this by saying: 'Tuskegee' (ibid, p. 32), which refers to the Tuskegee Syphilis Experiment, conducted between 1932 and 1972 by the United States Health Public Health Service, in which hundreds of Black men who accepted being part of the study in exchange for the promise of free medical care were denied life-saving treatment long after the beneficial effects of penicillin had been established.

The play equates medical injustice towards Black people with violence against Black bodies:

Henrietta: Like George Floyd was calling
        Like Sandra Bland was calling
        Like Stephen Lawrence was calling

(ibid, p. 34)

This is followed by medicine and violence coming together in Lacks's plea for the creation of a vaccine that will end racism, in which case she agrees to give away her uterine cells for free. She is represented as an agent in the projected uses of her uber-performing uterus:

Henrietta: If you can create a vaccine for racism,
        Find a cure for white supremacy,
        An immunization from discrimination for all of your children
        You can have my permission
        You can take my cells!
        And my eyes and my ears and my tongue and my lungs
        Have it all!
        For free!
        What do you say?

(ibid, p. 35)

Uterine extraction is later on equated with the concept of Black death, where Black bodies who have undergone violence and whose uteruses have been either thought of as raw material, to be exploited and mined for capitalism or cut out as a result of losing a child:

Oshun: They cut a piece from you, Henrietta, cut up Lucy, Betsey and Anarcha, cut short Ain, Bibi and Lyn, cut out the womb of Fannie Lou Hamer, cut down the offspring of Doreen Lawrence.

(ibid, p. 59)

At one moment, Lacks confesses, 'I'm just *speculating* from my little petri dish' (ibid, p. 39, italics in original). Offering yet another instance of a (splintered) uber-performing uterus and of a play that formally performs uterine cancer, what is 'talking' is Lacks in the shape of her multiplying cells. So, the uber-performing uterus is given a voice. Cancer talks. Cancer interacts. That is exactly what many people with cancer want other people to understand: that cancer is a result of the interaction and our relationship to what is inside and what surrounds us and by extension everything. Another crucial interaction with cancer is generated when the character of Henrietta holds, looks at and even stares at a female pelvis model on stage. We cannot know what she imagines, but the image itself is resonant performatively because she seems to be reflecting on her very uterus's performance. Upholding permaculture visually, we are simultaneously in a theatre and in cell land, in an orchard and a cemetery, a wake and a party that celebrates life.

The festive approach to Lacks' life traverses the play – 'Don't the dead deserve a party?! Especially when they're still alive!' (ibid, p. 21) – and it is nowhere more explicit than at the end when Lacks has a feast organized in her honour. At the centre of this gathering, not in the margins or hidden, and blessed by Oshun, the Yoruba deity whose attributes include love, fertility and water, Lacks (and her uber-performing uterus) is transformed into the 'Orisha of Cells' (Adebayo, 2023, p. 60). This is based on the African tradition of the orishas and the loas, who 'are cosmic forces in the universe – sometimes personified, sometimes thought of as deities, but always divine' (Dorsey, 2020, p. 12). The end of the play signals a metaphoric wished for death of racism and white supremacy through the burying of the Smoking Man by the three dead nurses and is a celebration of the uber-performing uterus that lives on, offering the possibility of life and love (for instance, a section of Toni Morrison's *Beloved* is read by Bibi in Scene Five) to others.

Eve Ensler's *In the Body of the World*

The explicit connections between agriculture, colonialism, capitalism, medicine, gynaecology, climate change, violence towards women, Black people and migrants and of course cancer make *Family Tree* a good example to be considered alongside Eve Ensler's *In the Body of the World*.[5] Lacks says:

> *Henrietta:* We were their harvest!
> And they reap what they did not sow!
> Reaping and raping and reaping and raping,
> stealing and slicing, and stitching us up
> When does it STOP?!
>
> (Adebayo, 2023, p. 25)

As stated, *In the Body of the World* (2016) is a one-woman show about Ensler's lived experience of uterine cancer, based on her eponymous memoir from 2013. This chapter uses them both as the play is a concentrated version of the memoir rewritten for the stage as a monologue. It largely offers a 'quest narrative' (see Frank, 1995), where the narrator transforms as a result of the illness experience and shares that learning. Divided into very short chapters/scenes (scans), the result is that the memoir/play ends up having a form shaped by a medical instrument/test. The 'medical technology' form of the play also makes the spectator's experience more straightforward, approachable and perhaps detached. After all, uber-performing uteruses is a topic societies have been avoiding for thousands of years.

Shortly after the beginning of the work, Ensler informs the audience that:

> I spent time with women in colleges, sex clubs, refugee camps, and war zones. Then in 2007, I was invited to the Democratic Republic of Congo by Dr. Denis Mukwege [2018 Nobel Peace Prize winner], a Congolese gynaecologist who was literally sewing up the vaginas of rape survivors as fast as the militias were tearing them apart.

(2019, p. 5)

In the Congo, Ensler 'met an 8-year-old girl who couldn't stop peeing on herself because huge men had shoved themselves inside her' (2019, p. 6). In 2010, while in the Congo, she found out she had uterine cancer and needed to urgently get treatment. As the cancer 'scans' progress, through Ensler's narration and descriptions, the body of women, and her body in particular, is woven with the body of the Earth. See, for instance, the paradigmatic moment in the work when she states: 'The raping of the Earth. The pillaging of minerals. The destruction of vaginas. They were not separate from each other or from me' (2016, p. 14). Then there are the numerous analogies between her cancer and destructive human activities: 'The tumor moved like an irrepressible army, like CO_2 through the atmosphere' (Ensler, 2016, p. 22).

In this sense, although I think the service her work does to women's bodies and lives is above the following observation, my response to *In the Body of the World* encapsulates a combination of discomfort and admiration. Despite the numerous ecological analogies that she makes in the work and the alignment with the book's thesis, they feel sometimes far-fetched. For one, the climate emergency, the dirty side of the fight for economic gain and conflict (and all in combination) affects parts of the world asymmetrically. Besides, no matter how much she emphasises her privilege, it is problematic to compare vaginas and the vaginal traumas of people with different backgrounds and experiences. One of the analogies I find less palatable is the one between her atrocious experience with a doctor's objectifying and impersonal way of communicating about her treatment choices and the feeling of a Pakistani bride seeing her husband blown to pieces by a drone bomb. In fact, one of the main critiques of her work has been that '[r]ather than using Ms. Ensler's illness to illuminate the world's, it too often borrows from the world's suffering in an effort to legitimize her own' (Green, 2018: online).

I think, however, that Ensler sometimes powerfully invokes a radical ecological approach. For instance, the women in the community she has extensively worked with are mainly raped by militia members so that those populations leave the land, with the subsequent exploitation of the soil in those areas in order to extract materials which end up being used mainly in the manufacturing of technological devices. So, *In the Body of the World* writes and stages Ensler's uber-performing uterus and verbalises thoughts that I think are not clearly expressed elsewhere: the idea of trying to feed the hunger of the uterus with work commitments, promiscuity, anorexia and even performance art, or the idea of 'trauma baby' (Ensler, 2016, p. 37) - or growing cancer as a response to the inability and/or indisposition to grow life, which connects to deeply ingrained traumatic experiences related to rape and parental estrangement in her case- are but a few of the rich, daring and necessary ideas and metaphors she offers. I also align with her idea that the illness process is the result of the separation from the body and that the healing work can only happen when we allow the body back: 'Cancer, a disease of pathologically dividing cells, burned away the walls of my separateness and landed me in my body' (Ensler, 2016, p. 15).

There are other suggestions that may be well known to people familiar with mind-body-spirit medicine but that her reader or spectator may not have encountered before. Without hiding the genetic connections (Ensler's mother has suffered from several bouts of cancer in different places in her body), she explains cancer as '[a] flesh creature birthed out of the secrets of brutality, each blood vessel a ribbon of story' (2016, p. 26). Here she is echoing the principle in mind-body-spirit medicine that blocked emotions and past traumas as well as our perceived connections to those traumas create the favourable conditions for the manifestation of illness, and of course an uber-performing uterus. A moment in the memoir that many may feel dismissive and sceptical about made me stop on my tracks, as I am familiar with the intricacies of illness manifestation and the meaning matter inscribes in our lives. In other words, how we process meaning matters to matter. We are what we think and what we do, the law of attraction gurus would say. Speaking of listening and caring for rape survivors as the source of her own fistula, she claims that 'the cancer had done exactly what rape had done to so many thousands of women in the Congo. I ended up having the same surgery as many of them. Dr. Handsome . . . said, "These findings are not medical, they are not science. They are spiritual"' (Ensler, 2016, p. 35; see also p. 63). *In the Body of the World* is an extreme piece of work, but so are uber-performing uteruses. A beautiful way in which the idea of ecologies of the womb extends into the world is that the surgeon that performed surgery on Ensler has collaborated in the theatre so-to-speak with Denis Mukwege in the Republic of Congo (see Ensler, 2018), creating new gynaecological communities of care.

Conclusion: material and immaterial legacies

'The narratives about women's health in public discourse have material consequences precisely because we act in the world based on the perspectives and identities offered to us in the stories that make up our lives' (Dubriwny, 2013, p. 6), so I hope this chapter has humbly contributed to improving the health of uteruses by creating visibility and terminology to discuss women's health and representations of it.

Legacies also matter. Lacks's statue in Bristol is not only 'the first public statue of a Black woman made by a Black woman to be permanently installed in the UK' (University of Bristol, 2021) but also the first one in the UK to celebrate a Black woman in the medical sciences.[6] Ensler's activist contribution to women's health, including the centre City of Joy, is also testament to the importance of continuing work on the improvement of women's health.

Despite their difficult subject matter, both plays make explicitly hopeful points. *Family Tree* gestures towards a fairer and more positive future – Adebayo has spoken about 'Black futures' and the play being 'hopeful' and 'celebratory' (see 2021), and Ensler's final thoughts on the City of Joy conclude: 'It is the metaphor for a new beginning, for building a new world' (2016, p. 143). For Adebayo, Lacks's (deadly) cancer becomes a healing force. For Ensler, her cancer is figured as a sort of manifestation of all the abuse that women/vaginas experience and of the abuse of the planet. Both plays discuss (cellular) reproduction as both malignant and potentially healing, which is conveyed in the plays' content and form in crude as well as creative ways.

Uber-performing uteruses, belonging to patient, healer or both, albeit potentially problematic, dis-eased, complex and traumatised, matter and leave their mark on the world. In these two works, the uber-performing uterus is understood, upheld and celebrated rather than punished, disbelieved and disciplined. The uber-performing uterus is a uterus that brings knowledge, life and the divine with it, for other uteruses and for the world to never feel unloved again. These uber-performing uteruses experience and are deeply affected by the world and come out of their cages (their issues and their tissues) to be seen, listened to and become part of the world. Not hidden, not sorry, just temporarily broken. After all, the uterus is considered 'the second heart' in Chinese medicine. Creatively walking down and up the uterus vessel that connects the heart and the uterus, called *bao mai*, now I understand what the expression 'from the bottom of my heart' means. Surging and pumping, filling and empty-ing, breathing and feeling, this uber-performing uterus would like to tell you: We will be healed.

Note: This chapter has been written with respect and in solidarity to all people experiencing cancer and discrimination and disbelief in medical settings and beyond and with gratitude as well as in homage to Henrietta Lacks, Lacks's family and her material and immaterial legacies.

Acknowledgements: Many thanks to Andrew Smaje and Ameera Conrad from Actors Touring Company for the outstanding research support they have provided me with over these years. Warm thanks to Eve Ensler and Mojisola Adebayo for speaking with such clarity and brilliance about women's bodies. This article was supported by 'Gender, Affect and Care in Twenty-First Century British Theatre,' a research project funded by the Spanish Ministry of Economy and Competitive-ness (FFI2016–75443-P). See www.ub.edu/cbtbarcelona.

Notes

1 Recipient of the 25th Alfred Fagon Award 2021 for Best New Play of the Year, the most recent production of *Family Tree* took place at Brixton House, London, UK, in 2023 in a co-production of Actors Touring Company and Belgrade Theatre Coventry in association with Brixton House. The discussion of the play in this chapter is based on the 2023 co-production.
2 See, respectively, V-Day and One Billion Rising websites: www.vday.org/; www.onebillionrising.org/.
3 See James M. Henslin and Mae A. Biggs's (1971) article 'Dramaturgical Desexualization: The Sociology of the Vaginal Examination'. See also, Kelly Underman's book *Feeling Medicine: How the Pelvic Exam Shapes Medical Training* (2020).
4 A seminal book about the medical experimentation on Black Americans is Harriet A. Washington's *Medical Apartheid: The Dark History of Medical Experimentation on Black Americans from Colonial Times to the Present* (2008), also quoted in Adebayo's publication of *Family Tree* (2023, p. 20).
5 Besides, the metaphor of the tree also connects both plays. Ensler has stated that realising that the tree she could see outside through her hospital room window was 'a tree' and her interaction with it felt as a turning point in her cancer treatment (see Ensler, 2018).
6 Importantly, and in connection to *Family Tree* itself, J. Marion Sims's statue was removed in 2018 from Central Park, New York.

Reference list

Adebayo, M. (2021) *Family tree and leaves – my latest work performed in London and Berlin this August, 2021*, 14 July. Available at: https://mojisolaadebayo.co.uk/2021/07/14/family-tree-and-leaves-my-latest-work-performed-in-london-and-berlin-this-august-2021/ (Accessed: 14 November 2021).

Adebayo, M. (2023) *Family tree*. London and New York: Methuen Drama.

Conrad, A. (2021) *Family tree research pack*. London: Associate Director Actors Touring Company.

Cuomo, C.O. (1998) *Feminism and ecological communities: an ethics of flourishing*. London and New York: Routledge.

Daly, M. (1978) *Gyn/ecology: the metaethics of radical feminism*. Boston: Beacon.

DeShazer, M.K. (2005) *Fractured borders: reading women's cancer literature*. Michigan: University of Michigan Press.

Dorsey, L. (2020) *Orishas, goddesses, and voodoo queens*. Newburyport: Weiser Books.

Dubriwny, T.N. (2013) *The vulnerable empowered woman feminism, postfeminism, and women's health*. New Brunswick, New Jersey and London: Rutgers University Press.

Encyclopaedia Britannica (2022) *Conversion disorder*. Available at: www.britannica.com/science/conversion-disorder (Accessed: 7 September 2022).

Ensler, E. (1996) *Vagina monologues*. London: Virago.

Ensler, E. (2016) *In the body of the world*. London: Virago.

Ensler, E. (2018) 'Eve Ensler on her play, "in the body of the world"', *Build Series*. Available at: www.youtube.com/watch?v=mSHTjyHkEA (Accessed: 7 October 2021).

Ensler, E. (2019) *In the body of the world*. New York: Dramatists Play Service.

Fernández-Morales, M. (2020) 'Postmillennial cancer narratives: feminism and postfeminism in Eve Ensler's in the body of the world', *Feminist Theory*, 21(2), pp. 235–252.

Frank, A.W. (1995) *The wounded storyteller*. Chicago: University of Chicago Press.

Furse, A. (2020) 'Augustine (big hysteria)', in *Performing nerves*. London and New York: Routledge, pp. 34–77.

Green, J. (2018) 'Review: Eve Ensler goes deep "in the body of the world"', *New York Times*, 6 February. Available at: www.nytimes.com/2018/02/06/theater/in-the-body-of-the-world-review-eve-ensler.html (Accessed: 7 October 2021).

Henslin, J.M. and Biggs, M.A. (1971) 'Dramaturgical desexualization: the sociology of vaginal examination', in Henslin, J.M. (ed.) *Studies in the sociology of sex*. New York: Appleton-Century-Crofts, pp. 243–272.

Kapsalis, T. (1997) *Performing gynaecology from both ends of the speculum*. Durham and London: Duke University Press.

Lorde, A. (1984) 'An open letter to Mary Daly', in *Sister outsider*. Berkeley, CA: Crossing, pp. 67–71.

Monagle, C. (2019) 'Mary Daly's gyn/ecology: mysticism, difference, and feminist history', *Journal of Women in Culture and Society*, 44(2), pp. 333–353.

Nezhat, C., Nezhat, F. and Nezhat, C. (2012) 'Endometriosis: ancient disease, ancient treatments', *Fertility and Sterility*, 98(6), pp. 1–62.

Sprinkle, A. (1991) *A public cervix announcement*. Available at: https://vimeo.com/184135882 (Accessed: 4 November 2021).

Steingraber, S. (1998) *Living downstream: an ecologist's personal investigation of cancer and the environment*. London: Virago.

Underman, K. (2020) *Feeling Medicine: How the Pelvic Exam Shapes Medical Training*. New York: New York University Press.

University of Bristol (2014) 'Henrietta lacks and her cell line inspires "a brush with immortality"', *News and Features*, 6 October. Available at: www.bristol.ac.uk/news/2014/october/a-brush-with-immortality.html (Accessed: 4 December 2021).

University of Bristol (2021) 'Statue of Henrietta lacks unveiled at university of Bristol', *News and Features*, 4 October. Available at: www.bristol.ac.uk/news/2021/october/henrietta-lacks-statue.html (Accessed: 5 October 2021).

Washington, H.A. (2008) *Medical apartheid: the dark history of medical experimentation on black Americans from colonial times to the present*. New York: Harlem Moon Broadway Books.

Witze, A. (2020) 'Wealthy funder pays reparations for use of HeLa cells', *Nature*, 29 October. Available at: www.nature.com/articles/d41586-020-03042-5 (Accessed: 6 February 2022).

4

PLACES TO (MIS)CARRY

Scoring diffracted narratives of multiple miscarriage

Joanne 'Bob' Whalley

This chapter is offered to the reader as a reflection upon the strategies I developed to navigate the process of multiple miscarriages. Over a seven-year period, I experienced six miscarriages at various stages of the foetus' development. What follows is an attempt to capture the performance process I started to manage a variety of medical interventions. When left in recovery suites, either in advance of the clinical intervention, or while I waited for various drugs to take effect, I began sketching a variety of the medical objects around me and those I imagined would soon be pressed into service in theatre. These actions, the marking of paper with crude representations of medical ephemera, were never about the creation of the image. Instead, it was always the act itself, the moving of pen across paper, that was important. Perhaps because of my training (although my first degree was in fine art, I consider myself to be a body-based performance maker), these behaviours felt much more like performance than like sketching. Here, the term 'performance' is indebted to the writings of Richard Schechner, as these site-specific actions were much less about display than they were in dialogue with the understanding that performance and ritual are woven closely together. These 'twice-behaved behaviours' (Schechner, 2013, p. 28) were more about my own management of the situation I found myself in, than in making 'sense' to an external eye. I have come to think of the artefacts as 'performance drawing', a document of a thing done more than the production of a piece of artwork. In the performances I enacted, often swiftly under the sheets in a variety of recovery suites, the act of mark-making was always more important than the marks made, an outcome of embodied actions rather than the generation of objects in and of themselves. José Esteban Muñoz suggests 'performance studies, as a modality of inquiry, can surpass the play of interpretation and the limits of epistemology and open new ground by focusing on what acts and objects do in a social matrix rather than what they might possibly mean' (1996, p. 12). The marks made, the images produced were clearly intended to be representations of medical equipment, but the context of their development, my body cocooned beneath the sheets of hospital beds, far outweighed the images themselves. Their meaning lies not in what is represented but in the fact they were generated by this body, in that space, in that moment. As such, they function as documents of sited action, emotionally freighted with locations and events that outstrip any possible singular meaning.

DOI: 10.4324/9781003036500-6

The approach (only when you're certain of the direction you're going in)

Geographer Derek Gregory extends Henri Lefebvre's 'practico-sensory realm' in *The Production of Space*, where Lefebvre foregrounds sensations of bodies through space and time. Gregory frames a 'corpographic' approach and acknowledges a corpography: a 'different way of *knowing*, *ordering* and *navigating* the space' (2015, p. 33, original emphasis). If I gingerly approach the term 'corpographic', staying on the balls of my feet and making as little noise as possible, I can hold the ideas of the body alongside its mapping. Further, choreographer Vida Midgelow uses the term '(auto)corpography' to describe individual acts of refusal, where the materiality of the body is in tension with its inscribed surfaces (2010, p. 56). The body, my body, is finding its way through words and images which are mappings of the stochastic process of recurrent miscarriage. My body, which through the experience of multiple miscarriage, has been made and unmade, each time depositing sticky residue for me to wade through.

In this it has offered me the chance to explore the diffracted-self that occurs before-during-after miscarriage. If, as Karen Barad suggests, '[m]atter is a sedimented intra-acting, an open field' (2014, p. 168) then both the pregnant body and un-pregnant body are points of flux. Experiences, sensations, thoughts, negotiations, enter the body and leave, and these pages are an attempt to find space to read the body diffractively. I imagine this chapter, 'snapshot of practice', as a brief illumination, revealing a kind of 'phosphenic knowledge'. Phosphenes are visual phenomena that suggest seeing light without there being a light source, and they can be created by applying pressure to the eyeball whilst the eyelids are closed.

Barad continues and takes a neologistic turn, bringing together the terms 'space', 'time', and 'matter' into a single word. This portmanteau speaks directly to how I feel, and I find a comfort in her attempt to point to this fundamental entanglement. In my 'spacetimemattering' (Barad, 2014, p. 168) as I sit in between the moment-to-moment experience of miscarriage, I realise that my 'bodily capital' (Dworkin and Wachs, 2009, p. 104) is not of high value, in its state of flux and its uncertain articulation of knowledges. Sitting in the twilight state of miscarriage, my body is no longer my own. It has ceased to house the child I thought would reside there, and it becomes instead an empty vessel. Something to be handled, dealt with, cleaned up, and sorted out.

Within this partial, marginal, and sedimented understanding of miscarriage is, however, an opportunity for finding new articulations of the dramaturgies of medical humanities and to say something about 'difficult' bodies. But this requires labour, and the irony of this is not lost on me. I need to explain, to explicate. Even here, in this chapter, years after the events I remember, I find myself plunging down to fathom the right words. I want to offer clarity to you as reader but recognise this comes at a cost to me. And I write these words on the same day that another friend sends another set of scans, of another child growing in another womb. And my scratchings, made beneath the covers in recovery suites, bring some comfort, even as I chill remembering the pen in my hand. This snapshot of practice, handheld and intimate, is an attempt at a mobile articulation of difficult and dark ecologies (Morton, 2016). By applying a little pressure, it sees light where there is none.

Aim to make your steps small

In the time spent waiting for the pessaries to dilate my cervix, I often consider the 'and' situated in between the procedure that followed: 'dilation' and 'curettage'. Two words, a polite elision. But rather than omit sounds or syllables, the whole process is tidied from view. Even more so the shorthanding of 'D&C' that comes so easily off the tongue and covers me in expertise. I wield

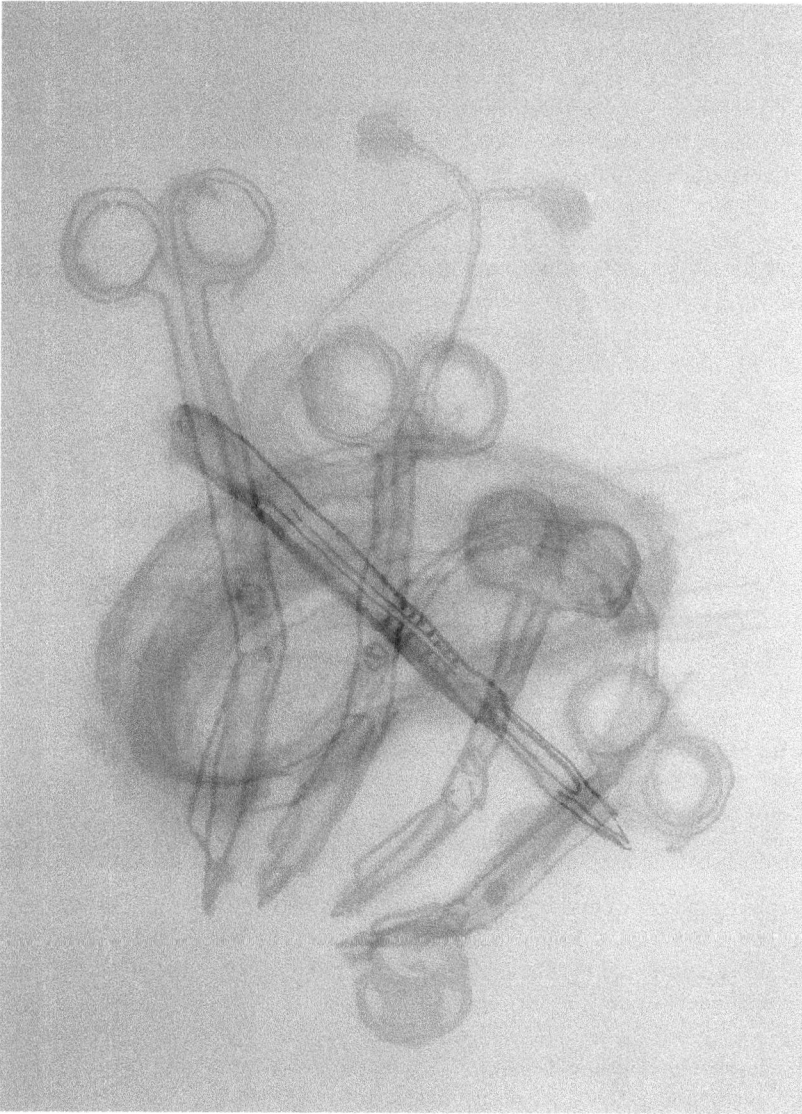

Figure 4.1 'Secure in this warm gloaming I draw the objects around me'. Performance drawing by Joanne 'Bob' Whalley ©2022. Reproduced with permission from the author.

the phrase like words I know. Which I do. The ampersand that lies between dilation and curettage is a reminder of an 'and', and 'and', and 'and'. To promote dilation, the medication softens the cervix, and every time I imagine a slow and lazy smile. Opened and hollowed out. In the three- to four-hour wait, I create a pocket of space by pulling the tightly tucked hospital blankets over my head.

Secure in this warm gloaming, I draw the objects around me, real and imagined. Scissors, scalpels, stainless-steel bowls, blue waffle blankets, a hospital corner, a stethoscope. Some are included with this writing, overlaid on top of one another, repeated and repeating. An object is a tangible thing; it is something that can be perceived, experienced, encountered by the senses. From the mediaeval Latin *objectum*, it is the 'thing put before', it is an interface with the world. An object intervenes, comes between the body and the world. A mode of encounter can be altered by the mediation of the object. But what of the thing it meets? What if that thing is another thing like me? A thing of flesh. What does the object become then? Does it cease to be a mediator and become a bridge, or is it the thing that holds this other thing, this like-me but not-me thing, in place? And what of the thing itself? The object? What of the agency it holds? To the posthuman, this object is no less vibrant than the things it bridges and/or separates. If I allow myself to remember this, perhaps I can wonder not only about its agency but about how it feels. Not just in my hand but in terms of its own affective state.

And then I might find myself asking how it is feeling.

Things we carry

To examine this thing I am, have become, I turn to another 'snapshot': Katharine A. Tillman's list in her article 'Pathological Fracture: 50 Lessons from the Medical/Surgical Floor'. This sparse list offers its reader fifty 'lessons', exchanges captured by Tillman which reflect on the lived experience of female patients and family members and drawn from their experience of clinical environments. As a performance maker, it functions much like a performance score for me, those prompts to action that grew first from Dada, then through Fluxus, and are now a staple of contemporary performance making. I read her words and I urge myself:

stand, sit, lean, listen, remember, forget, think, eat, drink, reach, rest, relax, walk, wash, dress, ask, and decide. To do these things nonstop all day without looking like she's doing them nonstop all day.

(Tillman, 2020, p. 231)

This list forms a kind of 'woundscape', a term used by audio artist Gregory Whitehead as a strategy for beginning to articulate how significant injuries create a complex and multilayered opening. Whitehead takes on the role of 'vulnerologist' in his radio play *Display Wounds* to examine the meaning of individual wounds:

Sensing its *emotion*. Sensing its *quality*. Getting the *feel* of the wound.
Sensing its emotion. Sensing the deeper nature of its experience.
Sensing the implications of the *kinds of wounds* that can be expected.

(1999, p. 135)

Whitehead develops both of these terms as playful means of reclamation. 'Woundscape' repositions the injured body, returning it from the status of object situated in the territory of the clinician and giving agentic control to the patient. 'Vulnerologist' similarly seeks to explore the expertise those who occupy the 'woundscape' have developed. These two terms offer agency to Whitehead in a way similar to my own use of Barad's 'bodyspacematter'.

Gender and sexuality scholar Jennifer Terry develops Whitehead's 'woundscape' to identify 'polytrauma', where the 'tone of the discourse is methodical, objectifying, and impersonal. Its structure is symptomatically bullet-point-like' (2017, p. 59). These soundings echo through my flesh, reverberate against my attempts at articulation of recurrent miscarriage in my body.

Tillman, Terry, and Whitehead offer simultaneously terms of anchorage and also the impossible burden of the 'vulnerologist'. The sensation held in the body of multiple miscarriage over time ceases to have edges and the experience of 'no absolute boundary between here-now and there-then' (Barad, 2014, p. 168), but as 'vulnerologist', I can layer my thin and resistant insights, extending Barad's diffracted methodology and attending to a series of miscarriages through time. Even in the lack of a visible woundscape, with my organs tucked away, 'being vulnerologist' functions through a kind 'haptic visuality'. A concept developed by Laura U. Marks, it describes a visuality that both touches and functions like the sense of touch (2014). Describing knowledges that are 'local', situated, and embodied: knowledges that form a strange loop, a Möbius strip:

> [w]hen you trace your finger along a Möbius strip, you find yourself weirdly flipping around to another side – which turns out to be the same side. The moment when that happens cannot be detected. The twist is *everywhere* along the strip. Likewise beings are intrinsically twisted into appearance, but the twist can't be located anywhere.
>
> (Morton, 2016, pp. 108–109)

From the spaces left vacant by errant foetuses, my twisted woundscape also acknowledges the 'double wound' of Cathy Caruth's traumatic event, where the initial trauma is haunted by secondary reverberations, and 'the reality of the way that its violence has not yet been fully known' (1996, p. 6). A return, and also a 're-turning as in turning it over and over again' (Barad, 2014, p. 168). Repeated entanglements of body–space–matter, from the spaces left vacant. Remembering that I might forget.

And-and-and

And I am thinking about closing the gaps between bodies.

And I am thinking about bodies in the margins, between the ridges of my fingernails.

And I am thinking about Zhang Huan, who carefully collects burnt incense ash from Buddhist temples to use in his drawings and sculptures.

And I am thinking about the suspension of invisible bodies in prayers.

And I am thinking about when he says '[l]ife is a process of transmigration, [and] I want to express and record this process' (Huan, 2009).

And I am thinking about performing dust.

And I am thinking about inviable things.

And I am thinking about being effected/affected/infected by bodies.

And I am thinking about being effected/affected/infected by my own body.

And I am thinking about how to find my lungs, my corporeal soul.

And I am thinking about.

And I am thinking about.

And I am thinking about Roland Barthes when he says '[t]he Pleasure of the text is that moment when my body pursues its own ideas – for my body does not have the same ideas I do' (1990, p. 17).

And I am thinking about permeable entities.

And I am thinking of Sara Ahmed, who suggests '[d]epending on which way one turns, different worlds might even come into view' (2006, p. 15).

And I am thinking about typing with dirty fingerprints.

Knots knot knots

My body as 'an open system . . . as pure potential, pure virtuality' (Massumi, 1992, pp. 70–71) curls around narratives of diffraction. This conceptual principle emerges from the quantum physics of Niels Bohr and Werner Heisenberg in the 1920s and then subsequently developed by Donna Haraway and Karen Barad. All four were asking questions about being in the world – questions of ontology spring from the initial two-slit experiment of Bohr and Heisenberg and emerge with what Haraway defines as 'worlding-with' (2016, p. 58). This initial recognition that particles behave differently under observation and an attendant shift in perspective has led to a recognition that how we know something is reliant on what the thing is. A miscarriage is both me and not me, it is a worlding-with par excellence. It may well be that the pull toward the posthuman is an act of resistance. By embracing a philosophical perspective that moves beyond the primacy of human narratives, it allows me to shuck off the singularity of the narratives I might otherwise inherit as a means to frame my experience. When the diffracted self is encouraged, the binary logic of success/failure so often ascribed to the maternal body can be elided so that while the binary still exists, it is diffracted through the lens of more complex systems. The diffraction that occurs as cells divide in a process of becoming, which is then arrested (in my case for a wide range of unconnected reasons), is central to my understanding of miscarriage as nonetheless generative: of experience, of cellular material, of changes in my body, of grief, of unlimited potential. A miscarriage, seen through diffraction, is not only an ending. It is a boundary into becoming. Haraway notes, as she extends the ideas of social anthropologist Marilyn Strathern:

> It matters what matters we use to think other matters with; it matters what stories we tell to tell other stories with; it matters what knots knot knots, what thoughts think thoughts, what descriptions describe descriptions, what ties tie ties. It matters what stories make worlds, what worlds make stories.

> (2016, p. 12)

The and-and-and, and an entangled beginning.

Reference list

Ahmed, S. (2006) *Queer phenomenology: orientations, objects, others*. Durham: Duke University Press.

Barad, K. (2014) 'Diffracting diffraction: cutting together-apart', *Parallax*, 20(3), pp. 168–187.

Barthes, R. (1990) *The pleasure of the text*. Oxford: Basil Blackwell Ltd.

Caruth, C. (1996) *Unclaimed experience: trauma, narrative, and history*. Baltimore: John Hopkins University Press.

Dworkin, S.L. and Wachs, F.L. (2009) *Body panic: gender, health and the selling of fitness*. New York: NYU Press.

Gregory, D. (2015) 'Corpographies: making sense of modern war', in Lambert, L. (ed.) *The funambulist papers. Vol. 2: curated*. New York: Punctum Books, pp. 36–45.

Haraway, D.J. (2016) *Staying with the trouble: making kin in the chthulucene*. Durham: Duke University Press.

Huan, Z. (2009) *Rebirth: between spirituality and tradition*. Interview with Zhang Huan. Interview by Elena Guena for *ProjectB contemporary art*. Available at: www.zhanghuan.com/ft/info_78.aspx?itemid=1170 (Accessed: 26 July 2023).

Marks, L.U. (2014) 'Haptic aesthetics', in Kelly M. (ed.) *Oxford encyclopedia of aesthetics*. 2nd edn. Oxford: Oxford University Press.

Massumi, B. (1992) *A user's guide to capitalism and schizophrenia: deviations from Deleuze and Guattari*. Cambridge, MA: MIT Press.

Midgelow, V. (2010) 'Reworking the ballet: stillness and queerness in Swan lake, 4 acts', in Carter, A. and O'Shea, J. (eds.) *The Routledge dance studies reader*. 2nd edn. London and New York: Routledge, pp. 47–57.

Morton, T. (2016) *Dark ecology: for a logic of future coexistence*. New York: Columbia University Press.

Muñoz, J.E. (1996) 'Ephemera as evidence: introductory notes to queer acts', *Women & Performance: A Journal of Feminist Theory*, 8(2), pp. 5–16.

Schechner, R. (2013) *Performance studies: an introduction*. 3rd edn. London and New York: Routledge.

Terry, J. (2017) *Attachments to war: biomedical logics and violence in twenty-first-century America*. Durham and London: Duke University Press.

Tillman, K.A. (2020) 'Pathological fracture: 50 lessons from the medical/surgical floor', *Women & Performance: A Journal of Feminist Theory*, 30(2), pp. 231–236.

Whitehead, G. (1999) 'Display wounds: ruminations of a Vulnerologist, radio play', in Burns, B., Busby, C. and Sawchuk, K. (eds.) *When pain strikes*. Vol. 14. Minneapolis: University of Minnesota Press, pp. 132–138.

5

DANCING WITH IMAGINED MEMORIES

Variant identities and new rehabilitative forms

Sarah-Mace Dennis

The following scenes are from a film that I have been writing and editing for fourteen years but that has never been produced.

Interweaving autobiography, neuroscience, theatrical writing and speculative philosophy, these scenes recall the many different versions of my identity that I performed after sustaining a very severe traumatic brain injury in 2008. In its attempt to make sense of how my internal thoughts and feelings relate to the descriptions recorded in my medical records, this performative hallucination integrates autobiographical, neuroscientific and speculative dialogues. Thinking across and beyond these languages, I attempt to find new ways to 'perform' the subjective reworldings that I have experienced in my encounters with neurotypical and rehabilitative procedures. Speculating on events that I will never completely remember, I interweave my embodied impressions of a near-fatal car crash – during which I sustained severe brain trauma – into philosophical, scientific and dramatic accounts of neurological variance. What results is 'a complex layering of potential experience that continually shifts between the plane of thought/feeling and the plane of articulation' (Manning, 2008: online).

The voices that emerge here are not necessarily the ones I heard but the ones I might have heard, had I been allowed the space to think outside of the clinical routines that re-languaged my modified brain/body – directing me to eat, sit, stand up and speak with predefined patterns of language and movement.

On the outside, I was performing the part that I needed to play to be discharged from the hospital. On the inside I was enlivened by the dance of the non-dancer. This is a dance that does not respond to the repetitions set out in predefined medical choreographies. Rather it 'trips, flails, mindlessly repeats', it 'happens not on a stage but in a shower stall' (Fujii, 2019: online). These freefalling, unpredictable movements enabled me to explore the world through elusive and magical forms of becoming.

Although the clinical languages used by medicine to rehabilitate damaged brains instinctually rebuild a patient's identity according to socially acceptable behavioural norms, another sort of dance *is* possible when we embrace the new forms of experiential plasticity that emerge from sudden neurological change. Exploring unlanguaged states of being, this writing uses the performative potential of speech utterances to imagine rehabilitative procedures as practices that instruct neurologically modified bodies to organise themselves through predefined patterns of movement.

DOI: 10.4324/9781003036500-7

What if, rather than directing the movements of body parts, medical dialogues could open themselves to the power of plasticity, creating space for subjective performances that provide insight into new ways of 'approaching and conducting life' (Spandberg, 2018: online)?

Isolated dirt road in regional Australia – night. One year before the accident

The performance began in around June, 2007. The following scenes were not recorded to camera. Although many of them have been speculated upon by police, ambulance drivers and doctors, there is no evidence that they were ever acted out.

One night, while sleeping in the middle of an old village in an old house with the man she thought was the love of her life, the protagonist of the film experienced a dream that was as cold and as hard as ice. When she woke up shaking in the early hours of the morning, these are the things that she had learned: when you lose control of your car at high speed, the Earth begins to spin. It is 'an uncanny process of amplification and thickening', as if the event of being unable to stop the vehicle is 'already existing behind itself', is 'already active beyond itself, to infinity' (Foucault, 1977, p. 55).

In the height of such momentum, your thoughts begin to double. As they fold over the event that is emerging in real time, you sense an image of what is happening before it even takes place. You know that the rough, empty paddock will not stop skating in circles around you. You know that the car will continue to slide until it collides with the tree. As your chest thrusts into the empty space above the wheel, the ground below you erupts and turns. Terrified and relieved that you aren't quite dead, you open the car door and look down at the hard, dry Earth as you fall toward it.

When she woke up, the story's protagonist struggled to make sense of the vision that had just consumed her. Was it a dream? Or was she rehearsing a script for a performance yet to happen?

Brain injury ward – morning. Three days after the accident

On 20 January 2008, a nurse was sitting at her desk writing a report about a woman, who a year earlier had dreamt that she was in a near-fatal car accident on her way home to the remote village where she lived. In the nurse's report it was noted that the woman she was treating had 'sustained a very severe traumatic brain injury as a result of a single motor vehicle accident on the 17 January 2008. She had been driving back to her home in Hill End (about 1.25 hours drive from Bathurst in New South Wales, Australia) and was only about 15 kilometres from home when she crashed'.

Although she had survived a car accident that she would never remember, she had sustained:

an extremely severe traumatic brain injury, incorporating subarachnoid haemorrhage, extradural hematoma, right lateral ventricular bleed and right thalamic contusions. The Glasgow Coma Score was 9 at the scene and the period of post-traumatic amnesia was of 19 days duration. Other injuries included a small pneumothorax, pulmonary contusions, and pneumomediastinum.

The nurse's patient now had mild right hemiparesis, dysconjugate gaze, ataxia and cognitive impairment.

When the brain injured body written about in that report started to regain consciousness, I/she was somehow estranged from the person they had been before. Rebuilding my/her character in response to medical directions acted out inside hours of rehabilitative scenarios, the protagonist began to feel/observe (and forever cross check) her performances – both those that were spoken to an audience and those that were played out entirely inside their head. Their newly acquired neurological variance would now demand that I/she perform an identity that was forever coming and going: narrated by an unfamiliar voice that would always transition between the experiences of me, her, them and I.

In learning these performances of alterity, I/she could no longer remember the voice that I/she thought with before the performance began. Nor could I/she always ascertain which thoughts were my/her own and which ones belonged to the voices of the doctors.

Living room in a cramped London apartment. Thirteen years after the accident

On her second tequila and soda, it started coming back.

This wasn't the way it was supposed to happen, was it? There was that one neurologist who told her/me that drinking was no longer allowed. I/she poured another glass, mentally replaying the conversation:

Her/I:	What. Do you mean never as in ever?
	Close-up of the Doctor's eyes. He is examining the expressions on her face.
I/She:	No you mean I *can* drink, just not very much don't you?
Doctor:	I wouldn't be drinking at all if I were you. Well, perhaps half a glass, on very special occasions.
Them/Us/Me:	What the fuck is a special occasion?
	The protagonist swallows. The Doctor is writing notes.

Now I am/she is thinking of her oldest friend Jimmy. I am/she is remembering a meeting they had about a year after the accident. When I/she closes my/her eyes, I/she can still hear the conversation.

Bench in a quiet inner city park – Brisbane. One year after the accident

Her/I/The Protagonist:	Now you have known me forever, so you have to tell me how it really is okay?
Jimmy:	I have to tell you what?
Her/I/The Protagonist:	How it really is. Even if it is different than how my brain thinks it is.
Jimmy:	What are you talking about?
Her/I/The Protagonist:	*listening to the voices of the Doctors* I need you to tell me if I'm the same.
Jimmy:	If you are the same as what?
Me:	The same as I was before.
	A beat.
Her/I/The Protagonist:	In the hospital they kept asking if I was speaking louder and faster than I used to. They wanted to know if I'd lost my inhibition.
Jimmy:	You always spoke louder and faster and over the top of everybody else. You had a lot to say. And you didn't let anyone stop you saying it.
	She looks him in the eye. She is trying to make out if he is lying.

Jimmy: You know the shittiest thing Sarah-Mace Dennis. You don't drink any-more. You used to be the coolest person in the world to get drunk with.

Gold mining village – regional Australia. Six months before the accident

Ten years after Jimmy and Sarah-Mace Dennis finished school, this film's protagonist found her-self in an old house that a hundred years earlier had been built in the middle of Hill End – a historic village in regional Australia. She had gone out there to find a man called X. She had discovered in her research that he had a similar lifestyle to her character's love interest. Although she told herself she needed to find him in order to research for her role, it soon became clear that she was rehearsing a different kind of performance.

Cut to

VHS video montage. We see the film's protagonist at age 16. Dressed in knee high pvc boots and a short tartan kilt, she is in a squat with a man in a leather jacket smoking cigarettes. Now she is filming herself dancing and reading books in the university library. These flashbacks to the past are intercut with hand-held mobile phone footage. She is driving up an isolated dirt road toward regional Australia. We see shots of the expansive landscape at dusk: paddocks, vintage farm-houses, trees that are broken with drought, locals drinking at the pub, a cattle dog running in an isolated paddock.

WOMAN'S VOICE (narration over video sequence)

The first time she met X, his mystical outwardness pulled her into a world that was beyond the reality that contained in the performances of some of her more recent past lives. *That* girl who got good grades at university, *that* girl who presented her honours research at an international arts conference, *that* girl who, after spending her youth kissing the necks of men with syringe marks in their arms, became transfixed by Michel Foucault's writing on knowledge and power. It wasn't long before she found herself at home, even able to hold her own, in conversations with people that years before she didn't have the vocabulary to interact with.

Did she go out there to find X because she was somehow ready to leave that language behind? His was a world of slower rhythms and gestures: the open fields where she walked their dog, the hours that were evaporated by the river on a nearby farm, the sound of their footsteps walking underneath the expansive night sky. Although it may have been possible to indicate its 'location in reality', the place she found out there was 'outside of all places' (Foucault, 1984: online).

Sometimes she would close her eyes and see pictures in her head: scenes of fog enclosing mountains; vast, drought-stained landscapes dotted with broken eucalyptus trees; the sky at dusk. She thought about what kind of critical language could describe the embodied affect of moving through these places.

Cut to

The words 'Michel Foucault, Of Other Spaces (*1967*) Heterotopias' appear in bold font over the image sequence.

*THE PROTAGONIST (*narration over video sequence*)*

In cosmological theory, there were the supercelestial places as opposed to the celestial, and the celestial place was in turn opposed to the terrestrial place. There were places where things had been put because they had been violently displaced, and then on the contrary, places where things found their natural ground and stability (Foucault, 1984: online).

Brain injury ward – morning. About a month after the accident

Now everything around her/their comatose body drifted in a glared haze: blurred outlines only occasionally beginning to materialise inside conscious awareness. For the rest of the time, their thoughts moved around the room like waves rolling in the ocean.

During this unbecoming, her/their world was sensed through undefined constellations of time and space. Sometimes she/they could direct their shifting energy into contemplative frameworks that intellectualised their relationship to the shadows in the room. These were always intense moments of focus where she/they experienced philosophical ideas, even if only in an embodied way. For the rest of the time, her/their energy resonated with Antonin Artaud's writing on the Body without Organs (BwO)[1]:

> When you will have made him a body without organs
> then you will have delivered him from all his automatic reactions
> and restored him to his true freedom.
> Then you will teach him again to dance wrong side out
> as in the frenzy of dance halls
> and this wrong side out will be his real place.
>
> (Artaud, 1976, p. 571)

What was she/they, in that comatose state, when she/they could not summon the cognitive momentum needed to understand the things around her/them? Unable to think or move, her/their body and skin was a glacial site of corporeal intensities 'where the alluvions, sedimentations, coagulations, foldings and recordings that compose an organism – and also a signification and a subject', were yet to reoccur (Deleuze and Guattari, 1987, p. 159).

Freed from the habitual routines that 'she' had once used to navigate the world, this Brain without Organs (BwO) began to form the moment she/they drove their car off the road. It was then that the world started to be experienced in ways that were not organised through any kind of embodied logic or semiotic reason. 'She' no longer had 'a brain or nerves or chest or stomach or guts'. All that was left was 'the skin and bones of a disorganised body' (Deleuze and Guattari, 1987, p. 150). As the opposite of psychoanalysis, which converts everything into phantasy, the Body without Organs was what remained when the rest of her identity was taken away:

> What you take away is precisely the phantasy, and significances and subjectifications as a whole. Psychoanalysis does the opposite: it translates everything into phantasies, it converts everything into phantasy, it retains the phantasy. It royally botches the real because it botches the BwO.
>
> (Deleuze and Guattari, 1987, p. 151)

She/they had experienced this kind of unbecoming before, in the house in the village on the hill with X: cradling, cussing, coming in and out of the room. Now his hand was on their back, on their body, on another body, in another time, in another place. There they were bathing in the river, their thoughts inspirited by the banks around: the banks that always were, that always will be, Wiradjuri Country. There they were watching the Chinese migrants who had territorialised those banks in the 1800s, their ambitions now nothing but ghosts still hunting for gold. In another time, in another place, they were there with a second man, laughing. There she/they were laughing, trying to explode every trace of their history. History 'with its themes of development and of suspension, of crisis, and cycle, themes of the ever-accumulating past, with its great preponderance of dead men and the menacing glaciation of the world' (Foucault, 1984: online).

In that awakening her/their/our organs became unmediated experiences: 'matter where no gods go; principles as tones, essences, substances, elements, remissions, productions; manners of being or modalities as produced intensities, vibrations, breath, Numbers' (Deleuze and Guattari, 1987, p. 158).

Brain injury ward – evening. About a month after the accident

Now X was sitting beside her/them/us in the hospital room, talking about the house and their dog: how he had spent days sitting ghost-like in the corner, waiting for her return. The temperature started to change. The pitch and volume of the heart machine became louder.

Her/Them/Us: Puppy. Baby, come here.

Westmead brain injury ward – evening. About two months after the accident

During those early rehabilitative rehearsals, she/her/they sensed that doctors and nurses, not always able to comprehend disorganised brains, tried to organise them into neurotypical routines so that they could prevent them straying toward undesirable performances of delusion. Even her/their organs, freed from their sanctification inside time and space, sensed that they would soon be refolded by the medical procedures that were there to redirect her/their actions into morally acceptable patterns of thought and movement.

The Protagonist's Mother: Come on Sarah, time to wake up.

She/they wanted to stay in bits and pieces. Her/their heart was in the ceiling. Her/their hands were on the floor. Her/their hands were on his ribs, on his body, on another body, in another time, in another place. She wasn't looking at the road. She dreamt about the tree before she drove toward it.

She/their mother bent down and lifted her/their hands from the floor. Then she was holding their right hand in hers, in theirs. Beside them the nurse was calling out the names of body parts and functions. Then the nurse was moving her/their limbs. Then she was training her/our movements, was teaching them/us how we/they would *have* to move toward *her* neurotypical survival.

Nurse: (reading a list of pre-written instructions):
>   1. Step into the shower at eight o'clock in the morning and wash your legs and then your face and then your hair. 2. Step out of the shower and onto the mat. Dry yourself completely before putting your clothes on. 3. Eat breakfast and then brush your teeth before

rinsing the residue from your mouth with a glass of water. Rinse your mouth thoroughly, even if you have never done it this way before.

The therapists at the hospital gathered around her/them each day, training her/them in the correct techniques for reforming their personality. Years after she/they were released, she/they would continue to habitually re-enact these daily routines.

'You will be signifier and signified, interpreter and interpreted – otherwise you're just a deviant' (Deleuze and Guattari, 1987, p. 159).

Isolated dirt road in regional Australia – late afternoon. Nine months after the accident

She/they/us were walking the dog to the lookout when they first sensed *her* – their previous identity who had walked that road hundreds of times before the accident. This other woman was running: both toward and away from the person she would become. She/they/us were now distributed throughout time and space. Still, she/they/us were trying to reach out and clutch on to fragments of that woman we had been before the accident.

Who was she? Did she even exist? Why did the Doctors insist they/she reform their identity to match the reflection of another woman's image?

Note

1 Artaud refers to the Body without Organs in his 1947 radio play *To Have Done with the Judgement of God*. The unbodied, corporeal impulses explored in this explosive and 'mystical rant' (Granade, 2017) are taken up by Gilles Deleuze and Felix Guattari in *Capitalism and Schizophrenia* (1987). Here they use this concept to describe a corporeal intensity that is not organized through any kind of semiotic logic or agency. I learnt about the BwO during my undergraduate studies in critical theory (1999–2004). When I emerged from coma, unable to sense or make sense of my surroundings, some part of my intuition understood that I was a Body without Organs. This embodied knowledge allowed me to mentally shield myself from, and gradually come to terms with, the rehabilitative discourses that demanded I re-language my 'self' according to what felt like repressive organisational structures. From this point on, I have used the term to describe the spatially distributed movements between self, space and other that have defined my world post injury. Deleuze and Guattari's articulation of the BwO has provided me with new approaches for describing the potential that neurological variance offers for reimagining the Judeo-Christian concepts of time, space and subjectification adopted by Western rehabilitative practices.

Reference list

Artaud, A. (1947/1976) 'To have done with the judgement of god, a radio play', in Sontag, S. (ed.) *Antonin Artaud: selected writings*. Berkeley: University of California Press, pp. 555–576.

Deleuze, G. and Guattari, F. (1987) *A thousand plateaus: capitalism and schizophrenia*. Translated by B. Massumi. Minneapolis: University of Minnesota Press.

Foucault, M. (1977) 'Language to infinity', in Bouchard, D. (ed.) *Language, counter-memory, practice: selected essays and interviews by Michel Foucault*. New York: Cornell University Press, pp. 53–67.

Foucault, M. (1984) 'Of other spaces, heterotopias', *Architecture, Mouvement, Continuité*, (5), pp. 46–49. Available at: https://foucault.info/documents/heterotopia/foucault.heteroTopia.en/ (Accessed: 19 December 2021).

Fujii, M. (2019) 'Dancing with Claire Denis', *The New Yorker*, 5 April. Available at: www.newyorker.com/culture/cultural-comment/dancing-with-claire-denis (Accessed: 4 January 2020).

Granade, R. (2017) *Body without organs*. Los Angeles: Ochi Gallery. Available at: www.ochigallery.com/info/ (Accessed: 28 February 2022).

Manning, E. (2008, May) 'Creative propositions for thought in motion', *Inflexions: How is Research Creation*, (1). Available at: www.inflexions.org/issues.html#i1 (Accessed: 28 February 2022).

Spandberg, M. (2018) *Spandbergism*. Available at: https://spangbergianism.wordpress.com (Accessed: 4 January 2020).

6

OVERCOMING STIGMA

Performing the workplace experiences of people living with epilepsy in France

Brenda Bogaert

This chapter details a theatre piece showing how people living with chronic illness may overcome stigma through performance. It will discuss a theatre show created by a group of people living with epilepsy in France in 2018. The show made use of forum theatre, an interactive methodology invented in the 1970s by Augusto Boal, that engages non-professional actors and audiences to articulate and rectify oppressions experienced in their daily lives (see Boal, 2008). The subject matter of a forum theatre show is usually one that is of direct relevance to the audience so that they can relate to the central character who is being oppressed. In the methodology, the audience is first shown a short play in which a character encounters a form of oppression that they are unable to overcome. The play ends at this point, and then it is replayed with an invitation for an audience member to step up onto the stage and replace one of the characters (becoming what Boal calls a 'spect-actor'). The audience member deviates from the script, trying different ways to resolve the oppression faced by the main character. More than one attempt can be made (including by different audience members), generating creative debate among the actors, spect-actor(s) and audience members. In the play discussed in this snapshot, a group of adults living with epilepsy used forum theatre methodologies to engage a range of audiences in addressing workplace stigma associated with this condition. The creative debate brought about by the methodology highlighted the importance of recruiting support persons in order to reduce workplace-related stigma.

The theatre troupe

The forum theatre troupe comprised seven individuals, six persons with epilepsy and one person interested in learning about epilepsy (myself as researcher). The group was made up of three women and four men; three of them were successfully employed, two were retired, and two were unable to work due to their condition. I had come to know the team while conducting ethnography on experiences of epilepsy with an independent patient group in Lyon, France, that held their monthly meetings at an epilepsy research centre. I was invited to participate in the theatre project not specifically as a researcher but as a fellow actor. However, I was also interested in using theatre as a research methodology, both in order to better understand the lived social experience of epilepsy through play and also as a way to 'give back' to the epilepsy community, a way of helping to rectify the stigma I had uncovered in my research. Participating directly in the play's development

DOI: 10.4324/9781003036500-8

and acting in the play gave me precious research insights, notably helping me to better understand the value of support persons in reducing stigma (Bogaert, 2020).

In terms of the play's development, only two people (myself and another) had already done forum theatre, but none of us were professional actors or writers. Therefore, in order to develop the play, we did a workshop with an expert in forum theatre. She used theatre games to help the group to identify the most salient issues relevant to epilepsy stigma and then proposed a preliminary script which was further refined through a group discussion. While the role of the expert was pivotal in helping the troupe develop the script and acting skills, it was the actors themselves who identified what the themes would be and how to play these themes based upon their difficulties of living with epilepsy in society. In particular, the decision to focus on workplace stigma emerged directly from the workshop and the personal experiences of the participants.

Audience for the show

As the aim of the play was to build awareness and combat epilepsy stigma in society, a diverse audience was invited to see and participate in the show. The play was shown four times (twice in February 2018, once in June 2018 and once in February 2019). First, as a test run, it was shown to an audience of about forty people living with epilepsy, their families and neurologists during an epilepsy awareness day at a local epilepsy centre. A week later, we played to an audience of about thirty people at a local church, attracting a diverse public who were not necessarily informed about epilepsy. We also played to a group of about thirty medical students from France, Canada and China as part of an international summer programme at the local medical school in order to help future doctors better understand the quality-of-life issues facing people living with epilepsy. Finally, at another epilepsy awareness day the following year, we played in the main street of the city in order to show our play to a wider audience.

Why talk about stigma in epilepsy?

Epilepsy is a serious chronic condition that is defined by recurring seizures. As the most common neurological condition after migraine, it affects up to fifty million people worldwide. The various manifestations of epilepsy – and seizures themselves – are highly individual and dynamic. Some manifestations of seizures, in particular tonic-clonic seizures, are seen as 'impressive' and 'frightening' by outsiders, especially when the witness does not know how to help the person. Despite affecting various groups and people of all ages, having epilepsy has led to stigma throughout history, and unfortunately it has been hard to shake even today.

Epilepsy stigma dates back to Antiquity. The Greeks coined the word epilepsy (*epikgwia*), coming from the verb *epilambanein*, meaning 'to seize, to possess'. They considered epilepsy the effect of a miasma (bad air) that was thrown on the soul of sinners, and this understanding led to stigmatisation on the assumption that those with epilepsy were immoral (Magiorkinis, Sidiropoulou and Diamantis, 2010). In the Middle Ages, it was associated with witchcraft. In the nineteenth century, more 'scientific' theories were formed, often drawing on the emerging field of psychoanalysis. These were no less stigmatising, for example, the belief that there was such a thing as an 'epileptic personality' and that it was due to bad family character traits, such as alcoholism. The mistaken belief that epilepsy was a psychiatric condition also led to people with epilepsy being among the first patients when asylums were created. Nevertheless, this period also saw the emergence of neurology and epileptology, leading to successful treatments (Patel and Moshé, 2020). While this gradually helped both the medical community and society to recognise epilepsy as a neurological disorder (and helped many to better manage their seizures through successful treatment), it did not make epilepsy stigma entirely disappear.

Indeed, diverse misunderstandings persist in the popular imagination today, including seeing it as a psychological condition, psychiatric disorder or even contagious disease. For this reason, epilepsy stigma remains a problem worldwide and has a significant effect on the person's quality of life, including in social relationships, in education, and in the workplace (de Boer, 2010). Although certain professions are prohibited to persons with epilepsy due to the safety risks associated with seizures, in general, seizure-related work accidents and absence rates are not substantial problems, and most people living with epilepsy can integrate into normal working environments (Krumholz, Hopp and Sanchez, 2016). In spite of this, numerous studies have linked epilepsy with higher rates of unemployment and underemployment, as well as greater difficulties in job retention (Smeets *et al.*, 2007). Having epilepsy has also been correlated with job layoffs, being declared 'unfit to work', feeling shame for having the disease and depression (de Souza *et al.*, 2018). This is largely due to epilepsy stigmatisation and continued misunderstandings about the condition.

Identifying the problem and a potential solution through performance

How epilepsy stigma impacts the person in the workforce can best be seen through recurrent discussions in patient groups. For instance, at the support group in France that created the play, a heated topic was the decision of whether to tell one's future employer about their condition. This is a real issue for persons with epilepsy, as many find that when they disclose their condition at the interview, they are not hired. This remains hard for them to prove, as potential employers will not state this reason in their refusal letter and non-discrimination legislation such as the 2000 European Union directive on equal treatment and the French labour code explicitly forbid this; however, it remains a reality for many persons with epilepsy. Whether or not they disclose their condition at the hiring stage, it is often necessary for persons with epilepsy at some point to discuss how their role may need to be adapted. These included padding sharp corners so the person would not hurt themselves if they had a seizure; allowing rest breaks or time off for doctor appointments; or adapting tasks and deadlines due to the side effects of medication, which may cause tiredness or concentration problems. In general, however, these changes are relatively minor, and the person is usually able to continue doing their job well. However, even when employers were able or willing to adapt a post, this was often not well accepted or understood by their colleagues. Fellow colleagues frequently perceived that the person was receiving 'special treatment' or 'exaggerating' the seriousness of their condition, in particular because of recurring misperceptions of epilepsy as psychological. This made it difficult for these persons to do their jobs well but also integrate into the workplace with other colleagues, and they often felt isolated. According to the experiences of persons in the patient group, this stigma was particularly aggravated in lower-status, administrative jobs in the private sector which demanded a high level of efficiency. In higher-status jobs, and/ or in the public sector, some persons said employers were more willing to 'adapt', but this still took a willing and understanding supervisor. All in all, whatever the educational background or job status, persons in the patient group all faced some form of stigma in access to and inclusion in the workplace.

As problems with employment came up at nearly every meeting, some group members decided that it was not enough to discuss these issues among themselves, among those who already knew, understood or experienced it. They decided instead to do something about the stigma they experienced in the workplace. Their solution was the forum theatre show.

The epilepsy and prejudice show

The plot of the ten-minute theatre show takes place around a birthday celebration for Pierre, a person living with epilepsy. Two of his family members (Suzanne and Emma) and two work colleagues (Nathalie and Pascal) have come to his house party, where Pierre has just had a seizure and is resting in a chair. The first part of the theatre piece shows Emma advising Pierre on how to manage his epilepsy in a rather paternalistic manner. It is the second part of the play that addresses stigma in the workplace, when Nathalie and Pascal confront Pierre about the 'special treatment' he receives at work. Nathalie tells Pierre that 'everyone thinks you're a slacker' for taking sick days, while Pascal jokes that 'even when you're present, you have absences!' When Suzanne comes to his defence, Nathalie dismisses his illness as 'purely psychological, all of that stuff. Get out a bit more, you'll see, it will do you good'. A little later the two work colleagues confront Emma about their problems with Pierre.

Pascal: Well, he's acting strange, that Pierre!

Emma: Yes, how unlucky, on his birthday . . .

Nathalie: I think it's more of a mental problem, those seizures . . .

Emma: What?

Nathalie: Well, it's obvious something's not right. We're his colleagues,
we see him every day at work, and sometimes, he seems crazy. He says weird things . . . and then he doesn't even remember saying them! It's some kind of delusion. When it's like that, you should go see a psychiatrist. There are hospitals for that kind of thing.

Pascal: Now wait a minute, you're exaggerating a bit . . .

Emma: But it's not that . . .

Nathalie: You know before, they used to think they were possessed, those . . . *(she mimics someone who is convulsing)*. Personally, I don't believe it, but maybe there's some truth in it . . .
When Pierre and Suzanne rejoin the group, Natalie and Pascal reveal their naïve belief that epilepsy might be contagious:

Nathalie: Ah, you see, when you want to . . . but wait, it's not contagious, is it? your thing? Because I looked it up on the Internet and I also asked some friends. They told me it could be contagious . . .

Pascal: Really, it's contagious? Oh no . . . I catch anything and everything that's going around. Here, Pierre, your gift . . .
He throws the gift at Pierre and runs away, putting his hands over his mouth.

In these excerpts from the theatre piece, we can understand how workplace stigma is perpetuated by Pierre's colleagues. First of all, there is the misperception that Pierre is inefficient, as he sometimes has to take sick days or work flexible hours. Even though Suzanne explains that the management have used these adaptations as an excuse to give him the 'dirty work', his colleagues continue to give him a hard time about this 'special treatment'. Rather than trying to understand why he may need reasonable adjustments they accuse him of being lazy, or that his condition is 'in his head'. By doing so, they perpetuate the idea that his condition is psychological rather than neurological, however, they also perpetuate ongoing misrepresentations of epilepsy as contagious. This may seem surprising, but several members of the theatre troupe reported experiencing this in their real life. In this theatre piece, we can therefore understand how living with stigma affects the person's wellbeing in the workplace, in particular by isolating them from their colleagues.

Audience interaction and engagement

As noted, in forum theatre, the audience does not passively watch the show but also has the opportunity to become 'spect-actors', actively intervening to try to change the conflictual situation by replacing one of the characters. While the spect-actor in this case was not permitted to replace Pierre (the person oppressed) or the main oppressor (Nathalie), they were able to change places with either Suzanne, Emma or Pascal. In the showings, audience members brought several new ideas about how to combat stigma in the workplace. In one case, an audience member replaced Pierre's relative, Suzanne. In the scene when Nathalie makes a damaging statement about his moods and absences, rather than getting frustrated, the spect-actor decided to patiently explain to the two colleagues the side effects of seizures. She explained that they can cause fatigue and that was the reason that he is sometimes very tired at work. She also told them that Pierre had found coping mechanisms after seizures occurred, such as deciding to do easier tasks while he recovered. Through this educational approach, the new Suzanne was able to show Pierre's colleagues that he was capable of working well despite his condition. This helped resolve the conflictual situation, and the colleagues responded afterward in a more supportive way toward him.

In a second approach, Pascal was replaced by an audience member who took a different tactic. In the play, Nathalie is the vector of misunderstandings, notably by reinforcing the idea that epilepsy is a psychiatric condition, is contagious or is simply 'in his head'. Pascal is more ambivalent, as he has not yet heard much about epilepsy. Therefore, rather than agreeing with or joking with Nathalie at each stage of the conversation, the new Pascal took the opportunity to ask Pierre about his epilepsy to better understand it. This immediately forced Nathalie to stop harassing Pierre. As a result, they both started to empathise with him about being given the 'dirty work'. The conversation then moved from teasing Pierre to discussing their problems with their jobs in sympathy with Pierre. They left the conversation understanding that epilepsy is a neurological condition that is not contagious and that Pierre is their colleague, who also had a hard time at the office despite his need for reasonable adjustments.

Conclusion

In both of the solutions proposed by the spect-actors in the forum theatre piece, it was possible to resolve the conflictual situation and to overcome stigma in the workplace. It also gave new inspiration for those working to combat epilepsy stigma. In particular, the audience interventions showed that it was vital to involve a support person who could actively be involved in educating others about epilepsy. As the spect-actors showed, this resource person could either be a family member or a friend or those 'figures in the middle' who could also become supporters if they better understood the condition. Although this risks reducing the agency of the oppressed person themselves, making them passive, it also turns the reduction of stigma into a social responsibility rather than that of the individual. This case study shows that methodologies such as forum theatre can help raise awareness of the difficulties of living with chronic disease, but they can also bring forth creative change to entrenched problems.

Reference

Boal, A. (2008) *Theatre of the oppressed*. New edn. London: Pluto Press.

Bogaert, B. (2020) 'Untangling fear and eudaimonia in the healthcare provider-patient relationship', *Medicine, Health Care and Philosophy*, 23(3), pp. 457–469. https://doi.org/10.1007/s11019-020-09956-1

de Boer, H.M. (2010) 'Epilepsy stigma: moving from a global problem to global solutions', *Seizure*, 19(10), pp. 630–636. https://doi.org/10.1016/j.seizure.2010.10.017

de Souza, J.L. *et al.* (2018) 'The perceived social stigma of people with epilepsy with regard to the question of employability', *Neurology Research International*, pp. 1–5. https://doi.org/10.1155/2018/4140508

Krumholz, A., Hopp, J.L. and Sanchez, A.M. (2016) 'Counseling epilepsy patients on driving and employment', *Neurologic Clinics*, 34(2), pp. 427–442. https://doi.org/10.1016/j.ncl.2015.11.005

Magiorkinis, E., Sidiropoulou, K. and Diamantis, A. (2010) 'Hallmarks in the history of epilepsy: epilepsy in antiquity', *Epilepsy & Behavior: E&B*, 17(1), pp. 103–108. https://doi.org/10.1016/j.yebeh.2009.10.023

Patel, P. and Moshé, S.L. (2020) 'The evolution of the concepts of seizures and epilepsy: what's in a name?', *Epilepsia Open*, 5(1), pp. 22–35. https://doi.org/10.1002/epi4.12375

Smeets, V.M.J. *et al.* (2007) 'Epilepsy and employment: literature review', *Epilepsy & Behavior*, 10(3), pp. 354–362. https://doi.org/10.1016/j.yebeh.2007.02.006

7

NATURALIST HAUNTINGS

Staging psychiatry in *Anatomy of a Suicide, People Places Things* and *Blue/Orange*

Leah Sidi

The late 2010s saw a cluster of mental health plays hitting UK stages, part of a dramatic increase in discussion of mental health across the country. Everyone from the prime minister to the media, the National Health Service (NHS) and service users seemed to agree that the UK faced a 'mental health crisis'. Prime Minister Theresa May's first speech of 2017 addressed the 'burning injustices of mental health and inadequate treatment' (PMO, 2017). It reflected new public attention to mental health issues that had grown over recent years due to sustained campaigns by the NHS and service-user groups to highlight the under-resourced nature of psychiatric and mental health services. May's speech marked a tacit acknowledgement that economic austerity had severely damaged mental health service provision. However, as groups such as the National Service User Network were quick to point out, it fell short of reversing cuts to essential services (NSUN, 2017).

This chapter considers theatrical representations of mental health services at this moment of crisis. It suggests that mainstream contemporary theatre continues to be haunted by an entanglement between medical and theatrical gazes embedded in a Naturalist approach to theatrical space. 2016–2017 saw a trio of high profile and critically acclaimed plays thematising psychiatry on the London stage: Alice Birch's *Anatomy of a Suicide* (dir. Katie Mitchell, Royal Court, 2017), Duncan Macmillan's *People, Places, Things* (dir. Jeremy Herrin, National Theatre, 2016) and the restaging of Joe Penhall's *Blue/Orange* (dir. Matthew Xia, Young Vic, 2016). Each of these productions deliberately experimented with the legacies of theatrical Naturalism to speak to the 'mental health crisis'. At the same time, their engagements with mental health narratives are additionally haunted by Naturalism's limited representational strategies and rely on domestic space as a binary opposite of institutional care. In this context, haunting refers to an unwilled influence, carried alongside more deliberate appropriations of historical forms.

Psychiatry does not constitute a unified, monolithic discipline in the UK. Mental health care is delivered via a network of services composed of the NHS, the third sector and private providers. In 2016, the Independent Mental Health Taskforce noted 'mental health services have been underfunded for decades, and too many people have received no help at all, leading to hundreds of thousands of lives put on hold or ruined, and thousands of tragic and unnecessary deaths' (p. 3). The report painted a picture of decentralised, underfunded and chaotic mental health services which struggled to meet the needs of service users, who were themselves often in precarious living situations. It highlighted that people who were poorer, from marginalised communities, in prison

DOI: 10.4324/9781003036500-9

or precariously housed have a higher prevalence and severity of mental health problems and struggle to access adequate care. The report demonstrated that the mental health crisis was rooted in a crisis of housing, of care and of social responsibility.

Crises are declared as much as they are created. They have discursive as well as material dimensions, which are not strictly separate from each other. On the one hand, the material conditions of resource scarcity and institutional chaos in the 2010s drove campaign groups to raise the public profile of mental health service cuts, providing impetus and urgency to the work of activists and advocates for better service provision (Kritsotaki, Long and Smith, 2016). On the other hand, the increased use of mental health discourses in a range of public settings (not least the wide adoption of the language of mental health and wellbeing by a generation of social media users) has shaped the ways in which mental health is discussed and approached in and beyond health care provision. The intertwining of the material and discursive aspects of crisis provides a cultural and social fabric from which theatre-makers create work pertaining to mental distress. New works of theatre which we might describe as 'mental health plays' further contribute to this fabric.

The discursive landscape of the mental health crisis is complex. Whilst acknowledging this complexity, it is possible to identify a dominant trend in mental health speak emerging in the late 2010s. Hannah Jane Parkinson summarised this trend as 'a transformation in the way we talk about mental health . . . as depression and anxiety went from unspoken things to ubiquitous hashtags' (2018). Parkinson notes two major threads in 2010s mental health discourse. First, the destigmatisation of certain forms of mental distress leaves little room for addressing complex and severe experiences:

> Tend[ing] to focus on depression and anxiety, or post-traumatic stress disorder. It is less comfortable with the mental illnesses deemed more unpalatable – people who act erratically, hallucinate, have violent episodes or interpersonal instability.
>
> (ibid, p. 2018)

Second, dominant mental health discourses present psychiatric help as easily accessible and an efficient fix to mental distress. The emphasis on 'talking about it' and 'asking for help' are frustrating if help is difficult to access and includes facing months of waiting lists, lack of medication, displacement due to unavailability of psychiatric beds and housing precarity. What Parkinson identifies as the shortcomings of 'The Conversation' about mental health are precisely a blindness to the material and emotional complexities of living with mental distress in a moment of crisis.

This chapter explores the role that theatre has had to play in these cultural mental health discourses. I examine how the mechanics of theatrical production – especially its spatial organisation – contribute specific understandings of the construction and experience of mental health and illness to a wider cultural field. The focus here is on the theatrical mainstream. It is true that there are many performance artists and small theatre companies across the UK working on innovative, service user–led projects which explore the ways in which theatre might provide sites of resistance or self-making outside of dominant mental health discourses.[1] At the same time, 'major' theatre productions in London's West End constitute a theatrical mainstream which reflects and contributes to the cultural discourses of a given moment. By examining the role of three 'high profile' theatrical productions in the late 2010s, I offer a critique of theatre's legacy in engaging with and even shaping discourses surrounding 'mental health'. I argue that there is a trace of theatre's historical relationship with psychiatry to be found in contemporary productions – one that may actually distance us from the realities of many mental health service users.

Naturalism and the medical gaze in 'mental health' plays

Anatomy of a Suicide (*AoS*), *People, Places and Things* (*PPT*) and *Blue/Orange* (*B/O*) each innovated in distinctive ways with Naturalist forms to stage unusual narratives of mental illness which question the idea of recovery. Created by writer Alice Birch and director Katie Mitchell, *AoS* explores the (unscientific) idea that suicidality 'could be passed on through our DNA' by staging the stories of three generations of suicidal women simultaneously on stage (Hoggard, 2017). The stage is split into three areas, each representing a different decade, with the stories running in parallel. In the 1970s, Carol comes home from hospital after a failed suicide attempt. She struggles with her life as a housewife; buys a new house; and has a daughter, Anna. Carol raises Anna for sixteen years, undergoes electroshock therapy and eventually commits suicide by drowning. Her suicide is not staged but is narrated by her husband John. In the 1990s, her daughter Anna struggles with addiction and suicidal feelings. She meets documentary-maker Jamie, who is making a film about addiction. They fall in love and move back to the family house, eventually having a daughter, Bonnie. Anna feels haunted by her mother's presence and struggles to care for Bonnie. She is hospitalised and treated with electroconvulsive therapy (ECT). On returning from hospital, she kills herself by electrocuting herself in the bath, onstage. In the 2030s, Bonnie is an Accident and Emergency doctor, treating Jo – a patient who has cut her wrist. Bonnie and Jo fall in love and have a strained relationship, as Bonnie struggles to deal with the legacies of her mother's and grandmother's deaths. We discover that her father remarried and now has grandchildren. In the end, Bonnie leaves Jo and decides to pursue sterilisation to end the maternal family line and sells the family house. Images and phrases are repeated from one time zone into the other, especially in relation to water, swimming and electricity – the materials of Carol and Bonnie's suicides.

PPT is also centred around a mentally unwell woman and her psychic inheritance. The play stages the experiences of Emma, an actress in her 30s who experiences addiction and goes through two rounds of rehabilitation before returning to her toxic parental home. *PPT* begins with a high Emma collapsing in the middle of a production of Chekhov's *The Seagull*. She signs into a state-funded rehabilitation centre, experiences intense dissociation as she detoxes, refuses to accept the Alcoholics Anonymous programme, leaves early and then relapses. In rehabilitation she provides false identities and histories for herself, variously calling herself, Nina, Emma and Sarah. In the play's second half, Emma returns to rehab and tries again, opening up about the death of her brother and attempting to re-learn a monologue which she had practised with him and which becomes her version of the serenity prayer. She returns to her parental home to find her mother has preserved all her drugs and that neither of her parents believe that she is sincere about her recovery. The play ends with Emma auditioning with her corporate monologue, a queue of identical actresses waiting on stage to go next.

B/O was a revival of Joe Penhall's 2001 play, which stages the experiences of Christopher, a Black man who is being held in an acute facility under a section order. The action takes place over twenty-four hours in a psychiatric consulting room in an NHS hospital and is centred around a disagreement between two psychiatrists, Bruce and Robert, about the future of Christopher's treatment. The senior doctor, Robert, is eager to discharge Christopher into the 'care of the community' and uses anti-psychiatric language to justify a position which is motivated by resource scarcity. Bruce, younger, more idealistic and more biomedically minded, believes that Christopher requires inpatient care. The play is largely structured around the two white doctors debating the nature of psychiatric treatment, using their Black patient Christopher as a pawn in their debate. As Rachel Clements puts it, by the time Christopher is discharged at the end of the play, 'it is unclear whether anyone has Christopher's best interests in mind, let alone at heart' (Clements, 2013, p. xli).

All three plays deliberately build on and subvert theatrical forms associated with nineteenth-century Naturalism. The plays highlight the intertwining of the theatrical and the medical gaze, pointing to a deep historical relationship between theatre and the 'psy' disciplines (psychiatry, psychology and psychoanalysis). The development of modern biomedicine in the late 1800s provided a crucial context for the emergence of Naturalist theatre. Emile Zola's Naturalist Manifesto declared in 1881 that literary Naturalism's 'impetus was given by new scientific methods' (Schumacher, 1996, p. 70). Scholars of Naturalism have identified a fundamental epistemological shift shared by theatre and biomedicine at this moment, characterised by the primacy of the medical gaze (Rebellato, 2019, 2020; Shepherd-Barr, 2016). The medical gaze in the late nineteenth century is essentially concerned with exposing anatomical features as diagnostic information. Under this gaze, there is no separation between medical theory and anatomical fact. Sufficiently exposed, the body speaks for itself – Zola went so far as to describe his play *Thérèse Raquin* as an autopsy: 'I simply carried out on two living bodies the same analytical examination that surgeons perform on corpses' (Rebellato, 2019, p. 186). Strindberg famously released his Naturalist manifesto as the author's note to *Miss Julie* and used it to give a detailed explanation of the causes of his emotionally unstable heroine's behaviour. The audiences of Naturalist theatres are positioned in both cases as audiences of a public dissection, having ills of contemporary society exposed and revealed to them. This is compounded by the 'descriptive density . . . of putting real objects on stage', generating a 'representational surplus' which leaves little room for alternative speculation (ibid, pp. 181–182). Writing in 1911, Reimer's survey of German theatre noted the extent to which the presence of real domestic objects and solid sets had become an expectation of audiences, who believed that 'the world of illusion must always offer a heightened reality . . . the actor has to open the door himself with a wooden handle' (Schumacher, 1996, p. 125). Even within the illusions of theatre, the objects of the Naturalist gaze were expected by the 1910s to be 'real'.

This kind of representational density is drawn on and deliberately heightened in the three twenty-first–century plays under discussion. The 2016 production of *B/O* was staged in the round using a simple, functional set to represent the consulting room. Beneath the stage was a full reconstruction of an NHS waiting room which the audience had to walk through to reach their seats. The waiting room was visible through windows beneath the stage during the performance, providing a form of representational surplus contrasting with the more open staging in the round. Above ground, the theatricality of the play was highlighted by the audience's ability to see one another whilst also looking into an enclosed, 'real' waiting room below. This set builds on what Penhall describes as a 'heightened Naturalism' in his playwriting, exaggerating the polyvocality of human speech by integrating a range of linguistic registers in his work: in this case 'medical jargon, cultural references, colloquialisms, and the language of anti-psychiatry' (Clements, 2013: xliii). Similarly Katie Mitchell, director of *AoS*, is famous for her intensification and subversion of Naturalist modes – a process which Ben Fowler calls a '*hyperbolic* realism' (2020, p. 5). This involves focusing on the minutiae of performance to create representations which are as 'real' as possible. In rehearsal for *AoS*, for example, Mitchell spent half an hour working with actress Hattie Morahan 'on "making concrete" the simple direction in which her character (Carol) peels apples for a crumble' (Fowler, 2020, p. 6). This generates a psychological equivalent of Naturalism's representational surplus, anatomising the motivations and movements of the actors on stage and scrutinising them for their veracity.

Whilst Penhall and Birch and Mitchell exaggerate Naturalism's claims to representational veracity within the world of the play, Macmillan undermines them by literally overlaying his twenty-first–century play with Naturalist ones. The play opens with Emma failing to complete her role as Nina in Chekhov's *The Seagull* and being ushered offstage, to be replaced by an understudy. Later in group therapy, Emma avoids providing her personal history, instead giving the story of Ibsen's *Hedda Gabbler*. Where Ibsenite and Chekhovian Naturalism would insist on the 'realness' of objects and emotions on stage, Macmillan's play highlights replaceability – nothing in Emma's life is authentically 'real'; everything is a stand-in for something else. This excessive theatricality is heightened through doubling in casting. Emma repeatedly tells her doctor and then her therapist that they 'look like my mother', even as the audience sees that the mother, therapist and doctor are all played by the same actor. Emma herself is represented through a pattern of replacements and doubles. When she goes through benzodiazepine withdrawal, her dissociation and pain are represented through the emergence of multiple 'Emmas' on the stage, writhing and shaking under flashing lights. These 'Emmas' are also her understudies and the actresses who audition for the same part as she at the end of the play. Through this use of doubling, *PPT* makes its audience hyper-aware of their spectating practice, highlighting and then undermining Chekhovian and Ibsenite claims to authenticity. In *AoS*, Mitchell achieves a similar effect by having the main actors carry out costume changes on stage. Lead actors Hattie Morahan, Katie O'Flynn and Adelle Leonce moved to the front of the stage in between scenes, where they were stripped to their underwear and re-dressed by male dressers in suits. In this sense, Macmillan and Birch and Mitchell undermine Naturalism's claims to authenticity by replacing it with *metatheatrical* form of representational surplus – an over-insistence on the theatricality of the event.

By exaggerating Naturalist claims to veracity in psychiatric settings, these productions make explicit the shared assumptions embedded by the theatrical and the medical gazes. The relationship between theatre and late nineteenth-century psy- and neuro- disciplines is best understood not as mono-directional but as *entangled*. The notion of entanglement is derived from feminist technology studies and has been important in developing the field of critical medical humanities. 'Entanglement' is an epistemological stance which suggests that two areas which seem separate are in fact deeply embedded within one another (Fitzgerald and Callard, 2016). This relationship is multi-directional, with theatricality and performance shaping the founding assumptions of theories of the mind, even as theatre draws on the psy- and neuro- disciplines to cultivate an objective, psychological gaze. For example, Jean-Martin Charcot's foundational work on neurology was underpinned by close clinical observation of the symptoms of neurological disease. Lisa Appignanesi notes that Charcot 'prided himself for his talent for observation, his eye for detail, his rigorous method' (2008, p. 145). Charcot incorporated theatricality into his diagnostic and teaching methods, famously holding lectures at La Salpêtrière in which he hypnotised patients in front of a clinical audience. Theatricality and objective observation were intimately linked in Charcot's practice. Whilst Charcot displayed his patients in a performative spectacle (Bartleet, 2003), Freud used a structure derived from tragedy to underpin his spatialisation of human consciousness and unconsciousness. Jean-Michel Rabaté goes so far as to suggest 'that the edifice of psychoanalytical concepts is founded on literary' – we might better say theatrical – 'texts from a well-known play by Sophocles to Shakespeare's dark prince' (2014, p. 27).

At the centre of this entanglement is the figure of the (female) hysteric. As Elin Diamond identified in her landmark work of feminist theatre criticism, *Unmaking Mimesis*, 'Ibsenite realism' (or Naturalism more broadly) is structured around the detection and revelation of the pathologised inner life of a hysterical heroine (1997). Through a careful arrangement of objects and perspectives, Ibsenite theatre 'reinforce[s] the pleasures of perspectival space' whilst giving the appearance of exposing incidental, objective reality (1997, p. 5). Kim Solga builds on Diamond's work to stress that this form of drama 'relies for its signifying power on a closed, carefully self-selected world and the promise that its spectators will eventually see all that world has to offer' (2007, p. 355). The illusory nature of this promise only makes Naturalism more insistent on the revelatory nature of its frame:

> Of course, we know there is a world outside the drawing room/kitchen/bedroom we see onstage, just as we know that we are watching a theatricalization of the real rather than the 'real' itself. But the promise of realism is that all we need know will be contained within this closed room. . . . All this means, of course, that realism is not really obsessed with the visible at all; in fact, it is more deeply, neurotically, concerned with what can no longer be seen, with the stuff it has had to shove beyond its frame in order to instantiate that frame as the container of all relevant truth and knowledge.
>
> (Solga, 2007, p. 356)

Following Solga's formulation, we might say *B/O, AoS* and *PPT* expose Naturalism's neurosis about the unseen, insistently bringing the mechanisms of theatre into the representations of clinical space on stage.

Naturalist haunting?

So far, I have theorised an explicit connection between late 2010s 'mental health plays' and Naturalism's preoccupation with diagnosis and visibility. I would like now to suggest that these productions also carried with them a set of implicit (possibly unwilled) representational politics inherited from their Naturalist predecessors. This inheritance can be understood as a mode of haunting – the ghosts of past forms lingering uninvited in present (theatrical) spaces. The language of haunting has been deployed in literary studies in contrasting ways, either to theorise states of ontological uncertainty following Derrida's 'hauntology' (Rabaté, 2014; Foley, 2017), uncanny encounters with otherness (Lipson Freed, 2017) or (as I will use it) as a politically significant mode of forgetting and endurance following Avery Gordon (Gordon, 2008; Frosh, 2013). For Gordon, 'haunting describes how that which appears to be not there is often a seething presence, acting on and often meddling with taken-for granted realities' (2008, p. 8). These twenty-first–century 'mental health plays' carry forms of blindness inherent to nineteenth-century theatre, obscured by their more visible critiques of Naturalist theatricality. This haunting is present first in the structures of (gendered) revelation in relation to pathology and second in the plays' relationships to domestic and clinical space.

All three plays follow the structure of pathology and revelation which Diamond critiques. Each play stages a stereotypical, 'othered' madperson – a psychotic Black man in *B/O* and mad, unruly women in *PPT* and *AoS*. In Diamond and Solga's analyses, Naturalism's epistemological work parallels the work of the early psychoanalyst or psychiatrist: wading through the plethora of experiences and behaviours to create a narrow frame of symptoms and tells through which the hysteric can be understood and displayed. Solga suggests

> that realism relies for its truth-effects on the figure of the hysterical woman with a past, whose previous transgressions must be both confessed and translated onto her body in order for audiences to enjoy the ocular proof of the play's positivist inquiry and receive the payoff of the reality effect.
>
> (2007, p. 357)

PPT is structured around a series of false revelations about Emma's identity which structurally mirror the revelations surrounding the pathologies of naturalist heroines. In this play, as Harpin notes: 'the mechanism of truthfulness operates as an authenticating discourse in recovery' (2018, p. 164). Emma's complete refusal to tell the truth throughout the play positions her as a proto-hysteric within an addiction narrative. In the penultimate scene of the play, just as we think we have learned all there is to learn about Emma's identity, her mother reveals that her real name is Lucy. Coming from Emma/Lucy's mother, this final (re)naming reinserts a discourse of authenticity into what has become a heavily illusory theatrical field. What is more, it casts Emma/Lucy even more firmly in the role of the malingerer. The trajectory towards authenticity which Emma/Lucy appears to have followed in the second half of the play by opening up about her brother's death as the 'real' trauma behind her addiction is thrown into doubt by her failure to reveal her true name.

B/O contains a similar moment of revelation between the doctors, who are debating the status of Christopher's belief that Ugandan dictator Idi Amin is his father. In an effort to clear bed space, psychiatric consultant Robert attempts to convince Bruce that there is reasonable doubt that he may in fact be the son of Idi Amin and that it is racist to assume this is a delusion. The turning point comes as Bruce reveals that previously Christopher has believed himself to be the son of other internationally renowned figures, such as Muhammad Ali:

Robert: Don't you think you're being a bit arbitrary?
Bruce: What?
Robert: Why should he put [a newspaper cutting about Idi Amin's wives and children] away?
Bruce: Why?

    . . .

    Because he cut it out of *The Guardian* on Saturday. I watched him. Where do you think he got a pair of scissors from?
    Pause.
    Robert snatches the article from Christopher and examines it.
Robert: So . . . ?
Bruce: Three weeks ago it was Muhammad Ali. He'd seen Muhammad Ali on the television winning 'Sports Personality of the Century' and put two and two together (Penhall, 2000, 97).

Having explored some ambiguity as to the reality of the patient's beliefs through the conflict between Robert and Bruce, the play now confirms the psychotic, 'unreal' nature of Christopher's fantasy parentage. In differing ways, both plays reinstate the boundaries between what constitutes fact (as mental health) and fiction (as mental illness) into their dramatic universes.

In all three plays, this reality effect is haunted by an approach to space which is inherited from Naturalist forms. All three plays are structured around a medical-domestic binary, which seeks to explain mental pathology through the exposure of domestic space. In *PPT* and *AoS*, the result is the location of aetiology in a domestic sphere which is problematically haunted by a toxic mother. In *B/O* the absence of such a domestic location contributes to the opacity of Christopher's character to his doctors and the audience. Each of the story lines of *AoS* begins with a medical institution: Carol returning from hospital, Anna arriving in hospital and Bonnie working in hospital. The clinical and the domestic are constantly overlaid and interwoven in this play. Carol's experience of ECT, for example, is repeated first in Anna's more humane ECT treatment and then in Anna's brutal onstage suicide by electrocution in the bath – the bath positioned in the exact location and orientation of Anna's earlier hospital bed. This act in turn takes place at the moment when Anna's daughter Bonnie, in another time zone, is in a doctor's surgery contemplating sterilisation.

In the 2017 production, Mitchell worked with set designer Alex Eales to literally layer these spaces on top of each other. As Fowler summarises:

> Eales situated Birch's timelines in a simple boxed room with seven access doors: two in each side wall and three in the upstage wall . . . finished with a bruised concrete effect. . . . Each of the co-terminously unfolding but temporarily distinct narratives occupied a third of the stage from front to back. . . . Behind the back wall, Eales had also designed a detailed hallway the entire width of the stage including a side-view of a balustrade staircase, based on his and Mitchell's realisation that multiple scenes take place in a family home passed between the generations.
>
> (2020, p. 230)

The front section of the set was evocative of stereotypical imagery associated with medical or disciplinary institutions. Bare and grey, the rigidity with which the different generations remained in their sections of the stage evoked the spatial arrangement of beds in a ward. Throughout the play, the stage has hospital style strip lights above it. At the end of the play, after deciding to go ahead with sterilisation, Bonnie sells the house which has been haunted by her mother's and grandmother's suicidal presences. In this production,

> a striking *coup de théâtre* preceded this final scene as the upstage wall flew out, yielding a clear view of the staircase and transforming the stage into a unified naturalistic space: a bare front room in a Victorian house with bright sunlight flooding its bay windows.
>
> (Fowler, 2020, p. 233)

This moment of revelation offers a clear scenographic indication of a release from previous generations' mental pathologies, triggering a slow-motion sequence with Carol and Anna 'breaking out of their confinement in distinct temporal lanes and making physical contact with Bonnie as they passed' (ibid).

In both *PPT* and *AoS*, then, the plays reach an (arguably unsatisfying) resolution through a striking *coup de théâtre* in which a woman's mental pathology is exposed in and explained by the maternal relationship in the bourgeois family home. *PPT* also layered the medical and domestic sites within the scenography. The 2017 production used a versatile open box set designed by Bunny Christie, with two walls, ceiling and floor made up of starkly lit white panels and audience members sitting on either side of the stage. The associations of a stereotypical 'medical' imagery of a blank, sterile and constantly observed environment were unmistakable. When Emma/Lucy returns to her parents' house, her room in the rehabilitation ward is replaced on stage by her childhood bedroom, and her doctor is replaced by her mother. In the final scene the bed moves away, and Emma is left standing on a bare stage, finally correctly reciting the corporate monologue as though in an audition – a heavily metatheatrical move in which all is revealed to be theatre. This underpinning of psychopathology in domestic space is itself an engagement with Naturalism – one which is much less ironic than the earlier references to *The Seagull* and less explicit than Mitchell's hyperbolic attention to detail.

In Naturalist theatre, we peer into the mind of the hysteric by peering into the bourgeois home, and we understand the home via the revelations of the hysteric. The home provides a stable container for the hysteric's instability and ultimate revelation. As Rebellato notes, *localisation* is an essential function of the Naturalist/medical gaze:

> At one point, Foucault summarises the change from the eighteenth to the nineteenth-century as a move from 'what is the matter with you?' to 'where does it hurt?'. The Naturalists similarly moved away from the metaphysics of tragedy to the socialisation and localisation of moral crisis. To the question, where does it hurt?, the Naturalist will answer, in the mines and laundries . . . and above all in the bourgeois home.
>
> (2019, p. 180)

This impulse to identify the location of the source of an ill in a physical place is a foundational area of conflict and debate in the history of the psy- disciplines. Katja Guenther has demonstrated the extent to which concerns with localisation at the end of the nineteenth century were essential to the development and subsequent divergence of both psychoanalysis and neuroscience. Freud debated and then rejected the idea of mental illness as localised – of a direct relationship between symptoms and brain regions. Nevertheless, his own associative approach to mental illness in psychoanalysis 'was informed by insights from the very tradition he attacked, and consequently his formulation of psychoanalysis was not so much a break from earlier brain science, but rather can be more productively understood as a radicalization of its principles' (Guenther, 2019, p. 72). Freud's departure from neurology and localisation introduces the domestic interior as the locus of mental life. We might say that Freud's response to the question 'where does it hurt' moves from 'in the brain' to 'in the ego' or even 'in the family home'. Freud maintains a spatialised understanding of the psyche in his development of psychoanalysis, even if it was a very different one from those found in neurology and later neuroscience.

The bourgeois home in *AoS* and *PPT* clearly repeats this spatial dynamic. In the context of the late 2010s 'mental health crisis' outlined in the introduction, in which poverty, housing precarity and scarcity of services are widespread and urgent issues, the ubiquity of this spatial binary in mainstream cultural representations of mental illness is troubling (MHT, 2016). The medical space is a relatively stable, accessible site in these productions and in this respect differs starkly from the reality of contemporary mental health service provision. As a reviewer in *The Lancet* medical journal noted of *PPT*:

> The thorny issue of who's paying for the treatment Emma refuses is never tackled. In this cash-strapped world it's almost touching that Macmillan thinks that a person could refuse to participate in a treatment programme and yet keep a place.
>
> (Ginn, 2015, p. 1125)

What's more, these journeys are represented as entirely personal, with 'home' a toxic but nonetheless economically stable, middle-class house, reliably available to its adult daughters. This suggests first, and predictably, that the cultural (especially theatre) sector remains dominated by middle class theatre-makers and producers, for whom a kind of ongoing financial and domestic stability can be written as a given into a dramatic universe.[2] This assumption of some measure of personal family wealth is a dangerous one that has underwritten multiple policies relating to poverty, housing and mental health and disability under post-2013 austerity policies (Ryan, 2019). Second, it points to the extent to which the idea of the institution as a long-stay or residential site of care and, as the counterpoint or opposite of home, continues to have a powerful hold on the way in which mental illness figures in the public imagination – one which I think theatre has had a role in constructing and maintaining.

Unseen experiences

The bourgeois home continues to be the staged site *par excellence* in theatrical representations of mental illness, forming a counterpoint to medical space and haunting our discipline's assumptions about mental illness. The prevalence of this staging limits the kinds of stories which theatre is able to tell. If mental distress is largely rendered legible in mainstream theatre through the overlaying of psyche and home, then those forms of distress that cannot be rooted in the home for socio-political reasons become much more difficult to express. Stephen Frosh proposes that:

> To be haunted is . . . to be influenced by a kind of inner voice that will not stop speaking and cannot be excised, that keeps cropping up to trouble us and stop us going peaceably on our way. It is to harbour a presence that we are aware of, sometimes overwhelmed by, that embodies elements of past experience and future anxiety and hope, and that will not let us be.
>
> (2013, p. 7)

Haunting is a kind of repetition or disturbance caused by a deliberate *not looking at* the conditions of the present – and therefore a repetition of the political and social oppressions that are obscured by this refusal of history. By generating a set of representational limits, this haunting becomes 'a social phenomenon, an index of oppression' (Frosh, 2013, p. 241).

This is clear in *B/O*, which engages directly with the conditions of mental health service provision whilst also exposing a representational limit in mainstream 'mental health' theatre. Rather than giving us access to Christopher's inner life, this play emphasises the extent to which he is defined from the outside exposing 'the bureaucratic doublethink of mental healthcare' (Watson, 2008, p. 199). What we do know about Christopher by the end of the play is that he is erratic, sometimes psychotic, challenging and precariously housed. He has experienced violence and threats beyond the walls of the hospital, but these experiences are not given validity. Instead, as Penhall described in an interview, *B/O* is

> saying that in this country we pay too much attention to the well-spoken well-educated individual. . . . *Blue/Orange* is about the conspiracy of the professions against the laity, the educated establishment against those who have no status at all.
>
> (Clements, 2013, p. xl)

The action of the second half revolves around the question of his release into the (non-existent) care of the community, but the space outside the medical setting is never staged. Christopher's conditions are much closer to those of many contemporary mental health service users insofar as he has no stable home to return to, no community to provide him with care. Yet Penhall's play can only stage his story insofar as he remains in the medical space and under the diagnostic gaze. Christopher becomes invisible once he is discharged, and the play ends not with his life post-institution but with doctors making complaints about one another.

Discharged into homelessness, Christopher moves out of mainstream theatre's visual field. Penhall's play might thus be understood to reveal the gap left by Naturalism's representational politics, which is embedded in *PPT* and *AoS*. The resurgence of the image of the institution-home binary in contemporary theatre may contribute social blindness to everything that contributes to mental illness outside of the family drama and biological determinism: to poverty, housing precarity, racism, sexism, neoliberalism. The spatial politics of theatre thus keeps alive in the mainstream a version of the experience of mental distress which is not only limited but potentially actively obscures the real conditions that most mental health service users exist in today.

Notes

1 Readers wishing to explore these avenues might look to recent studies on theatre and madness by Jon Venn (2021) and Anna Harpin (now anna six) (2018).
2 Katie Beswick, for example, demonstrates the consequences of this in relation to the cultural 'creation' of the image of the council estate in theatre (2019).

Reference list

Appignanesi, L. (2008) *Mad, bad and sad: a history of women and the mind doctors from 1800 to the present.* London: Hachette UK.

Bartleet, C. (2003) 'Sarah Daniels' hysteria plays: re-presentations of madness in ripen our darkness and head-rot holiday', *Modern Drama*, 46(2), pp. 241–260.

Beswick, K. (2019) *Social housing in performance.* London: Bloomsbury Methuen Drama Publishing.

Birch, A. (2017, 4 July) *Anatomy of a suicide.* Directed by Katie Mitchell. London: Royal Court Theatre.

Clements, R. and Penhall, J. (2013) *Blue/Orange.* London: Bloomsbury Methuen Drama Publishing.

Diamond, E. (1997) *Unmaking mimesis: essays on feminism and theater.* New York: Routledge.

Fitzgerald, D. and Callard, F. (2016) 'Entangling the medical humanities', in Whitehead, A. and Woods, A. (eds.) *The Edinburgh companion to the medical humanities.* Edinburgh: Edinburgh University Press, pp. 35–49.

Foley, M. (2017) *Haunting modernisms: ghostly aesthetics, mourning and spectral resistance fantasies in literary modernism.* Basingstoke and London: Palgrave Macmillan.

Fowler, B. (2020) *Katie Mitchell: beautiful illogical acts.* Abingdon: Routledge.

Frosh, S. (2013) 'Hauntings: psychoanalysis and ghostly transmission', *The American Imago; A Psychoanalytic Journal for the Arts and Sciences*, 69(2), pp. 241–264.

Ginn, S. (2015, September) 'Transgression and redemption', *The Lancet*, 386, p. 1125.

Gordon, A. (2008) *Ghostly matters haunting and the sociological imagination.* Minneapolis, MN: University of Minnesota Press.

Guenther, K. (2019) *Localization and its discontents: a genealogy of psychoanalysis and the neuro disciplines.* Chicago: Chicago University Press.

Harpin, A. (2018) *Madness art and society: beyond illness.* Abingdon: Routledge.

Hoggard, L. (2017) 'Alice Birch: I'm interested in whether trauma can be passed on through DNA', *The Guardian*. Available at: www.theguardian.com/stage/2017/jun/04/alice-birch-anatomy-of-a-suicide-play-interview (Accessed: 23 February 2022).

Kritsotaki, D., Long, V. and Smith, M. (2016) *Deinstitutionalisation and after post-war psychiatry in the western world.* London: Palgrave Macmillan.

Lipson Freed, J. (2017) *Haunting encounters: the ethics of reading across boundaries of difference.* Ithaca, NY: Cornell University Press.

Macmillan, D. (2016) *People, places, things.* Directed by Jeremy Herrin. London: National Theatre, Recording Viewed Courtesy of National Theatre Archive.

Mental Health Taskforce to the NHS in England (MHT) (2016) *The five year forward view for mental health.* London: NHS England.

National Service User Network (NUSN) (2017) *Theresa may's first speech of 2017 focused on mental health.* Available at: www.nsun.org.uk/news/theresa-mays-first-speech-of-2017-focused-on-mental-health (Accessed: 12 November 2021).

Parkinson, H.J. (2018) ' "It's nothing like a broken leg": why I'm done with the mental health conversation', *The Guardian*, 30 June. Available at: www.theguardian.com/society/2018/jun/30/nothing-like-broken-leg-mental-health-conversation (Accessed: 12 November 2021).

Penhall, J. (2000) *Blue/Orange.* London: Metheun Drama.

Penhall, J. (2016, 27 May) *Blue/Orange.* Directed by Matthew Xia. London: Young Vic Theatre.

Prime Minister's Office (PMO) (2017) *The shared society: prime minister's speech at the charity commission annual meeting*. Available at: www.gov.uk/government/speeches/the-shared-society-prime-ministers-speech-at-the-charity-commission-annual-meeting (Accessed: 23 February 2022).

Rabaté, J. (2014) 'Freud's theater of the unconscious: Oedipus, hamlet, and "hamlet"', in *The Cambridge introduction to literature and psychoanalysis*. Cambridge: Cambridge University Press, pp. 25–47.

Rebellato, D. (2019) 'Sightlines: Foucault and naturalist theatre', in Fisher, T. and Gotman, K. (eds.) *Foucault's theatres*. Manchester: Manchester University Press.

Rebellato, D. (2020) 'Objectivity and observation', in Shepherd-Barr, K. (ed.) *The Cambridge companion to theatre and science*. Cambridge: Cambridge University Press, pp. 12–25.

Ryan, F. (2019) *Crippled: austerity and the demonization of disabled people*. London: Verso.

Schumacher, C. (1996) *Naturalism and symbolism in European theatre, 1850–1918*. Cambridge: Cambridge University Press.

Shepherd-Barr, K.E. (2016) 'The diagnostic gaze: nineteenth-century contexts for medicine and performance', in Mermikides, A. and Bouchard, G. (eds.) *Performance and the medical body*. London: Bloomsbury Methuen Drama Publishing, pp. 37–50.

Solga, K. (2007) 'Blasted's hysteria: rape, realism, and the thresholds of the visible', *Modern Drama*, 50(3), pp. 346–374.

Venn, J. (2021) *Madness in contemporary British theatre*. London: Palgrave Macmillan.

Watson, A. (2008) 'Cries of fire: psychotherapy in contemporary British and Irish drama', *Modern Drama*, 51(2), pp. 188–210.

8

PERFORMING DEATH ON THE STAGE AND IN THE HOSPITAL

Emily Russell

Modern studies of death and dying typically begin by arguing that as medical authority over the body has risen, our everyday encounters with death have fallen to almost non-existent. Contrary to past eras when illness and death took place at home and were attended by family and religious figures, it is almost impossible to be terminally ill in the Global North today without falling under medical authority. Although historian Philippe Ariès most influentially laments this loss of domestic ceremonies of dying, contemporary critics have focused not only on the loss but on the new forms of ritualised behaviour that have been scripted in their place. These new scripts allow individuals – from patients, to family, to medical professionals – to make sense of frightening and painful experiences.

With this secreting away of death in the professional space of the hospital, art and media now play a stronger role in shaping our understanding of death and dying. Without direct encounters, the public is more likely to take cues about how dying 'should' unfold from scripted performance (Tercier, 2002). Staged death, then, offers an influential set of social scripts by which dying individuals and their caretakers make meaning from loss and cement expectations about the correct way to behave.

Death in the hospital or hospice setting is similarly influenced by notions of enactment and ritual. Doctors, patients, and loved ones use props, costuming, and ritualised exchange to make death meaningful. In the face of such profoundly disorienting information and experiences, routine social scripts can confer a powerful and reassuring familiarity (Hart, Sainsbury and Short, 1998; Timmermans, 2005).

The performance of death on stage and in medical settings mutually construct a new shared understanding of the proper way to die. In the past fifty years, the hospice movement has been highly influential in constructing a popular ideology of the 'good death'. The principles of this ideology include 'dying with dignity, peacefulness, preparedness, awareness, adjustment, and acceptance' (Hart, Sainsbury and Short, 1998, p. 72). In his 1981 article on contemporary drama and mortality, Donald Duclow argues that a new art of dying is in the making, in which staged death reinforces and constructs emergent social values that include 'a renewed emphasis on truth telling, the values of autonomy and control, a myth outlining the journey of dying, and ritual of terminal care' (1981, p. 212). This era of redefinition of the normalised behaviours and beliefs surrounding death and dying shines a brighter spotlight on the moments where we enact death both on stage and in life.

DOI: 10.4324/9781003036500-10

The push and pull between medicalised norms of death and the hospice alternative shows up in the opposing paths by which models of dying are developed on stage between the 1970s through the end of the twentieth century. The principles of a good death as outlined by the death and dying movements of the last fifty years have largely gone uncontested by medical drama produced during that time. Playwrights diverge, however, in whether they arrive at those principles by way of negative or positive models. The plays discussed here share a vision of what constitutes a good death but differ in whether they depict a negative critique of patient experience or an aspirational vision of a better way to experience dying. Margaret Edson's *Wit*, which premiered in 1995, offers a sharp critique of medicalised death. In taking a more aspirational approach, Michael Cristofer's 1977 Tony and Pulitzer Prize–winning play, *Shadow Box*, directly dramatises the principles of 'proper' death and grieving: autonomy, acceptance, and family reconciliation. Tony Kushner's *Angels in America* (1993, Broadway premiere), on the other hand, introduces ambiguity into the consensus vision of the good death and cautions against redemptive cultural fantasies of dying. Taken together, these examples of staged performance and their real-life counterparts confirm and create the dominant scripts for the contemporary enactment of death.

Enacting death in the hospital

Both on stage and in life, the setting, rituals, and props associated with death have undergone a profound shift since the middle of the twentieth century. The dying – now classified as 'patients' – are often heavily sedated, carefully monitored, and 'dependent on death-prolonging technology' (Duclow, 1981, p. 211). As Pamela Renner writes, death on stage has undergone a similar shift. She reviews 1990s productions by Lisa Loomer and Margaret Edson which include dialogue marked by 'the polysyllables of medical lingo and . . . property lists [that] groan beneath the burden of hospital beds, morphine drips, and IV poles' (Renner, 1999, p. 34). The rituals and ceremonies commonly found in the at-home death – stopping clocks, covering mirrors, wrapping the winding sheet, and keeping vigil at the bedside – have fallen away or been recast in the hospital setting. In their place, clinical protocols emerged as a way to govern and make sense of death and dying.

In addition to pushing scenes of death into the hospital, the medicalisation of dying reveals a new understanding of death itself. Where once we accepted death as familiar, natural, and inevitable, it is now 'seen as something that can be controlled, postponed, and potentially reversed, its timing elective, planned and managed' (Muller and Koenig, 1988, p. 354). This belief that death can be managed leads to reimagined scripts for delivering diagnoses, interpreting vital signs, and prescribing treatment. If death is no longer understood to follow an inevitable and natural course, then the clinical setting becomes an opportunity to enact death and to work out core questions about its meaning. What should a 'good death' look like? When is it permissible for a physician to 'let' a patient die? How can families' expectations and wishes be appropriately met?

Scholarly observers in modern intensive care units have documented the way that physicians understand their work within a heroic narrative. This self-concept becomes important in determining the course of treatment for individuals with terminal diagnoses. In his article 'Death Brokering: Constructing Culturally Appropriate Deaths', Stefan Timmermans argues that physicians can attribute 'tremendous – bordering on magical – powers' to managing death (Timmermans, 2005, p. 997). Observers of clinical settings report that medical staff demonstrate a strong bias toward active intervention, a desire for self-absolution upon a patient's death with the ability to say, 'I did all I could' (Tercier, 2002, p. 316). Metaphors of 'fight' and 'battle' against death overwhelm discourse in curative medicine. Under this ideology, interventions can be more about performing in the fight against death than they are about changing the course of disease: 'Medical interventions, offered as "gifts of life," take on symbolic meaning for physicians that extends beyond the individual patient to represent medicine's battle with death. It is the "fight" itself that becomes important as physicians struggle to find out what is wrong with a patient and to stop or alter the course of disease' (Muller and Koenig, 1988, p. 368). This focus on giving a patient 'a chance', however, can swamp other realities, including the fact that a procedure or course of treatment might be futile, might extend a patient's life for only a short time, or might entail significant discomfort or pain (Muller and Koenig, 1988, p. 368). Professional guidelines from diverse organisations clearly state that physicians are under no obligation to provide futile medical treatment (American Medical Association, 2016; General Medical Council, 2010; World Health Organization, 2020), but the same organisations acknowledge that such decisions are ethically and emotionally charged for all parties. These complexities account for the wide borderlands between curative and palliative medicine. In this space of uncertainty, the symbolic performance of this fight offers a reliable script for managing death. Physicians and families understand the heroic (if ultimately unsuccessful) role they are expected to play and can place treatment decisions within this predictable unfolding of scenes.

As death has shifted from the back bedroom to the hospital room, one particular prop has come to dominate both the real-life setting and the public imagination. The beeping peaks, valleys, and the dreaded flat green line on the heart monitor screen have become a universal symbol of medicalised dying. The prop is so powerful in our understanding of death that it has become a verb – 'She's flatlining!' – and is synecdochic with death itself. This externalisation of a patient's life-or-death status carries complex implications for families and clinical staff. The monitor screen can become an anchor for anxious families, a way to gain information in an uncertain time. Both Hans Hadders and Janet Harvey describe families' increased reliance on the bedside heart monitor and clinical staff's feeling of ambivalence toward this phenomenon. Although the tubes, wires, and monitors of the modern hospital room can feel frightening, families of sedated patients will often learn to 'read' the monitor screen, mimicking the action of hospital staff. In contrast to notions of a 'good death' that would reject technological intervention, Hadders describes how 'observing medical technological enactment of the life of their loved one becomes just as important an ontological mooring for them as seeing or touching him/her' (2009, p. 581).

Nurses are likely to believe this reliance is excessive and will go so far as to turn off monitors and alarms as death approaches so that relatives will redirect their focus exclusively to the patient. Janet Harvey reports similar beliefs among clinical staff, with one nurse telling her: 'The worst time is [when] . . . you've told the relatives nothing else can be done and the heart will just fail. They sit waiting and watching the monitor' (Harvey, 1997, p. 728). Although the nurses described here give voice to a common belief that technology interrupts interpersonal connection and compromises the 'natural' trajectory of death, the ubiquity of the heart monitor as a prop in modern death scenes suggests that any tool for gaining insight into a patient's physical condition has value for the audience. The flatline offers a reliable enactment of the dreaded event, a secure signal that announces the end of 'dying' and the arrival of 'death'.

The same impulses that would exclude technological intervention from definitions of a 'good death' might also recoil at the notion that human interaction surrounding death and dying is highly scripted. To suggest that clinical staff are performing pre-established roles or that patients' and family members' expressions of grief follow predictable scripts might seem to indicate a lack of sincerity. In highly individualist cultures like the US and Western Europe, each terminal diagnosis and the 'why me?' agony that follows initiates a private tragedy. But despite an emphasis on patient autonomy within death and dying movements, there is an accompanying understanding that ritual and familiarity can make meaning from seemingly senseless misfortunes. In particular, the rise of Elisabeth Kübler-Ross's model of five stages of grief has provided a guiding mythology for clinicians, families, and the public. To the extent that death has taken on elements of staged performance – like props, costuming, and routine dialogue – these elements make up the rituals by which we understand contemporary death and grieving.

David Sudnow describes a series of ritualised moments surrounding death and dying in his 1967 study of two urban hospitals, *Passing On: The Social Organization of Dying*. The language of performance repeatedly surfaces in his writing, such as when he describes the surgical and waiting rooms as having a 'clear front stage-backstage boundary' (Sudnow, 1967, p. 120). In a memorable anecdote, Sudnow illustrates how doctors use the techniques of performance – in this case, costuming – to manage their interactions with patient families. He describes a case in which a surgeon completed an operation and then removed his cap, mask, and shoe covers before taking an extended break in the doctor's lounge. After chatting with colleagues for about half an hour, he put his cap and mask back on, 'with the mask hanging around his neck in that position which suggests it was just taken off' (ibid, p. 121). He returns to the waiting room and talks with the family. This act of resuming his costume was intentional; 'With the cap and mask on, he reported afterwards, it appears as though he has just put down the needle and suturing thread and carries exceedingly fresh news' (ibid, pp. 121–122). By self-consciously restoring his surgical costume, the surgeon demonstrates an awareness of his role and its performative elements. While one interpretation of this event could accuse the surgeon of calculated callousness, another reading would be that he uses the staging techniques available to communicate to his audience the urgency he knows they desire and to allow himself a period of decompression before delivering news.

Sudnow observes that performative rituals extend as well to the death announcement, when a doctor must tell the family of their loved one's demise. He writes that the conversation follows a 'general ceremonial structuring' (ibid, p. 151), with regular rules that are predetermined and understood even by individuals who have never participated in such exchanges. One reason for this predictability is that popular media has staged versions of this dramatic event countless times. Sudnow's observations lead him to the counter-intuitive claim that in these conversations, the content is less important than the structure, which consists of a back-and-forth exchange of conversational units. He argues that mutual respect for the other's position subordinates the specifics of the death itself as each 'agree[s] to sustain a little piece of sociable talk' (ibid, p. 151). Such exchanges are often likely to end with the family thanking the doctor in a moment of politeness that might seem out of step with the event. Despite this strangeness, these scripted but 'empty' exchanges are another way that we manage death. Once the crucial information has been conveyed, the participants can retreat to the ceremonial structure without needing to call upon higher orders of mental processing. They find security (if not comfort) in playing mutually recognisable roles and falling into the familiar scripts of conversational exchange – greeting, news, query, response, thank you, farewell.

Sudnow's 1967 characterisation of the death announcement as highly ritualised and 'empty' may reflect broader attitudes toward 'breaking bad news' characteristic of medicine in the middle of the twentieth century. Surveys conducted during this period reveal that when prospects for cancer patients seemed bleak, most physicians 'considered it inhumane and damaging to the patient to disclose the bad news about the diagnosis' (Baile *et al.*, 2000, p. 302). Consistent with the death and dying movements that emerged as interventions in the decades following this period – most notably in principles like preparedness, awareness, and truth telling – new techniques have been developed to reimagine communication with patients. While more honest, these forms of communication are also bound up in performance. Both scripted and unscripted role-playing, for example, is widely used in medical education, even at the undergraduate level (Nestel and Tierney,

2007). The SPIKES method, first published in *The Oncologist* in 2000, offers a stepwise strategy for breaking bad news to patients. This method is also attentive to elements crucial to performance such as setting, audience, and sample scripted dialogue (Baile *et al.*, 2000).

The hospital on stage

Shifting from these examples of real-life performance, contemporary stage dramas offer another site for developing shared social scripts for dying. Margaret Edson brings the hospital setting to the stage in an openly didactic critique of curative medicine. In *Wit*, Edson uses performed rituals of clinical exchange and metatheatrical elements to critique hollow attempts to find meaning in suffering. By the play's end, Edson has wholly rejected doctor-centred medical scripts for managing death and instead embraces hospice principles of simplicity, humanity, kindness, and autonomy.

Wit unfolds without intermission, telling the story of Professor Vivian Bearing through her diagnosis of Stage 4 ovarian cancer, experience of aggressive and experimental chemotherapy treatment, and eventual death. In addition to winning the Pulitzer Prize for Drama in 1999, the play has been taken up by medical educators as required reading for their students. Although *Wit* is perhaps as scathing about the loss of humanity within 'humanist' studies of literature, its resonance with audiences lies in its dramatisation of medical practitioners' failure to see the person under their care.

The play's opening line, 'How are you feeling today?' – addressed rhetorically to the audience in this instance – inducts viewers into the play's medical setting. Bearing goes on to describe the irony of this banal question:

Vivian: I have been asked 'How are you feeling today?' while I was
        throwing up into a plastic washbasin. I have been asked as I was emerging from a four-hour operation with a tube in every orifice, 'How are you feeling today?'
        I am waiting for the moment when someone asks me this question and I am dead.

(Edson, 1999, p. 7)

In this context, 'How are you feeling today?' does not seek an answer but serves as a rote social performance (Belling, 2013, p. 482). This clinical exchange operates very much like the ritualised conversations that David Sudnow describes structuring the notification of death in the hospital. Where Sudnow's assessment of this ritual is largely neutral in its description of trading empty conversational units, Edson calls out these routine moments as a failure of curative medicine. She acknowledges the elements of performance that direct clinical exchange but argues that such routines obscure the emotional life and humanity of the patient.

The earliest moments of the play also announce its self-conscious theatricality, a key device through which Edson communicates the ways in which we understand death and dying through the elements of performance. From her first lines of direct address to the audience, to calling out her hospital gown as 'costume', and the startling declaration, 'I think I die at the end' – we are immediately inducted into performance as the central frame by which the character makes sense of her experience. Characteristic of a literature professor, Bearing is attentive not only to the broadly theatrical elements of her experience, but also to the *genre* of her dying: 'I would prefer that a play about me be cast in the mythic-heroic-pastoral mode; but the facts, most notably Stage 4 metastatic ovarian cancer, conspire against that. *The Faerie Queene* this is not' (Edson, 1999, p. 8).

Critic Jacqueline Vanhoutte is particularly attentive to questions of genre in her reading of *Wit*. Drawing from her own experiences as both a scholar of Renaissance literature and a cancer patient, Vanhoutte reveals the way that tragic conventions can repeat and endorse moralising public fantasies about illness. Tragedy would seem to be the appropriate choice to structure a tale of dying. Playwrights like Edson, however, wade into morally tricky territory when they mine tragic conventions. Such conventions can reproduce the central assumption of tragedy that the protagonist is ultimately responsible for their fate. Drawing from Susan Sontag's discussion of the social and symbolic dimensions of illness, Vanhoutte surfaces the ways in which *Wit* trades in moralising stereotypes about cancer, particularly what Sontag calls 'the cancer-prone personality' (Sontag, 1978, p. 36): dry, closed-off, repressed, and cold. Most devastatingly, Vanhoutte charges that by deploying the tragic mode, Edson reproduces both the notion that cancer is somehow a punishment for personal failures and that suffering offers a path to redemption and enlightenment. Although Edson wants to offer an indictment of the dehumanising practices at the centre of medicine, her genre choice, according to Vanhoutte, ends up perpetuating the very stereotypes about cancer and illness that provoke such treatment (2002, p. 400). Vanhoutte's incisive critique exposes the dangers of using cultural scripts as a tool for making meaning in the face of profoundly destabilising diagnoses. Such scripts will inevitably direct heterogeneous individual experiences into more narrow channels, useful perhaps in their familiarity and coherence, but potentially dangerous because they come laden with sometimes painful preconceptions. Vanhoutte's analysis demonstrates that it can be difficult to adopt theatrical conventions in a piecemeal form; once patients, physicians, and authors begin to understand death and dying according to a generic vein like tragedy, their imaginations become freighted with a host of associated tropes.

Wit's self-conscious theatricality persists through Bearing's final speech. In what Bearing names 'her last coherent lines', she attempts a recitation of the final line of John Donne's 'Death, Be Not Proud', the poem that has been at the centre of the play's meditations on both literary interpretation and death. In these moments, Edson reveals another trap of drawing from cultural conventions, like poetry, to make sense out of death and suffering: attempts to make meaning can fall short, expectations can go unmet, and redemption can remain out of reach. The stage directions here capture the attempt of the dying patient to wrest control over her last moments and construct meaning from them: '*Vivian concentrates with all her might, and she attempts a grand summation, as if trying to conjure her own ending*' (Edson, 1999, p. 57). In this metatheatrical attention to the expectation for closure, Bearing attempts to use the tools of the theatre to cast herself as a valiant heroine in the battle with death (Gottlieb, 2015, p. 332). She immediately acknowledges, however, that the figure of the tragic protagonist 'doesn't work' and '*looks out at the audience, . . . shakes her head and exhales with resignation*' (Edson, 1999, p. 58). In this moment of self-conscious performance of John Donne poetry, Edson illustrates the ways in which we use art to 'conjure' meaningful deaths and the fact that such attempts may fail.

Bearing's performance as tragic heroine in this brief play-within-a-play 'doesn't work' because her choice of poetic phrase places her within the heroic school of curative medicine locked in adversarial battle with death. In announcing, 'Death – *capital D* – thou shalt die – *exclamation point!*' (Edson, 1999, p. 57), Bearing has not only failed to learn the literary lesson in punctuation offered by her mentor but also fails to express the humanist revelation that unfolds in the play's concluding scenes of medical dialogue and death. In contrast to the hollow, seeming-victories of the traditional heroic medical model, *Wit's* ending advocates for the hospice principles of autonomy, kindness, and simplicity. Although the unyielding stickler in Bearing rejects the 'maudlin' and 'corny' displays of care between patient and her nurse, Susie, she also acknowledges that when death moves from the abstract to the material and personal, 'now is not the time for verbal swordplay [or] metaphysical conceit. Now is a time for simplicity. Now is a time for, dare I say it, kindness' (Edson, 1999, p. 55).

Following Bearing's 'last coherent words', the play shifts from a metatheatrical comment on the self-conscious attempt to use art to make meaning from illness to offering a didactic model for effective caretaking. These lines of inquiry overlap when, after giving up her final attempt to conjure her climax with the Donne recitation, Bearing gives herself over to the palliative care of her nurse, rejects the fight to extend her life with a Do Not Resuscitate order, but still achieves redemption following death: '*The instant she is naked, and beautiful, reaching for the light – Lights out*' (Edson, 1999, p. 66).

The value of palliative care is ultimately symbolised in the play through the pump that delivers patient-controlled analgesic. This prop, introduced by the nurse who serves as the moral centre of the play, relocates medicine from the exclusive authority of the physician and instead elevates patients' self-assessment of their needs. When she introduces the pump in the scene, Susie says, '(*Importantly.*) It's very simple and it's up to you' (Edson, 1999, p. 56). The stage direction, '*Importantly*', rejects subtlety in arguing for patient autonomy and kindness in end-of-life care. It is Susie who successfully assumes the role of active heroine at the play's conclusion (not Bearing and not her doctors). In this chaotic scene, Susie insists to the assembled medical staff that the patient is 'no code' and struggles to be heard against their routine performance of the heroic medical model in a violent attempt at resuscitation. As presented in the play, attempts to extend the patient's life against her express wishes represent a clear violation; Susie's ironic act of heroism in advocating for her patient's death exposes the failures of the medical model.

Scripting death with dignity

Where *Wit* delivers a powerful critique of the medical model, Michael Cristofer's *The Shadow Box* offers an affirmative vision of the good death. The play, which premiered at the Mark Taper Forum in Los Angeles during the 1975–76 season, takes place over twenty-four hours in the lives of three terminally ill patients: Joe, Brian, and Felicity. The patients and their families have agreed to spend their final days living in identical cottages on the grounds of a large hospital and to be interviewed as part of a psychological study. The nested forms of medical setting demonstrated in the play – psychological study, the hospital grounds, and the hospice-centre–like distance of the cottages – underscore the complex web of medical professionalisation that structures care of the dying. The play showcases the diversity of emotional responses to terminal diagnosis and the experience of illness. Characters range in their attitudes between denial, dark humour, sentiment, fear, and weariness. In this work, Cristofer dramatises the alternative philosophy of the hospice movement that became popular through the late twentieth century and asserts the patient-centred values of autonomy, community, and acceptance.

The death and dying movements of the last half century – including hospice, alternative funeral, and right to die movements – have offered various and important critiques of the curative model of medicine and its inadequacies in care for those with terminal diagnoses. For these critics, death has become bureaucratic, mechanical, dehumanised, and lonely (Ariès, 1981; Glaser and Strauss, 1965; Hart, Sainsbury and Short, 1998; Kübler-Ross, 1993, Sudnow, 1967). The hospice movement, most notably, emerged as an alternative to what they saw as the isolated and dehumanising medical death. Hospice philosophy seeks a holistic model of treatment that considers the social and emotional needs of the patient alongside the physical demands of the dying body. Although hospice workers are also commonly medical professionals, their model of treatment is explicitly patient centred, a feature they share with many depictions of death and dying on stage. Despite the fact that hospice care offers a rebuke to the mid-century practices of death in the hospital, both types of medical care use performative elements to construct scripts for managing death.

In *The Shadow Box*, Cristofer uses a strategy of simultaneity in his staging to emphasise what he understands as the universal dynamics of grief and dying. Although his central characters do not directly interact, the uniform cottage setting jumps between one family grouping and another, and shared delivery of lines in the final scene offer a vision of a single compelling script for dying. In the play's coda, this strategy of simultaneity reaches its height as all the characters – both patients and their families – pick up lines from each other mid-sentence:

Brian: Someone should have said, this living . . .
Mark: . . . this life . . .
Beverly: . . . this lifetime . . .
Brian: It doesn't last forever.

(Cristofer, 2008, p. 249)

In her introduction to the play, Angela Belli uses phrases like 'identical experience', 'equal intensity in affirming the same truth', 'unity', and 'all the characters come together simultaneously' (Belli, 2008, p. 193). Despite variations, the play dramatises the convergence of its characters to advocate for a single, compelling model of dying and grief.

Cristofer's unified vision for making sense of dying follows the cultural reception of Elisabeth Kübler-Ross's theory of the stages of grief (denial, anger, bargaining, depression, and acceptance). Her theory gave a 'tangible script' for death and dying that allowed patients, families, and clinicians to understand their reactions and channel their behaviour (Hart, Sainsbury and Short, 1998, p. 68). Although her stage theory is often critiqued for seeming too linear and prescriptive, it was the very possibility of understanding grief as a unified phenomenon that made the work so culturally powerful. In *The Shadow Box*, Cristofer distributes Kübler-Ross's stages of grief among his characters, ultimately ending with a simultaneous expression of acceptance in repeating the word 'Yes' a dozen times. Despite the sad circumstance of its characters' impending deaths, the message of the play is to affirmatively dramatise the hospice principles that were just beginning to gain public notice in 1960s and 70s America. The play's critical success – winning the 1977 Pulitzer Prize for Drama and Tony Award for best play – and its Emmy-nominated television adaptation by Paul Newman in 1980, suggest that the values expressed caught hold of public attention as a compelling way to understand dying and grief.

Rethinking the redemptive script of the good death

Tony Kushner's *Angels in America: A Gay Fantasia on National Themes* reminds us that severe illness and dying are inherently theatrical experiences. First appearing on Broadway in 1993, this Pulitzer Prize–winning play stages a complex interweaving between the material demands of the ill body; AIDS as a national crisis; and the social, religious, and political networks of meaning that such embodied experiences are tied up in. Despite its subtitle 'A Gay Fantasia', Kushner also puts the physical realities of death and illness at the centre of the stage. The play opens with a coffin and funeral scene. The central characters, Prior Walter, Roy Cohn, and Harper Pitt, are all struggling with different stages of serious illness. Actors playing these roles must make a series of choices throughout the production for how to physically manifest the rising pain and debilitation their characters experience. The play's most direct engagement, though, with the demands of the ill body are in Prior's blunt descriptions of his physical symptoms. In contrast to the oblique jargon that serves to mask harsh realities in a medical context, Prior's dialogue is direct. His lines centre the experience of the patient, not the coded language insular to the physician; he describes lesions, nausea, pure-liquid bowel movements, a chapped butt, leg pain, a fuzzy tongue, and 'glands like walnuts' (Kushner, 1995, pp. 45, 103). By surfacing the physical realities of the ill body through performance and dialogue, Kushner reminds his audience that while the play engages with 'national themes' and a socio-political response to AIDS in the 1980s, such considerations should not sidestep the uncomfortable realities of the individual body in pain.

In addition to this performative manifestation of internal symptoms, *Angels in America* shows how role-playing can direct behaviour surrounding death. As Donald Duclow argues, the destabilising experience of terminal diagnosis may lead patients to 'take on the roles of resisting hero, wailing sufferer, accepting stoic, or penitent Everyman' (1981, p. 210). Such roles are not only assumed by the diagnosed patient but are occupied by friends and family as well. One of the more grounded (and devastating) plotlines in the play is Louis's failure to appropriately perform loyalty and support when his lover's, Prior's, symptoms become more severe. Although Louis's dialogue makes his failures in the role of loving boyfriend both realistic and legible to the audience, Kushner is also unflinching in dramatising the emotionally brutal consequences of Louis's choices for Prior. Louis himself is openly guilty about his failures; for example, very early in the play he asks a rabbi in barely veiled third person, 'what does the Holy Writ say about someone who abandons someone he loves at a time of great need?' (Kushner, 1995, p. 31). He goes on, 'maybe that person can't, um, incorporate sickness into his sense of how things are supposed to go. Maybe vomit . . . and sores and disease . . . really frighten him, maybe . . . he isn't so good with death' (Kushner, 1995, p. 31). This reference to frightening vomit, sores, and disease creates a frame for placing Prior's subsequent blunt enumeration of his painful symptoms into context. Unlike the positive model of ultimate acceptance staged in *The Shadow Box*, Louis cannot properly assume the role of the steadfast caretaker. Neither Kushner nor Cristofer deny the fear felt by both terminally ill patients and their loved ones, but the play also does not absolve Louis for praying 'please let him die if he can't return to me whole and healthy and able to live a normal life' (Kushner, 1995, p. 58). The loving care and unflinching support shown by Belize, a nurse and former lover of Prior's, place Louis's choices in ever sharper relief. For a play that ends with Prior insisting, 'I want more life' (Kushner, 1995, p. 285), Louis's prayer for death for his suffering loved one suggests a profound moral failure. This contrast offers a challenge to the virtues of acceptance and individuality celebrated in death with dignity movements. Prior's desire for more life and the communal vision at the play's close suggest that for a population twice marginalised by severe illness and the social stigma of AIDS, finding a pathway to living with AIDS is a profound act.

Although the play centres on illness and several scenes take place in the hospital, the only character to die on stage is Roy Cohn. Here, again, Kushner uses a negative example to offer a cautionary tale against cultural belief in terminal diagnosis and death as inherently ennobling. Even through his final moments, Cohn behaves in ways that are consistent with his characterisation as a vengeful, exploitive, and closeted power broker. Kushner exposes the audience's fantasy death-bed script by having Cohn stage a false emotional conversion in the moments before he dies. Mistaking the ghost of Ethel Rosenberg for his Ma, confessing his fear, offering a blanket apology – these lines conform to our public fantasies of a redemptive death scene. In the following beat, however, Cohn jubilantly denies this conversion script, insisting 'I fooled you . . . I can't believe you fell for that ma stuff' (Kushner, 1995, p. 266). In a political context where living with AIDS is a radical act, Kushner cautions against excessively romantic visions of reconciliation with death.

Like the anatomy theatres of the eighteenth century in which surgeons dissected corpses for a rapt audience, moving death to the stage educates the public on profound questions about medical authority and 'proper' attitudes and conduct. By using performance as a frame to understand attempts to manage death in a medical context and, conversely, by looking at scenes of hospital death on stage, we can see how scripts have been revised to make sense of life's most profound losses. As curative and palliative medical professionals grapple over the vision for a good death, contemporary drama enters into these debates, staging the complex moral and human dimensions at the heart of the matter. Patients and families, in turn, take cues not only from their physicians but from scenes absorbed out of art and culture. Collectively, these roles, mythology, dialogue, props, and costumes come together to reflect and construct a compelling script for contemporary death and dying.

Reference list

American Medical Association (2016) 'Withholding or withdrawing life sustaining treatment', *AMA Principles of Medical Ethics*, 5(3). Available at: https://code-medical-ethics.ama-assn.org/ethics-opinions/withholding-or-withdrawing-life-sustaining-treatment (Accessed: 26 July 2023).

Ariès, P. (1981) *The hour of our death: the classic history of western attitudes toward death over the last one thousand years*. Translated by Helen Weaver. New York: Vintage Books.

Baile, W.F. *et al.* (2000) 'SPIKES-A six-step protocol for delivering bad news: application to the patient with cancer', *The Oncologist*, 5(4), pp. 302–311.

Belli, A. (2008) 'Introduction', in *Bodies and barriers: dramas of dis-ease*. Kent, OH: Kent State University Press, pp. 193–196.

Belling, C. (2013) 'Begin with a text: teaching the poetics of medicine', *Journal of Medical Humanities*, 34(4), pp. 481–491.

Cristofer, M. (2008) 'The shadow box', in Belli, A. (ed.) *Bodies and barriers: dramas of dis-ease*. Kent, OH: Kent State University Press, pp. 193–250.

Duclow, D.F. (1981) 'Dying on Broadway: contemporary drama and mortality', *Soundings*, 64(2), pp. 197–216.

Edson, M. (1999) *Wit*. New York: Dramatists Play Service Inc.

General Medical Council (2010) 'Treatment and care towards the end of life: good practice in decision making', *Ethical Guidance for Doctors*. Available at: www.gmc-uk.org/-/media/documents/treatment-and-care-towards-the-end-of-life–english-1015_pdf-48902105.pdf (Accessed: 26 July 2023).

Glaser, B. and Strauss, A. (1965) *Awareness of dying*. Chicago: Aldine Publishing Company.

Gottlieb, C. (2015) 'Pedagogy and the art of death: reparative readings of death and dying in Margaret Edson's *Wit*', *Journal of Medical Humanities*, 39, pp. 325–336.

Hadders, H. (2009) 'Enacting death in the intensive care unit: medical technology and the multiple ontologies of death', *Health: An Interdisciplinary Journal for the Social Study of Health, Illness, and Medicine*, 13(6), pp. 571–587.

Hart, B., Sainsbury, P. and Short, S. (1998) 'Whose dying? A sociological critique of the "good death"', *Mortality*, 3(1), pp. 65–77.

Harvey, J. (1997) 'The technological regulation of death: with reference to the technological regulation of birth', *Sociology*, 31(4), pp. 719–735.

Kübler-Ross, E. (1993) *On death and dying*. New York: Collier Books.

Kushner, T. (1995) *Angels in America: a gay fantasia on national themes*. New York: Theatre Communications Group.

Muller, J.H. and Koenig, B.A. (1988) 'On the boundary of life and death: the definition of dying by medical residents', in Lock, M. and Gordon, D. (eds.) *Biomedicine examined*. Dordrecht: Kluwer Academic Publishers, pp. 351–374.

Nestel, D. and Tierney, T. (2007) 'Role-play for medical students learning about communication: guidelines for maximising benefits', *BMC Medical Communication*, 7(3).

Renner, P. (1999) 'Science and sensibility', *American Theater*, 16(4), pp. 34–36.

Sontag, S. (1978) *Illness as metaphor*. New York: Farrar, Strauss and Giroux.

Sudnow, D. (1967) *Passing on: the social organization of dying*. Englewood Cliffs, NJ: Prentice-Hall, Inc.

Tercier, J. (2002) 'The lips of the dead and the "kiss of life": the contemporary deathbed and the aesthetic of CPR', *Journal of Historical Sociology*, 15(3), pp. 283–327.

Timmermans, S. (2005) 'Death brokering: constructing culturally appropriate deaths', *Sociology of Health & Illness*, 27(7), pp. 993–1013.

Vanhoutte, J. (2002) 'Cancer and the common woman in Margaret Edson's *Wit*', *Comparative Drama*, 36(3/4), pp. 391–410.

World Health Organization (2020) *Palliative care*. Available at: www.who.int/news-room/fact-sheets/detail/palliative-care (Accessed: 26 July 2023).

PART 2

Diagnosis

Introduction

Russell's discussion of the scripting of health care professionals' words and behaviours, at the end of Part 1, leads us into Part 2 of this volume. This focuses on how health care professionals are represented and how they perform, both on and off the theatrical stage. It analyses performances of health care professionalism enacted in a range of contexts, including medical school ceremonies, hospital bedsides, patients' homes, the maternity ward, operating theatre, in public demonstrations taking place on the streets and in the media and in rehearsal rooms, as well as in theatre playscripts and on stage. In encompassing such a broad array of clinical, educational, political and artistic settings, we propose an equivalence and continuity between the fictional performances of the stage, the cultural representations and media depictions of health care workers and the real world of clinical practice, even in the life-or-death context of cardiac surgery. This is not to say that doctors and nurses are 'faking it' when they are treating patients. Rather, the fulfilment of health care roles involves skills that are not dissimilar to those of the performer, and analysing real-world clinical interactions through a dramaturgical lens can reveal some of the complex factors that go into the effective acquisition and portrayal of medical professionalism. Nor does this suggest, of course, that theatre performances or media accounts provide accurate depictions of how health care professionals behave 'in real life'. Our claim instead is that they can reveal insights into public perceptions of the medicine, the hopes and anxieties that surround a set of professional roles that have immense impact on our health and happiness. In all, the dramaturgical approach to health care professionalism that is adopted in this section addresses the question of what it means to be a health care worker, especially at historical moments when the institution of medicine undergoes radical change.

Our first two chapters discuss plays about doctors performed at such moments of disjuncture. First, Katherine Burke offers a close analysis of Jules Romains' 1923 satire *Dr. Knock, or the Triumph of Medicine*. Burke argues that the enduring popularity of this satirical play reflects some of the anxieties provoked by scientific, increasingly professionalised and hospital-based medicine that first emerged in Paris from the turn of the eighteenth century. She draws on Foucault's seminal archaeology of medicine to explain how this anatomo-clinical medicine endowed physicians with new forms of power and authority. As she puts it, the play 'holds a funhouse mirror' to the form

DOI: 10.4324/9781003036500-11

of medical practice described in *The Birth of the Clinic*, with its eponymous doctor – a charlatan who gets rich quick by promoting his own brand of remedies for invented diseases – manifesting long-standing fears of medical abuse and capitalist exploitation. The second chapter focuses on the adaptation of *Professor Bernhardi* by Arthur Schnitzler, a contemporary of Romains (the play was first performed in 1912). As Judith Beniston describes, Robert Icke's 2019 version, *The Doctor*, follows a very similar plot to the original, tracking the scandal that ensues after the eponymous doctor refuses to allow a Catholic priest to attend to a young woman dying of sepsis following an illegal abortion. That this story needs little updating reflects what Beniston calls an 'unfortunate continuity' in concerns around the role of the doctor, notably 'tensions between the self-regulating character of the medical profession and its embeddedness in broader institutional, political and social structures'.

The next three chapters turn a dramaturgical or performative lens on how medical students and qualified doctors navigate the social, institutional and political factors that pertain to medical professionalism in the present moment. Observing their subjects in their clinical habitats, our contributors reveal how their micro performances in front of their patients, peers or educators respond to the particular mix of expectations and performance pressures that now circulate around the role of the doctor. James Dalton and Claire Hooker give an insightful overview of the cumulative challenges posed by patient groups (and, we would add, activists and commentators) to the medical authority and objectivity associated with contemporary versions of Foucault's 'clinic'. Similarly, Alan Bleakley and Robert Marshall describe how medical professionalism now encompasses 'courtesy towards patients and awareness of safety, inclusivity, and lack of discrimination, and, most recently, looking after one's own physical and mental wellbeing'.

Through a series of vignettes drawn from fieldwork in an Australian teaching hospital, Dalton and Hooker's chapter reveals how 'medical students must construct a version of 'professionalism' that holds on to their expertise and (some) authority while being simultaneously committed to patient autonomy and patient care'. How, they ask, might students 'meet professional expectations *and* care for patients, when these ends are not always aligned?' Gretchen A. Case's analysis of students in her own institution in the US hones in on the costumes and props associated with medical authority: the white coat, scrubs and the stethoscope. These, she says, 'might be status symbols, but they are not static symbols' and, after an historical overview of medical dress, she tracks the way staff and students adapt how they are worn, improvising in relation to the specific context as they negotiate and evolve their medical identity. Bleakley and Marshall also draw attention to the improvisational nature of medical performance, drawing an analogy between the 'oral performance' of the doctor, for example, while giving a case history, and that of the ancient Homeric tradition of epic storytelling.

Case notes how performance studies 'crosses so productively into fields such as cultural studies and anthropology'. We would also suggest that these chapters align with the related tradition of medical sociology which seeks to understand the highly specialised cultures that make up the medical domain, often using ethnomethodological approaches such as the observational fieldwork used by our contributors. Sociology analyses the behaviours of 'actors' (as research subjects are called in sociological analyses) for how they are determined by social context. In doing so, they often use theatre as a metaphor. Talcott Parsons, for example, described the social status of patients in terms of a 'role', while Erving Goffman's notion of impression management, the presentation of self in everyday life, saw professional behaviours understood as a form of performance. What these chapters do is take the theatrical metaphor more seriously and more expansively. Steve Reid, Laurie Rauch and Alp Numanoglu examine minimally invasive surgery as a form of performance in their chapter. Their argument is that both performing arts and surgery involve physical skill and mental preparation to optimise effectiveness while under performance pressure. Thus, the analogy to performance enables us to recognise not only the social dimension of health care practices but also the psychological and the physical dimensions.

Christina Lammer, Tamar Tembeck and Wilfried Wisser also focus on the highly specialised field of advanced surgery. Surgeons, they say, 'penetrate into the total reality of human existence. They change the composition of the viscera in order to support the body's capacity to heal'. Their explorations included observation of a surgery but also creative experiment, as they brought a cardiac surgeon into their rehearsal studio, engaging with action painting, experimental film and Decroux's mime corporeal. These performance forms are employed within a research methodology that allows microanalysis of the way surgeons engage their whole bodies as 'healing instruments', of the gestural, inter-corporeal and material aspects of surgery, and that reveals 'the ways in which the body of the operator and the patient's heart are intimately entangled'. Another insight into practice is provided by Lucinda Coleman, who describes a similar performance-based, aesthetic and imaginative investigation of health care practice, in this case focusing on the reported experiences of nurses and midwives. Their account of this collaborative project argues for greater recognition for 'epistemological art-making within the health humanities' and demonstrates how such approaches can expose under-recognised aspects of healthcare practice. This includes playfully challenging 'stereotypes of nurses and midwives through authentic, reflexive storytelling' and revealing the fleshly, affective and aesthetic aspects of health care practice in general. 'Although the choreographic intention was not social transformation' they tell us, 'artistic ephemeron has potential to shift, disrupt, delight, provoke, and transform at the intersection of the performing arts and health field'.

We stay with this topic of interdisciplinary exchange between performing arts and health care for the next chapter, by dramaturg Pauline Bouchet. Here Bouchet offers three case studies of theatre projects conducted in collaborations between the Department of Performing Arts at the University of Grenoble-Alpes and the University Hospital Centre in France: the involvement of performing arts students in simulation-based communication skills education for medical students, the creation of verbatim theatre with cancer patients and a version of Goethe's *Faust* that reimagines Faust as a haematologist. In each case, Bouchet argues, the practice of dramaturgy is 'the ideal place for mediation in projects linking the world of theatre and the world of medicine' because of its ability to 'mediate interdisciplinary dialogues between artists, caregivers and doctors, patients and the audience in order to build common fictions in medical performances'.

Like a theatrical performance, Part 2 closes with a round of applause. Giskin Day offers a detailed case study of the 'clap-for-carers' phenomenon that briefly flourished during the COVID-19 coronavirus epidemic, reminding us that the 'act of clapping as an expression of communal appreciation takes its cue from theatre' and that 'its function is far from straightforward'. For example, she points out the potential for 'emotional dissonance' between 'celebratory atmosphere centred on the ethos and pathos of gratitude' and 'the contextual atmosphere of fear, anger, grief and shame engendered by the pandemic'. In debating this and other aspects of this performance of public gratitude towards health care workers, the chapter encompasses the social, political and affective within the public discourse pertaining to the health care profession.

9

IT'S FUNNY BECAUSE IT'S TRUE

Dr. Knock, Michel Foucault, and the birth of a satire

Katherine Burke

The Birth of the Clinic, published in 1963 by French philosopher Michel Foucault (1926–1984) is an examination of a rapid shift in medical epistemology and the emergence of teaching hospitals in post-Revolutionary France. In it, Foucault examines the scientific and cultural changes that led to new methods of practicing and teaching medicine, as well as the transformation of medical language. Foucault focuses particularly on the late eighteenth and early nineteenth centuries, a period in which a French national discourse on disease was prominent. This time brought about new ways of observing patients and the science of correlating symptoms with specific pathologies (Osborne, 1992). To better visualise how this transformation was experienced by French citizens during this transition, we can turn to Jules Romains' 1923 satire *Dr. Knock, or the Triumph of Medicine*. About a scam artist doctor who rapidly transforms a country town into a centre of medical tourism, the play holds a funhouse mirror to *The Birth of the Clinic*. Romains provides us with satirical examples of the elements Foucault describes, including the medical gaze, the use of signs and signifiers to diagnose conditions, and the swift way in which hospitals developed.

Michel Foucault's father was a surgeon and obstetrician who taught at a medical school in Poitiers, providing Michel Foucault with the basis of an interest in French medical history. *The Birth of the Clinic* is Foucault's second major book, preceded by *Mental Illness and Psychology* in 1954. His writings do not follow traditional philosophical norms in which one searches for truth or proposes guidelines for ethical living. Instead, as Lynn Fendler writes, he attempts 'to provoke in us new questions about who we are and how we think', calling his method 'problematization' (Fendler, 2014, p. 6). *The Birth of the Clinic* is known as one of Foucault's 'archaeological' studies (the subtitle is *An Archaeology of Medical Perception*); in it he strives to excavate the reasons that things are the way they are in French clinical medicine (Philo, 2000).

That both Foucault and Romains examined the evolution of French medicine is no accident, as their mutual home of Paris had become a locus of medical industry and innovation. Reconstruction of the city following the Revolution allowed for spaces to be built specifically for science and medicine, and medical and anatomy schools proliferated. The early 1900s saw the building of twenty modern hospitals in Paris, and what became known as the Paris School of Medicine was born in this climate, expanding upon the practice of studying, conducting, and teaching of anatomy, physical examination, and medicine (Weiner and Sauter, 2003). Examining the rapidly changing landscape of French medicine around the Revolution is helpful for understanding Foucault's interest in the clinic.

DOI: 10.4324/9781003036500-12

French hospitals and medical practice

The end of the eighteenth century was a time of transition in Paris, with tremendous population growth, Revolution, and governmental change. The vigorous intellectual post-Revolutionary climate made Paris an ideal spot for medical innovation (Weiner and Sauter, 2003). Foucault describes pre-Revolutionary health care institutions as charitable and religious institutions that were essentially poorhouses, doing nothing to alleviate the root causes of illness, suffering, and poverty (Foucault in Philo, 2000). In the early 1600s, France had been home to several *hôspitaux-générales* (general hospitals) staffed by Augustinian nuns, Brothers of Charity of St. John of God, and Sisters of Charity. In Paris and other larger cities, the medieval *Hôtel Dieu* (God's hostels) served as welfare houses. By 1700, Paris had forty-eight charitable religious hospices, able to care for only 20,000 of Paris' 300,000 residents. These institutions relied on donations from the faithful, but with a decline in religious practices in the eighteenth century came a marked reduction in tithing and charitable giving. By the start of the French Revolution the population of Paris more than doubled to 700,000, with many coming to Paris from country provinces (Risse, 1999). The small, religious-run medieval hospices were insufficient, and they came under scrutiny. The Enlightenment brought ideals about improved physical health, and the possibility of curing illness across all social strata (Risse, 1999).

Further illustrating the insufficiency of medical care in the late 1700s, we can examine the Paris *Hôtel Dieu*, a medieval building located on both sides of the Seine, with 112 wards connected by a system of narrow corridors. It housed 3,500 patients in 1,200 beds, with patients lying head-to-toe. The Encyclopaedist Denis Diderot described it after a visit:

> Imagine every kind of patient, sometimes packed three, four, five, or six into a bed, the living alongside the dead and dying, the air polluted by this mass of sick bodies, passing the pestilential germs of their afflictions from one to the other, and the spectacle of suffering and agony on every hand.

> (Risse, 1999, p. 295)

A week-long fire in December 1772 damaged the structure so much that Louis XV ordered its demolition. His untimely death from smallpox and the ascension of Louis XVI delayed the demolition, with an eventual plan emerging to reconstruct the hospital, led by physician Jean Colombier. In 1787 Colombier set out to codify procedures at the *Hôtel Dieu*, transforming it into a medical and surgical institution (Risse, 1999).

Revolutionaries then quickly uprooted the old medieval medical system in France, seizing all of Paris' 48 religious hospitals and shutting them down. By the early 1800s, Paris was the largest city on the European continent, with 6,000 indigent and ill who still needed public health care. Revolutionary reformers innovated in the arts and sciences; doctors, scientists, and revolutionaries all connected and mingled. The clinicians of the Paris School of Medicine created modern medicine in Paris, teaching new methods of physical examination and 'anatomo-clinical' diagnostic methods, thanks in part to the Revolutionary government making bodies of unclaimed deceased patients available for dissection (Weiner and Sauter, 2003).

Jules Romains, *Dr. Knock,* and satire

Jules Romains, born Louis Farigoule in 1885, was raised in Paris, and studied philosophy. After changing his name at the age of eighteen, Romains became a professor of philosophy

(Wilson, 1958). Through his plays, poetry, and prolific fiction writing (he is largely remembered for his 27-volume novel *Men of Good Will*), he developed and expressed his philosophy of 'unanimism', a theory of group consciousness (Walter, 1936). Romains originally coined the term 'l'unanimisme' to mean the literary portrayal of collective actions and emotions (Norrish, 1958). Many of Romains' works, including *Knock*, feature the concept of unanimism as a central theme.

The plot centres around the title character of Knock, a mostly autodidact doctor who comes to the rural French town of Saint-Maurice to buy the medical practice of Dr. Parpalaid, who intends to open a new practice in Lyon. Years prior, Knock had talked his way into a job as a ship's doctor, a position for which he was entirely unqualified at the time, but through which he learned some of the tricks he would eventually employ in Saint-Maurice. He later completed his training at a medical school. Knock, who received his degree only a year prior, had expected that Parpalaid's practice would be financially lucrative, but upon arriving comes to understand that Parpalaid had not run the business well. In fact, patients only paid their medical bills once a year on the Catholic feast day of 'Michaelmas', which, conveniently for Parpalaid, has recently passed when Knock arrives. Moreover, Knock has no money to pay Parpalaid, but he senses an opportunity to convert the village's residents into a unanimised community of patients. As they stand waiting for Parpalaid's driver to fix his rattletrap jalopy, Knock expresses the beginnings of his plan to turn individual village denizens into a collective under his spell of medicine, declaring that 'the Age of Medicine can begin' (Romains, 1984, p. 14). Knock makes a deal with Parpalaid that within three months he will turn the quiet country practice into a bustling enterprise and that Parpalaid will receive his money then. Knock concocts a scheme to enrich himself that involves slide shows of microbes, copious medical jargon, and, in the end, the birth of a bona fide clinic. Under Knock's spell, the villagers become unanimised, developing group consciousness around medicalisation.

The characters and actions within *Knock* are exaggerated and comical, and the title character, while an actual doctor, is a con man who illegitimately applies his skills to enrich himself. Still, the success of the play leads one to believe that audiences recognised the essential truth within the satire. *Knock* was Romains' greatest commercial success, first staged at the *Comédie des Champs-Élysées* in December of 1923 (Boak, 1974). The play became a long-running source of funding for the theatre, which revived it whenever money was running low (Fratto, 2021). Some considered it to be the greatest French comedy of its day, playing the *Athénée* theatre more than 800 times (Whitman, 1972). Since its debut, it has been staged around the world and has had multiple film renditions.

Satire is a particularly apt tool for understanding and analysing politics and society. Featuring absurdity, exaggeration, irony, and humour, satire lies at the intersection of entertainment and critique (DeClercq, 2018). The form takes its name from ancient Greek theatre, in which satyr plays, performed as a part of dramatic competitions, often poked fun at public figures, featuring choruses of mythical satyrs who served as bawdy comic relief (Shaw, 2014). Just as a broadcast of *Saturday Night Live* combines sociopolitical criticism and comedy, Romains' play mixes judgment and entertainment to reveal cultural truths, keeping the audience engaged with the play's humour while simultaneously scrutinising the field of medicine (Greenberg, 2011). Satire is effective precisely because the audience recognises something familiar. In fact, the play's original producer and star Louis Jouvet, himself a former pharmacist, was concerned that *Dr. Knock* landed too close to the mark and feared that the public may react negatively and shut the play down. It turned out that Jouvet was wrong, and *Knock* became a hit, making Romains a fortune (Boak, 1974).

The epistemological shift

In the preface to *The Birth of the Clinic*, Foucault compares two doctors, about a century apart from each other. In the mid-eighteenth century, Pomme described a treatment for hysteria, in which the patient soaked for ten to twelve hours a day in water for many months. As a result, the patient shed skin and tissues, inside and out. It is not the treatment in which Foucault is interested, but the way in which Pomme describes the tissues with metaphor. Pomme writes that the tissues resemble 'damp parchment', or 'tunics', and describes the physical reactions and sensations of the patient as the tissues peeled off 'with some slight discomfort', or vomited some tissues up (Foucault, 1973, p. ix).

Less than a century later, the second physician, Bayle, a member of the Paris School of Medicine, wrote about a patient with chronic meningitis, detailing observations about colours and thicknesses of brain lesions: 'The false membranes are often transparent, especially when they are very thin; but usually they are white, grey, or red in colour, and occasionally, yellow, brown, or black' (Foucault, 1973, p. ix). The passage Foucault quotes does not mention whether the tissues described are connected to or came from a person, nor does it mention any symptoms or narrative history of the patient (Foucault, 1973). Instead, Bayle described the details of the images he saw through his microscope, neither understanding nor interpreting the meanings of the colours and textures.

In the years between the two doctors' writings, something changed substantially in the way doctors saw and described patients, the body, symptoms, and illness. Pomme's gaze is to the exterior of the patient, focusing on behaviour, symptoms, and larger portions of tissues. Bayle peers into the interior, engaging with microscopic fragments of the body (Rajchman, 1988). Neither doctor practiced what we today would consider evidence-based medicine, but Bayle's language contains the trappings of something science-like. Foucault notes that the ability to see into the body, through microscopy and dissection of corpses, allowed Bayle to see and describe things that Pomme could not. '[T]he relation between the visible and invisible – which is necessary to all concrete knowledge – changed its structure', argues Foucault, 'revealing through gaze and language what had previously been below and beyond their domain. A new alliance was forged between words and things, enabling one to see and to say' (1973, p. xii).

Microscopy, photography, and magic lanterns

The new technologies Foucault describes, such as the microscope and stethoscope, feature comically and prominently in *Dr. Knock*, demonstrating their newfound prevalence in medical practice and public health education surrounding germs and hygiene, thanks in large part to the invention of the microscope. Prior to the acceptance of the germ theory of contagion, people were aware that some invisible substance emanated from the ill, capable of transmitting disease, a belief often referred to as 'miasma theory'. In the 1700s, there was little understanding of disease or cellular biology, and the use of microscopes was not yet fully embraced by medicine. Marie-Francois Xavier Bichat (1771–1802), a surgeon and anatomist at the Paris *Hôtel Dieu*, classified and distinguished tissues such as nerves, arteries, veins, and glands by manipulating them through boiling, baking, soaking, or exposing them to acids (Simmons, 2002). Foucault writes that Bichat refused to use a microscope, favouring a more 'natural' way of seeing things: 'In a way that seems strange to us . . . the analysis of pathological tissues dispensed, over a period of several years, with even the most ancient instruments of optics' (1973, p. 167).

Advances in microscopy in the seventeenth and eighteenth centuries led to greater under-standing about the causes of communicable diseases. Dutch spectacle maker Hans Janssen (c. 1580–1638) is credited with inventing a compound microscope in the 1590s, a straightforward instrument with a lens at each end of a tube, which could magnify objects three to nine times (Masters, 2008). German physician and pathologist Rudolf Virchow (1821–1902), who advocated the use of the microscope in his book *Cellular Pathology*, showed that diseases are associated with the disruption of normal cellular processes (Masters, 2008). In the late 1870s German physi-cian Robert Koch proved that microbes were linked with disease, leading to the identification of bacteria that were responsible for cholera, tuberculosis, gonorrhoea, typhoid, and scarlet fever (Tomes, 1998).

Around the same time, medical photography was becoming increasingly important in a vari-ety of medical spaces. In the late 1800s, along with the growing acceptance of the germ theory of disease, photo-microscopic imagery grew in popularity, and became more common in public lectures, print media, and medical education. Robert Koch established criteria for photographing microscopic specimens, and French physician Alfred Donné (1801–1878) and his assistant Léon Foucault (1819–1868) showed microphotography of bodily secretions at the French Academy of Sciences in 1840. (Curtis, 2012). The combined technologies of photography and microscopy facilitated a new way of seeing in the nineteenth century. The capacity to observe physiology, asserts Foucault, was central to this practice.

> Nineteenth-century medicine . . . formed its concepts and prescribed its interventions in relation to a standard of functioning and organic structure, and physiological knowledge – once marginal and purely theoretical knowledge for the doctor – was to become established (Claude Bernard bears witness to this) at the very centre of all medical reflexion.
>
> (1973, p. 35)

The technology of microscopy is featured in *Dr. Knock*, introduced through the use of magic lantern projections for public hygiene education. The invention of the magic lantern is credited by some to Roman Catholic priest Athanasius Kircher in the eighteenth century, first using hand painted slides projected onto a screen for popular entertainment (Shepard, 1987). The germ theory of disease led to a new profession of public hygienist (Weiner and Sauter, 2003), who would edu-cate the public, sometimes with the use of magic lantern slides, about the dangers of microbes. At a 1934 speech, German Physician Bruno Gebhard praised the value of lantern slides for pub-lic health education and described the popular use of the Deutsches Hygiene Museum's slides throughout Europe.

> The Lantern Slide Service alone has more than 100 series, and each has from fifty to sixty slides concerning all branches of public health. They are employed in schools and for special lectures. One can hire or buy them, and they can be used in any country no matter what its language.
>
> (Gebhard, 1934, p. 1151)

Romains' Dr. Knock values microscopic imagery and photographic projections as tools through which he can wield power over the inhabitants of Saint-Maurice. On the day of his arrival at his new practice, he summons the local schoolteacher, Monsieur Bernard, a queasy, modest man. Knock presents Bernard with his plan to employ the teacher to educate the public on hygiene, just as Gebhard described in his speech:

Knock: I have here the material for several popularized lectures: very complete notes, good slides, and a projector. Take, to begin with, a little lecture – all written out, I promise you, and very agreeable – on typhoid fever: the unsuspected forms it takes, the innumerable ways of transmission – water, bread, milk, shellfish, vegetables, salads, dust, breath, etc., the weeks and months during which it incubates unsuspected; the fatal accidents that it suddenly causes; the fearful complications it leaves in its wake. And all embellished with lovely pictures; bacilli enormously enlarged, details of typhoidal excrements, infected ganglions, perforations of the intestine – and not black and white, but in color! Reds, browns, yellows, and the greenish white you can only imagine

(Romains, 1984, p. 25).

It is easy to see here the comparison between Knock's description of the imagery on the slides and Bayle's description of the 'white, grey, or red . . . and occasionally yellow, brown, or black' tissue (Foucault, 1973, p. x)

If Knock is akin to Bayle in his description of precise and colourful imagery, then Parpalaid, from whom Knock bought the practice, is akin to the earlier physician Pomme, who had little diagnostic capacity and prescribed folk remedies. Knock interviews the Town Crier, an illiterate but eager fellow, about his predecessor. The Town Crier expresses his disappointment in Parpalaid:

Town Crier: When someone came to see him, he didn't find . . . what you had. Nine times out of ten he would send you away, saying 'It's nothing at all. You'll be on your feet tomorrow my friend . . .' and then he would suggest some remedy that cost four sous; sometimes a simple herb tea.

(Romains, 1984, p. 18)

In Romain's physician characters we see Foucault's description of the epistemic change theatrically personified. As the character of Knock takes over from Parpalaid and proceeds to medicalise Saint-Michel, we see the villagers rapidly fall under the spell not only of Knock's magic lantern technology, but of the way in which he wields language and the medical gaze.

Power, language, and the medical gaze

A theme in all of Foucault's works, including *The Birth of the Clinic*, is power, even though Foucault does not explicitly name 'power' frequently in the text (Bolanos, 2010). *The Birth of the Clinic* examines the relationship between language and power in medicine, arguing that disease is only understood because the doctor can see it and subsequently name it. Foucault asserts that the changes in medicine were made possible not only because of changes in technology and science, but by changes in language (Foucault in Osborne, 1992). Much of the text focuses on the doctor and the nature of expertise, and the right and ability to use medical language (ibid.). Foucault recognises the power of the doctor, 'supported and justified by an institution . . . endowed with the power of decision and intervention' (1973, p. 89). Romains picks up on this theme as well, as the character of Knock insists to the Town Crier that he be referred to by his professional title:

Knock: Call me 'Doctor'. Answer 'Yes, Doctor' or 'No, Doctor . . .' And when you speak of me to others, never fail to express yourself thus! 'The doctor has said', 'The doctor has done . . .' I attach importance to this.

(Romains, 1984, p. 17)

Parpalaid, on the other hand, was referred to informally by several nicknames (including, strangely, 'Jack the Ripper'), according to the Town Crier, and was not highly respected:

Town Crier: We used to say, 'he's a good man, but he's not very smart'.

(Romains, 1984, p. 17)

Foucault examines what doctors see when they look at a patient and dubs the act of seeing, interpreting, and naming the 'medical gaze' (Fendler, 2014). Language and seeing are intertwined, writes Foucault, and as the epistemic shift progressed, '[t]he medical field was . . . open[ed] on to something which always speaks a language that is at one in its existence and meaning with the gaze that deciphers it – a language inseparably read and reading' (1973, p. 96). Later in his book *The Archaeology of Knowledge*, Foucault critiques his own concept of the gaze, which, in the original French publication, is written as *regard médical*, as it seemed to suggest that the one doing the gazing or regarding commanded knowledge. Nevertheless, the term 'medical gaze' synthesises the way in which knowledge, vision, and language come together, articulating in one phrase 'what the doctor can see, feel, say, teach, or know' (Osborne, 1992, p. 79).

In 1816, René-Théophile-Hyacinthe Laennec, a French physician and musician, invented the stethoscope while teaching and practicing at Paris' *Hôtel Necker*. Accustomed to carving his own flutes, Laennec carved a tube that, when applied to the patient's chest, amplified the sounds within the body (Scherer, 2007). Prior to the invention of the stethoscope, physicians would have to put their ears directly on the patient's chest; the stethoscope allowed some modesty for female patients. Laennec used his invention first to auscultate (i.e., examine a patient by listening) heart sounds and then lung sounds. He became so expert at associating sounds with specific diseases that he could use percussion and auscultation to diagnose the various stages of pneumonia (Weiner and Sauter, 2003). At a lecture at the *Collège de France*, Laennec foresaw a time when:

> there could be signs in patients who were asymptomatic and symptoms in patients without perceptible signs – a disturbing admission in the world of pathological anatomy with its reliance on ascertainable proof of disease.
>
> (Weiner and Sauter, 2003, p. 37)

Foucault credits Laennec's invention and use of the stethoscope with augmenting the medical gaze: 'The stethoscope, solidified distance, transmits profound and invisible events along a semi-tactile, semi-auditory axis' (1973, p. 164). Foucault incorporates the technology of the stethoscope, as well as physical touch, into the medical gaze:

> The sight/touch/hearing trinity defines a perceptual configuration in which the inaccessible illness is tracked down by markers, gauged in depth, drawn to the surface, and projected virtually on the dispersed organs.
>
> (ibid, p. 64)

Foucault is especially interested in the language Laennec uses to describe what he perceives (Osborne, 1992), declaring that it has 'extraordinary formal beauty' (1973, p. 169).

The character of Knock employs the medical gaze and the power of medical language to establish his practice, hoodwinking wealthy clientele into believing that they are ill when in fact they are not. After sending the Town Crier out to advertise free examinations, Knock's waiting room fills with patients eager for consultations. First in line is the Lady in Black, a wealthy

111

landowner who makes do with a staff of 'three farm hands, one maid, and the extra hands for the busy season' (Romains, 1984, p. 30). She complains of worry about her extensive lands, and exhaustion as a result of worry. Knock seizes the opportunity before him and examines her, 'finding' a devastating condition, which he convinces her is the result of a fall from a ladder when she was young:

Knock: I shall explain it to you in one minute on the blackboard. . . . Here is your spinal cord in cross section, very roughly, of course. You recognize here your Turck's fascicles and here is your Clarke's column. You follow me? Well, when you fell from the ladder, your Turck and your Clarke slipped in inverse direction of several tenths of a millimeter. You will tell me that this is very little. Obviously. But it is very badly located. And then here you have a continuous pulling or jarring of the nerve cells.

(Romains, 1984, p. 31)

Here Knock takes advantage of the Lady in Black's trust, using what Foucault calls 'a grammar of signs', in which the physician looks to minute 'elements of corporal space', such as the colours and textures described by Bayle, rather than to the larger constellation of the patient's experiences and symptoms (Foucault, 1973). The Lady in Black of course has no discernible symptom for this invented condition; Knock manipulates her imagined symptoms into signs. Here, and throughout the script, Knock wields symptoms, real and invented, as signs that only he as a doctor has the capacity to interpret. In this way Knock justifies his profession and practice, as the one who first discovers a symptom, crafts it into a sign for a condition, diagnoses the condition, and then treats the patient.

Knock repeats this pattern with wealthy patient after patient, including the Lady in Violet, who suffers from insomnia. Again, he employs the jargon of medicine and anatomy:

Knock: Insomnia can be due to essential trouble in the intra-cerebral circulation, particularly to an alteration of the vessels called "pipe-stem." You have, perhaps, madam, these pipe-stem cerebral arteries.

(Romains, 1984, p. 36)

For both the Lady in Black and the Lady in Violet, Knock prescribes rest and medicine and promises that he will provide frequent and expensive home consultations.

Doctors, hospitals, and the free field

Foucault devotes a great deal of *The Birth of the Clinic* to the role of the doctor and credits the Paris School, through the study of anatomy, dissection, the invention of the stethoscope, and the development of physical examination, with the advancement of clinical medicine in Paris (Wilson, 2007). Public opinion about medical professionals and hospitals in late eighteenth-century France was mostly unfavourable, due in large part to the poor state of hospitals and high mortality rates; public calls for oversight of physicians increased (Risse, 1999). In 1803, a law was enacted regulating medical practitioners, many of whom had entered into their professions in the *Ancien Regime* or during the Revolution. Doctors of medicine or surgery were only allowed to practice at state medical facilities, of which there were three after 1815, after completing four years of study, passing five examinations, and writing a thesis. Health officers were licensed by juries of physicians after lengthy apprenticeships with doctors, through military service, or at medical school

(Sussman, 1977). The character of Dr. Knock, who began his autodidactical medical education on a ship, completed his education when he realised that a 'medical degree is an indispensable formality' (Romains, 1984, p. 12).

Foucault envisioned a future with two roles for physicians, and a dual medical structure. The 'free field', as Foucault named it, would consist of 'a continuous supervision of the social space' (1973, p. 42), with doctors traversing France to serve the sick (Philo, 2000). The free field could preserve the 'natural locus of disease', that is, the home, as a place where a sick person could ideally convalesce, with the family offering 'gentle, spontaneous care, expressive of love' (Foucault, 1973, p. 17). At the same time, Foucault recognised the need for medical specialists who would be housed at teaching hospitals, where scientific discovery and acute care would take place.

Romains' character of Dr. Knock incorporates both the free field and the institutional hospital into the life of Saint-Maurice. After three months, Knock's practice outgrows his little office. He expands 'the hotel of the county seat' into a 'Medical Hotel'. Romains' stage directions describe the scene: 'the nickel plate, the white enamel, the white linen of modern asepsis appear' (Romains, 1984, p. 40). The previous maids and bellboys are now employed as nurses and aides, frantically taking temperatures and collecting specimens. This state-of-the-art hospital is so bursting with patients who have come from far and wide that they have no more beds available, and an extension to the hospital is under construction to house more patients. Knock is of course in charge of the entire hospital but also maintains his role in the free field, as described by the maid-turned-nurse Madame Remy:

> We see him passing through the whole country, spending ten francs worth of gasoline and stopping in his beautiful car before the hut of some poor old woman who hasn't even a goat cheese to give him.
>
> (Romains, 1984, p. 44)

For Foucault, the ideal medical framework incorporates 'a generalized medical consciousness, diffused in space and time, linked to each individual existence, as well as to the collective life of the nation' (1973, p. 31); Romains' concept of unanimism embraces this idea of collective life, actions, and emotions. By the play's final scene, Knock has succeeded in unanimising the village of Saint-Maurice with a culture of medicalisation. Parpalaid returns to collect what Knock owes him and is astonished at what he finds. The entire village and surrounding countryside are now patients under Knock's care. Knock revels in his success, describing his triumph to Parpalaid as they look out the window of the hospital over the landscape, now:

> *Knock:* entirely impregnated with medical science, enlivened by the subterranean fire of our art, which runs through it. . . . In two hundred and fifty of these houses . . . there are two hundred and fifty bedrooms where someone professes his faith in medical science. Two hundred and fifty beds where a recumbent body testifies that life has a direction and, thanks to me, a medical direction.
>
> (Romains, 1984, p. 50)

In the end, Knock convinces Parpalaid himself that he is not well and should not endure the railroad journey back home; Parpalaid becomes one of Knock's patients in the new hospital. Romains ends the play with eerie stage directions in which the hospital staff, carrying medical instruments, file across the stage, illuminated by the 'glow of the Light of Medical Science' (Romains, 1984, p. 56).

The wild popularity of *Dr. Knock* at its premiere in 1923 indicates not only that Romains had a talent for farce but that the Parisian audience found the characters and plot familiar. To this day, a century after its debut, the themes the play satirises, including the medical gaze, language, power, medical technology, and epistemology, are strikingly relatable. In his descriptions of the ways in which doctors see and speak, the history of the development of the teaching hospital, and the ways in which patients interact with medical professionals, Foucault lays out observations that Romains corroborates comically in *Dr. Knock*. Turning to Romains' satirical depiction of the speedy birth of a fictional clinic can give us insight into the ways in which the French population of the time may have experienced and reacted to the rapid transformation of the institution and practice of medicine in post-Revolutionary Paris. Medical care centres quickly developed from small and simple religious hostels to large institutional clinics with advanced technology and equipment, just as in Romains' fictional town of Saint-Michel. The relationships between doctors and patients quickly shifted from ones similar to those with Parpalaid, who encouraged his patients to merely rest and drink tea, to interactions with physicians like Knock, who employed stethoscopes, microscopes, projections, complex medical jargon, and lengthy and expensive treatments. Moreover, this play can help us to critique our own clinical experiences in the twenty-first century. How do we as patients interact with physicians? How do we as health care practitioners translate technology and treatment plans to patients? Can we use language not to obfuscate but to illuminate? Is more expensive technology always the way to better care? The satirical nature of this play allows us to think about these questions and Foucault's archaeology from an aesthetic distance, giving us the space to examine these issues with more clarity. It is said that art imitates life. If that is so, then Romains' satire clearly imitates the rapid change in medicine that 1920s Parisians found familiar, and Foucault's *The Birth of the Clinic* is likewise an accurate depiction of the shift to, as Dr. Knock declares it, 'the Age of Medicine' (Romains, 1984, p. 14).

Reference list

Boak, D. (1974) *Jules Romains*. New York: Twayne Publishers.

Bolanos, K.A. (2010) 'Kelly, Mark G.E., the political philosophy of Michel Foucault: review of the book', *Kritike: An Online Journal of Philosophy*, 4(1).

Curtis, S. (2012) 'Photography and medical observation', in Anderson, N. and Dietrich, M.R. (eds.) *The educated eye: visual culture and pedagogy in the life sciences*. Hanover, New Hampshire: Dartmouth College Press, pp. 68–93.

Declercq, D. (2018) 'A definition of satire (and why a definition matters)', *The Journal of Aesthetics and Art Criticism*, 76(3), pp. 319–330.

Fendler, L. (2014) *Michel Foucault*. London: Bloomsbury Methuen Drama Publishing.

Foucault, M. (1973) *The birth of the clinic: an archaeology of medical perception*. Translated by A.M. Sheridan. London: Tavistock Publications Limited.

Fratto, E. (2021) *Medical storyworlds: health, illness, and bodies in Russian and European literature at the turn of the twentieth century*. New York: Columbia University Press.

Gebhard, B. (1934) 'Health education in Germany', *American Journal of Public Health and the Nations Health*, 24(11), pp. 1148–1151.

Greenberg, J. (2011) *Modernism, satire and the novel*. Cambridge: Cambridge University Press.

Masters, B.R. (2008) 'History of the optical microscope in cell biology and medicine', in *Encyclopedia of life sciences (ELS)*. Chichester: John Wiley and Sons.

Norrish, P.J. (1958) *Drama of the group: a study of unanimism in the plays of Jules Romains*. Cambridge: Cambridge University Press.

Osborne, T. (1992) 'Medicine and epistemology: Michel Foucault and the liberality of clinical reason', *History of the Human Sciences*, 5(2), pp. 63–93.

Philo, C. (2000) 'The birth of the clinic: an unknown work of medical geography', *Area*, 32(1), pp. 11–19.

Rajchman, J. (1988) 'Foucault's art of seeing', *October*, 44, p. 88.

Risse, G.B. (1999) *Mending bodies, saving souls: a history of hospitals*. New York: Oxford University Press.

Romains, J. (1984) *Knock, or, the triumph of medicine: a comedy in three acts*. Translated by B. Scherr Sacks. New York: Vantage Press.

Scherer, J.L. (2007) 'Before cardiac MRI: Rene Laennec (1781–1826) and the invention of the stethoscope', *Cardiology*, 14(5), pp. 518–519.

Shaw, C. (2014) *Satyric play: the evolution of Greek comedy and satyr drama*. Oxford: Oxford University Press.

Shepard, E. (1987) 'The magic lantern slide in entertainment and education, 1860–1920', *History of Photography*, 11(2), pp. 91–108.

Simmons, J. (2002) *Doctors and discoveries: lives that created today's medicine*. Boston: Houghton Mifflin.

Sussman, G.D. (1977) 'The glut of doctors in mid-nineteenth-century France', *Comparative Studies in Society and History*, 19(3), pp. 287–304.

Tomes, N. (1998) *The gospel of germs: men, women, and the microbe in American life*. Cambridge, MA: Harvard University Press.

Walter, F. (1936) 'Unanimism and the novels of Jules Romains', *PMLA*, 51(3), pp. 863–871.

Weiner, D.B. and Sauter, M.J. (2003) 'The city of Paris and the rise of clinical medicine', *Osiris*, 18(2), pp. 23–42.

Whitman, A. (1972) 'Jules Romains, man of letters, dies in a Paris hospital at 86', *The New York Times*, 18 August. Available at: www.nytimes.com/1972/08/18/archives/jules-romains-man-of-letters-dies-in-a-paris-hospital-at-86-jules.html (Accessed: 18 October 2021).

Wilson, A. (2007) 'Porter versus Foucault on the "birth of the clinic"', in Bivins, R. and Pickstone, J.V. (eds.) *Medicine, madness and social history*. London: Palgrave Macmillan.

Wilson, D.S. (1958) *L'ame diffuse: the ethics of Jules Romains*. Graduate Student Theses, Dissertations, & Professional Papers, The University of Montana.

10

ROBERT ICKE'S *THE DOCTOR*

Exploring modern medicine through Arthur Schnitzler's *Professor Bernhardi*

Judith Beniston

Perhaps somewhat surprisingly, the one work by Austrian doctor-writer Arthur Schnitzler (1862–1931) that long-time *Guardian* theatre critic Michael Billington includes in his compendium of *The 101 Greatest Plays* is not the endlessly adaptable daisy-chain of sexual encounters that is *Reigen* (*La Ronde*) but the medical drama *Professor Bernhardi* (1912). Billington thereby professes to admire Schnitzler not primarily as 'a writer about sex' but as 'a major social dramatist' (2015, p. 260). Set in Vienna around 1900, *Professor Bernhardi* tells the story of a scandal: the Jewish title figure, a respected clinician who heads a charitably funded hospital, denies a Catholic priest access to a young woman who is dying of sepsis following an illegal abortion. He does so not for religious reasons but because he regards it as his professional duty to spare the patient an anguished death. The play tracks the fallout from this action, which polarises opinion amongst his medical colleagues, in parliament and in the wider public sphere, resulting in a two-month prison sentence for Bernhardi and near bankruptcy for the hospital. *Professor Bernhardi* is not merely a medical drama but also potentially a state-of-the-nation play. The word 'sepsis' means putrefaction: there is something rotten in the state of Austria that the play and its title figure can diagnose but not remedy.

Billington's endorsement is all the more unexpected as *Professor Bernhardi*, in which Schnitzler draws on his experience of antisemitism in turn-of-the-century Vienna and on aspects of his and his father's medical careers, had by 2015 been revived only once on the London stage since a 1936 production directed by Schnitzler's son Heinrich. That revival was a 'new version' by Samuel Adamson, which retained the historical Viennese setting and was directed by Mark Rosenblatt at the Arcola Theatre in 2005 (Beniston, 2017, pp. 40–42). In the German-speaking world, by contrast, *Professor Bernhardi* can boast numerous stage and (since the 1960s also) television productions (Nuy, 2010). There, as elsewhere, post-war realisations of the play have necessarily engaged with its depiction of medicine, politics and race *c.*1900 from a post-Holocaust perspective, with the result that what Schnitzler designates as a comedy has come to seem darkly prophetic. In recent decades, high-profile modern-dress productions by Dieter Giesing (Burgtheater, Vienna, 2011) and Thomas Ostermeier (Schaubühne, Berlin, 2016) have updated Schnitzler's exploration of the social and political contexts in which medicine is embedded by casting women in some of the play's twenty-two male roles. Two adaptations premiered in 2019 – Olga Helen Bach's *Dr. Alici* (Kammerspiele, Munich) and the subject of this chapter, *The Doctor*, written and directed by

DOI: 10.4324/9781003036500-13

Robert Icke (Almeida Theatre, London) – have gone further. Both switch the gender of the title figure, with Bach also making her Muslim rather than Jewish, and relocate the action – to contemporary Munich and London, respectively. There the similarities end: while Bach dispenses with the medical thematic, Icke keeps the doctor's performatively constituted identity at the centre of his play, using it to explore the nature and limits of the social licence that is afforded to modern medicine and, like Schnitzler before him, to reflect (on) broader societal ills.

Icke bills *The Doctor* as 'very freely adapted from Arthur Schnitzler's *Professor Bernhardi*', which underlines his creative input and implicitly discourages comparative readings. Icke has made his name as a writer-director who reboots classic texts: volume one of his *Works*, issued by Oberon Books in 2020, presents *The Doctor* alongside his versions of the *Oresteia*, Chekhov's *Uncle Vanya*, Schiller's *Mary Stuart* and Ibsen's *The Wild Duck*. Three of these projects have earned him Best Director awards – including *The Doctor*, which also drew plaudits for Juliet Stevenson in the title role. A sell-out run at the Almeida, opening on 10 August 2019, was followed by a stint at the Adelaide Festival in early 2020 and transfers to London's West End in September 2022 and to New York's Park Avenue Armory in June 2023 (both delayed by the coronavirus). *The Doctor* has also been restaged several times, notably in Dutch at the Internationaal Theater Amsterdam, in Japanese at the Parco Theater in Tokyo, in Estonian at the Ugala theatre in Viljandi, in Hungarian at the Átrium theatre in Budapest and in German at the Burgtheater in Vienna. Icke has commented that he is drawn to works that were 'profoundly troubling' when they first appeared (Allfree, 2015), and the return in January 2022 of a reimagined *Professor Bernhardi* to the city in which Schnitzler wrote and set his play is not without irony: it was initially banned from performance in Austria due to Schnitzler's unflattering depiction of Austrian public life and consequently premiered in Berlin in November 1912. Extensively debated in the Austrian press, the ban was only lifted in 1918, after the collapse of the Habsburg Empire.

Although *Professor Bernhardi* has become a post-war repertoire staple in the German-speaking world, of Icke's five adaptations listed above, *The Doctor* is the one where British theatre-goers are least likely to have prior knowledge of the source text, which he is said to have described as a 'weird old Schnitzler play' (Lewis, 2020, p. xx). Therefore Michael Billington, who praises *The Doctor* as 'a brilliant expansion of the original's themes' (2019) and is familiar with both the performance history of *Professor Bernhardi* and the translation by Q.M.J. Davies for the Oxford World's Classics series (2015, p. 260), is not the average (or perhaps even the intended) spectator, and neither am I, since I am the lead editor of *Professor Bernhardi* in *Arthur Schnitzler digital*, the online historical-critical edition of his works (1905–1931), and have detailed knowledge of the play's genesis, its original Viennese context and its reception history. I am consequently aware that my responses to *The Doctor*, like Billington's, are atypical, that for many audience members the pleasure of encountering the play does not reside in an experience of repetition with variation. I would nevertheless echo Linda Hutcheon's view that an adaptation should ideally appeal both to knowing and unknowing spectators and that a parallel reading can be enriching, if carried out not in a spirit of nit-picking fidelity criticism or with the intention of declaring one play better or worse than the other but in order to engage analytically with both the result and the process of adaptation (2012: especially pp. 120–128). The relationship between *Professor Bernhardi* and *The Doctor* will be explored in this spirit, showing that Icke draws more extensively than one might expect on the 'weird old Schnitzler play'. Both scandals play out against the background of cutting-edge research and, while Schnitzler's comedy highlights the canker of antisemitism spreading through Austrian public life, *The Doctor* follows Peter Nichols's *The National Health* (1969) and Alan Bennett's *Allelujah!* (2018) in drawing attention to some of the perils facing both the NHS and the polity that created and sustains it.

Comparative anatomy of a scandal

Medical scandals are a perennial problem, most obviously attributable to tensions between the self-regulating character of the medical profession and its embeddedness in broader institutional, political and social structures. This unfortunate continuity allows Icke to follow Schnitzler very closely in how he establishes and escalates the crisis of *The Doctor*. The five acts of *Professor Bernhardi* become five 'days', each explicitly announced to the audience. They play out on a slowly revolving stage designed by Icke's regular collaborator Hildegard Bechtler, a clinical white space lit from above by flickering fluorescent tubes, and the action is accompanied by the heartbeat-like rhythms of a lone drummer. The first act/day takes place in an area adjoining a hospital ward where, offstage, a young woman, aged eighteen in Schnitzler's play and fourteen in Icke's, is succumbing to sepsis. The act/day culminates in a verbal and physical confrontation between the title figure, in Icke's play Professor Ruth Wolff, and a Catholic priest, which erupts when the doctor refuses to allow the priest access to the dying patient. The precise nature of the contact – 'Was it a touch or a shove? Or a push? Did it have force?' (Icke, 2019, p. 13) – is disputed in both plays, and Icke recommends that *'[p]robably this shouldn't be naturalistically dramatized: that is, we shouldn't be shown exactly what happens'* (ibid, p. 12). In *The Doctor* as in *Professor Bernhardi*, the title figure and several of the other doctors explicitly identify as Jewish or of Jewish descent and the hospital, of which Ruth Wolff, like Bernhardi, is founder-director, is substantially funded by Jewish philanthropists. Schnitzler's Elisabethinum, named after Austria's Empress Elisabeth, wife of Emperor Franz Joseph I, morphs effortlessly into London's Elizabeth Institute, named for the British monarch, and the medical scandal is easily updated: sepsis is still life-threatening without early diagnosis and treatment, online pharmaceutical sites offering abortion pills by post are barely safer than the backstreet practices of old and the Roman Catholic Church remains implacably opposed to procured abortion.

Icke's cast list is somewhat shorter than Schnitzler's, and roles are doubled up in the TV debate that constitutes the fourth 'day'. The ten department heads, two assistants, one medical student and one nurse representing the Elisabethinum become six named doctors, a hospital public relations manager and a nameless junior doctor. The secondary roles that change least are the deputy director and scheming antagonist Ebenwald/Roger Hardiman and the title figure's devoted ally Cyprian/Brian Cyprian; the rest take on selected characteristics of Schnitzler's medical personnel, likewise ranging themselves on the side of protagonist or antagonist. Icke also retains key features of the doctor-turned-politician Flint but switches the gender, thereby complicating his depiction of women in public life. As the surname suggests, Health Minister Jemima Flint is a hard-headed careerist who, like Schnitzler's character, initially supports her former colleague but then reneges on that commitment in order to protect her own position. In neither play is Flint's precise political affiliation clear: instead both represent a politics of spin and morally compromised pragmatism that is diametrically opposed to the principled stance of the title figure.

In its time, *Professor Bernhardi* was distinctive in presenting no doctor–patient interaction, instead offering audiences the unfamiliar experience of eavesdropping on doctors talking to doctors. Nowadays, by contrast, medical documentaries and reality series, as well as hospital soaps incorporating a behind-the-scenes perspective, have long been popular television fare, including a 2022 dramatisation of Adam Kay's bestselling memoir, *This Is Going to Hurt: Secret Diaries of a Junior Doctor* (Kay, 2017). Just as the fictionalised Adam's performances on the labour ward are characteristically framed by carpark and locker room scenes, with the mechanised dispensing of scrubs, so the original production of Icke's *The Doctor* began with the medical personnel entering the stage in everyday clothes, donning white coats and collecting props. In so doing they assume roles within a complex hierarchical structure that is constituted by performative repetition and can readily be analysed using Erving Goffman's dramaturgical model of social interaction (Hooker and Dalton, 2019, pp. 207–208). While, in Schnitzler's text, rituals of greeting and farewell and minutely differentiated honorifics and address forms help to maintain both collegiality and hierarchical distinctions (Beniston, 2017, pp. 42–44), Icke starts with the extremes: Hardiman pompously introduces himself as 'senior consultant, deputy director –' (2019, p. 1) and sets off a sad running gag by giving the play's junior doctor no chance to reciprocate. Dubbed 'BB = Big Bad' by her colleagues, Ruth Wolff presents a formidable figure, immediately taking directorial control of the performance space in both clinical and dramaturgical terms as she briskly dispatches colleagues to their work and reports on the sepsis patient. Her authoritative persona is encapsulated in the oft-repeated phrases 'I'm a doctor' and 'I am crystal clear', but there are tensions from the outset. The sparkling lucidity of the clinical gaze, generating scientifically founded diagnoses, is mocked as an otherworldly 'Jedi perception' (ibid, p. 2) and the ostensibly affectionate soubriquet 'BB' brings with it the unspoken question, 'Who's afraid of the big bad wolf?'.

In both plays the stand-off between doctor and priest indeed opens up existing institutional faultlines attributable to differences of race, religion and, in *The Doctor*, also gender. In the second act/day, the male, non-Jewish, Catholic deputy director Ebenwald/Roger Hardiman leaks the story to his political contacts and immediately begins to machinate, with the result that the hospital's backers desert it and matters come to a head in a tumultuous management meeting that constitutes the third act/day. This meeting is interrupted in Schnitzler's play by the news that Bernhardi is to be charged with obstructing religious observance (*Religionsstörung*), a criminal offence under the Austrian Penal Code of 1852. While Schnitzler's fourth act takes place on the evening of Bernhardi's trial, after he has been given a two-month prison sentence, Ruth Wolff is tried in the court of public opinion, a television show called 'Take the Debate', in which she faces aggressive questioning from a panel of experts representing a range of different interest groups. This sequence, in which she endeavours to maintain her medical persona on a very different stage, concludes with a ministerial announcement that the incident will be formally investigated. The fifth act/day of both plays is a coda, taking place after Bernhardi's release from prison and after Ruth has been found guilty of bringing discredit upon the profession and effectively struck off. A significant difference is that, whereas Bernhardi has been convicted on the basis of false testimony and is poised to return to medical practice and research following a retrial, Ruth's career is over, and her earlier observation that 'Open-ended isn't great in medicine. Usually means someone's about to enter the past tense' (ibid, p. 18) becomes ominously prophetic as the play closes.

Much of the intellectual freight of Schnitzler's play is carried by a series of highly charged duologues, in which Bernhardi spars with Ebenwald, Flint and the Priest, defending his initial action and his refusal to engage with the subsequent politicisation of his case. Icke retains this feature of *Professor Bernhardi*. He has two confrontations between doctor and priest, with the second, which comes in Schnitzler's fourth act, taking up most of the final 'day' in *The Doctor*. Like Schnitzler's second act, Icke's second 'day' includes a private conversation between the institute's director and her deputy, Hardiman, in which she rejects the proposal that they should appease public opinion by appointing a less qualified, black, Catholic man to a vacant post in preference to a well-qualified, white, Jewish woman. This scene is followed by one between the title figure and Flint, who quickly goes from urging compromise and contrition to promising support. A moral reckoning between this pair, around which Schnitzler builds his final act, becomes a much briefer encounter towards the end of Icke's fourth 'day', after Jemima Flint, like her male namesake, has made a U-turn and ordered an inquiry. It is arguably in the cut and thrust of these duologues, debating the play's key questions, that Schnitzler's voice can be most clearly heard in *The Doctor*. For the knowing spectator, the palimpsestic quality of the adaptation highlights the intractable nature of debates around such principles as appointment purely on merit and personal integrity in public life, as well as the need for constant renegotiation of the relationship between medicine and faith(s).

Searching for a cure

Reflecting on the experience of reading a complete translation of *Professor Bernhardi*, Michael Billington exclaims 'my God, the play is long!' (2015, p. 260). And a well-known actor in the audience for press night at the Almeida was supposedly overheard at the interval to say of Icke's play, 'It's a lot, isn't it?' (Lewis, 2020, p. xvi). Both have a point: *The Doctor* has a running time of approximately two hours and forty-five minutes, while Schnitzler's comedy is always abridged in performance (Schnitzler himself made extensive cuts for the premieres in Berlin and Vienna) and remains even then a substantial, demanding work. Icke's approach is all the more remarkable because, rather than streamlining Schnitzler's play, his version is arguably even more complex and intricately detailed in its presentation of the multiple ways in which modern medicine is entangled in society, politics and life.

Whereas Schnitzler's title figure has no private or family life beyond his affectionate relationship with his son and loyal assistant Oskar, Icke's play reminds its audience forcefully that a doctor is 'a person too' and that their life outside work may be complicated and emotionally draining (2019, p. 105). *The Doctor* is punctuated by scenes between Ruth Wolff and her partner Charlie. The character's gender is not specified in the text, and the role can readily be cast as non-binary. Charlie is a somewhat ghostly figure – in the play's final moments quite literally so – who announces the start of each 'day' to the audience and otherwise exists only alongside Ruth in the domestic sphere, where tea is 'the currency of love' and the sound of a metonymic kettle boiling marks the shift of setting (ibid, p. 17). Charlie acts as a private sounding board for Ruth, thereby further underlining the performative nature of her professional interactions, but never shares the stage with any other character. This demarcation of Charlie as not entirely 'there' in terms of the live theatrical event derives from both Ruth's rigorous compartmentalisation of her life and, increasingly, from the character's cognitive decline: Charlie has dementia. Although it is at first unclear why Ruth has labelled her kitchen cupboards, as early as the second 'day', Charlie struggles to find both objects and words. As memory loss becomes more severe, the lyrics of a favourite song evade recall and, when required to announce the fifth 'day', Charlie no longer knows what 'day' it is. Only when Ruth and Charlie briefly dance together and bodily communication takes over does Charlie seem fully present on stage. This addition to Schnitzler's plot becomes all the weightier as it culminates in Charlie's suicide, using a so-called 'exit hood', so as not to implicate Ruth. Her subsequent explanation of this asphyxiation device – a large plastic bag with an elastic band at the opening – to the priest opens up questions about euthanasia and dementia.[1]

As Elinor Fuchs has observed, dementia seemed in 2017 to become 'the theatre season's "in" disease' (2017a). Featuring in several new plays, it tended to be part of a tragedised narrative of ageing, typically involving a daughter who sacrifices her life to care for an increasingly dependent parent. Although Fuchs was writing about New York, similar observations could be made about London. Florian Zeller's *The Father* (2012), which exemplifies many of the dementia stereotypes, had impressed London audiences before its Broadway transfer in 2017 (Fuchs, 2017b); Terry Johnson's *Prism* (2017) celebrates renowned cinematographer Jack Cardiff through the lens of his Alzheimer's-affected memory; and Lucy Kirkwood's *Mosquitoes* (2017) has a dementia sub-plot involving the once-brilliant mother of particle physicist Alice. By continuing this trend and making dementia part of Ruth Wolff's personal experience, Icke gives his play a bitter underlying irony because the research focus of the Elizabeth Institute is Alzheimer's disease.

The political and institutional machinations of *The Doctor* are thus presented as threatening world-leading, possibly Nobel Prize-winning research into 'a brutal, ugly, merciless disease' (Icke, 2019, p. 102). This context has an analogy in *Professor Bernhardi* for, just as Alzheimer's is incurable and a major cause of social anxiety today, so, in the early twentieth century, was syphilis, to which Schnitzler's play repeatedly alludes (Beniston, 2019, pp. 205–206). Amongst the staff of the Elisabethinum is a professor of dermatology, a specialism that in the early twentieth century included the treatment of sexually transmitted diseases, which characteristically have rashes or skin lesions as primary symptoms. Whenever he is called out 'zu einem ang'steckten Fürsten' [to treat a prince who's caught a dose] (Schnitzler, 2024, p. 18), he is replaced, like the ailing Professor Cresswell in *The Doctor*, by his Jewish assistant, whose latest research output is a 'Serumarbeit' [academic paper on serum] (ibid, p. 28) that Bernhardi regards as 'außerordentlich, richtunggebend' [exceptional, pioneering] (ibid, p. 87).[2] These and other details imply that the topic is syphilis: the causative bacteria were identified in 1905; a reliable serologic test for the disease was developed in 1906; and the first effective treatment, Salversan, came onto the market in 1910. The background of cutting-edge research not only ups the stakes in both plays but also makes available an idealised image of the doctor as an unequivocal force for good. Whereas admiration for the medical profession is not seriously undermined in *Professor Bernhardi*, Icke simultaneously conveys public mistrust of a seemingly closed world of privilege, both in the TV debate and in allowing the dead patient's father to intrude on the back-stage deliberations of the hospital meeting. Furious at being made to wait 'because I don't wear a white coat when I do a day's work' (Icke, 2019, p. 58), he tells them: 'You all protect each other, you people. A little fucking cabal. I've seen it on the TV, incompetence and you kill someone and then it all gets covered up' (ibid, p. 59). It is typical of late twentieth- and twenty-first-century medical drama for patients to have a stronger and more critical voice (Shepherd-Barr, 2016, p. 49). However, one might also observe that, in allowing Ruth to reflect so movingly on Charlie's decline and death, Icke's play simultaneously pleads for greater empathy towards doctors.

'Who gets to choose'

Alongside the figure of Charlie and the resulting personalisation of the socio-medical context, Icke's other substantial (and, in the view of some commentators, unnecessary) addition to *Professor Bernhardi* is the introduction of Sami, a transgender teenager whom Ruth befriends. Their sporadic conversations form the second strand of Ruth's private life, adding depth and complexity to Icke's characterisation of his title figure and to the overall design of *The Doctor* as a meditation on the principle of choice, a topic that brings medicine into conflict not merely with religious faith but with identity politics more broadly.

At the heart of *The Doctor*, as of *Professor Bernhardi*, is the question of patient choice. By refusing the Catholic priest access to the unseen patient, who in Schnitzler's play is barely characterised, Bernhardi imposes his secular definition of 'ein glückliches Sterben' (Schnitzler, 2024, p. 45, literally 'a happy death') as one that is free of fear, pain and distress. This approach generates an ironic role reversal between doctor and priest: the former behaves in the paternalistic manner often regarded as characteristic of a clerical elite, while the latter treats the dying woman as an autonomous human being (Robertson, 1999, p. 109). Ruth Wolff's attitude resembles Bernhardi's: the patient is fourteen years old and semi-conscious. As her parents cannot be contacted, full responsibility lies with the doctor whose name is above her bed,[3] and she endeavours, in an inversion of Schnitzler's phrase, to protect the young woman from 'an unpeaceful death' by denying access first to her boyfriend, whom she has asked for, and then to the Catholic priest who arrives at the behest of her parents. While Ruth effectively assumes the patient's identity in asserting, 'It's my name above her bed', the Priest refers to her by her own name, Emily, and insists that 'she has the right to make her own choice' (Icke, 2019, p. 10). Although it is stressed that Ruth follows General Medical Council guidelines, her actions, like Bernhardi's, generate an ethical dilemma. One way of thinking about it is suggested by the Hippocratic injunction 'first, do no harm', which is printed on the back cover of both playtext and programme, but the play itself complicates matters when Brian Cyprian observes that, in modern medicine, the Hippocratic oath is merely a guideline: 'the thing that really counts is patient choice' (ibid, p. 22), respecting the patient's right to be involved in decisions made about their health care.

While Schnitzler's audience would have been familiar with the significance of the last rites, Icke has the patient's father spell out in graphic terms that for Catholics abortion is a mortal sin and that, because of the doctor's actions, his daughter has died without absolution and gone to hell (ibid, p. 59). For Ruth Wolff, following regulations to the letter, it is, however, not enough that she comes from a Catholic family. She needs incontrovertible proof that the patient has freely chosen that identity rather than merely being born into it. Ruth herself is Jewish but hers, like Bernhardi's, is not a religious identity: 'my Jewishness is cultural if it's anything at all: it's not about believing anything' (ibid, p. 43). Schnitzler observed (around 1912) that it was 'not possible, especially not for a Jew in public life, to ignore the fact that he was a Jew; nobody else was doing so, not the Gentiles and even less the Jews' (Schnitzler, 1971, p. 6). By contrast, Ruth regards it as the positive legacy of the Holocaust that 'we now get to choose what defines us' (Icke, 2019, p. 31). Her choice is to be a doctor, medicine is her God, and the phrase 'I'm a doctor' tellingly concludes her first speech in the play and her last. That she is white, Jewish, well-educated and a woman comes a distant second to her professional identity, and she stonewalls queries about her sexuality, saying 'I don't go in for badges' (ibid, p. 44). Both title figures indeed subscribe to a notion of progress rooted in the values of liberal Enlightenment and conceptualise medicine as a scientific discipline and a humanitarian practice that stands above identity politics: no accommodation between medicine and religious or cultural identities is necessary because 'progress beats identity every single time' (ibid, p. 27). It is a thought-provoking continuity that these secular, humanist values make both Bernhardi and Ruth Wolff into reactionary figures, radically out of step with their time.

The self-identification of Icke's title figure is challenged from every possible angle in the TV debate, as five panellists put it to Ruth that her professional judgement and behaviour towards the patient and priest were informed, perhaps unwittingly, by facets of her own identity and biography – by her 'religious belief' or 'belief about religion' (ibid, p. 80), by the fact that she had an abortion as a teenager and by unconscious bias. As the questioning intensifies, inconsistencies emerge: for example, she defends abortion on the basis of patient choice but denies Emily the right to choose the manner of her death; she advocates appointment on merit but is comfortable with positive discrimination towards women as counteracting 'a systemic imbalance in our field' (ibid, p. 83). In an attention-grabbing directorial intervention, Icke illustrates how unconscious bias might work by creating deliberate dissonances between the identity of the actors and the characters they play: 'the acting should hold the mystery until the play reveals it. The idea is that the audience are made to reconsider characters (and events) as they learn more about who the characters are' (ibid: unnumbered page). Most importantly, the priest is played by a white actor but it emerges that the character is Black. Recorded snatches of the first 'day' are replayed during the TV debate and, in a very Brechtian moment, the audience is asked along with Ruth to reconsider the significance of her calling him 'uppity'. The effect of this unrelenting attack, which has no parallel in Schnitzler's *Professor Bernhardi*, is that Ruth's confidence in her ability to stand above identity politics and be nothing but a doctor is severely eroded. Unlike Bernhardi, who consistently refuses to engage with the politics of his actions, she ultimately acknowledges 'that there is a context bigger than this single incident' (ibid, p. 92).

Schnitzler's play is a comedy; in correspondence and in private reflections on its journalistic reception, he denied that it was a politically tendentious drama pitting medicine against religion, preferring to call it a 'Charakterkomödie' [comedy of character] (Beniston, 2019, p. 197). Bernhardi is likeable, charismatic and retains absolute moral purity. He becomes comic above all because he is naïve, stubborn and constitutionally unsuited to politics. Icke's title figure has wit and verbal dexterity, but her 'trademark disdain' (2019, p. 66) is considerably less appealing than Bernhardi's trademark irony. Her management style is autocratic, and she is admired as a 'woman of integrity' (ibid, p. 42) rather than liked. The points when Ruth acts as 'language police' (ibid, p. 17) may get a sympathetic laugh, especially when she unpicks Sami's teen sociolect, but her linguistic pedantry is also a means of belittling a junior colleague and, as the specialist in postcolonialism points out, identifies her as a member of the educated elite claiming the right to determine what words mean and '[w]ho gets to choose' (ibid, p. 89).

Furthermore, in one key respect, Ruth Wolff fails to maintain her moral integrity. In *Professor Bernhardi*, Flint and the priest have in common that both throw Bernhardi under the metaphorical bus in order not to harm what they perceive as the greater good: Flint's plans to improve medical training and public health, and the priest's continued Christian ministry, both of which would have been endangered had they publicly declared their solidarity with him. Bernhardi, by contrast, retains an aura of moral purity; he is their victim. Icke's minister and priest behave in much the same way as their models: Jemima Flint tells Ruth that there are 'things more important than you' (ibid, p. 94), and the priest privately admits that both acted correctly in their institutional roles but refuses to jeopardise the Church's mission 'for one person's benefit' (ibid, p. 98). However, Icke's title figure cannot claim the same purity of victimhood as Bernhardi. At the end of the TV debate she tries to demonstrate her respect for the choices of others by talking about Sami:

Ruth: I'm – I have a little friend, comes to my house some nights in the week to do her homework, a friend of mine, she was born a boy but now, since I've known her, at this point, for her, she's a she, as far as she's concerned, you know, she wears female clothes: it's what you're saying: she gets to choose. And that is fine by me –

(ibid, p. 90)

Ruth's betrayal of Sami – outing her on national television – disqualifies her from claiming the moral high ground; in an attempt to save herself, she has chosen on behalf of Sami. Whereas she had consistently refused, like Bernhardi, to apologise for her treatment of the dying sepsis patient, the fourth 'day' closes with Sami's rejection of her heartfelt apology. Ruth Wolff is arguably a more flawed character than Bernhardi but, in acknowledging those flaws and suffering more grievously, she acquires a grandeur that even the most philosemitic post-Holocaust stagings cannot give Bernhardi.

The ending of Icke's play is much darker than Schnitzler's, raising the likelihood that, bereft of her career, her partner Charlie, and the 'little friend' who at one point even calls her 'Mum' (ibid, p. 73), Ruth makes the ultimate choice and takes her own life, that the 999 call with which *The Doctor* opens and closes is prompted not by Charlie's death but by her own. This reading is supported by Ruth's reassurance to Sami, as the witch-hunt against her intensifies, that she is not suicidal: 'Don't be scared. If I get there, I'll call the ambulance first, there's no danger of you being the one that finds me. No, I promise you, if I kill myself, I won't leave the clear-up to you' (ibid, p. 74). *The Doctor* is a play in which language is far from innocent or neutral: it looks both backwards and forwards. Words have histories that can reveal unconscious bias and latent meanings that can anticipate futures unbeknown to their speakers: 'When the end comes, it shows itself first in the language' (ibid, p. 73). With the benefit of hindsight Ruth's clinical mantra that 'It's not over 'til there's a body' (ibid, p. 6, 19) speaks of more than merely her patient's fate, just as Sami's furious outburst, 'I hope you fucking literally DIE' (ibid, p. 95), for once does not confuse the literal with the figurative.

Conclusion: medical drama as diagnostic performance

As Ruth Wolff explains to Sami in one of her mellower moments, diagnostic medicine is a 'process of looking at someone, at something about them. Extrapolating evidence. Guessing what will happen to them next' (ibid, p. 18). For all its analytical rigour, it is as much an art as a science, a performance akin to fortune-telling. Social drama may be said to enact a comparable diagnostic process, confronting the spectator with material that is symptomatic of a current concern, attempting to anticipate future developments and perhaps also suggesting remedies. Like their title figures, both *Professor Bernhardi* and *The Doctor* confidently diagnose a septic rottenness in the body politic, one that, once it takes hold, admits no cure. In Schnitzler's Austria, the Enlightenment values that had underpinned the development of nineteenth-century medicine as a scientific discipline and a clinical practice were under threat, challenged by ideologies founded on class, race and religion. With the creation of the NHS in the aftermath of the Second World War, Britain made an emphatic commitment to strengthen social cohesion and build a universal health care system based on rational humanist principles, a consensus project that, *The Doctor* suggests, is undermined by the fragmentation of society into multiple communities and groupings.

Just as there is a sense of lateness in Schnitzler's *Professor Bernhardi*, with the founders of the Elisabethinum looking back nostalgically to the youthful idealism that brought the hospital into being, so there is a moment of wistful reminiscence in Ruth Wolff's final conversation with the priest that goes far beyond the personal: 'I feel things are ending. The post-war institutions, the post-war ideals. The public good that blossomed after peace. All the things they fought for. Starting to crack'. For the priest, whose empathy and emotional intelligence make for a moving crepuscular scene, faith too is 'shedding a skin' (ibid, p. 101), a metaphor that speaks of loss and uncertainty but also of growth and transformation. It is this character to whom Icke gives the play's final insight into the complexities of identity: 'Every person is a city full of people. We all contain a thousand different selves, and – they can't all be equally important. We choose which selves we want to put in charge' (ibid, p. 99). Not to acknowledge this richness and the tensions it generates, to play a single role to the exclusion of all others, is to harm and impoverish the self – a diagnosis of what ails not only the play's title figure but perhaps also the modern polity.

Notes

1 Although Icke was apparently unaware of the parallel at the time of writing, Schnitzler explores the theme of euthanasia in unpublished sketches and drafts that are part of the lengthy genesis of *Professor Bernhardi*. See '*Professor Bernhardi* Entstehungsgeschichte', in *Arthur Schnitzler digital*.

2 References to *Professor Bernhardi* in German are to the reading text in *Arthur Schnitzler digital*, which is based on the first print, published by the Fischer Verlag in Berlin in 1912. Translations are my own.
3 The 'name above the bed' policy, to which *The Doctor* alludes, stipulates that every hospital patient should have a named doctor responsible for their care. It was introduced in the UK in 2014, in the wake of a public inquiry into failings at the Mid Staffordshire NHS Foundation Trust.

Reference list

Allfree, C. (2015) 'Greek hero: how Robert Icke made his three-hour courtroom drama *Oresteia* as relevant as ever', *Evening Standard*, 10 December.

Beniston, J. (2017) 'Doctors talking to doctors in Arthur Schnitzler's *Professor Bernhardi*', in Brodie, G. and Cole, E. (eds.) *Adapting translation for the stage*. London and New York: Routledge, pp. 39–55.

Beniston, J. (2019) 'Schnitzler and the place of tendentious drama: *Professor Bernhardi*', *Austrian Studies*, 27, pp. 195–209.

Billington, M. (2015) *The 101 greatest plays: from antiquity to the present*. London: Guardian Books.

Billington, M. (2019) 'The Doctor review – Robert Icke offers brilliant diagnosis of modern ills', *The Guardian*, 21 August.

Fuchs, E. (2017a) 'Dementia: the theater season's "in" disease, part 1', *The Theatre Times*, 16 January. Available at: https://thetheatretimes.com/dementia-theater-seasons-disease-part-1/ (Accessed: 26 July 2023).

Fuchs, E. (2017b) 'Dementia: last spring, dementia made it to Broadway! part 2', *The Theatre Times*, 4 February. Available at: https://thetheatretimes.com/last-spring-dementia-made-broadway/ (Accessed: 26 July 2023).

Hooker, C. and Dalton, J. (2019) 'The performing arts in medicine and medical education', in Bleakley, A. (ed.) *The Routledge handbook of the medical humanities*. London: Routledge, pp. 205–219.

Hutcheon, L. (2012) *A theory of adaptation*. 2nd edn. London: Routledge.

Icke, R. (2019) *The Doctor: very freely adapted from Arthur Schnitzler's 'Professor Bernhardi'*. London: Oberon Books.

Kay, A. (2017) *This is going to hurt: secret diaries of a junior doctor*. London: Picador.

Kay, A. (2022) *This is going to hurt*. BBC TV Miniseries.

Lewis, H. (2020) 'Introduction', in Icke, R. *Works one*. London: Oberon Books, pp. vii–xxvi.

Nuy, S. (2010) 'Vom Komödienspiel der Politik: *Professor Bernhardi* im Fernsehen', in Aurnhammer, A., Beßlich, B. and Denk, R. (eds.) *Arthur Schnitzler und der Film*. Würzburg: Ergon Verlag, pp. 297–316.

Robertson, R. (1999) *The 'Jewish question' in German literature 1749–1939: emancipation and its discontents*. Oxford: Oxford University Press.

Schnitzler, A. (1912) *Professor Bernhardi*. Berlin: Fischer.

Schnitzler, A. (1971) *My youth in Vienna*. Translated by C. Hutter. London: Weidenfeld and Nicolson.

Schnitzler, A. (2024) *Professor Bernhardi*. Ed. by Beniston, J. with Babelotzky, G. *et al.*, in Lukas, W., Scheffel, M., Webber, A. and Beniston, J. in collaboration with Burch, T. (eds.) *Arthur Schnitzler digital. Digitale historisch-kritische Edition (Werke 1905–1931)*. Wuppertal, Cambridge, Trier 2018 ff. Available at: https://www.cam.ac.uk/Schnitzler-Edition

Shepherd-Barr, K.E. (2016) 'The diagnostic gaze: nineteenth-century contexts for medicine and performance', in Mermikides, A. and Bouchard, G. (eds.) *Performance and the medical body*. London: Bloomsbury Methuen Drama Publishing, pp. 37–49.

11

THE EXCESS AND THE ERASED

Dramaturgical notes on performing care in medical education

James Dalton and Claire Hooker

In medical education, students experience pressures from the norms of professional socialisation (such as sometimes suppressed emotion, a highly disciplined body and ruthless time management). They are also invited, and often deeply desire, to authentically care for their patients. How does one meet professional expectations *and* care for patients when these ends are not always aligned? In this chapter we consider how students do this by illuminating the negotiation as both performance and performative. We address our question by examining specific experiences of final-year medical students who are learning to enact professional care in the high-pressure setting of a major metropolitan teaching hospital in Australia.

Illuminating the socialisation of medical students through performance is of interest as we consider now a time of significant transition. A shift, perhaps a culture change, is taking place. Doctors were formerly considered to hold unchallenged medical authority and exercise it over patients, students and other practitioners in the inflexible hierarchy of the hospital (Willis, 2020). The social hierarchy of the hospital reflected an epistemic hierarchy in which the 'biomedical model' of disease dominated diagnosis as treatment, largely excluding patient experience and values as well as other forms of knowledge and therapeutic practice (Carel and Kidd, 2014). But now, old hierarchies and norms are being questioned, doctors increasingly need to work in multidisciplinary teams, and we aspire to health care that is values based and patient centred in its delivery (Thistlethwaite, 2012; Kitson *et al.*, 2013; Delaney, 2018). We say more about this transition in the following section. Hierarchical relations, however, continue alongside team interactions in hospital and other health care settings; patients may experience both disempowerment and agency in their interactions with their clinicians, and medical students must work out, through their practice, how to navigate the tensions between the new ideals and the persistent pressures, between older and newer ways of knowing, being and doing (Scott *et al.*, 2015).

How do they do this, and how can they find their way to the ideals of patient-centred care? To explore medical student experience in this transitional context, one author, Dalton, undertook nine months of fieldwork in 2019. Dalton is a theatre-maker and researcher who applies theatre and performance methodologies to understand medical socialisation and learning. His fieldwork included following a cohort of final-year medical students as they interacted with peers, superiors and patients in an Australian major metropolitan teaching hospital, observing as they learned to perform as doctors. We applied a dramaturgical lens to Dalton's fieldwork observations, analysing

DOI: 10.4324/9781003036500-14

for performances of professionalism and performances of care. We share moments where these align, or diverge, in this chapter. In Australia, senior medical students experience a clinical phase in teaching hospitals and participate in treating real patients under the guidance of senior doctors. This is a complex time: students may conduct procedures under supervision and attend ward rounds as if already doctors while also engaging in more structured pedagogical practices. These practices include 'bedside tutorials', where a consultant teaches a class of students with patients in the hospital, and a 'long case history', a specific form of medical interview between a single student and consenting patient. Students apply their knowledge and skills with patients, each interaction offering a moment for the student to perform one 'way' to the exclusion of potential others. How students perform in these moments reveals flickers of their emergent 'identities' – as medical professionals and moral agents – amid the contradictory pressures of patient-centred ideals and constrained and hierarchical health services.

To highlight the particularity of moment-to-moment events, we present our analysis through *ekphrasis*: vignettes written to draw a reader's senses, emotions and attention into an otherwise absent experience. Each vignette amplifies a moment where students enacted their becoming doctors, written to draw attention to how students negotiate specific relationships while enmeshed in the limited institutional affordances of professional expectations and appraisal from their supervisors. Our hope is to encourage reflection and to imagine how future performances may show embodied, attentive and particularist 'radical performativities of care' (Hamington, 2015).

The following sections serve as a primer. Readers may look for signs in each vignette that a performance, of professionalism or of care, comes at the expense of the other: something is offered but ignored and becomes 'excess' to the clinical encounter, or something occurs but is actively 'erased'. By 'excess' we mean elements present in an experience construed as unnecessary to clinical judgement. Doctors and students bracket these out when perceiving, discussing and responding to interactions with patients as medical practice. By 'erased' we refer to a conscious, intentional masking of elements by doctors and students – such as withholding information or diverting attention. In the past the excess and erased have been prominent features of medical authority in clinical consultations – doctors were notorious for failing to listen to patients, for example, often interrupting them in medical history taking (Menz and Al-Roubaie, 2008; Danczak, 2015) or withholding information, such as a terminal diagnosis. We were therefore sensitised to them in our analysis. Today, 'patient-centred' practice should in theory not contain or produce either excess or erasure. But to what degree is this the case?

A time of transition

Medical schools are required to produce graduates who have learned 'professionalism', 'the cornerstone for safe, effective and ethical health care practice' (Kirk, 2007; Australian Medical Association, 2015; Monash University, no date). Professionalism is a complicated, slippery concept; it encompasses the maintenance of both ethical and clinical standards. In the twenty-first century, treating patients with respect, empathy and compassion is seen as central to medical professionalism. Instead of considering patients lay people whose narratives contain excessive information unnecessary for diagnosis, patients are now discursively positioned as 'experts' in their own lived experience.

In the introduction, we thumbnail-sketched the transitions in medical culture and practice in terms of shifts in social and epistemic authority. But the transition could be expressed in other terms as well. For example, as others have commented, until recently, medicine has instantiated and reproduced the ideologies and power relations of modernity (Pringle, 1998): dualistic, it discursively opposed mind and body, subject and object, active and passive, the knower and the known, (hard) reason and (soft) emotion; by corollary, male and female, doctor and patient. In this ideological and social system, physicians held (explicitly) 'God-like' status. They held almost unquestionable epistemic authority in invulnerable bodies – failure was inadmissible – and ethical patient care was constructed in the terms of patronage: it was the doctor's ethical responsibility to know, and enact, what was best for the patient.

Decades of challenge to medical power from patient groups have slowly eroded this paradigm and sought to replace it with 'values-based medicine', 'shared decision making' and 'patient-centred care' and, in the process, have laid bare all the social and discursive foundations of medical power. This has finally brought *doctors themselves* into discursive view. No longer all-knowing brains, very recently, doctors have become *situated* (Haraway, 1988), fallible and vulnerable people with bodies and families. They are faced with navigating still vertiginously hierarchical, competitive and demanding health service institutions in which patients are positioned as consumers. Medical students must construct a version of 'professionalism' that holds on to their expertise and (some) authority while being simultaneously committed to patient autonomy and patient care.

A senior medical student in the past was expected to cope with teaching by humiliation, the distress of witnessing suffering and death and excessive workload without comment or complaint or stumbling (Scott *et al.*, 2015). A senior medical student today is required to both build and demonstrate technical competencies *and* show empathy and experience failures and learning moments. They must demonstrate certain professional qualities *while also* navigating relationships across peers, patients, institutions, teaching and non-teaching supervisors, senior health care workers in other disciplines and hospital management. The resulting performances are unavoidably complex.

Performances by medical students

Here we follow Alex Mermikides's term 'medical performance', a constellation of practices emerging in the twenty-first century which interrelate health care, medical professions, patients, social interests and artistic projects across a panoply of sites and agencies traditionally siloed to either artistic or medical experiences (Mermikides, 2020). Performances are 'events' separated from others by demarcating time and space, presenting 'human activity' by at least one human to another, performative in their 'intention . . . to make something happen, to change what the participants and those who view them know, feel, understand and might do as a result' and are 'live encounters' seeding a reciprocal potential in the relationship between the humans involved in the performance (Mermikides, 2020, p. 4). This definition resonates with a transition in medical education from encoding students with a boilerplate 'professionalism' to a nuanced theory of students developing their own 'medical identity' (Monrouxe, 2016). Every medical student is a specific doctor-in-training, learning through study and experience to 'become' a doctor who is authentic to themselves while also maintaining a standard of professionalism for patient and community wellbeing (Hafferty, 2016, pp. 56–57).

Not only do medical students enact professionalism for their peers and supervisors, but we suggest they become doctors in the teaching hospital through performances of *care*. Care-as-performance emerges out of the moral theory of feminist care ethics. Early feminist theorists developed care ethics as a normative morality based in the specific needs of people cared for in interpersonal relationships rather than universal principles or abstract equations. It is a morality of the lived experiences of caring labour, grounded in the 'feminine' realm of the family and home (Gilligan, 2003, p. 19; Noddings, 2013, pp. ix–xvi). Care ethicists claim this as a distinct moral theory, capable of challenging oppressive structures, including in settings where caring labour occurs – in health care institutions, for example (Held, 2005, p. 10). Maurice Hamington has extended this line of thinking to argue that care is both radical and, key to our analysis, performative (2015). He argues that care is a *doing* more than it is a virtue, disposition or value. In this chapter, attending to the tenuous navigation of medical performances in a clinical setting illuminates Hamington's performative qualities of care:

> *Care is a political embodied performance, every iteration of which has the potential to contribute to our dynamic sense of moral identity, adds to our disruptive knowledge of the other, and supports the notion that ethical understanding is a mind-body activity that is ripe for autopoetic development.*

> (2015, p. 280, original emphasis)

Medical students in this time of patient-centred and values-based medicine embody a *moral identity* through their performances in clinical events. How they personally enact the ethics and values of their training towards care (primarily for patients but also for themselves and others in the hospital) is core to their 'becoming' doctors, and beyond, to how their actions constitute professionalised medicine here and now. It is the subtle, sometimes ephemeral, transient ways in which this occurs that we set out in this chapter.

How do students negotiate what is most appropriate to perform in becoming a doctor? How *is* and how *might* a more compassionate health care be *performed*? Our vignettes are one approach to answering this, proposing Hamington's radical performativities of care as the key register of change. By combining observed performances – the 'how *is*' – with an ekphrastic mode of writing, we stimulate readers to respond towards the 'how *might*'. Our method for collecting such diverse student performances in a complex Australian teaching hospital was 'negotiated interactive observation', a mode of ethnographic fieldwork developed specifically for health care settings (Wind, 2008). Dalton, being neither medical personnel nor patient, could not participate directly in the daily experiences of the hospital; his role as observer was always in a process of negotiation. Specifically, theatre-makers in a hospital site pose uncertain risks in an already compromised environment (Brodzinski, 2010, p. 18). For this reason, Dalton was not present when students, supervisors and patients withheld consent.

Our heuristic for analysing medical performance for tensions of professionalism and care was to look for instances when something emerges as *excess* or becomes *erased*. We recognise that the excess and erased are contextual and mutable. The narrative medicine movement, for example, introduced physicians to analytical tools from literature studies, which encourage observing how a patient describes their illness, including the types of words used and narrative structure of their medical history, and considering these as part of a medical diagnosis (Charon, 2006). A post-narrative-medicine medical student will find less about their patient's account clearly definable as 'excess'. A similar distinction between a contemporary medical student and their equivalent in the twentieth century is the improvement in patient rights for access to information about their diagnosis.

Yet, despite these and other changes to medical authority and practice, doctors and medical students remain time-poor, health systems remain complex and patients remain diverse in their preferences and the amount of information they want, among other things. Hence observing, or feeling for, the excess and erased guides our chapter. Moment-to-moment, students perform something that *is* medicine and represent medical authority through embodying professional sensibility, communication and comportment. How students and their supervisors excise or erase elements moment-to-moment adumbrates medicine in that particular event. It may be the case that twenty-first century medicine is becoming more patient centred and values based, but specific events and their circumstances afford performances messier than abstract principles.

Dramaturgy and *ekphrasis*

In the jointly clinical and pedagogical setting of the teaching hospital, our excess/erased heuristic balances on the tension between professionalism-as-performance and care-as-performance. This is not to say professionalism and care are necessarily antonymous. Rather, this is a tension of relational affordances – in a given moment, for example, does a medical student focus on the specific, radical needs of a patient or a colleague in distress, or do they focus on the pedagogical framing of the relationship? How possible is it to attend authentically to all relationships in a clinical event? In framing the teaching hospital as a site of multiple performances stretched across complex events, we sit in a fuzzy space – a student leaves a patient having experienced a 'learning moment', one amid many during the day; that patient experienced an encounter with a person of medical authority, another chapter in their unique health care history.

The following vignettes respond to these complexities as dramaturgical potential, re-presenting the complex affect and affordances of observed student experiences. We are guided by Hamington's conception of care ethics as radically performative in their construction. First, care ethics recognises the importance of emotion as moral guide. Our use of affect to prompt response reflects this. Second, care ethics centralises relations of interdependence and dependence and the ethical qualities of these relations, performed through the elements of attentiveness and responsiveness to the other and of competence and responsibility in one's self. Our analysis is sensitive to how students accrete their professional identity through relational performances – embodied, ethical and entangled with others (Hamington, 2015, p. 280). Third, caring is particularist. It is experienced individually and, crucially, through and in the body: 'if care is indeed performative, then . . . understanding care is tied to attending to physicality, bodily comportment, and proximity as well as cognitive consideration of morality' (Hamington, 2015, p. 280). Physicality, proximity and bodily comportment emerge as central motifs in our vignettes, centring unique, embodied actors. This includes two categories of actor who are discursively rarely recognised as embodied (usually only patients have bodies): medical students and Dalton, the researcher.

Hamington argues that a key aspect of care-as-performance is that it reveals *disruptive knowledge*, 'the kind of information about the other that is compelling and disrupts our lives to the point of motivating emotion and action' (2015, p. 280). Care is a knowledge-disruptor of 'how things have been' and the 'how *is*', requiring medical students to be present and navigate what is excess, or should be erased, in every new moment. For Hamington, after Butler, the moral identity of a carer – here medical students becoming doctors – is instantiated through a 'stylised repetition of acts' (Butler, quoted in Hamington, 2015, p. 282). How students become doctors and how they care for patients, peers and selves moment to moment will in the longer term constitute their 'dynamic sense of moral identity' (Hamington, 2015, p. 280), alongside their socialised professional one (Hafferty, 2016; Monrouxe, 2016).

Theatre and performance-makers, no strangers to the immediate, compelling or disruptive, can offer a dramaturgy for medical student performance in clinical settings. Developing the following vignettes as *ekphrasis* is one means of delivering this. As a mode of writing, *ekphrasis* approximates the experience of an absent image or object to bring a reader into a sensorial, emotive relationship with it. More than narration, *ekphrasis* represents embodied, material elements (Zeitlyn, 2014, p. 343). Each vignette is an exercise in applying Dalton's theatrical sensibility, a perception 'characterized by a sensitivity and consciousness to the *dramaturgy* of lived and represented experience' (Mermikides, 2020, p. 29, original emphasis), to draw a reader's attention to where he felt something excised or erased. Dalton's observations, analysis and representations remain partial, with their own excesses and erasures; therefore these vignettes are purposefully open, seeking to disrupt and encourage a reader's own attentive care to what they find strange, imagining how else these performances might be.

I. Interruptions

I join a group of medical students for their weekly bedside tutorial session, led by a consultant at the hospital. Tradition calls for students to dress conservatively when on the wards and to 'not dress better than the consultants'; we are a chorus of whites, greys, blues and beige to the consultant's tailored purple suit and antique cowboy boots. Today we visit a patient in a single-occupancy room on the oncology ward, carrying spare chairs with us like gifts to a party. Student faces and torsos relax into a polite stillness from which they might smile in encouragement or furrow in compassion when required. I mirror their rehearsed comportment of 'detached concern'. The eight of us fan around the perimeter of the spacious room. Do their pulses thud as much as mine?

The patient greets us from a bed below a bright canopy of flowers: banksias, grevillea and callistemon. A single fan rattles, smudging hot, muggy air across the patient's torso. They are as topless as a sunbather, their face beaming with beachside enthusiasm. At the patient's side sits their sister knitting woollen green and white, skilled hands moving in patterns, her attention saved for her sibling. She brought a picnic: honey, nuts and fresh fruit, in sealable glass tubs arranged on a small bedside table. Such virile pleasance cannot mask the preservative tang of antiseptic chemicals, nor the patient's physical condition. The broad anatomy of their skeleton, the deep hollows, their stretched skin, all the craft of voracious tumours demanding more than one metabolism can give. Every student writes a word, one I will not hear spoken in this room: *cachexia*. Medical cant, from the Greek 'bad condition'.

The consultant kneels close at the patient's elbow while the students and I sit with our chairs in a horseshoe-shaped audience. Peacock-suited and naked chest, the strange pair lean towards one another as co-conspirators, the floral bed a mystical, private moment the rest of us are desecrating. The consultant has a 'detached concern' as bespoke as his suit; his warmth towards the patient feels genuine to me; and when he invites the group to introduce ourselves he winks at the patient, promising them he has not given away any hints. Consultant and patient already know their diagnosis, so why does this patient consent to the demands of a bedside tutorial? They already have a visitor. There is no journal at their side for taking notes.

For the students, this bedside tutorial is an exercise in applying academic knowledge under real circumstances to correctly diagnose a patient's illness. Students 'take lead' in turns, week to week, one interviewing a patient while their peers silently observe. Under the consultant's guidance they will translate this conversation into a medical case history, which the group will debrief on afterwards, out of the patient's earshot. Today's lead is new to the class, having only met the consultant minutes earlier, and this is his first time interviewing a real patient in front of an audience. He pulls his chair out of the horseshoe, closer to the foot of the bed. The patient, propped against pillows, straightens their posture in a playful attention. There is a pause.

'So, what happened that has brought you here today?' the lead asks.

The patient relays a story they would have told to many others since arriving at the hospital. They were swimming in the ocean, something they did all their life, but a wave caught them hard and broke one of their arms. The lead nods encouragement to the story, leaning forward in their chair.

'I tumbled about like in a washing machine', the patient recalls.

'Wow, that sounds like quite the experience', the lead replies, 'can I ask you a question about your –'

'That would've been scary', the consultant interrupts. He gently clasps the patient's arm, drawing their attention back to him.

'I've never been so frightened in my life', the patient says.

The consultant and lead make eye contact. Now the lead asks about the patient's experience in the ocean. This part of the story feels less rote, the patient paddling through a memory, struggling back to shore. A second time the consultant cuts through the lead's attempted follow-up question.

'Yes, I'm interested now though in whether or not you have enough information about what the acute issue is – if you were in emergency what questions would you be asking here?'

The lead pauses, perhaps to visualise being in the hospital's emergency department, perhaps to process his mistake in focusing on the ocean. He asks now about the broken arm, and this line of questioning runs uninterrupted until the patient shares their experiences with cancer.

Again the consultant squeezes a pause at the patient's wrist, the two leaning back into their eye-to-eye conference. The patient seems to speak only with the consultant now, whose listening face settles into a soft sobriety, the comfort one might find in a warm mug after escaping rain. Their focused intimacy lulls me, until the consultant cleaves a sentence with a sharp turn to a different line of questioning. Without waiting for response, he pulls away and brings the rest of us back.

'It is important to know when to interrupt your patient, to find important detail in what they're saying, and go deeper', he tells the lead.

The lead and some other students make a note.

'Can I interrupt?' the patient asks, their finger raised.

'Of course!' the consultant says, smiling at the patient.

'I've a side note to make', the patient says to the students, 'that through diet alone, no extra medication, I shrunk the tumour in my [organ]'.

No one says or writes a word this time.

'I just want you all to take note of that', the patient says.

The consultant nods. Still, no students record this observation, despite their eager note-taking throughout the interview.

Once the lead solves the puzzle of diagnosis, the consultant asks the patient, 'What do you want? What do you want to be able to do after all of this?' He emphasises 'all of this' with a circular wave of his hand, polishing an invisible mirror in our direction.

They plan to return to the ocean. A surfing trip, three months from now.

The students all write this down. I do too.

'It's your task to hear this', the consultant instructs the class, 'and think about what will help your patient achieve this, as well as what is going to fix their condition'.

Returning to the patient's gaze, the consultant presses their wrist a final time.

'Thank you, you've been so gracious with your time. We've kept you long enough'.

Today there is no time for a debrief, our session ran longer than usual. The consultant ends the session out in the corridor, offering only grave advice: 'When you hear the patient speak about what they want, you have to use your gut feeling and work out what is realistic for them'.

The following week the tutorial group and I do manage to debrief with the consultant about the patient beneath the flowers. He recounts being stopped by the sister as he left the room and her saying, 'Something's not right, no one gave me any sense of time'.

The consultant was not the patient's treating physician.

'It's not my place to say', he had replied, 'but I'd prepare myself'.

II. Bullshit

'Brogue' already knows he wants to be a surgeon and makes it no secret that he thinks long case histories are 'bullshit'. He models himself on 'The Fat Man', a character in Samuel Shem's 1978 satirical novel *House of God*: street-wise, cynical and filled with aggressive axioms for surviving as a junior doctor. Bullshit or not, long case histories are part of his final year assessments, and in two hours he must present one to his supervisor. Interviewing and physically examining a patient will easily take one hour of this narrow window.

We find today's patient perched at the edge of their bed, one of four in the room, and they've drawn the curtain for some privacy. Brogue greets the patient, his hand held out, a manilla folder tucked under his arm. He is cheerful but business-like. Brogue introduces me as a PhD student without any medical experience.

'This is my medical history, all of the medications I'm on', the patient says, handing a piece of paper to Brogue.

'Oh thank you, but the exercise is for me to get this out of you', Brogue replies, pushing the sheet back.

A nurse on the ward had suggested this patient to Brogue, referring to them as 'interesting'. The patient tells us they have qualifications in physics and biomedicine.

'That means doctors can't bullshit me', the patient says.

Usually students commence their interview with a standard question, such as 'Please tell me what brings you here today', but the patient initiates instead with an account of their career, running alongside their decades-long convoluted medical history, punctuating key events with finger taps on the rejected sheet of paper.

'Woah, hold up, you're giving me all your secrets before I start', Brogue says, raising his hand to stop the patient. 'Let's go to the beginning'.

'Nah, it's just my chit-chat', the patient replies.

'So tell me, this visit, why are you in today?' Brogue asks. His demeanour is friendlier than his words suggest, but I feel like he is trying to close a deal.

The patient sits back, looks at Brogue, and says with cool brevity: 'Well, I had to come in and change the battery for my IPG'.

Brogue nods at the acronym, making a note on the manila folder, and gestures at me across the bed.

'Just so James can keep up with the conversation, could you please tell him what IPG means', Brogue says.

'Implantable pulse generator', the patient tells me. I thank them, making a note of it. Brogue later vents to a classmate in the student common room, asking if they had heard of an IPG before. The classmate responds by throwing their arms up in mock disgust, walking away and yelling, 'Get that away from me!'

I think the patient wants Brogue to grasp a pattern in their medical history, twisting back and forth along the injuries and medical interventions across the decades of their life. Brogue interjects throughout, light-hearted with flecks of urgency in the speed and volume of his voice. There is a methodical structure to the long case questions he needs for his assessment, but the patient is a tenacious storyteller.

'This is important, because you see I was given only months to live', the patient says, raising their volume above one of Brogue's interruptions, 'and that meant I could be a guinea pig for the implant in its PMA phase'.

Brogue quietens down to listen but prompts the patient to 'let James know what PMA means'.

We *both* learn it means 'pre-market approval', and the patient sees Brogue writing this down after they've explained it. They pause for Brogue to finish, and then say, 'It's good you have to do this'. The patient reminds me of a tough but fair teacher, especially when Brogue attempts another misdirection, this time in response to the patient describing a particular medical crisis. They ask Brogue, 'This was fight/flight, and what happens then?'

Brogue asks them to explain the mechanism to me.

'You're the doctor', the patient says, 'you tell me'.

'You're teaching me more than I'm teaching you', concedes Brogue, 'please, go on'.

Brogue must conclude with a physical examination; otherwise, his supervisor will mark him 'not yet competent'. He and the patient continue to talk, Brogue asking questions to collect information at the same time as he examines the patient. Other physical examinations I've observed are quiet, soft moments of tender interaction; Brogue and the patient crack jokes at one another and move like siblings trying to win at tickling.

'So many injuries', Brogue laughs, 'you've been busy!'

He pushes at the patient's arms. For a moment the pair look like they are wrestling. Their eyes fixed, hands locked, both exerting force against the other. Four arms wobble with the tension.

'It's good to do this with a patient who's so much stronger than me for once', Brogue says.

Letting go, the patient replies, 'You need to go to the gym more'.

Brogue scoffs, 'You'd be surprised how little time in the day there is for that'. He looks down at his watch and asks, 'Think I've got enough of the history? This is going to take hours to decipher now!'

We all laugh and Brogue thanks the patient, shaking their hand and immediately applying hand sanitiser from a pump by the bed. Once beyond the patient's view, Brogue all but jogs ahead of me. He has just under an hour to condense his notes into something he can sufficiently deliver to his supervisor. Usually students take the stairs, but today he needs the elevator. Just before the doors open, I catch a Fat Man glint in his eye.

'That's the problem with a patient who is medical', he says, 'who is in a medical field, that is. They assume they know more'.

Conclusion: *ekphrasis* of an excessive body

The previous vignettes illuminate enactments perhaps anticipated from teaching hospital fieldwork; students interact with patients, peers and supervisors in a formal activity. However, care is a radical performativity. The corporeal reality of medical students, and all health care workers, is rarer to grasp in a professional environment that provides little affordance for their care needs. This final vignette serves as a conclusion by drawing attention to the complexity of presence when serving between professional expectations and patient care. A dramaturgy for medical education towards more compassionate performances of health care attends also to that which we erase of ourselves, how we exclude our being in moments of care for others. What follows comes from before the COVID-19 pandemic and is of a researcher's embodied experience.

We leave you, reader, to what it foreshadows.

The corridors choke today. Our tutorial group moves single file, sidestepping flocks of hospital staff administering perpetual triage. Patients lie prone on couches, some with IV bags jury-rigged beside coffee tables. They call it Category Three. The hospital has more patients than beds.

'Bad influenza season', the tutor says, 'the GPs are so busy, they're sending their patients to Emergency'.

We stop at a door marked with an alarming orange sign: Contact Precaution. A student hands me a bundle of blue plastic personal protective equipment, though the tutor voices his preference for 'the white ones'. They're cooler apparently. What I have is a torso-shaped garbage bag, a long-sleeved apron made from impermeable plastic that clings by a loop stretched around my neck. The patient has a vicious bacterial infection, so I need not worry about a face-mask, just a pair of thick latex gloves. Already I'm sweating. The latex puckers around my fingers, too small for my hands, but everyone else is already in the room.

The tutor has us stand in a line to face the patient at a safe distance, a parade of blue soldiers, and I am vigilant to the slightest fidget I make, each one farting a loud squeak from the PPE. It is a busy day. The air is broth. Usually we would sit, but this patient has the luxury of a single-bed room only because of the infection risk. There's only one chair anyway, pushed out of the way against the wall.

Note-taking is a struggle in the gloves. I cannot feel the pen and my handwriting wilts illegibly on the page. The conversation has become too medical, too dense for me to follow. I try to jot the details of the room. I yawn. I abandon my notes. I pretend to listen. Whenever someone speaks I look them in the eyes. My puckered gloves are slick from my repeated brow-wiping. I cannot stop yawning. My mouth feels gummy. Sweat marbles my arm hair in swirls against the PPE's transparent sleeves.

My faint begins as curious architecture: why did I not notice this room had a slant? Then, a cold tingle from my forehead cascades down, its icy granules hiss through cheeks and the back of my head. I hear a loud clatter, someone's dropped their pen. A student looks at me. I leer back at him. 'This is a joke, I'm making a joke', I think I try to say. People try to say something to me, but all I hear is deep whale song below a buzzing frequency. Lights too bright. Hands at my shoulders. I tumble backwards down a hill that was not there before.

When I later apologise to the tutor for interrupting the class, he smiles.

'Oh god no, you're fine. There isn't a week that goes by that someone doesn't faint around here. Happens all the time', he says, 'don't eat much, don't sit down; we're just so bloody awful to ourselves'.

Reference list

Australian Medical Association (2015) *Medical professionalism – 2010. revised 2015.* Available at: www.ama. com.au/position-statement/medical-professionalism-2010-revised-2015 (Accessed: 12 September 2022).

Brodzinski, E. (2010) *Theatre in health and care.* London: Palgrave Macmillan UK.

Carel, H. and Kidd, I.J. (2014) 'Epistemic injustice in healthcare: a philosophical analysis', *Medicine, Health Care and Philosophy*, 17(4), pp. 529–540.

Charon, R. (2006) *Narrative medicine: honoring the stories of illness.* Oxford: Oxford University Press.

Danczak, A. (2015) 'British GPs keep going for longer: is the 12 second interruption history?', *British Medical Journal*, 351, p. h6136.

Delaney, L.J. (2018) 'Patient-centred care as an approach to improving health care in Australia', *Collegian*, 25(1), pp. 119–123.

Gilligan, C. (2003) *In a different voice: psychological theory and women's development.* Cambridge, MA: Harvard University Press.

Hafferty, F.W. (2016) 'Socialization, professionalism, and professional identity formation', in Cruess, R.L., Cruess, S.R. and Steinert, Y. (eds.) *Teaching medical professionalism.* 2nd edn. Cambridge: Cambridge University Press, pp. 54–67.

Hamington, M. (2015) 'Politics is not a game', in Engster, D. and Hamington, M. (eds.) *Care ethics and political theory.* Oxford: Oxford University Press.

Haraway, D. (1988) 'Situated knowledges: the science question in feminism and the privilege of partial perspective', *Feminist Studies*, 14(3), pp. 575–599.

Held, V. (2005) *The ethics of care: personal, political, and global*. New York: Oxford University Press.

Kirk, L.M. (2007) 'Professionalism in medicine: definitions and considerations for teaching', *Baylor University Medical Center Proceedings*, 20(1), pp. 13–16.

Kitson, A. *et al.* (2013) 'What are the core elements of patient-centred care? A narrative review and synthesis of the literature from health policy, medicine and nursing: core elements of patient-centred care', *Journal of Advanced Nursing*, 69(1), pp. 4–15.

Menz, F. and Al-Roubaie, A. (2008) 'Interruptions, status and gender in medical interviews: the harder you brake, the longer it takes', *Discourse & Society*, 19(5), pp. 645–666.

Mermikides, A. (2020) *Performance, medicine and the human*. London: Bloomsbury Methuen Drama Publishing.

Monash University (no date) *Definition of professionalism*. Available at: www.monash.edu/medicine/study/student-services/definition-of-professionalism (Accessed: 12 September 2022).

Monrouxe, L.V. (2016) 'Theoretical insights into the nature and nurture of professional identities', in Cruess, R.L., Cruess, S.R. and Steinert, Y. (eds.) *Teaching medical professionalism*. 2nd edn. Cambridge: Cambridge University Press, pp. 37–53.

Noddings, N. (2013) *Caring: a relational approach to ethics & moral education*. 2nd edn. updated. Berkeley, CA: University of California Press.

Pringle, R. (1998) *Sex and medicine: gender, power and authority in the medical profession*. Cambridge: Cambridge University Press.

Scott, K.M. *et al.* (2015) '"Teaching by humiliation" and mistreatment of medical students in clinical rotations: a pilot study', *Medical Journal of Australia*, 203(4), pp. 185–185.

Thistlethwaite, J.E. (2012) *Values-based interprofessional collaborative practice: working together in health care*. Cambridge: Cambridge University Press.

Willis, E. (2020) *Medical dominance*. London and New York: Routledge.

Wind, G. (2008) 'Negotiated interactive observation: doing fieldwork in hospital settings', *Anthropology & Medicine*, 15(2), pp. 79–89.

Zeitlyn, D. (2014) 'Antinomies of representation: anthropology as an ekphrastic process', *HAU: Journal of Ethnographic Theory*, 4(3), pp. 341–362.

12

HIDDEN DRESS CODES

Wearing the role of physician

Gretchen A. Case

Despite sustained efforts by many health care systems in the United States to flatten hierarchies and move toward a paradigm in which every member of the health care team (including the patient and patient's family and support network) is equally important, the physician holding a medical degree remains the primary icon of medicine in the US. This iconic status comes with a physical representation of the physician that is hard to remove from the public imaginary. Dress codes for physicians are both symbolic and functional, with at least two explicit goals: making the physician recognisable as a member of their profession and allowing optimal performance of their professional tasks. However, just as medical education recognises an informal or 'hidden' curriculum, in which trainees learn by observation (rather than by being instructed formally) how to comport themselves as physicians, there is also an informal or 'hidden' dress code. This hidden dress code often begins with a formally regulated or traditional dress code but includes important variations performed by individuals and subcultures of physicians that symbolise identity and inclusion to those who recognise them. Here, I address wearable symbols, the white coat, scrubs, and stethoscopes, which are strongly identified with the image of a physician.

I have an unusual perspective on the ways physicians present themselves, as a non-medical member of the faculty at the University of Utah School of Medicine, on a health sciences campus at a large, regional academic medical centre in the western United States. As a scholar steeped in performance studies from my early university days through to my PhD, I emerged from my education acculturated fully into a way of knowing that begins with performance. My primary lens on the world assumes that humans perform multiple roles, wear costumes, use props, and respond to cultural scripts not only on recognised stages but as part of everyday life. Because performance studies crosses so productively into fields such as cultural studies and anthropology, I have been pulled in my work toward understanding how culture and performance inflect each other. I am intrigued and confused by medicine as culture, an interest sparked by my own significant experiences in the patient role and by studying the experiences of other people who interact with medicine. This is a confusion that matters; a better understanding of both broadly drawn and highly localised cultures of medicine is potentially productive for both patients and clinicians.

For fifteen years, keeping a lens of performance firmly in place, I have been observing the costumes and props that physicians wear and use every day. These observations are not part of the work I am paid to do, which is to teach the arts and humanities as part of a medical curriculum.

DOI: 10.4324/9781003036500-15

I was not hired to be an observer, but I cannot help but observe learners acculturating into their new habitus as they study medicine. When I began teaching in medical schools after years in performance studies and theatre classrooms, I was plunged into an extraordinarily different milieu, one in which analyses of everyday performance are not taught or valued in the same way as scientific findings or treatment algorithms. In the medical world, 'costume' and 'prop' sound diminishing to anyone who does not hear these words used as part of a larger lexicon of performance, in which they are essential elements.

However, I have realised that I have been using these terms to mean attire and objects that have been assigned to a character, with no agency on the part of the character to change them. Designers for theatrical or other performances create costumes and props for performing bodies and expect them to be used as designed and directed. Physicians and trainees significantly and continuously alter their costumes and props, in ways unlikely to be tolerated in formally staged performances. The white coat, scrubs, and stethoscope might be status symbols, but they are not static symbols. Here, I will establish the importance of applying a lens of performance to the attire and artifacts of the medical profession. Avoiding the temptation to force a theatrical framework, I use the existing academic literature in medicine and health care, rather than performance and theatre studies, to present a brief history of dress codes and traditions as well as current approaches to dressing the part of physician.

From black to white coats

A white laboratory coat, worn as safety equipment to protect both skin and everyday clothing, is referred to in medicine as simply a white coat. The end of the nineteenth century saw a move away from the black 'frock coats' worn as markers of gentlemanly class and reputation, as white coats began appearing on surgeons in many countries associated with Western medicine. While this change to white coincided with new scientific interest in antisepsis – and certainly the rarely, if ever, washed black coats were reputed to hide significant stains from blood and other bodily fluids – historians Hardy and Corones argue that white was more important because it *symbolised* cleanliness and health rather than because it helped achieve it (Hardy and Corones, 2016, p. 38). The white coat went through many iterations between 1860 and 1920 before settling into common use. Its adoption by surgeons, a group that has been historically considered separate from other medical doctors in some countries (in the US they are referred to as 'Dr' and receive the postgraduate medical degree), was not without controversies. The same is true of surgical garments other than the coat, which moved from the dark-coloured everyday work dress of a gentleman to white clothing that matched the idyllic white space of the operating room. The garments known as 'scrubs' (so named because of the association with scrubbing of hands and arms before entering a surgical space) first were white but then began appearing in muted green and blue during the twentieth century. Hardy and Corones argue that this change was not primarily for reasons of asepsis or sartorial preference, but in large part because these colours avoid the eye strain surgeons suffer due to the stark contrast of blood and harsh reflection of electrical light on white clothing (Hardy and Corones, 2016, p. 43). Since the early twentieth century, the white coat has been a key identifier of a physician in the US. In the late twentieth century, medical schools in the US began to include a ceremonial recognition of this meaning-filled piece of clothing.

'The White Coat Ceremony'

The White Coat Ceremony is the formal initiation into medical education for almost every allopathic medical school in the United States as well as nineteen other countries (The Arnold P. Gold

Foundation, 2022). Boosted into existence in 1993 by the Arnold P. Gold Foundation and the Robert Wood Johnson Foundation, the White Coat Ceremony has become a recognisable rite of passage, centred on one of the most recognisable symbols of the physician. Over thirty years, the ceremony has developed to include other symbols, including a lapel pin from the Gold Foundation emblemising humanism in medicine and a stethoscope. The students receive each item in a meaning-laden presentation. At the school of medicine where I teach, each student is enrobed in the white coat by two members of the faculty, often designated mentors, welcoming them into the fold. The student's new coat is 'pinned' by a member of the Gold Humanism Honor Society, which is supported by the Gold Foundation, marking them as dedicated to humanism. The stethoscope is presented by alumni of the school, predicting their advancement to proficient use of this medical instrument.

For those who participate and witness it, the White Coat Ceremony can be a poignant initiation, a confirmation of entry into a new way of life. Students take an oath, usually a version of the Hippocratic Oath, alongside the faculty and staff who are their future colleagues. Although schools can choose the timing, most medical schools hold this ceremony during the earliest days of the first year of medical education, often before students have ever entered a classroom or encountered a patient in a clinical setting. The timing of this induction is the most controversial aspect of the ceremony; students are vested with these powerful symbols before they likely understand the responsibility that goes along with the perceived authority that has been conveyed (Wear, 1998). Undeniably popular, White Coat Ceremonies are rapidly expanding to schools of nursing, pharmacy, and physician assistant programmes. Formal initiation into health care professions matches the received wisdom that these people are more than simply students in an academic programme or beginners at a job. Responding to a calling, they are chosen and ritually marked as part of a special culture. Thus, they are newly costumed and have been handed their first prop.

The hidden dress code of stethoscopes

Although the white coat and scrubs may be more obvious aspects of physician attire, it is the varying styles for wearing of stethoscopes that inspired my thinking about hidden dress codes. Physicians enjoy making broad categorisations about how each medical specialty wears or carries stethoscopes: for example, 'Surgeons always have their stethoscope in their white coat pocket' or 'Psychiatrists never have a stethoscope with them at all, and they never wear white coats'. These kinds of comments tell me that they recognise the existence of unofficial, 'hidden' dress code requirements, including how a stethoscope should be worn, to further identify and differentiate exactly what sort of physician one is.

While dress codes for surgical specialties regularly include detailed instructions on when and how to wear scrubs and white coats, how to wear one's stethoscope is not included. Yet, although it is not a requirement, it would be very unusual to see a surgeon with a stethoscope draped around their neck instead of in the pocket of their white coat. The stethoscope has become part of a hidden dress code and a way for members of this subculture (surgeons) to recognise each other. Surgical trainees put their stethoscopes in their pocket when they observe – or sometimes are told informally, including through ridicule – that surgeons carry their stethoscopes in their pockets. Psychiatrists are perceived to hold to a different hidden dress code requirement for stethoscopes than their surgeon counterparts, although all are equally physicians and an observer outside of medical cultures might not note this difference. Psychiatrists in outpatient practice do not wear scrubs, white coats, or stethoscopes on a daily basis, but they are more likely to wear this attire in a hospital setting. Psychiatrists do need stethoscopes for their work with patients and may have one nearby in an examination room or office rather than on their person. Thus, the stethoscope as signifier of identity in a physician subculture is tempting but is an oversimplification of the performance of a hidden dress code. The certainty of identifying medical specialties by their stethoscope-wearing style alone is appealing, but, as with white coats and scrubs, the style depends on the circumstances. Not only does the wearing of the stethoscope vary among physicians, but also because there are other health professionals who regularly wear scrubs, white coat, and stethoscope.

The explicit work of dress codes

Dress codes are established for both inclusion and exclusion; in health care, emphasis is placed on distinguishing each member of the health care team by role and, in particular, distinguishing physicians from other members of the health care team such as nurses or technicians. The current health care dress code at my institution was established in 2010 and included a 'crackdown' on how and when scrubs are worn by providers (University of Utah Health, 2022). As scrubs became popular attire for health care workers in all roles because of their comfort and utility, 'patients were never sure who was a nurse and who was a custodian' (Richards, 2010). This institution-wide health care worker dress code does not mention white coats and in doing so distinguishes the white coat to be a symbol worn only by the physician or physician trainee:

> Nurses in the emergency department will wear white with red, navy or black bottoms. Pharmacists will wear olive. EMTs [Emergency Medical Technicians] and certified nurse assistants will wear red, black or navy. A [colour]-coded chart in each patient's room will help keep track of the [colour] assignments. . . . The new policy does not apply to the hospital's physicians or medical students.
>
> (Richards, 2010, n.p.)

The public communications explaining this new dress code, which was developed with the input of employees, directly linked professional role and conduct to attire. The exclusion of physicians and physician trainees from this colour-coding is significant, as it emphasises that physician attire is likely to change based on function. Physicians in the emergency room at our hospital wear black scrubs to distinguish them from other providers. In our hospital's operating rooms, all surgical staff, including physicians, wear blue scrubs. At another major hospital system in our region, all surgical staff in the operating room wear green scrubs (Intermountain Healthcare, 2022; University of Utah Health, 2022). Surgeons wear white coats over their blue or green scrubs when they are with patients outside of the operating room to signify their status as a physician, a rule which is included in formal dress codes created for physicians and trainees by individual departments and programmes (University of Utah Department of Neurology, 2022; University of Utah School of Medicine, 2021).

Required attire for physicians is formalised in dress codes, with the level of detail varying by department and institution. Dress codes for physicians routinely describe when and how to wear scrubs and white coats but also what other attire is acceptable, to include not only clothing but also footwear, jewellery, tattoos, and other aspects of appearance. Descriptions of appropriate professional dress may be highly specific (for example, no open-toed shoes) or provide general guidelines, such as 'respectful' and 'reflect the dignity and standards of the medical profession' (University of Utah School of Medicine, 2021). As long as the specifics of formal dress codes are met, hidden dress codes can flourish within those generalities.

Patient perceptions of physician attire

While hidden dress codes can allow insiders to cultures of medicine to identify and categorise each other, formal dress codes are created for patients and other outsiders. Physicians have a vested interest in dressing so that they are recognisable and appear both respectful and respectable. Physicians are keenly interested in how their patients regard their attire, with notable attention to white coats, and the medical literature abounds with studies trying to determine patient preferences. Many of these studies quote a version of the Hippocratic Oath, which refers to the appearance of the physician but not specifically what they should wear. For instance, a large 2018 study by Petrilli *et al.* involving patients at ten academic medical centres in the US confirms that, while physician attire matters to a majority of patients, how it matters depends on context. This study illustrated a significant correlation between physician attire and patient perception of physician professionalism but leaves open the question of how the patient forms notions of what a doctor should wear. At a minimum, immediate location and circumstances (emergency room, surgery centre, clinic) and geographical region influences patients' preference for physicians wearing scrubs, white coats, formal, or casual dress. While this study did address gender by showing patients photos of both male-presenting and female-presenting physicians, it did not address other elements of identity such as race or ethnicity. In the limitations of the study, the authors note that they used professionally photographed images of 'young, slender, Caucasian' physicians with 'identical postures and facial expressions' to minimise bias expressed in earlier studies, although considering 'young, slender, Caucasian' neutral imagery reveals its own bias (Petrilli *et al.*, 2018).

The scholarly literature on patient preferences for physician attire frequently addresses the specificity with which clothing such as scrubs and the white coat are read, depending on the given cultural circumstances. In one study, for example, Brazilian patients, physicians, and medical students all strongly preferred physicians wearing white coats, or at least white clothing, in all clinical settings, although the authors were careful to note that their study only applied to the urban setting of Sao Paulo and not all of Brazil (Yonekura *et al.*, 2013). Patients in South Korea who were asked to view photographs of physicians identified as practicing 'Western medicine' or 'Oriental medicine' [sic] preferred those wearing white coats, regardless of medical tradition, even though the white coat is strongly associated with Western medicine (Chang *et al.*, 2011). A large, multi-centre study in Japan in 2020 also found a strong preference for white coats across groups of patients. Like the Petrilli study in the United States, this Japanese study found that geographic location, clinical setting, and elements of identity (such as the age of the patient) play a significant role in patient preferences for physician attire (Yamada *et al.*, 2010).

In each study, the authors conclude something along the lines of 'it all depends'. Studies of what patients or physicians think is appropriate or preferred clinical attire cannot be separated from culture, identity, and the immediate circumstances. To their credit, these studies, which ask their participants to respond to professionally staged photographs of providers, regularly note that the appearance of the models in their images are a weakness because they likely affect the way viewers respond to the images. But even with this limitation noted, there is no real way to separate all the elements included in the viewers' response to a photo nor to come up with an objective standard for dress. So much is contingent when anyone makes decisions about who is professional, or even who is a physician. White coats matter, except when gender or race matters more. White coats matter, except when the patient is older or when they are younger. White coats matter, except when the clinical setting is rural, or culturally distinct in dress, or when business or casual street clothes are preferred. White coats are not worn in some medical specialties (paediatrics is most often cited as eschewing white coats) because they cause 'white coat syndrome', an additional cause of stress to patients, except when they *are* worn and are *not* correlated with increased levels of stress in patients. Children and their parents do not express clear preferences regarding white coats, although many paediatricians do not wear one out of concern that they will appear threatening (Walker and Tolentino, 2007). When parents and guardians can identify physicians treating their children, it is far more likely because the doctor has introduced themselves rather than based on anything they are wearing (Brewer, Key and O'Rourke, 2004). Paediatric patients had no preference for colours or patterns for nurses wearing scrubs, but their parents and guardians showed a preference for nurses in white (Albert *et al.*, 2008). Some doctors wear their white coats every day, while others are not sure in which closet theirs is hanging. The white coat matters, except when it does not, and identifying predictors for when it will matter, and when it will not, is an elusive goal.

Physicians are aware that they have limited control over how others read their style of dress. Patients do notice what physicians wear, but it is not always the white coat or scrubs that the patient regards as a symbol – it might be a pair of fanciful socks that confirms the humanity a patient seeks in their doctor (Yavorkovsky, 2020). Physicians are not above making fun of themselves and their own concerns about what they wear, not only for reasons of style, but because of ongoing controversies regarding sanitary and antiseptic best practices. Responses to guidelines and dress codes based on best practices have included suggestions of naked surgeons and cartoon superhero costumes (Bartek, Verdial, and Dellinger, 2017; Spiegel, 2010; Clement, 2012). More seriously, physicians struggle with dress codes not only when they conflict with function or comfort but also when they conflict with deeply held values. Muslim women physicians, for example, can face significant challenges in finding surgical garb, especially headwear and arm coverings, that meets religious expectations of modesty and sanitary standards (Malik *et al.*, 2019).

Hierarchies and dress codes

The public imaginary of what a physician looks like apart from their attire has been slow to shift. Women, particularly women of colour, report consistent misrecognition or refusal of recognition as a physician even when they are wearing the symbols of their profession. This phenomenon means that the sartorial choices are extremely important for those who do not 'look like' a physician or surgeon. Scrubs are a style industry of their own, designed to improve upon the unisex, pyjama-like garments provided by hospitals, and are as recognisable as any other fashion label to those who pay attention. Health care workers can order scrubs that not only provide comfort and easy sanitising but also offer a flattering fit, often reflecting broader fashion trends and referencing popular culture, such as the scrubs line trademarked with the name of the popular television show *Grey's Anatomy*. White coats come in a variety of styles and can be customised like any other item of clothing. Both scrubs and white coats can be unintentionally deceptive, not only causing confusion about professional roles among health care providers but also about who is medical and who is a non-medical observer or visitor (but dressed in scrubs) in a clinical setting (Myers and Volpe, 2017). A carefully chosen set of scrubs or white coat, tailored to the individual physician, indicates an understanding of the power of attire, both affecting and affected by explicit and implicit dress codes.

While working in Chicago-area hospitals at the beginning of my teaching career, I quickly noticed the different lengths and different colours of coats worn and asked a colleague what they meant. I was informed that coats got longer with the years in practice, and that grey, light blue, and pink coats signified both specialty and rank. A white coat in Chicago was standard but not special. Although it is not clear how much this practice was ever institutionalised and whether it has/will persist, and when I asked about it, more than fifteen years ago, it was clear that the practice was part of an 'old guard' dress code. Certainly, some decisions are made at institutional levels, determining the meaning of a certain kind of white coat in a localised medical culture. The medical school where I teach is one of only a few that gives long coats to first-year medical students at their White Coat Ceremony. Received wisdom is that this decision was made to afford trainees the same respect as experienced physicians. However, students doing 'away rotations', where they learn for weeks or months at another institution, find themselves acquiring a short white coat to show that they recognise their role and that they respect the local understanding of medical hierarchy.

The pandemic era and white coats

Trainees are constantly negotiating hidden dress codes as they form their identities as physicians and as the world around them demands adjustments. Eighteen months into the coronavirus (COVID-19) pandemic, when I asked second-year students to 'dress as they would for clinic' for an off-campus activity, I realised belatedly that they might not yet have seen their clinical educators in anything other than scrubs. At the beginning of the pandemic, in March 2020, dress codes at hospitals and clinics shifted radically as part of infection containment protocols. COVID-19 put physicians around the world back into scrubs due to stricter sanitation requirements, even if they had left them behind long ago, and changed their meaning of this symbol (Walsh and Creamer, 2020). Patients and other physicians were surprised to see physicians in scrubs when their specialty (for example, family medicine) or health care setting (for example, outpatient clinic) had previously excluded scrubs as professional attire. Some physicians no longer looked like a physician because their attire had changed so radically. Some physicians continued to wear the scrubs and white coats that they had always worn even when interacting with patients through virtual interfaces. The unfamiliarity of meeting with a neurologist through a videoconference platform could be mitigated by the familiar sight on the screen of that neurologist in scrubs and white coat.

Ubiquitous masks and personal protective equipment (PPE) have further shifted the public's idea of what a physician looks like and have complicated the reading of scrubs, white coats, or other professional attire. More than ever, patients and health care workers alike need ways to identify each other. Recent campaigns to label bonnets and caps worn in surgical settings with the name and role of each person are potentially helpful for communication (Brodzinsky *et al.*, 2021). PPE portraits are photos of providers worn on the chest in situations where no identifying attire is visible and are another way, like the cap labels, to help patients recognise their providers during the pandemic (Brown-Johnson *et al.*, 2020). COVID-19 is as much a historical disrupter of health care dress codes, formal and hidden, as antisepsis or electrical lighting more than a century ago.

On (not) cracking the (dress) code

The quixotic goal of my research and observation since I arrived in this medical world was to crack the secret code of medical attire, understood only by insiders and mystifying or invisible to those on the outside. I imagined a kind of field guide to stethoscope-wearing or white-coat length that would offer insight to the physician role as performed, more than simply identifying medical specialty or seniority. However, signifiers like white coats, scrubs, and stethoscopes are slippery, dependent on given circumstances, in no way as definite as a dress code might suggest. The sheer number of medical cultures precludes any definitive guide; for example, with few exceptions, this manuscript addresses only allopathic medicine as practiced at academic medical centres in the United States.

Further, I had been thinking of the performance of medicine as a stage play, heavily scripted and designed, with performers confined to that script and design. I was fooled by White Coat Ceremonies and dress codes to think that I could identify physician-like characters as in a staged play, by how they wore and used these items. Instead, performers (physicians) are not characters in a play so much as improvisateurs who respond to their practical needs (easily washable, pockets, and so on) and to what others around them with whom they want to identify are wearing, and to fashion trends, like anybody else.

More important than being able to identify a physician by how they wear a white coat, stethoscope, or scrubs is acknowledging that clinical spaces remain so inscrutable for many of us. This urge to identify and categorise stems not only from curiosity but also from real needs, including preservation of health, establishment of professional identity, and efficiency and safety in the clinic. Any solution toward meeting these needs – for patients and health care providers – will be highly localised, even within an institution, and always already incomplete. As important as dress codes and posted charts of scrub colours are, the meanings ascribed to attire are often subverted by other markers of identity, such as race and gender, as well as by behaviours, including the simple act of being in a clinical space. A person in scrubs, in a white coat, or wearing a stethoscope is likely to be recognised as a physician, no matter what their badge says or what they themselves explain themselves to be (Myers and Volpe, 2017). A dress code embodied means variations for comfort, function, or preference and is unlikely to be truly uniform. Rather than a single code that can be cracked, physician attire is a performance.

Reference list

Albert, N.M. *et al.* (2008) ' "Impact of nurses" uniforms on patient and family perceptions of nurse professionalism', *Applied Nursing Research*, 21, pp. 181–90.

The Arnold P. Gold Foundation (2022) *White coat ceremony – the Arnold P. Gold foundation.* Available at: www.gold-foundation.org/programs/white-coat-ceremony/ (Accessed: 13 March 2022).

Bartek, M., Verdial, F. and Dellinger, E.P. (2017) 'Naked surgeons? The debate about what to wear in the operating room', *Clinical Infectious Diseases*, 65, pp. 1589–1592.

Brewer, T.L., Key, J.D. and O'Rourke, K. (2004) 'Identification of resident and attending physicians: do parents know who is caring for their hospitalized child?', *Ambulatory Pediatrics*, 4, pp. 257–259.

Brodzinsky, L. *et al.* (2021) 'What's in a name? Enhancing communication in the operating room with the use of names and roles on surgical caps', *Joint Commission Journal on Quality and Patient Safety*, 47, pp. 258–264.

Brown-Johnson, C. *et al.* (2020) 'PPE portraits – a way to humanize personal protective equipment', *Journal of General Internal Medicine*, 35, pp. 2240–2242.

Chang, D.S. *et al.* (2011) 'What to wear when practicing oriental medicine: patients' preferences for doctors' attire', *The Journal of Alternative and Complementary Medicine*, 17, pp. 763–767.

Clement, R. (2012) 'Is it time for an evidence based uniform for doctors?', *BMJ*, 345, p. e8286.

Hardy, S. and Corones, A. (2016) 'Dressed to heal: the changing semiotics of surgical dress', *Fashion Theory*, 20, pp. 27–49.

Intermountain Healthcare (2022) *Your hospital care team | intermountain healthcare.* Available at: https://intermountainhealthcare.org/health-information/about-your-hospital-stay/your-hospital-care-team/ (Accessed: 13 March 2022).

Malik, A. *et al.* (2019) ' "I decided not to go into surgery due to dress code": a cross-sectional study within the UK investigating experiences of female Muslim medical health professionals on bare below the elbows (BBE) policy and wearing headscarves (hijabs) in theatre', *BMJ Open*, 9, p. e019954.

Myers, K.R. and Volpe, R.L. (2017) 'Unintentional subterfuge', *Annals of Surgery*, 265, pp. 656–657.

Petrilli, C.M. *et al.* (2018) 'Understanding patient preference for physician attire: a cross-sectional observational study of 10 academic medical centres in the USA', *BMJ Open*, 8, p. e021239.

Richards, M. (2010) *New dress code for U hospital workers.* Available at: www.ksl.com/article/10066516/new-dress-code-for-u-hospital-workers (Accessed: 13 March 2022).

Spiegel, J.H. (2010) 'Wearing white-right or wrong? A satirical analysis of medical attire', *Journal of Hospital Medicine*, 5, pp. 120–123.

University of Utah Department of Neurology (2022) *Professional attire standards*. Available at: https://medicine.utah.edu/neurology/residencies/adult/residency-policies/professional-attire.pdf (Accessed: 13 March 2022).

University of Utah Health (2022) *About your hospital stay*. Available at: https://healthcare.utah.edu/locations/hospital/services/stay.php (Accessed: 13 March 2022).

University of Utah School of Medicine (2021) *University of Utah school of medicine student handbook*. Available at: https://medicine.utah.edu/students/current-students/files/som-student-handbook.pdf (Accessed: 13 March 2022).

Walker, D.M. and Tolentino, V.R. (2007) 'White coat versus no white coat: the pediatrician's dilemma', *Ambulatory Pediatrics*, 7, pp. 201–202.

Walsh, S. and Creamer, D. (2020) 'A very peculiar practice: dermatology in the era of COVID-19', *British Journal of Dermatology*, 183, pp. 940–941.

Wear, D. (1998) 'On white coats and professional development: the formal and the hidden curricula', *Annals of Internal Medicine*, 129, pp. 734–737.

Yamada, Y. *et al.* (2010) 'Patients' preferences for doctors' attire in Japan', *Internal Medicine*, 49, pp. 1521–1526.

Yavorkovsky, L.L. (2020) 'The importance of physician attire-the socks with the bulls', *JAMA Oncology*, 6, p. 1169.

Yonekura, C.L. *et al.* (2013) 'Perceptions of patients, physicians, and medical students on physicians' appearance', *Revista da associacao medica Brasileira*, 59, pp. 452–459.

13

DOCTORS AS SINGERS OF TALES

Medical performance in the Homeric tradition

Alan Bleakley and Robert Marshall

In this chapter, we draw an analogy between certain contemporary medical practices and an ancient oral performance tradition that dates to around 700C BC, prior to written texts. We justify the analogy between these historically disjunctive activities on the basis that they can both be conceived as forms of performance involving the following features: an interplay between scripted text/behaviour and improvisation, reliance on rhetorical devices designed to facilitate the act of memory (for example, repeated and visually arresting phrases) and other oral performance techniques such as improvisation and style of delivery. While there are limits to the analogy, this chapter reveals the ways in which medical education can be framed as engaged with performativity generally and specifically with 'impression management' (Goffman, 1956) – how a doctor comes across to patients and colleagues.

We will show how the structures of Homer's epics as performed songs or lyrical poems relate to key aspects of the daily work of doctors. Medical students gain identities through such performances as forms of 'professionalism' (Merlo, 2021). Here, communication is treated as a clinical skill, choreographed early in medical education through formulaic simulation training (Bleakley, Bligh and Browne, 2011). Such impression management includes frontstage sets of behaviours and semiotics such as dress code (Bleakley, 2020) and informal backstage activities such as use of slang (Bleakley, 2017). Even where behaviour goes off script, as in physician burnout or substance abuse, there is a scripted response from the wider medical education community, such as promoting 'resilience' (Peterkin and Bleakley, 2017).

We use the term performativity to describe doing things with words, where sentences are also actions ('you'll just feel a small scratch') (Austin, 1955). We expand this to inter-actions through a dramaturgical model, metaphorically treating life as theatre. Performativity is now commonly framed in terms of specific identifications such as those of gender (Butler, 1990) and ethnicity (Spivak, 1993), especially as these are performed under conditions of oppression or structural inequity and inequality. For Butler, where performativity is a stylised repetition of acts and a reproduction of dominant conventions, the question is how this can be turned from a situation of oppression into one of revolution. For example, surgical education is currently going through a revolution based on more women entering surgery who 'perform the feminine' in the face of an entrenched masculine culture (RCS, 2020). Such surgical dramaturgy embraces, for example,

DOI: 10.4324/9781003036500-16

collaborative rather than competitive activity – a net gain as better teamwork reduces surgical error and increases worker satisfaction (Bleakley, 2014).

We recognise Lyotard's (1986) view that, within dominant capitalist ideological interpellation, performance is legitimated in terms of countable outputs (productivity) subject to performance review. Lyotard sees opportunities for resistance through alternative performances that destabilise the system. A good example of this is the series of junior doctors' strikes (as withdrawal of labour) in the UK during 2016, where organised demonstrations took on elements of political theatre (Bleakley, 2021). Derrida (1988) extends Lyotard's view by suggesting that effects of performance (for example in academic medicine) can be judged by citations, as iterations and re-performances. Thus, academics gain performance credibility through volume of citations (where other academics refer to your work), as do actors through reviews.

While medical performance is largely scripted and demands conventional role adoption, medicine could not develop without breaking away from script or improvising within it. For example, rituals of hand washing have functional purposes – control of infection. But when Semmelweis introduced the idea of hand washing on obstetric wards to control infection in the mid-nineteenth century, he was ridiculed (Bleakley, 2020). The characteristic and ingrained performance of medical students was to pass straight from the autopsy room onto the wards, without infection control. Nagy notes that archaic pre-Homeric *rhapsodes*, well before the epics were written down as texts, would freely improvise around fixed themes (1996). We can assume this from ethnographic studies of epic singer traditions, such as those studied by Parry and Lord in Yugoslavia in 1933 and 1935 (Marshall and Bleakley, 2017). The key element here is sensitivity to audience reception of the performance – what in medicine we now call both patient-centredness and democratic clinical teamwork (Bleakley, 2014).

Aristotle made a distinction between *diegesis* or narrative and *mimesis* or dramatic re-enactment. In an era that has lionised temporal narrative medicine (Charon, 2011) such that it remains almost beyond critique as a dominant discourse, we place emphasis here on performance as poetics situated in space and place (Bleakley and Neilson, 2022). Nagy suggests that: 'both epic and lyric in ancient Greece were fundamentally a medium of mimesis' (1996, p. 4). Where so much of medical practice is now read temporally, as forms of narrative or story, we are wary of the narrative frame being projected back onto patient encounters to afford the status of 'story' to what may be seen as a lyrical, poetic encounter of intensively collapsed, fragmented and disjointed exchanges. Nagy suggests that mimesis: 'does not describe, narrate or offer argument, but dramatises and embodies human speech and action' (ibid, p. 4). A tradition of dramatic re-enactment stretches from pre-Homeric *rhapsodes* through Medieval and Renaissance traditions of the troubadour and can be found to have influenced clinical routines and associated professionalism in contemporary medical work.

There are two key elements to this tradition (ibid, p. 4). First, 'songs' are not simply performed by individuals but are collaborative productions between groups of singers and their audiences (as forms of reception). Second, a singer must have, and show, authority in performance. This is partly invested by initiation into a tradition (for example medical culture) and partly by the authorisation of the audience (in medicine, patients' responses). For the performer to gain credibility, she must first be able to re-enact previous performances (a re-creation, as competent practice in a medical specialty, for example) and then must be able to create or innovate, bending, questioning and re-framing the rules. Here, improvisation again is key.

An example of this is how doctors deal with a fluid historical tradition such as that of the Hippocratic corpus, re-created for successive generations of medicine initiates. Where the corpus has the phrase: 'I will abstain from all intentional wrong-doing and harm', and the Hippocratic

School says: 'either help or do not harm the patient', the better-known 'first, do no harm' was a seventeenth-century adaptation, subsequently popularised by the nineteenth-century English surgeon Thomas Inman. This tradition has now morphed into a set of standards known as 'professionalism' that embraces courtesy towards patients and awareness of safety, inclusivity and lack of discrimination, and, most recently, looking after one's own physical and mental wellbeing (Figley, Huggard and Rees, 2013; Peterkin and Bleakley, 2017).

In the spirit of corporate capitalism, where medical performance is characteristically lauded in terms of qualities grounded in an ethical notion of trust, such performance has now become quantifiable in terms of 'entrustable professional activities' (EPAs). As Ten Cate suggests: 'EPAs are units of professional practice, defined as tasks or responsibilities to be entrusted to the unsupervised execution by a trainee once he or she has attained sufficient specific competence' (2013, p. 157). We see that medical education has fully embraced the business model, so that performativity equates with productivity.

Medicine as oral performance

Medical students and doctors can transcend historical medical scripts through political acts of resistance (Bleakley, 2020), as echoes of the ancient singer's powers of invention and improvisation around traditional themes. We have noted such dramatic re-enactments in the concern with professionalism and through doctors' strike action and women changing the face of surgical education. We will approach medical work as performance in a Homeric key by drawing on the following four dimensions: the Art of Memory, a stitching together of tales, use of formulae and the aesthetic of Minimalism.

The Art of Memory and the use of dark metaphor. Our first element in performing medicine is memory of script. This feeds into embodied social activities as a 'carnal hermeneutics' (Kearney and Treanor, 2015), a way of knowing through activity. Homer's *Iliad* and *Odyssey* are epic poems – textual versions of songs originally sung with lyre accompaniment. Written down around 750 BC, they describe events occurring 300–400 years before in the Trojan War and its aftermath. The *Iliad* is around 15,000 lines and the *Odyssey* 12,000 lines. Depending on the stamina of the audience, if we started to recite the *Iliad* early on a Monday, we would be finished on Wednesday or Thursday – a durational performance.

Various aspects of the composition of the texts, both major themes and specific words and phrases, puzzled scholars for centuries until it was realised that the poems predated writing. They were part of an oral tradition, where 'oral epic song is narrative poetry composed in a manner evolved over many generations by singers of tales who did not know how to write' (Lord, 2003, p. 4). Such tales were re-invented and embellished on every telling, but core content was formulaic: coded and repeated such that singers could more easily recall their lines, putting less stress on memorisation. As Lord says: 'The singer of tales is at once the tradition and an individual creator' (ibid, p. 4).

An Art of Memory (Yates, 1966) aided the recall of epic songs. Such mnemonic devices are formalised, coded use of visual imagery, epithets and metaphors. These are used as heuristics, or mental short cuts, to a larger volume of information. Seen as a training device for the mind, mnemonic techniques originated with the ancient Greeks and peaked as a pedagogic instrument during the Renaissance. Our own capacity for memorisation is dismal by contrast and this is seen as a direct result of the invention of writing, eventually displacing word of mouth messaging by mass circulation of print, exacerbated by digital communication. In *Phaedrus*, Plato tells the story of an Egyptian sage introducing writing to his king. It will, he says, make the Egyptians wiser and improve their memories. The king disagrees, where writing will 'produce forgetfulness . . . because they will not practice their memory. . . . You have produced an elixir not of memory but of reminding' (Perseus Digital Library, n.d., p. 275).

The basic method of the Art of Memory is to associate a striking, often pathologised, image with the object or fact to be memorised. Both recall and recognition are stimulated by this twin image, acting as a metaphor that serves to intensify the value of the original image. Thus, I might remember a mundane object or fact by association with a striking or bizarre image such as a burning lake. I might remember my long-dead grandfather not for his kindness but for the distinct birthmark on his face. In a revision guide for diagnosing common conditions, Schwartz and Richards embed cases in well-known fairy stories to provide Art of Memory prompts (2019: passim). For example, Humpty Dumpty provides a memorable recall image for a skull fracture; and Little Red Riding Hood attacked by a wolf for advice about treating an infected wound.

The principles of the Art of Memory are also key features of medical performance as diagnostic work. Doctors make judgements through pattern recognition supported by heuristics such as aphorisms and resemblances (Levine and Bleakley, 2012). An aphorism is a wise saying such as 'when you hear hoofbeats, don't think zebras' – or, go for the most likely explanation. Common resemblances are fruits – where strep throat remains untreated in a child, it may turn into scarlet fever, a bacterial infection. This turns the tongue white at first and then red, where the tongue looks like a strawberry (Bleakley, 2017). Again, the healthy, succulent red strawberry is a second register for a symptom of pathology – infection, suffering and illness. The diagnosis is *performed*, like a card trick or an illusion. Or at least it seems this way to the patient or the naïve medical student.

The stitching together of tales. Our second element in performing medicine is telling tales, but we have already warned that we read such encounters with patients as largely place based rather than temporal. The tale is then a poetic 'tail' that we must pin and will lead us to the body of the issue, as formal diagnostic work. Medical diagnostic work can be immediate as pattern recognition (as described) but usually requires confirmatory reception of a history from a patient that includes an account of symptoms and a physical or mental examination that may be accompanied by tests such as scans or blood tests. But such histories are often fragmentary and do not necessarily present as coherent stories.

Patients become cases in medical education – symptom presentations abstracted from the consultation and re-presented in academic grand rounds (discussed in a lecture theatre setting, or a General Practice training day), a clinical ward round at the bedside, a multi-disciplinary team meeting (MDT), a surgical team de-briefing or a problem-based learning (PBL) case for students. Ratzan called this process of doctors working first with their patients and then passing on their insights to colleagues and students the use of 'winged words' (1992: passim). He was the first to argue that the traditional presentation of the medical case history is a legitimate form of oral recital, a performance or dramatic re-enactment. Such case presentation is central to the socialisation of medical students and junior doctors. Doctors and students tend to savour more challenging, abstruse patient presentations with multiple diagnostic possibilities or examples of rare diseases. Enticement and educational value for the medical world may, however, shadow terrible suffering for a patient.

Lingard and colleagues argue that there are identifiable genres of case presentation – particularly the difference between the 'medical school genre', where students seek to present without interruption for academic capital, and the 'workplace genre', where seasoned practitioners seek to use case presentations as a way of constructing shared professional knowledge and teaching juniors and students (2003: passim). Here, the focus is on identity construction (or *performing the role*) as much as accurate knowledge (the focus, again, of the medical school genre). As Ratzan argued, the case presentation can be compared to the archaic singing of songs or repeating of epic lore that sustains a culture (1992). Here again is a mixture of tradition (memorised or encapsulated knowledge) and improvisation (according to the unique patient and the context of case presentation).

The way the story is recounted, or 'sung', declares and defines confidence as one who 'stitches-the-song-together' (*rhapsodos*) (Dalby, 2006, pp. 174–175) – often bringing together several stories in a grand story or diagnostic triumph (revealing the character flaws of Achilles; paring a complex differential down to a definitive diagnosis). 'Stitching together' is a metaphor that runs through Homer with its reference point in crafts as diverse as boatbuilding and weaving and to the act of poetry itself as a stitching together of words (Dougherty, 2001). There is much literal stitching of course in surgery and medicine but also metaphorical stitching together. Senior doctors, especially under (common) conditions of ambiguity, improvise around the stitching together of facts, just as jazz musicians learn to improvise around chord structures, scales and melodies. Improvisation is not possible without formulaic building blocks. Students gain expertise in diagnosis by stitching together scientific knowledge with practical clinical knowledge in tacit or encapsulated information such as 'illness scripts' or 'semantic qualifiers' that also act as mnemonic devices, energising an Art of Memory.

Novices who do this well impress expert teachers and shift identity, from medical student to trainee doctor. Canny medical students soon learn the ropes as they compose clinical poems to impress their seniors. Self-presentation is key, where students can bluff in the face of lack of knowledge, winning the respect of their seniors for showing apparent courage (sometimes merely bravado). Here is a typical medical history that a junior doctor might relate to a senior member of the clinical team:

> Mr Smith is a sixty-year-old man who came to A&E with crushing, central chest pain, which radiated down the arm and up into the neck. The pain came on out of the blue while working in the garden. There has been no previous episode. His ECG showed ST elevation.[1]

In a twin process, Greek epic poetry (and then the tradition of medical case presentation or 'song') was not simply recited *but constructed and created during recital* where, again, improvisation was key to good performance. Students will often observe seniors improvising in such a manner. Performance memory is structured and coded not only by Art of Memory techniques discussed previously but also by formulaic scaffolding, explained in the following. Singers and poets share the same descriptor in ancient Greek – *aodoi* – the modern equivalent of which would be 'performing artists'. Again, the recitation of the epics was known as much for creation as re-creation, where a formulaic epic narrative would be re-storied through leaps of the singer's imagination against a predictable hexameter, six-beats to the line rhythm.

For medical students and doctors, an illness script is an encoded narrative structure (a mental map or a cognitive schema) used to recall key attributes of a particular case and compare this against a stored set of prototypes (Lubarsky, 2015). A script encompasses symptoms, possible causes, time course, tests and treatments. Novices build illness scripts through constant work-based exposure and parallel knowledge explanations. Experts – especially those who have developed adaptive expertise as the ability to improvise when faced with ambiguous or contradictory sense-based information – rely on rapid cognitive processing as habitual pattern recognition. This engages three processes: first, close noticing of cues and clues from patient presentations; second, matching against stored or encapsulated scripts as feedback; and third, feed-forward 'ecological perception'. In the latter, anticipatory and predictive processing feedback loops operate as the doctor makes sense of the patient's embodied presentation and narrative in an improvisatory way, adjusting judgements according to the flow of information from the context of the consultation and accepting intuitions that feed into prognosis as much as diagnosis.

In drawing on any illness script, doctors must simultaneously entertain predisposing conditions, what is often referred to as the 'pathophysiological insult' or presenting symptom, clinical consequences and emotional and psychological effects. Within specialties, as knowledge and experience build, so polished performances follow as specialist scripts are learned with depth, precision and differentiating power. Use of illness scripts is enhanced by the development of the cognitive strategy of formulaic semantic qualifiers. This is a broad-brush set of search terms that help to narrow the diagnosis, such as 'acute vs chronic', 'tender vs non-tender', 'sharp vs dull', 'proximal vs distal', 'insidious vs abrupt' and so forth. For example, a patient presents with a pain that came on suddenly in her knee and that she has had a couple of times before, now presenting as 'acute, recurrent, large joint pain'.

The use of formulae. Our third element in performing medicine is the use of formulaic phrases to take the strain off memorising. The extent to which the pre-Homeric singer and Homeric poets called on and reused a stock of words, phrases and sentences only became clear on detailed examination, through work carried out by two iconic figures in Homeric scholarship, mentioned previously: Milman Parry (1902–1935) and Albert Lord (1912–1991). For example, 'sent to Hades' is a formulaic line ending used by Homer (referring to the common fate of men around the walls of Troy as they fell in brutal, hand-to-hand combat) that would have been used by singers originally. Thus, when the poet has in mind to kill off one of his fighters in a battle scene, this gives him his formulaic (and readily recalled) line ending.

Whenever Achilles appears in the tale, the formulaic beat or metric of his name – 'ti-tum-tum' – allow it to be placed almost anywhere in the line. There is then a further set of formulae that allows the poet to fill the rest of the line while planning how to move the story forward. Parry (1971, p. 272) defines such a formula as: 'a group of words . . . regularly employed under the same metrical conditions to express a given essential idea' (later, we give an example of a radiologist viewing an image of an 'apple core lesion', where 'the edges give an undercut appearance'). For example, the same words are often combined throughout the poem to form pairs of noun and epithet, or even longer combinations, sometimes running to complete sentences. Achilles, around whose wrath and appeasement the *Iliad* revolves, very often has the epithet 'swift-footed' attached to his name. When dawn breaks, personified as a goddess, she often has the lovely epithet 'rosy-fingered' attached to her. Indeed, the whole line for the breaking dawn is used about twenty times in the *Odyssey*: 'When the child of morning, rosy-fingered dawn appeared'.

Parry and Lord extended their research to field accounts of oral poetic traditions modern at the time, particularly in Yugoslavia between the two World Wars (Lord, 2003). They found an equivalent use of formulae not just as aide-memoires to allow the poet simply to remember the poem and recount the tale verbatim but metrical combinations that allowed the poet to compose on the spot. Again, tradition and innovation mix, where, as we have seen, oral poetry is not simply recited but is constructed and created during recital. That is a wonderful concept, difficult for us to understand. Most modern speakers would not give even a short talk without notes or PowerPoint backup. The singer of the *Iliad* sang for six hours a day for three or four days, adapting to the audience and adding variations.

When a character has spoken in the *Iliad*, Homer's next line creates itself, with a formula to fit every circumstance in the form of epithets:

Answering him spoke forth *swift footed* Achilles.
Answering her spoke forth *white armed* Hera.

Answering them spoke forth Odysseus *of many counsels* (also 'wily Odysseus' or 'cunning Odysseus').

The doctor too calls on formulae to move through familiar territory as she also makes sense of a bodily event:

Examination of the . . . system . . . within normal limits
Us and Es . . . unremarkable (urea and electrolytes in kidney function tests)
Full blood count . . . no abnormality

The start of each sentence can reach any of the three endings given a suitable bridge. Equally important is that, in addition to the formula theory that affects word combinations and sentences, whole themes recur throughout both the *Iliad* and the *Odyssey* (Foley, 1988). Arranging a truce, preparing a meal, offering a sacrifice or sticking a spear in a member of the opposing camp occur several, often many, times. Such iterations, as protocols, are expected to progress in a certain way and a certain order whether in Homer or in medicine. Doctors thus respond to regular, themed occasions (taking a history, 'crash' scenarios, breaking bad news, inserting a central line) in practiced ways, but improvisation is always possible.

Before considering where this comparison of oral traditions might lead, we should consider the limits to the argument. Oral traditions now are less important as we have moved on, with the advent first of writing and then of electronic information, to what has been described as a 'secondary orality' (Ong, 1982), a product of the era of word-processing and the World Wide Web. There is a risk of regarding primary orality as primitive or folksy. Ong draws a parallel for the literate world, considering the previous oral world, of describing a horse to those who know cars but have never seen a horse (ibid, pp. 12–13). A horse is then a 'wheelless car', running on hay rather than petrol, and so on, where: 'In the end, horses are only what they are not'. Doctors now have portable, electronic sub-scripts to feed into ongoing dramatic re-enactments, such as patient records, test results, protocols and evidence-based guidelines, drug formularies and the Diagnostic and Statistical Manual of Mental Disorders (DSM-5).

Does the 'singer of tales' in repeating the same tale over and over get bored and habituated, a common condition for making errors? 'Crushing, central chest pain' is hugely dramatic and metaphoric; it is just that doctors have read it in textbooks, heard it as students and used it often early in their careers, and now they are inured to the phrase – the metaphor is 'tired'. Parry takes an objective view where he accepts that formulaic epithets can be wearing, but in general, '[t]hey flow unceasingly through the changing moods of the poetry, unobtrusively blending with it, and yet, by their indifference to the story, giving a permanent, unchanging sense of strength and beauty' (1971, pp. 426–427). Perhaps too, Lord's view of his singer of tales as journeyman applies even more to the doctor: 'expression is his business, not originality, which, indeed, is a concept quite foreign to him and one he would avoid, if he understood it' (Lord, 2003, pp. 44–45).

Tradition is fine, but there would be no medical advances without innovation. Improvising then plays its part in each telling of an epic poem and each medical dramatic re-enactment. The bard was not just remembering 15,000 lines using the techniques described earlier and repeating them verbatim. Rather, each recital created the story anew. As s/he sang, so s/he made the poem – s/he was not only the singer but also the song (on female bards, see Dalby, 2006). The poems of ancient Greece were performed in Panathenaic Games, in symposia and in public places, and were also sung to select audiences – the king and his court. Similarly, traditional song-poems of Yugoslavia were sung in coffee houses to an inclusive public audience but also exclusively to male guests at a

Moslem wedding. While medical tales are told to a select and critical audience – often in the case of junior doctors to an audience of seniors ready to pounce on mistakes – the public audience (patients) is enacted and embodied in the process (and not just kept 'in mind'). This recreation of the patient is slyly criticised by Ratzan as disembodying the patient who is present in bedside teaching through the case history convention (1992). Here, the patient is presented, says Ratzan, as a 'skeleton'.

Ambiguity abounds in dramatic re-enactments and can be taken as opportunity (Bleakley and Neilson, 2022). The junior doctor will tell the patient history more than once to different audiences. A different doctor on the same team might also repeat the same history. Is it the same? Does it matter? Parry and Lord had the opportunity to ask their Yugoslavian singers to repeat the same tale twice, sometimes with an interval of years between or to listen to a tale sung by another and then sing it themselves. They asked the bard if they were the same tale.

Q: Was it the same song, word for word and line for line?

A: The same song, word for word and line for line.

Said with a straight face, the singers of tales thus saw no apparent paradox or contradiction in melding conservative tradition and necessary improvisation (playing to a particular audience, refreshing the song, but the song 'remains the same').

The Minimalist aesthetic. Our fourth element in performing medicine is to embrace a Minimalist aesthetic of stripping down information to a bare minimum without losing form and beauty, where 'less is more'. Stitched-together 'songs' appear in hospital as routine medical work including 'thinking aloud' diagnostic reasoning. Routinisation in hospitals has embraced long-standing rituals that echo Homeric accounts, such as the exercise of unconditional hospitality and characteristically heroic interventions in emergency medicine and surgery (Marshall and Bleakley, 2017). Drawing on the *Iliad*, Ratzan compares oral traditions with the medical Grand Round in terms of 'professional, social, and pedagogical significance', where 'a singer of medical tales recites a medical case history that is judged by its skill in transmitting the story and, in some venues, by its performative excellence' (1992, p. 110). Ratzan, however, only looks backward to Homer to justify his claim, while we suggest also looking around to modern aesthetic forms such as Minimalism (Meyer, 2004) to find a genre or aesthetic home for the reflexive case presentation and its creative possibilities in performance.

Let us return to our earlier case:

Mr Smith is a sixty-year-old man who came to A&E with crushing, central chest pain, which radiated down the arm and up into the neck. The pain came on out of the blue while working in the garden. There has been no previous episode. His ECG showed ST elevation.

The case presentation is often depicted as both depersonalising and dehumanising for patients – where the case history acts as an irreversible translation device from the patient's felt 'illness' to a medicalised 'disease' (Kleinman, 1988). Rather, in acting as a medium for identity construction of the doctor as medical performance artist, learning how to recite the case history does not just provide a means for forming a professional identity within the medical culture but can sensitise doctors towards the public, as audience, offering a radical version of patient-centredness. The case history can be aesthetic and ethical (stressing qualities and values) as well as functional (stressing biomedical information).

The crisp and collapsed case presentation draws on aide-memoires that allow the junior doctor rapidly to present each of, say, the fifteen or so patients whose story she heard the previous night.

The power of the case presentation rests with its Minimalist aesthetic: brevity, pointedness and a striking link of word and image through metaphor (given extra power where it is pathologised, such as 'crushing pain'). Here indeed is an elegant convention: systematic and based on clarity and concision: 'Mr K is a 23-year-old who had an episode of bleeding two weeks ago. He was at a urinal when he noticed bleeding from the tip of the penis', while 'Mrs B presented at the A&E department with severe pain in the upper abdomen radiating to the back'.

There is apparent objectivity, or singular lack of affect, that irons out initially disturbing and graphic experiences. If there is a characteristic style, then it is in the condensed smoothness of the presentation. Aesthetically, again this can be compared with the presentation of smooth, industrially precise surfaces that characterises Minimalism in its sculptural forms since its heyday in the 1960s (Meyer, 2004). But there are depths in surfaces, where smoothness does not signify lack of deep affect in response. Just as highly stylised Minimalist art viewed in an antiseptic white cube gallery can get the heart rate of an enthusiast racing, so Ratzan notes that the heart rates of junior doctors increase as they enact the performance of the case presentation in a 'highly charged atmosphere' (1992, p. 94). Minimalism has a beating heart.

Minimalism also invites highly charged and focused sensory participation. 'Aesthetic' at root means 'sense impression', so an aesthetic medicine is sensible or makes the best uses of the senses, as it is also sensitive, relating to patients' needs. Here is a radiologist reading X-ray images as if practicing as a Minimalist (Bleakley *et al.*, 2003), introduced earlier:

> This is a double contrast barium enema. There is an area of narrowing in the sigmoid. The undercut edges give an apple core appearance. This is colonic carcinoma.
>
> This is a chest X-ray of an adult patient. Calcification is rounded and peripheral. With this degree of symmetry and also eggshell calcification in the right para-aortic region, the most likely diagnosis is sarcoid.

The phrasing is tight but also poetic, intensively collapsed. First, the observation embraces a metaphor (here, a simile): the 'apple core' appearance allows for instant pattern recognition. But then there is alliteration: 'an apple core appearance', 'colonic carcinoma', and consonance ('undercut edges'). There is spatial beauty ('Calcification is rounded and peripheral'). And there is the inevitable tension that such beauty (or sublimity) is set in suffering – these are symptoms of cancer and sarcoidosis.

The radiologist's comments too are both descriptive and charged but go further in offering a diagnosis. As the Minimalist sculptor Morris suggests: 'simplicity of form is not necessarily simplicity of experience', and Sontag echoes this sentiment:

> ours is a culture based on excess, on overproduction; the result is a steady loss of sharpness in our sensory experience. . . . What is important now is to recover our senses. We must learn to *see* more, to *hear* more, to *feel* more. . . . Our task is to cut back content so that we can see the thing at all.
>
> (2009, para. 9)

Postscript

Study of Homer leads to the thought experiments: what would medicine be like without writing? And what will happen when we have the universal electronic patient record where writing itself is re-inscribed? If we transform Mr Smith's agonising chest pain – with all that it means to him and his loved ones – into a myocardial infarct or heart attack, what is lost when he is reduced further to a T2800 M58000 (the code for an infarct in SNOMED, the Systematised Nomenclature of Medicine)? Havelock referred presciently to the move from orality to literacy as a 'crisis' (1986, p. 17). We are about to turn patients into avatars. Is that our crisis in medicine, or will suitable dramatic re-enactments follow?

Note

1 ECG is electrocardiogram; ST elevation is the trace on the ST segment of the cardiogram showing a significant spike, indicating a possible heart attack.

Reference list

Austin, J.L. (1955) *How to do things with words*. Oxford: Clarendon Press.

Bleakley, A. (2014) *Patient-centred medicine in transition: the heart of the matter*. Dordrecht: Springer.

Bleakley, A. (2017) *Thinking with metaphors in medicine: the state of the art*. Abingdon: Routledge.

Bleakley, A. (2020) *Educating doctors' senses through the medical humanities: 'how do I look?'*. Abingdon: Routledge.

Bleakley, A. (2021) *Medical education, politics and social justice: the contradiction cure*. Abingdon: Routledge.

Bleakley, A., Bligh, J. and Browne, J. (2011) *Medical education for the future: identity, power and location*. Dordrecht: Springer.

Bleakley, A. and Neilson, S. (2022) *Poetry in the clinic: towards a lyrical medicine*. Abingdon: Routledge.

Bleakley, A. *et al.* (2003) 'Making sense of clinical reasoning: judgement and the evidence of the senses', *Medical Education*, 37, pp. 544–552.

Butler, J. (1990) *Gender trouble: feminism and the subversion of identity*. London: Routledge.

Charon, R. (2011) 'The novelization of the body, or how medicine and stories need one another', *Narrative*, 19, pp. 33–50.

Dalby, A. (2006) *Rediscovering homer: inside the origins of the epic*. New York, NY: WW Norton.

Derrida, J. (1988) *Limited Inc*. Evanston, IL: Northwestern University Press.

Dougherty, C. (2001) *The raft of Odysseus: the ethnographic imagination of homer's Odyssey*. New York, NY: Oxford University Press.

Figley, C., Huggard, P. and Rees, C. (eds.) (2013) *First do no self-harm: understanding and promoting physician stress resilience*. Oxford: Oxford University Press.

Foley, J.M. (1988) *The theory of oral composition: history and methodology*. Bloomington, IN: Indiana University Press.

Goffman, E. (1956) *The presentation of self in everyday life*. New York: Doubleday.

Havelock, E.A. (1986) *The muse who learns to write*. New Haven, CT: Yale University Press.

Kearney, R. and Treanor, B. (eds.) (2015) *Carnal hermeneutics*. New York, NY: Fordham University Press.

Kleinman, A. (1988) *The illness narratives: suffering, healing and the human condition*. New York, NY: Basic Books.

Levine, D. and Bleakley, A. (2012) 'Maximising medicine through aphorisms', *Medical Education*, 46, pp. 153–162.

Lingard, L. *et al.* (2003) '"Talking the talk": school and workplace genre tension in clerkship case presentations', *Medical Education*, 37, pp. 612–620.

Lord, A.B. (2003) *The singer of tales*. Cambridge, MA: Harvard University Press.

Lubarsky, S. *et al.* (2015) 'Using script theory to cultivate illness script formation and clinical reasoning in health care professions education', *Canadian Medical Education Journal*, 6(2), pp. e61–e70.

Lyotard, J.-F. (1986) *The postmodern condition: a report on knowledge*. Manchester: Manchester University Press.

Marshall, R. and Bleakley, A. (2017) *Rejuvenating medical education: seeking help from homer*. Newcastle: Cambridge Scholars.

Merlo, G. (2021) *Principles of medical professionalism*. Oxford: Oxford University Press.

Meyer, J. (2004) *Minimalism: art and polemics in the sixties*. New Haven, CT: Yale University Press.

Nagy, G. (1996) *Poetry as performance: homer and beyond*. Cambridge: Cambridge University Press.

Ong, W.J. (1982) *Orality and literacy: the technologizing of the world*. London: Methuen.

Parry, M. (1971) *The making of Homeric verse: the collected papers of millman parry*. Oxford: Clarendon Press.

Perseus Digital Library (n.d.) *Plato. Phaedrus*. Available at: www.perseus.tufts.edu/hopper/text?doc=Perseus%3Atext%3A1999.01.0174%3Atext%3DPhaedrus%3Apage%3D275 (Accessed: 30 March 2023).

Peterkin, A. and Bleakley, A. (2017) *Staying human during the foundation programme: how to thrive after medical school*. Baton Rouge, LA: CRC Press.

Ratzan, R.M. (1992) 'Winged words and chief complaints: medical case histories and the parry-lord oral-formulaic tradition', *Literature and Medicine*, 11, pp. 94–114.

RCS (Royal College of Surgeons of England) (2020) *Women in surgery*. Available at: www.rcseng.ac.uk/careers-in-surgery/women-in-surgery/

Schwartz, E. and Richards, T. (2019) *Cases of a Hollywood doctor*. Baton Rouge, LA: Taylor & Francis.

Sontag, S. (2009) *Against interpretation and other essays*. London: Penguin Classics.

Spivak, G.C. (1993) *Outside in the teaching machine*. New York, NY: Routledge.

Ten Cate, O. (2013) 'Nuts and bolts of entrustable professional activities', *Journal of Graduate Medical Education*, 5, pp. 157–158.

Yates, F.A. (1966) *The art of memory*. London: Routledge and Kegan Paul.

14

THE PERFORMANCE OF SURGERY

Steve Reid, Laurie Rauch and Alp Numanoglu

Roger Kneebone, trauma surgeon and expert in medical simulation, asks what we might discover if we see surgery as a form of performance. For him, a shift of emphasis 'from performing *surgery* to *performing* surgery' reveals the stagecraft of the operating theatre and the skills of the surgeon as analogous to those of artists (Kneebone, 2016a, p. 67). Elsewhere, he draws on collaborations with magicians and puppetry practitioners to highlight 'close-up performance and dextrous team-work' as exploratory lenses for re-examining clinical practice and finds the comparisons mutually fruitful for the improvement of practice (Kneebone, 2016a, pp. 67–82). This chapter extends such explorations of the parallels between the performance of surgery and other types of performance, with a focus on minimally invasive surgery. Written from the perspectives of two surgeons with teaching responsibilities in this area (Reid and Numanoglu) and a researcher of the autonomic nervous system in sports science (Rauch), the chapter describes the specific demands that this advanced surgery makes on the performance of the surgeon. As will be discussed more fully, the high stakes and manual dexterity of minimally invasive surgery (MIS) require specialist training relative to the 'open' surgery described by Kneebone, as well as increased emphasis on physical and mental preparation, in order to achieve what we have called the optimal 'performance zone', a term taken from the field of sports science. This makes it a rich area for analysis through a performance lens.

Performance is not confined to the performing arts, but it is also defined as the action or process of carrying out or accomplishing an action, task or function. In the arts, 'to perform' is to put on a show, a play, a dance, a concert. In everyday life, 'to perform' is to show off, to go to extremes, to underline an action for those who are watching. It is also to do something up to a standard – to succeed, to excel (Schechner, 2006, p. 28). The chapter understands 'performance' in two ways. First, following Kneebone (2016b), we see surgery as a sort of performance, seeking to draw parallels between the education and practices of MIS and those of performing arts, which are planned, rehearsed, executed and repeated under controlled conditions, even including the common context of a 'theatre'. The operating surgeon, as a medical professional, adheres to a professional code of ethical conduct and therapeutic practice that appears far removed from that of actors on a stage. But the principles are in fact very similar. In the following, we describe what surgeons do when they train in and conduct MIS, adding comments that we hope will prompt readers with more expertise in performance to explore similarities with performing arts

DOI: 10.4324/9781003036500-17

practices. Second, we think of 'performance' in terms of optimisation, of achieving the most successful output. This is where the practices of surgery and theatre performance most clearly diverge, because the stakes are different. While performance scholars are sometimes sceptical of 'performance management' (see, for example, McKenzie, 2001), it is essential in the context of surgery, where the price of 'errors' is measured in patient's lives and physical well-being. In his book, *Better: A Surgeon's Notes on Performance* (2007), Gawande defines three core requirements for successful performance in medicine – diligence, doing right and ingenuity. He elaborates on the near-obsessive nature required not only to attain excellence but also to perpetually develop to stay ahead of emerging evidence in order to 'make a science out of performance' (2007, p. 11). In keeping with this, we also offer an account of what is going on neurobiologically when someone is in a physiological and mental state for optimal performance, or what we call the 'performance zone'.

Minimally invasive surgery

Although the history of surgery dates back to the Neolithic (4300 BCE to 2000 BCE) and Pre-classic ages (2000 BCE to 250 CE), we can consider the introduction of general anaesthetics the start of modern surgery. The first public demonstration of the use of ether as a general anaesthetic agent took place in 1846 at the Massachusetts General Hospital in Boston. Once the associated pain could be eliminated from surgery, surgical techniques for complex operations could be developed. Although all surgery is performative in nature, we will consider a specific type of surgery known as minimally invasive surgery as especially illustrative of the principles in common with performance in other spheres of activity such as the performing arts.

Minimally invasive surgery (also known as endoscopic, laparoscopic or 'keyhole' surgery) allows surgeons to perform operations through very small incisions, using specialised equipment and instruments, with significant post-operative advantages. For example, instead of a large incision to remove a diseased gall bladder, the same operation can be performed through an incision less than 5mm long. The first use of MIS to perform an appendicectomy was conducted by Kurt Semm in Germany in 1981 (Mettler, 2003). In the subsequent development of MIS, the surgical device industry worked with surgeons to develop new instruments that are as small as 2–3mm in diameter and imaging equipment that also uses 3–4-mm-diameter telescopes to allow high-resolution videos of the operative field in real time. Progression in these and many other technical developments today even allows robotic surgery to be performed utilising minimally invasive techniques.

There are many advantages of minimally invasive surgery. Post-operative pain is minimal compared to open surgery, which means analgesic requirements using potentially dangerous agents such as opioids can also be avoided after surgery. Patients are mobilised early post-operatively, which in itself significantly quickens recovery from surgery and prevents complications associated with long periods of bed rest, such as chest infections and clots in the veins. MIS also allows patients to eat sooner after surgery, which in turn helps with quicker recovery and early return of gut function. Many complex operations are done using MIS today and these patients are discharged home on the same day of their operations, which was unheard of a few decades ago. Early discharge from hospital also translates into early return to work, with significant economic gains both to the individual and society.

The disadvantages of minimally invasive surgery are few. The first one is the significant capital outlay required to equip operating rooms for safe surgery. Second is the steep learning curve of trainees to perform MIS. When open surgery is performed, the surgeon is able to feel the tissue, move and position the area that needs to be dissected or sutured as required. With MIS, the haptic feedback that the surgeon receives is significantly reduced. Procedures are performed with the surgeon looking at a monitor positioned above the patient displaying the operative field images obtained from the camera systems and telescopes within the patient's body. Three-dimensional actions such as mobilising and removing tissue and suturing are performed remotely while looking at a two-dimensional image positioned above the operating field.

While MIS has advantages over open surgery post-operatively, it still carries risk to the patient: it can be severely damaging if not performed correctly. This sets a high level of tension to each operation. With such high risks, mistakes need to be avoided at all costs, which places great significance on training, rehearsal, monitoring and feedback before the actual 'performance' with/on a live patient. The acquisition of all these skills requires the intense and systematic training of surgeons, which should ideally take place in a simulated environment outside of operating theatres before surgeons are allowed to perform these procedures on real patients. Training through simulation can be thought of as a sort of rehearsal, preparing the surgeon, as 'performer', to draw on their learned skill while having the confidence to improvise as necessary.

Learning MIS through simulation

The need to train surgeons in these new techniques to the level of competence that is required before operating on real patients created the need to develop new training methods. Traditionally, the basic principles of surgical technique regarding tissue handling were taught using the apprenticeship model of the Halstedian methods, which involve teaching surgery while operating on live patients (McGaghie *et al.*, 2010). There are now several simulation training methods available of various levels of complexity, from training in a simple 'black box' simulator to sophisticated virtual reality trainers with haptic feedback. These developments resulted in the establishment of surgical skills training centres, where surgery is simulated by trainees performing tasks in simulators designed to mimic minimally invasive procedures. The steps in this process are observed and evaluated by trainers who can monitor progress more objectively, away from the pressure of real patients.

Doing surgery is often termed 'performing' an operation, which describes it as accomplishing a procedural task. However, the techniques of MIS created the opportunity to train away from patients on specially designed training models, similar to rehearsals in the performing arts such as music and drama. The value of rehearsals is that they create a legitimate space for attempting something new, making mistakes and learning from them and trying again repeatedly (Ziv, 2005). Observations by mentors giving constructive feedback accelerates skills development.

For example, a complex task such as tying an intra-corporeal knot (i.e. after putting a suture through the tissues that require approximation, being able to tie the knot inside a cavity such as the abdomen) has a steep learning curve. The surgeon is expected to insert a needle into the abdominal cavity with access through 5- or 10-mm incisions and ports. Unable to see the tissue with the naked eye, but looking at the monitor, the operator must use instruments about 30cm long to accomplish the task of creating a knot, pulling it tight and securing it perfectly when finished so that it will not come loose. Every step in this task has been broken down into steps that need to be undertaken in a predictable fashion, similar to a scripted play or a piece of choreography. When mistakes happen, the steps are repeated until perfected. Mentors are able to observe the process and provide input when needed, which also often requires them to demonstrate the tasks in the correct format to the trainees.

Trainees need to achieve a certain level of competence when learning in the skills laboratory. There are four stages they need to go through, which were originally described by Broadwell as follows:

1. Unconscious incompetence (Ignorance): The individual does not understand or know how to perform a task and does not recognise the shortfall. The individual must recognise their own incompetence, and the value of the new skill, before moving on to the next stage. The higher their interest in learning the skills, the shorter period an individual stays in this stage.
2. Conscious incompetence (Awareness): The individual may not know how to do something, but he or she does recognise the deficit, as well as the value of a new skill in addressing the deficit. The making of mistakes is an integral part of the learning process at this stage.
3. Conscious competence (Learning): At this stage, the person understands and knows how to do the tasks. However, demonstrating the skill or knowledge requires significant concentration. Often the task is broken down into steps, and there is heavy conscious involvement in executing each step.
4. Unconscious competence (Mastery): This stage is entered when the person practises sufficiently for the skill to become 'second nature'. The individual may be able to teach it to others, depending on how and when it was learned (1969, p. 2).

MIS training in skills laboratories aims to bring the trainees to the consciously competent stage, where they are at a level to execute the tasks correctly. The process to reach this stage either from being a novice or from very little experience may take several days to achieve. It might be even more difficult if incorrect methods have been taught to the trainees prior to attending sessions in the training centres. It is also often this stage that gives them the greatest feeling of achievement when mastering skills such as suturing, using the MIS instrument with images displayed on a 2D monitor.

The transition from simulation or rehearsal to a first live performance is accompanied by the same level of anticipation and apprehension as in the performing arts, where a first night experience would be equivalent to the trainee surgeon's debut with a real patient. But by direct comparison to the performing arts, in which nobody could die, the stakes are higher in surgery, so here the similarities may diverge. McGaghie *et al.* (2010) reviewed the literature and identified the following twelve features of simulation-based medical education as best practices:

1. feedback
2. deliberate practice
3. curriculum integration
4. outcome measurement
5. simulation fidelity
6. skill acquisition and maintenance
7. mastery learning
8. transfer to practice
9. team training
10. high-stakes testing
11. instructor training
12. educational and professional context

Observing, monitoring and measuring each of these steps consecutively and systematically is likely to result in more consistent performance of surgical skills with a high degree of competence. These steps have direct implications for other fields of performance where, although known by other names, they may be more fluid and iterative rather than structured or sequential. It could be argued that surgical processes are more precisely choreographed and less open to individual interpretation than in the performing arts, resulting in a more clearly defined orthodoxy of 'correct' and 'incorrect' ways of performing surgery.

Physical and mental preparation for performing MIS

In addition to practising the components of tasks that are carried out to perform surgery such as mobilisation, dissection, resection and suturing of tissue, trainees are expected to practice the ergonomics of performing surgery. Ergonomics, the study of people's efficiency in their working environment, plays a significant role in many professions in fields as diverse as piloting, welding and brick laying. Surgery has been deficient in giving due importance to ergonomics, which focuses on complex interaction between the person performing it and the instrument and equipment used. Ergonomics plays a significant role in positioning a patient and equipment around the operative table, as well as positioning the monitors at the correct axis. These adjustments allow the surgeon to operate optimally using a two-dimensional monitor for surgery. Camera angles when a 30-degree telescope is used give significant advantage to the surgeon to visualise the corners that are difficult to see around. Tilting the telescope and allowing the angles to be changed is a task most new trainees struggle to perform. Repeated attempts, similar to doing many rehearsals, helps them to gain the muscle memory and reach a stage where it becomes a movement without thinking: the unconsciously competent stage.

It is most important for the surgeon to be in the correct position to perform the surgery. This is both for achieving the optimal ergonomic position to perform the task correctly but also for prevention of injuries. Often, standing in a static position for hours results in fatigue, and may adversely affect the surgical performance. Training sessions are used to allow the surgeons to practice the best ergonomic principles and utilise cognitive simulation to prepare themselves for the task ahead.

It is not only physical ergonomics that are important in the learning process: the mental preparation and state of mind of the operator are crucial to successful performance. Any type of human activity is associated with bodily arousal or stress, and any enhancement in performance necessitates an enhancement in bodily arousal (Prinsloo *et al.*, 2013; Rauch, Schönbächler and Noakes, 2013a). This means is that proficiency in MIS performance necessitates moving out of one's comfort zone and entering the 'performance zone'. The performance zone entails quietening of one's thoughts by heightening one's awareness yet maintaining a healthy tension in the body in order to teach the body the necessary neuromuscular coordination to perform MIS unconsciously (Rauch *et al.*, 2013b). A similar situation pertains in the theatre where an actor has to become attuned to their own internal state and that of the character respectively through interoceptive awareness, mental activity and emotion regulation (Moore, 1984). Heightened awareness must be focused on channelling the nervous tension into the spine by maintaining the correct posture and deep diaphragmatic breathing. Keeping an awareness of posture and breathing alive like this helps to keep intrusive thoughts at bay and keep the heart calm, thereby enabling the surgeon to acquire the necessary skills in a focused and calm state (Rauch *et al.*, 2013b).

Neurobiology of the 'performance zone'

The performance zone allows for optimal performance during surgery (or on stage), allowing 'unconscious competence' to emerge while under the pressure to achieve. Physiologically, the performance zone is associated with a ten-second rhythm in the heart and vasculature to bring about a slowing of the heart rate via the baroreflex to thereby dampen increases in blood pressure. The baroreflex is made up of pressure sensors in the vasculature that fire if the blood pressure is too high, which then signals nuclei in the brainstem to both lower heart rate and to decrease the vasoconstrictor drive to the vasculature. Engaging a state of heightened awareness will facilitate this baroreflex-mediated feedback regulation via the ventromedial prefrontal cortex, while over-thinking typically leads to engagement of the 'Fight and Flight' system that brings about increases in both blood pressure and heart rate, thereby over-riding the baroreflex mediated feedback regulation. (Fourie *et al.*, 2011; Rauch *et al.*, 2013b). Engaging a state of heightened awareness will enable the surgeon to stay calm yet have enough energy to remain composed and focused. This understanding of neurophysiology has direct implications for actors and performers in the creative and performing arts. For example, certain performance-related disorders such as focal dystonia (Currey *et al.*, 2020), a disabling persistent muscular incoordination during specific movements of instrument playing resulting from over practice, can only be successfully treated through such an understanding.

Key to remaining in the performance zone is maintaining the optimal brain chemical balance: enough norepinephrine for optimal attention but not excessive amounts that could set off fear perception, enough serotonin to facilitate timing of movements and to balance the autonomic nervous system and enough dopamine to maintain high levels of intrinsic reward that would be intricately linked to successful MIS performance (Jacobs and Fornal, 1999; Rauch, Schönbächler and Noakes, 2013a).

Apart from direct corticomotoneuronal control of movement, there are neuronal networks in the spinal cord able to directly control arm and leg movements (Frigon, 2017). Spinal cord control of movement, known as locomotor movement, is coordinated by the basal ganglia and executed via brainstem locomotor regions and central pattern generators (CPGs) in the spine. Locomotor patterns can be elicited in people with spinal cord injuries by direct stimulation of the lumbar spine (Dimitrijevic, Gerasimenko and Pinter, 1998), and electromyography (EMG) recordings show that precise motor programmes, which are not under cognitive control, are acti-vated to initiate walking at different speeds (Crenna and Frigo, 1991). Patterned control during many other types of movement has also been found, for instance, during swimming, jumping and arm reaching, which is indispensable for sporting and other performance (Lacquaniti, Ivanenko and Zago, 2012).

The distinction between cortically and spinally controlled movement is well demonstrated in a primate with a primary motor cortex lesion. Though the ape was unable to grasp a nail to open a box containing a peanut (fine motor control), it was nevertheless able to grasp a wire of the same thickness for the purpose of climbing (Pribram *et al.*, 1955). This finding may be explained by the fact that internally generated climbing movement is primarily coordinated by the basal ganglia (Jordan *et al.*, 2008; Grillner *et al.*, 2005), while grasping a nail is better described as a visually triggered movement requiring cerebellar and cortical input (van Donkelaar *et al.*, 1999).

For it to qualify as a performance rather than as a cognitive exercise, the fine motor control required for MIS would need to be performed via CPGs, although crucial additional inputs are needed, given that visually triggered movement requires precise temporal and spatial control of movement from the cerebellum (Sathyamurthy *et al.*, 2020). During the learning process leading up to performing the surgery on a living patient, inputs from the motor cortex are necessary to teach the subcortical structures how to execute fine motor control via direct corticomotor neurons.

Once a MIS procedure has been learned, however, direct cerebello-spinal neurons from the deep cerebellar nuclei enable the execution of skilled forelimb performance as well as continued skilled locomotor learning without cortical input (Sathyamurthy *et al.*, 2020). This would then free up the brain from conscious motor control to focus instead on performing the task at hand, much like an actor who has memorised their script can focus on a delivery able to captivate a theatre audience.

Measuring the impact of skills training

It is quite difficult to measure the true impact of skills training in the performance of MIS on real patients. Time and motion studies in the skills laboratory give an indication of progress based on the time taken to complete specific tasks to a specified degree of accuracy. However, the translation of these skills into performance in an operating theatre with a real patient, when the pressure is on and mistakes are no longer acceptable, creates a context similar to that of a live theatre performance.

One way of measuring the degree of success of this translation is to review the practice of trainees following the completion of a skills centre training course. Skills learned in the training centre are translatable to the operating theatre, and this has also been documented in a systematic review of randomised controlled studies (Vanderbilt, 2014). In a study performed by Westwood *et al.* (2020), career progression and use of MIS as a procedure of choice significantly increased in the group attending the course. The increased use of MIS techniques in operating theatres as a preferred technique following a skills lab training has been documented in many studies (Tejos, 2019; Torricelli, 2016; Westwood *et al.*, 2020).

Conclusion

The aims of this chapter align with the field of medical humanities, which considers the issues relating to medicine, health, healing and well-being from a wide interdisciplinary perspective including the social sciences and the creative and performing arts (Atkinson *et al.*, 2015; Puustinen *et al.*, 2003). There are an increasing number of educational initiatives in medical and health humanities, including those embedded in health sciences education (Reid, 2014). Using MIS as a specific example of the activities of surgery, we have illustrated the similarities to performance in any field that requires significant spatial coordination and dexterity while simultaneously maintaining conscious mental continuity for the bigger tasks at hand. The specific steps and principles developed for surgical training could be applicable in many of the creative and performing arts, as well as in competitive sports and other physically exacting activities. We hope that the brief insight into how surgeons are trained to perform MIS enables readers who are familiar with the performing artis to identify areas of similarity and difference relative to their own practice.

Reference list

Atkinson, S. *et al.* (2015). ' "The medical" and "health" in a critical medical humanities', *Journal of Medical Humanities*, 36, pp. 71–81. https://doi.org/10.1007/s10912-014-9314-4

Broadwell, M.M. (1969) 'Teaching for learning (XVI)', *The Gospel Guardian*. Available at: www.words fitlyspoken.org/gospel_guardian/v20/v20n41p1-3a.html (Accessed: 3 August 2023).

Crenna, P. and Frigo, C. (1991) 'A motor program for the initiation of forward-oriented movements in humans', *The Journal of Physiology*, 437, pp. 635–653.

Currey, J. *et al*. (2020) 'Performing arts medicine', *Physical Medicine and Rehabilitation Clinics of North America*, 31(4), pp. 609–632. https://doi.org/10.1016/j.pmr.2020.08.001

Dimitrijevic, M.R., Gerasimenko, Y. and Pinter, M.M. (1998) 'Evidence for a spinal central pattern generator in humans', *Annals of the New York Academy of Sciences*, 860, pp. 360–376.

Fourie, M.M. *et al*. (2011) 'Guilt and pride are heartfelt, but not equally so', *Psychophysiology*, 48, pp. 888–899.

Frigon, A. (2017) 'The neural control of interlimb coordination during mammalian locomotion', *Journal of Neurophysiology*, 117(6), pp. 2224–2241.

Gawande, A. (2007) *Better: a surgeon's notes on performance*. New York: Metropolitan.

Grillner, S. *et al*. (2005) 'Mechanisms for selection of basic motor programs: roles for the striatum and pallidum', *Trends in Neurosciences*, 28(7), pp. 364–370.

Jacobs, B.L. and Fornal, C.A. (1999) 'Activity of serotonergic neurons in behaving animals', *Neuropsychopharmacology*, (2 Suppl), pp. 9S–15S. https://doi.org/10.1016/S0893-133X(99)00012-3

Jordan, L.M. *et al*. (2008) 'Descending command systems for the initiation of locomotion in mammals', *Brain Research Reviews*, 57, pp. 183–191.

Kneebone, R.L. (2016a) 'Performing surgery', in Mermikides, A. and Bouchard, G. (eds.) *Performance and the medical body*. London: Bloomsbury Methuen Drama Publishing.

Kneebone, R.L. (2016b) 'Performing surgery: commonalities with performers outside medicine', *Frontiers in Psychology*, 7, p. 1233. https://doi.org/10.3389/fpsyg.2016.01233

Lacquaniti, F., Ivanenko, Y.P. and Zago, M. (2012) 'Patterned control of human locomotion', *The Journal of Physiology*, 590(10), pp. 2189–2199.

McGaghie, W.C. *et al*. (2010) 'A critical review of simulation-based medical education research: 2003–2009', *Medical Education*, 44(1), pp. 50–63.

McKenzie, J. (2001) *Perform or else: from discipline to performance*. New York: Routledge.

Mettler, L. (2003) 'Historical profile of Kurt Karl Stephan Semm', *Journal of the Society of Laparoendoscopic Surgeons*, 7(3), pp. 185–188.

Moore, S. (1984) *The Stanislavski system: the professional training of an actor*. New York: Penguin Books.

Pribram, K.H. *et al*. (1955) 'The effects of precentral lesions on the behaviour of monkeys', *Yale Journal of Biology and Medicine*, 28, pp. 428–443.

Prinsloo, G.E. *et al*. (2013) 'The effect of a single session of short duration biofeedback-induced deep breathing on measures of heart rate variability during laboratory-induced cognitive stress: a pilot study', *Applied Psychophysiology and Biofeedback*, 38, pp. 81–90.

Puustinen, R., Leiman, M. and Viljanen, A.M. (2003) 'Medicine and the humanities – theoretical and methodological issues', *Medical Humanities*, 29, pp. 77–80.

Rauch, H.G.L., Schönbächler, G. and Noakes, T.D. (2013a) 'Neural correlates of motor vigour and motor urgency during exercise', *Sports Medicine*, 43, pp. 227–241.

Rauch, H.G.L. *et al*. (2013b) 'Effect of Taijiquan training on autonomic re-activity and body position and postures during mock boxing: a feasibility study', in Balagué, N., Torrents, C., Vilanova, A., Cadefau, J., Tarragó, R., Tsolakidis, E. (eds.) *Book of abstracts, 18th congress of European college of sport science*. Barcelona: European College of Sports Science, pp. 25–28.

Reid, S. (2014) 'The "medical humanities" in health sciences education in South Africa', *SAMJ: South African Medical Journal*, 104(2), pp. 109–110.

Sathyamurthy, A. *et al*. (2020) 'Cerebellospinal neurons regulate motor performance and motor learning', *Cell Reports*, 31, p. 107595.

Schechner, R. (2006) *Performance studies: an introduction*. New York: Routledge.

Tejos, R. *et al*. (2019) 'Impact of a simulated laparoscopic training program in a three-year general surgery residency', *ABCD. Arquivos Brasileiros de Cirurgia Digestiva*, 32(2), p. e1436.

Torricelli, F.C., Barbosa, J.A. and Marchini, G.S. (2016) 'Impact of laparoscopic surgery training laboratory on surgeon's performance', *World Journal of Gastrointestinal Surgery*, 8(11), pp. 735–743.

van Donkelaar, P. *et al.* (1999) 'Neuronal activity in the primate motor thalamus during visually triggered and internally generated limb movements', *Journal of Neurophysiology*, 82(2), pp. 934–945.

Vanderbilt, A.A. *et al.* (2014) 'Randomized controlled trials: a systematic review of laparoscopic surgery and simulation-based training', *Global Journal of Health Science*, 7(2), pp. 310–327.

Westwood, E. *et al.* (2020) 'The impact of a laparoscopic surgery training course in a developing country', *World Journal of Surgery*, 44(10), pp. 3284–3289.

Ziv, A., Ben-David, S. and Ziv, M. (2005) 'Simulation based medical education: an opportunity to learn from errors', *Medical Teacher*, 27(3), pp. 193–199. https://doi.org/10.1080/01421590500126718

15

MATTERS OF THE HEART

The orchestration of hands in cardiac surgery

Christina Lammer, Tamar Tembeck and Wilfried Wisser

A man in white overalls paints on a large-scale paper canvas: puffy aerial structures, clouds and dark blue whirlwinds, drawn together by fine threads. He is working in an artist's studio, far away from his usual area of operations, the Cardiac Surgery Department at Medical University Vienna, Austria. Wilfried Wisser is a cardiac surgeon.

This moment took place in one of a series of painting and movement workshops at the artist-run centre OBORO in Montreal, Canada, where I, Christina Lammer, was artist in residence in May and June 2018. I am a sociologist and filmmaker. Also participating in these workshops was art historian, curator and performer Tamar Tembeck. This collaboration across art and medicine addressed questions about *Einfühlung* (empathy), care and the gestures of surgeons, and in these workshops we used theatrical methods, sensory ethnography and experimental filmmaking to explore the orchestration of hands in the operating theatre. The workshops formed part of a wider collaborative practice, dating since 2015, which employs artistic and ethnographic methods to investigate the gestures of surgeons. This has resulted in a series of artworks, videos and analogue films (Lammer, 2018, pp. 29–53).

Hands-on practice

My artist residency at OBORO, like the experiments in distributed simulation conducted by British surgeon Roger Kneebone, 'provided a framework for sharing experience, and a common ground on which to base discussion of possible connections' between surgery and the performing arts (Kneebone, 2016, p. 77). Whereas Kneebone tackled questions about surgery as performance by using the concept of simulation, 'inviting performers to *take part* in the activities of surgery' (ibid, p. 77), I involved a cardiac surgeon in the development of artworks. Wilfried Wisser accepted my invitation to spend a week together at OBORO's artist studios, where we combined physical theatre approaches and action painting – learning to listen to the heart through performative and filmic practices.

In this chapter, we focus on three aspects of surgical 'performance' that we explored through choreography: the hand washing and hygiene procedures which take place before surgery; drawings that surgeons do to explain procedures – in this case, a minimally invasive surgery of the mitral valve – which we explored through action painting; and gestures during operations – covering the body with sterile cloths and the making of surgical knots in the closing stages

DOI: 10.4324/9781003036500-18

of the same operation, which we investigated by making a 16-mm multiple-exposure short experimental film, *Stitches in the Heart* (2019). While the experiments we describe involved close collaboration, it has been a challenge to write this chapter collaboratively because the COVID-19 pandemic made personal meetings impossible. In order to find a common language that allows us to articulate our individual experiences, we use a framework of 'correspondences' (Ingold, 2021), each writing in the first person. Thus, this chapter includes sections of dialogue and transcripts of interviews we conducted with each other to make our distinct voices perceivable.

Washing hands

Before operations on the heart can begin, a number of preparations are necessary. Strict hygiene measures must be followed in order to be allowed to operate on a body. Among the precautions are surgical gowning procedures, using sterile garments and fabrics, masks and gloves, and hand scrubbing with soap and disinfectant. In the course of making *Hand Washing* (2018), a 16-mm multiple-exposure black and white short film, Tamar, Wilfried and I jointly explored the gestural dimensions of the surgical cleaning ritual. For this we spent a day together in the studio, reproducing the movement sequences of the hand washing procedures demonstrated by Wilfried. Tamar conducted the workshop, and after a Pilates warm-up she initiated us in some compositional principles drawn from her training in corporeal mime. In contrast to mime, where movement is employed in an illustrative manner to replace speech, corporeal mime is a form of physical theatre that situates the drama within the actor's body: changes in pressure, resistance, rhythm and weight convey struggle in the body's movements, which can be read as metaphors for the movements of thought. In the words of the founder of this practice, Étienne Decroux, '*Le corps est un gant dont le doigt serait la pensée*' (The body is a glove whose finger would be thought) (1963, p. 30, free translation). Here, Tamar explains the relevance of this performance tradition to the study of surgical 'scrubbing up':

Christina: Could you outline your concept for the workshop and your particular use of physical theatre approaches?

Tamar: I wanted to start from a movement vocabulary that is so engrained in the process of surgical practice that one would not even have to think about it. So I asked Wilfried to walk us through his daily ritual, before even entering the operating theatre. He showed us his extensive hygiene routine, which involves a very thorough washing of the hands, including digits, palms, wrists and lower arms, and an elaborate choreography using elbows and knees to avoid unnecessarily touching handles or dispensers. During his presentation, I was fascinated to be able to follow what appeared to be Wilfried's internal transformation over the course of this functional ritual. During the twenty-minute sequence, as the handwashing progressed, one could tell that Wilfried's focus was gradually becoming sharper. It was evident to me that his hygiene routine was accompanied by a form of mental preparation for the high-stakes operation that, in the real world, would follow. I was also very impressed by the seriousness he brought to our experiment, and the extreme precision that transpired through his gestures. This was not 'make believe', it was a faithful reproduction of a routine he is used to conducting on a daily basis. As such, Wilfried's gestural vocabulary was very much embodied; it was not something he was 'putting on'. I was delightfully surprised, and ultimately very grateful that he, as a cardiac surgeon, was willing to be 'all in' for our artistic experiment. He was fully committed to the process, and in that respect, I discovered a new, unsuspected connection between his line of work and the approach of many performing artists.

Once Wilfried completed his demonstration, Tamar directed our moving bodies. She asked Wilfried to repeat specific excerpts from his sequence so that we could also learn them. Gradually, we developed a few shared movement scores, all directly drawn from Wilfried's regular pre-operative hygiene rituals. Tamar trained in corporeal mime with a number of Étienne Decroux's students, including Thomas Leabhart, from whom she learnt to develop her movement research on the basis of real, quotidian actions, such as tying a shoe or buttoning up a shirt. Here, the raw source material for our joint movement research was Wilfried's handwashing ritual.

Extending movement

On the basis of these daily, repeated actions, a spatial and dynamic vocabulary unfolded between us. Our bodies began to take shape as expressive instruments. Tamar guided us in extending the movements from real actions to more expressive and gestural ones. The following exchange took place during this work:

Tamar: Can you do that same part fast, the way you actually do it in the preparation?
Wilfried: Okay, then it is easier. I take it, open it, put it away, rinse. . . . It is an easy task because if you are in a hurry you do it fast anyway.
Tamar: And if you just extend each movement a little bit more than natural. If you are reaching, you are reaching a little bit more.
Wilfried: Extending in the sense of orientation and stretching?
Tamar: Yes.
Wilfried: Not in the sense of time.
Tamar: Orientation and stretching.
Wilfried: Orientation in space. Interesting task.

We built on that by adding steps, extending the volume of each gesture. Wilfried would describe the materials and objects he uses when washing himself, for example, a transparent plastic box that contains a sponge. His verbal descriptions helped us to better understand how he would move:

Wilfried: You take the sponge out. Then you throw the package into the bin.
Tamar: Go back to the initial sequence and where it transitions into the next one. I mean, if you reach, how does this action of reaching change the way you get to your next position? . . . The arm movement contaminates the rest of the body, it gets expanded into the rest of the body.

Through the extension of each particular movement, we were able to analyse these ordinary actions, to uncover the bodily (as opposed to functional) logic that leads from one gesture to another. Magnifying the movements, changing their pace, their orientation in space or the resistance used to enact them were amongst the compositional techniques Tamar employed to explore Wilfried's functional movement score as raw matter for expressive material.

Tuning in

I had the opportunity to see this hand washing ritual in the context of real operations that Wilfried and other surgeons invited me to attend at the Medical University Vienna. I also witnessed Wilfried's preparation for surgery. Usually there is no time to warm up before the surgical intervention. There is never the opportunity for rehearsal; according to Lisa Cartwright, 'all cuts are a live performance' (2015, p. 261). Nevertheless, Wilfried would prepare for surgery. He would visualise the procedures in the scrub room while washing and getting ready for the operation. He would tune himself in physically and mentally. He described this process in our interview:

Christina: Could you describe in which way you visualise the operation while you are washing hands?

Wilfried: As soon as I start washing my hands, I somehow leave every other task or obligation behind. I automatically, sometimes actively, empty my mind. I am getting focused on the operation, putting myself in a contemplative state where everything around me diminishes. I can feel into the body of my patient, comparable with how an actor would embody the character he is playing on the stage. The more difficult an operation is going to be, the more actively and intensely I immerse and sense the patient as a whole person.

When I am washing my hands, I am experiencing two additional things beside the sole cleaning procedures and the already mentioned processes. The physical part is an activation of my working tools, my hands and forearms, comparable to warming up the respective parts of the body, muscles and fascia, in sports, music or singing. The second part is the visualisation of the operation. During these couple of minutes, the main parts of the surgery pass by like a time lapse film. However, I can stop it at any moment, slowing down the speed, zooming in, recapping.

In my ongoing research at the clinic, I explore how surgeons use their bodies as healing instruments.[1] Relational aspects, for example, how organs are touched, are tackled. The significance of hands in surgery took me back to Thomas Leabhart's descriptions of hands in the context of Decroux's *Mime Corporel.* Hands, according to Leabhart, only play a subordinate role in this practice. He outlines in *Etienne Decroux* (2019),

[e]ven if the hands did sometimes of necessity occupy space away from the center of the body, they needed strong energetic links to that center. While the hands hold the tool – often close to the center of the body – the body does the work.

(2019, p. 93)

Thus, meaning arises from the way in which the whole body moves in space, engaging with other bodies, instruments and material components.

Moving in space

In the operating theatre, the person who needs to be operated on is lying on the table, scrub nurses and an assistant surgeon wash the body of the patient and cover them almost entirely with sterile cloth, marking out the area of operation. Before that the anaesthesia is administered. The cloths that cover the patient during surgery help with keeping the surgical field hygienic. However, they also have an important social function. The patient's face, their persona, is made to disappear. Draping serves as a barrier that allows the surgeons to entirely focus on the carefully marked out field of operation.

Christina: Can you imagine seeing the face of the patient while you are performing an operation on his or her heart?

Wilfried: I personally have no problem, although it would be unusual to see the patient's face during an operation. However, we once tested a surgical draping which had a transparent coating in the area of the patient's head. With this wrapping one could see the head in the course of the entire surgery. The reason for fully covering the body with an opaque fabric is twofold: The bright operating lights are absorbed by the cloth. In this way any disturbing reflections are avoided. Furthermore, the surgical cover allows to fully draw the attention to the operating field. That's more important for the team than it is for myself. There is less distraction. I would agree with you that draping is a barrier which helps to focus, though for me the patient does not disappear as a person! I am feeling into the person during the operation. I am bearing in my mind his or her character, mindset, hopes, anxieties, everything I know from this particular patient, very much like an actor who slips into the role of the character he or she has to embody.

We explored the qualities and meaning of surgical drapes in our movement workshop at OBORO. For example, we set up a ritual in which Tamar and Wilfried unpacked and unfolded a large white piece of fabric over a wooden dining table we were using as operating table. Drawing on earlier arts-based research projects in which we analysed the social function of the sterile wrappings, we performed artistic operations. Among the questions we tackled were the negotiation of proximity and distance and the regulation of touch in the operating room. A white cotton fabric represented the layers of cloth by which the body of the patient is almost entirely covered during surgery. The package for the delicate textile material was designed by visual artist Barbara Graf, with whom I have been collaborating for more than two decades. Modes of wrapping and packaging in surgery are important issues in Graf's artistic oeuvre. In our long-term collaboration we are turning the artist's studio into an operating theatre in order to disclose the widely unseen social and cultural mechanisms which are at work in surgery.

Painting and filming surgery

My collaboration with surgeons drew my attention to the way in which they use hand drawing of operations when explaining procedures to patients. What I discovered during fieldwork was that although the purpose of these drawings was to mediate knowledge, they also had emotional impact for the people who were anticipating having surgery. In particular, it is an important component of how surgeons build trust with their patients (Lammer and Zmijewski, 2013). Wilfried and I adapted this practice with the intention to present his surgical drawings of a mitral valve operation to an artistic audience at OBORO's galleries. For this, the cardiac surgeon drew and explained the procedures as a form of reenactment, which I video recorded, for an imaginary public. Wilfried would magnify smaller images which he had already prepared. In order to better understand his (personal) working style, I asked him to use a paintbrush instead of the surgical instruments and make colour paintings of the procedures. Wilfried painted entirely abstract images of the mitral valve, using colours which do not correspond at all with those of the body's inside. I asked him why:

Christina: Why did you use shades of white and blue?

Wilfried: That's simple! On the day at OBORO, I tried to mentally get into a typical operation. Sometimes I am in the flow while performing a surgery. The procedures easily go from the hand. Surgery 'simply happens'. And then I painted. On this day I used white and blue. I did not intentionally choose those colours. The other day I might have applied green and ochre. For the painting session, I purposely avoided work with colours which exist inside of the body.

A mysterious landscape gradually took shape on a white wall. The surgeon turned his attention inwards in order to make abstract images of his intraoperative perception of a heart valve. His gestures and body language told a story of what it feels like being intimately entangled, physically and mentally, with the most delicate structures inside of the heart.

The 16-mm multiple-exposure short film of a mitral valve surgery, *Stitches in the Heart* (2019), is another example of the empathetic entanglement of Wilfried's gestures with the tissue inside of the body (Lammer, 2020, pp. 114–121). The dexterity of the surgeon's hands is technologically enhanced. He uses magnifying glasses, endoscopes and tools which allow him to enter the body through little openings. In minimally invasive valve surgery, the length of the surgical instruments corresponds with the size of the physical structures in the interior. Material components are transported through the channels and cavities by precise movements. Valve tissue needs to be removed and replaced. Fine threads are pulled through the physical fabric. The loose ends are clamped on a circular frame that is positioned around the field of incision. One is reminded of the strings of a musical instrument. Tension and release of the surgical suture material should be kept in perfect harmony.

Epilogue

In our collaborative work we apply physical theatre and gestural art practices with the intention to better understand the performance of cardiac surgery. The ways in which the body of the operator and the patient's heart are intimately entangled during minimally invasive valve operations are represented in the form of abstract paintings and experimental analogue films. Surgeons penetrate into the total reality of human existence. They change the composition of the viscera in order to support the body's capacity to heal. In our artistic practice we develop ways of piercing through the tubes, valves and cavities of the heart not only with the help of a scalpel but in the imagination, performing operations on the most delicate organic structures and strings under the skin.

Acknowledgements

This chapter was supported by the Austrian Science Fund in the Programme for Arts-based Research under the title Visceral Operations/Assemblage (2019–23). The financial support for this research is gratefully acknowledged [Grant Number AR515].

Note

1 Lammer, C. (2015) *Performing surgery*. Available at: www.corporealities.org/ps/. Lammer, C. (2019) *Visceral operations: assemblage*. Available at: www.corporealities.org/visceral-operations-assemblage/

Reference list

Cartwright, L. (2015) 'Visual science studies: always already materialist', in Carusi, A. *et al.* (eds.) *Visualization in the age of computerization*. New York: Routledge, pp. 243–268.

Decroux, E. (1963) *Paroles sur le mime*. Paris: Gallimard.

Hand Washing (2018) [16mm multiple exposure black and white film, 4 minutes, 18 frames per second]. Directed by C. Lammer. Montreal. Available at: https://vimeo.com/299176151, Vimeo password: corporealities (accessed 4 December 2023)

Ingold, T. (2021) *Correspondences*. Cambridge: Polity.

Kneebone, R. (2016) 'Performing surgery', in Mermikides, A. and Bouchard, G. (eds.) *Performance and the medical body*. London and New York: Bloomsbury, pp. 67–81.

Lammer, C. (2018) 'Performing surgery: exploring gestures in the operating theatre', *Interfaces*, 40, pp. 29–53.

Lammer, C. (2020, Spring/Fall) 'The camera is the massage', in Weinbren, G. (ed.) *Millennium film journal, numbers 71/72*. New York: Millennium Film Workshop, pp. 114–121.

Lammer, C. and Zmijewski, A. (2013) *Anatomy lessons*. Vienna: Löcker Verlag.

Leabhart, T. (2019) *Etienne Decroux*. 2nd edn. New York: Routledge.

Stitches in the Heart (2019) [16mm multiple exposure black and white film, 4 minutes, 18 frames per second]. Directed by C. Lammer. Vienna. Available at: https://vimeo.com/381168259, Vimeo password: corporealities

16

BECOMING

Lucinda Coleman

In 2020, I was commissioned as a choreographer by Edith Cowan University (ECU) to create a contemporary dance film to represent the work of health care professionals in celebration of the 2020 International Year of the Nurse and Midwife. My intention was to create an interdisciplinary piece which playfully challenged stereotypes of nurses and midwives through authentic, reflexive storytelling. The genre of screendance provided an innovative space to creatively engage with the voice of the health care worker from within their own profession. The unexpected outcome was that the opportunity for cross-disciplinary collaboration challenged conventions of dancemaking for the screen, shifted audience perceptions of nurses and midwives, and created an artefact for promotion of the health care profession in a new way to new audiences (Cook, 2021; Ritchie, 2021; Ng, 2021).

The dance film, *Becoming*, features six dancers performing a series of duos and solos in hospital wards, in a new mother's home, on the beach, in a dance studio, and accompanied by an original, devised soundscape. The film integrates movement composition with cinematic conventions to create dance for the screen and is freely available via ECU's YouTube channel.

Becoming was delicately shaped by the reflections of thirteen experienced registered nurses (RNs) and registered midwives (RMs), whose recorded words determined the form of dance and provided the basis for the film's soundscape. *Becoming* explores the situation of a health worker being alone with a patient in crisis, caring for a new mother and baby, and responding to the death of a patient: all moments described by RNs/RMs as significant in identity formation. As one nurse reflected, 'there's no way we can get rid of, or reduce suffering, but we can do something about it' (Nurse voiceover: 00:36–00:40).

The sounds and images of water have been used as a metaphor for the nurses becoming professional carers: from washing hands, to tears, to immersion in the ocean, as representative of the all-encompassing work of RNs/RMs. The spoken reflections offered insight into health professionals' roles and their experiences of managing birth, illness, pain, and death, illuminating stories of advocacy with honesty, humour, and sensitivity. The recorded voices, together with ambient sounds and musical composition, constitute the soundscape for dancers whose work offers a performative response to nuanced emotions of shared narratives of care.

DOI: 10.4324/9781003036500-19

The commission provided an opportunity to cross-pollinate performing arts with the health sector and develop contemporary dance which might yield insight into the health profession through performance. The cross-disciplinary space benefits from a collaborative 'insider outsider' perspective which challenges the conventions of a single discipline: disrupting, illuminating, questioning, and reinventing pathways for innovative practices and inviting new ways of seeing the work of others (Sabroe and Declercq, 2021, 21:51mins). As the project cinematographer/editor, Rakib Erick, observed, 'I did not have any idea what a nurse or midwives go through with their work life. Seeing and hearing made me realize there's a lot going [on in hospitals] than what we see generally' (2021).

Becoming illuminates the potential of the academy to support epistemological art-making within the health humanities, in the sense of inviting deeper engagement of knowledge systems within a disciplinary field whilst simultaneously rupturing conventions of habit that would not typically be challenged. As a dancer in the film, Sarah Chaffey, commented, an artistic representation of health workers reveals the significance:

of engagement that these professionals have in the life cycle of the general public/patients (from birth to death). As such, the emotional and physical challenges they face in their profession on a daily basis . . . offer audiences the opportunity to reflect and appreciate the work of these professionals outside of the context of needing to directly require their assistance.

(2021)

The complexities of cross-disciplinary collaboration are not unfamiliar for artistic practitioners seeking 'to discuss the fleshiness of shared affective experiences' (Barbour, Hunter and

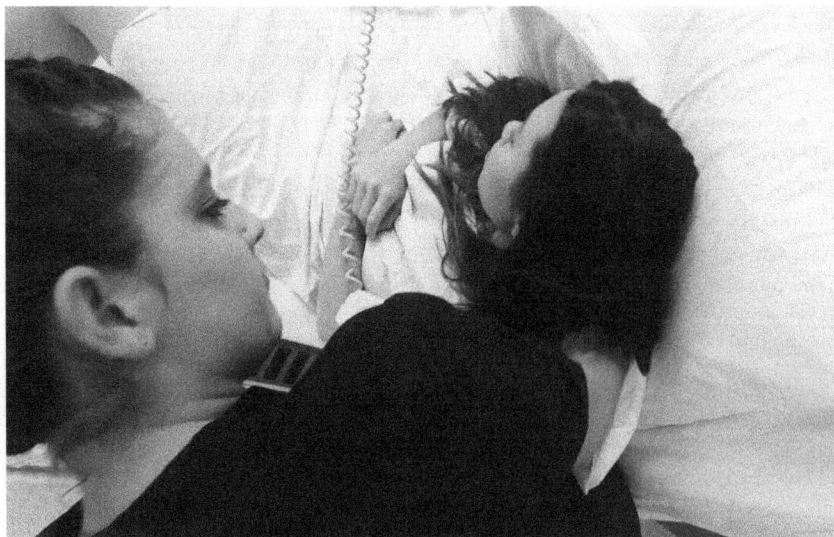

Figure 16.1 Becoming: A Contemporary Dance Film ©2020 (film still). The performers are Samantha Coleman (left) and Charity Ng.

Kloetzel, 2019, p. 109). Less common is translating the experiences of health practitioners into artistic artefacts to share stories perhaps unheard or unseen previously. Creative modes of meaning-making offer possibilities for affective engagement. As registered nurse and midwife, Emma Ritchie, observed of *Becoming*, 'the interpretation of words into dance was interesting, dramatic and entertaining' (2021), which ensured stories were heard, received, and remembered.

Process of becoming

And while she transitioned into motherhood, I felt transitioned from a student into a midwife.

(Nurse voiceover: 00:54–01:02)

Preparations for developing the contemporary dance film began when senior staff from the ECU School of Nursing and Midwifery invited and supported a select group of experienced ECU RNs/RMs to discuss how their professional experiences had shaped each to become a professional nurse and/or midwife. I was invited to record the stories of RNs/RMs managing a situation of pain/crisis on one's own for the first time, delivering and caring for a baby and new mother, and experiencing the death of a patient. RNs/RMs discussed moments in practices which unalterably shaped who they are as professionals. The impact of situations of caring for human beings were communicated through tears, gestures, and facial expressions, as well as through words. Through conversation, themes began to emerge, and it became clear that water (tears, sweat, liquids) was a fitting metaphor for RNs/RMs becoming fully seasoned and mature practitioners (from washing hands, bathing patients/babies, to immersion in the care of another person whose body is made mostly of water).

The descriptions of what it feels like to become seasoned RNs/RMs shaped the choreography. Spoken reflections became the heart of the film's soundscape, which also included sounds of running water, hospital noises, ocean waves, and composed instrumental music. I choreographed for the screen, in collaboration with professional contemporary dancers, in response to what, and how, stories were shared by the senior RNs/RMs. Text extracts were selected based on how common the experiences were for the health workers. Rather than a literal dramatic re-enactment of experiences, common emotions and reoccurring observations were interpreted through dance phrases, spoken text offering context for the dance. Through the process of developing dance material, project artists came to understand, in the words of one dancer, that 'cross-disciplinary work can be done well between both performing arts and health sectors, giving it time and space to allow each side of the stories to be heard. I think there is not much work that blends the arts with health' (Ng, 2021).

The choreographic structure for the film was determined by the commentary, observation, reflection, and stories communicated by the RNs/RMs. The establishing shot of the Indian Ocean moving off the coast of Western Australia (WA) and within a frame without horizon or shoreline cuts to water running from a tap in a hospital ward as student nurses demonstrate washing hands and voiceovers set the scene within the Australian context (Edith Cowan University, 2020: 00:00–00:58). While some experiences may be universally relatable, the work is 'Australia specific and cannot be generalised to other countries as the role and scope of these professions vary internationally' (Ritchie, 2021) and are visually represented as such through costuming and location in the dance film.

The first sequence of the film explores the emotional and physical challenges of coping with a patient in pain, as 'that's what nursing is all about: it's about getting rid of pain' (Nurse voiceover: 01:35–01:38). To capture the stress involved in responding to situations of crisis, reflective comments were layered as part of a soundscape that included emergency buzzes and hospital noises:

---

when I was a very, very junior nurse, um, and I was looking after a woman and she fell out of

bed and broke her hip. I was very, very junior and I just thought, oh shit, what have I done, and I
. this beautiful young lady, um, had no marks on her at all, apart from a big gash across the
just felt all this blame that came on me, and she's on the floor, like, oh my God, and I knew
back of her head which was really quite significant; it was very significant at the time, and
straight away that she had broken her hip, and I was just devastated
she was bleeding quite profusely from this wound across the head

. . . because of her clinical problems, sure enough, she went into heart failure

---

Figure 16.2   (Nurses' voiceovers spoken simultaneously: 01:57–02:57)

The second sequence represents the experiences of pregnancy, labour, and birth. One dancer performs as a midwife in danced phrases; another dancer who recently gave birth to a son, holds her newborn during the dancing, the two adults' movements representing shared care of the baby. The choreography emphasises symmetry, harmony, and strength of relationship through circular movement patterns, to create a sense of a bubble or nest: holding space through trust, because 'with midwifery, it's about *working with* pain, so we turn pain into a positive thing rather than a negative thing' (Midwife voiceover: 04:46–04:54).

---

the midwife
literally holds the woman,
y'know, on her face, and just
looks into her eyes, like, you
can do this: you're doing
really well and you
can do this

(Midwife voiceover: 05:38–05:49)

Death and dying is the focus of the third sequence. Spoken reflections are interspersed with sounds of wind, ocean waves, hospital noises, and water splashing in a bowl for bathing a dying patient: 'death makes you know yourself better, and it also puts into perspective, *life*' (Nurse voiceover: 08:43–08:49).

The transitions between film scenes were choreographed to be quick to represent the fast pace of health care. RNs/RMs described the need to walk out of one situation and immediately into a new situation of care, so doorways and circling movements are used to signal rapid shifts in focus between scenes. The transition from the hospital crisis scene to a midwife visiting a new mother and baby is represented by dancers spinning in sequence one, which then cuts to a new dancer spiralling outside a doorway to a home (03:48–04:21). The text bridges one scene to the next: 'we're in the most trusting profession and when we walk through the door, and whether you're a nurse or a midwife, you introduce yourself' (Nurse voiceover: 04:06–04:14). At the close of the second sequence, the camera circles the midwife and mother, then cuts to a doorway in a hospital ward, as the spoken text reminds us that 'sometimes there's no time to even think; I think it's just a skill that you learn. . . . It's literally like closing a door and then you open another one' (Nurse voiceover: 06:36–06:44). In the third sequence with beach and hospital bed scenes, the transition to an ending sees the dancer who has sat with a dying patient emerge from ocean waves to return to the hospital corridor, and again, the spoken reflection of a nurse is used to share the story of this struggle:

> you feel like you're proud, you're really proud of your profession; you feel like a duck under water, the legs are y'know, your patient could have been told they have cancer; another one might have just passed away, you still have to come out of them rooms and go into the next patient room and pretend nothing has happened.

> (Nurse voiceover: 10:51–11:18)

Becoming artefact

> If it doesn't affect you a little bit, you probably shouldn't be in that profession. We're in a caring profession. If you don't shed a tear, y'know . . .
> (Nurse voiceover: 10:38–10:48)

The benefits of artistic collaborations have been well documented in the performing arts (Barr, 2015; Bench and Ellis, 2015; Stock, 2014; Knox, 2017). In *Becoming*, the making of dance directed by texts provoked the manipulation of bodily shapes to communicate emotion. Movement dynamics were shaped by narratives of care, and as one dancer commented, 'I felt the responsibility to be more raw and genuine than I would normally be in my own specific discipline to convey a true scenario of a nurse and her emotional journey' (Scott, 2021).

As an artistic artefact, *Becoming* offers a glimpse into another way of learning, seeing, feeling, and understanding the work of nurses and midwives, because dance communicates emotion in a uniquely powerful way. As cinematographer/editor Erick noted:

> For me it's about creating a bridge between two worlds. Art speaks to millions therefore it is important. Not everyone is willing to hear or see what a nurse goes through (because it can be traumatising experience to hear) but portraying in a dance movement and capturing it is truly fascinating and comforting at the same time.

> (2021)

There is unsettling insight in receiving performed narratives in the language of contemporary dance. After the film screening to collaborating health care workers, artists, and invited guests at

Vin+Flower in Perth, WA, on 8 December 2020, one registered nurse and midwife reflected that 'I felt the negative or dark side of nursing and midwifery was well portrayed. The difficulty and challenges are often overlooked in other media' (Ritchie, 2021). Responses from audience members during and following the screening were overwhelmingly positive, excited, and affirming. The language of dance captured the emotional experience of RNs/RMs not often seen or understood by those outside the profession or even sometimes by those within the profession. Research questionnaires distributed to collaborating participants after the screening invited further reflection. As collaborating registered nurse and midwife Patricia Cook later wrote:

> The emotional burden nurses take on, push down, and get on with other tasks was a highlight for me. How we can become desensitised, because we have to. I felt really connected to other nurses/midwives when watching this film, supported in the knowledge that nurses have had similar experiences as I have and are still dwelling on incidents that happened many years ago, which has helped form the nurses/people that we are today.
>
> (2021)

The dance film is 'not necessarily a new concept but still a contribution to this area of cross-disciplinary practices involving dance' (Chaffey, 2021). As one dancer later reflected, 'personally, I don't think it developed any new experimental dance work for the screen. There's honestly nothing new anymore' (Khoo, 2021). Yet the cross-disciplinary space humbly ensures the

> dance film innovates by blending different sectors, ideas and styles. It has a balance of the narrative storytelling from the health professionals, the dancers moving and interacting with each other and the space, the cinematographic element and the composition of music to complement what's happening on screen.
>
> (Ng, 2021)

As such, the artefact becomes distinctive for 'offering the representation of new themes through dance – merging theatrical and abstract dance qualities into film' (Chaffey, 2021) and inviting new audiences to encounter the work of RNs/RMs with fresh perspectives. As an artistic product, distinct from a clinical instructional video, *Becoming* has application for situations of training, recruitment, instruction, and education, simply because, in the words of one of the dancers, 'the audience heard the stories and felt the journeys of the nurses and midwives' (Scott, 2021). The significance of a dance film about RNs/RMs, as Cook explains, is that:

> The film provided an opportunity for expression that goes beyond words. Rather than talking about feelings, it showed how various experiences felt – joy and happiness at a birth, numbness and fatigue (nurse supporting others), compassion and empathy (dying). The film showed the non-tangibles – the emotions, the situations, and was moving but not confronting. Film can help to release emotions which otherwise may be talked away.
>
> (2021)

Conclusion

I don't think you can do it cognitively and sometimes when you have that cup of tea half an hour later, it's too soon; you haven't processed it properly.

(Nurse voiceover: 11:24–11:31)

Becoming is an invitation to listen to what health practitioners are thinking and feeling as they care for human beings. Aesthetic tension generates affective experiences for audiences through embodiment:

> Watching the film was incredibly moving – the dance, the stories, the music were all incredible in their own right, and when brought together is fantastic. When I first heard of the project, I was bewildered at how nursing/midwifery could be represented by dance. I was delighted in viewing the film. The film highlighted the 'dance' or interactions we have with people when they are at their most vulnerable, or the biggest days in one's life.
>
> (Cook, 2021)

Artistic projects which interrogate the practices and experiences of those in the health profession invite collaboration, understanding, and curiosity across sectors, which 'improves networking and respect and awareness' (Ritchie, 2021). Cross-disciplinary conversations enlarge the capacity for exploration, inquiry, and change. The vulnerability of nurses and need for self-care revealed through an artistic medium invites (re)consideration of professional practices and approaches for managing care in the sector. The delicate revelation of porous boundaries between patient and nurse/midwife is evinced in the sweep of skin and circular turns of bodies dissolving boundaries through dancemaking. Although the choreographic intention was not social transformation, artistic ephemeron has potential to shift, disrupt, delight, provoke, and transform at the intersection of the performing arts and health fields.

Acknowledgements

Becoming was commissioned and funded by Edith Cowan Commissions for the *2020 International Year of the Nurse and Midwife*. Special thanks to the staff at the School of Nursing and Midwifery and the Western Australian Academy of Performing Arts, Edith Cowan University, Western Australia. In particular, the author would like to acknowledge and thank all participating collaborators and artists involved in making the dance film.

Reference list

Barbour, K., Hunter, V. and Kloetzel, M. (2019) *(Re)positioning site dance local acts, global perspectives.* Bristol, UK: Intellect.

Barr, S. (2015) 'Collaborative practices in dance research: unpacking the process', *Research in Dance Education*, 16, pp. 51–66. https://doi.org/10.1080/14647893.2014.971233

Bench, H. and Ellis, S. (2015) 'Editors' note: on community, collaboration, and difference', *The International Journal of Screendance*, 5, pp. 1–8.

Chaffey, S. (2021) *Research survey with S. Chaffey.* Interviewed by L. Coleman. *Becoming* [dance film]. Western Australia: Edith Cowan University.

Cook, P. (2021) *Research survey with P. Cook.* Interviewed by L. Coleman. *Becoming* [dance film]. Western Australia: Edith Cowan University.

Edith Cowan University (2020) *Becoming – a contemporary dance film.* Available at: www.youtube.com/watch?v=OGUrrJCTgLo (Accessed: 1 March 2022).

Erick, R. (2021) *Research survey with R. Erick.* Interviewed by L. Coleman. *Becoming* [dance film]. Western Australia: Edith Cowan University.

Khoo, S. (2021) *Research survey with S. Khoo.* Interviewed by L. Coleman. *Becoming* [dance film]. Western Australia: Edith Cowan University.

Knox, S. (2017) '"It's all of me there, all of the time": meanings and experiences of a holistic view of the individual within choreographic collaboration', *Journal of Emerging Dance Scholarship*, 5, pp. 1–31.

Ng, C. (2021) *Research survey with C. Ng*. Interviewed by L. Coleman. *Becoming* [dance film]. Western Australia: Edith Cowan University.

Ritchie, E. (2021) *Research survey with E. Ritchie*. Interviewed by L. Coleman. *Becoming* [dance film]. Western Australia: Edith Cowan University.

Sabroe, I. and Declercq, D. (2021) *Episode 9 – In conversation with professor Paul Crawford*. Conversations About Arts, Humanities and Health. Available at: https://open.spotify.com/episode/6DvEdsJPgfOVZ4dgzE2Mxh (Accessed: 1 November 2021).

Scott, E. (2021) *Research survey with E. Scott*. Interviewed by L. Coleman. *Becoming* [dance film]. Western Australia: Edith Cowan University.

Stock, C. (2015) 'Evoking poetics of memory through performing site: Naik Naik, a Malaysian Australian collaboration in the world heritage setting of Melaka', in Stock, C. and Germain-Thomas, P. (eds.) *Contemporising the past: envisaging the future proceedings of the 2014 world dance alliance global summit 6–11 July 2014*. Angers, France: Ausdance National, pp. 1–14.

17

BUILDING COMMON FICTIONS

Practising dramaturgy as mediation in three medical performances

Pauline Bouchet

This chapter analyses three projects that emerged from a collaboration, starting in 2016, between the Department of Performing Arts at the University of Grenoble-Alpes and the University Hospital Centre in France, which aimed to rethink the training of doctors. The three projects discussed here cover the field of 'medical performances' as discussed by Alex Mermikides (2020): simulation-based medical education, artistic projects with patients and performances that represent medical experiences. In these three projects, I found myself in the place of a 'tiers familiarisé', to use the term of Julie Henry (a professor of philosophy at the Ecole Normale Supérieure in Lyon), which can be translated as 'an acquainted third party'. I am neither an artist nor a medical practitioner but a teacher-researcher in theatre studies who works with the medical community and has two artistic practices (dramaturgy for several companies and improvisation in professional and amateur leagues). I am also a volunteer listener in palliative care in cancer departments who is trained in active listening. In these three contexts, I have occupied the position of a mediator: I served as an intermediary with a medical school and a trainer for performing arts students in simulated consultations (a project that has been running for five years at the time of writing); I facilitated playwriting workshops with cancer patients that led to a collaboration with a stage director who made them work with professional actors around a show based on the texts written in the workshop; and I am an artistic collaborator and dramaturg for the show *Si vous voulez de la lumière*, which represents Faust as an haematologist. Through the development of these projects in the medical humanities, I drew on my understanding of the field of dramaturgy in order to link interlocutors who do not have the same vocabulary.

My hypothesis is that the practice of dramaturgy is the ideal place for mediation in projects linking the world of theatre and the world of medicine because it is precisely the right tool for an interdisciplinary exchange. I would therefore like to turn to definitions of dramaturgy to show how this practice can mediate interdisciplinary dialogues between artists, caregivers and doctors, patients and the audience in order to build common fictions in medical performances.

The first definition of the term 'dramaturgy' refers to 'the art of composing plays' (Pavis, 2002, p. 55). This definition continues to endure and refers to the practice of playwrights. The second definition, which is the one given by Joseph Danan in particular, is the 'thought of the passage of plays to the stage' (Danan, 2010, p. 8). But with the disappearance of textocentrism on contemporary stages, other broader definitions have come to embrace more diverse dramaturgical practices.

DOI: 10.4324/9781003036500-20

We often return to Lessing's seminal work *The Hamburg Dramaturgy* (2010), a series of articles written between April 1767 and April 1768 for the Hamburg theatre, in which Lessing criticises performances, develops ideas about theatrical form and thus invents the function of today's drama-turg, who is often the director's partner, their literary advisor, the one who accompanies them in the elaboration of the thought of a performance: 'This is where Lessing's revolution comes in: his dramaturgy is not a (closed) system of rules about how plays should be written, but an (open) practice of questioning and producing thought' (Danan, 2010, p. 14).

Dramaturgy takes on its most traditional meaning in the first project discussed, which takes place in the context of simulated consultations in the Centre Hospitalier Universitaire Improvisa-tion (CHUI) at the Université Grenoble-Alpes. In the dual field of theatrical reflection and activ-ity, the concept of dramaturgy has undergone a notable semantic evolution: since Aristotle – and still recently – the term was limited to designating the stylistic composition, structural and formal composition of the dramatic text – in other words, 'the construction of the theatre text' (Martin, 2001, p. 82). Indeed, it is a question of composing small dramas through the collective writing of scenarios which make it possible to propose acting material for the simulated patients but also to construct the reception of the student doctors who participate in the device. We will thus see how, in the simulated consultations, the medical and performing arts trainers practise this dramaturgy together and how these dramatic objects push to return to an Aristotelian theatrical form[1] closed on itself, programming an empathetic reception and relying on the Stanislavski method for the patient-actors (Stanislavski, 2001).

Second, I will analyse the cancer project that took place through Résilience Assistée par le Travail Théâtral (RESISTT).[2] This was built around work on representations of cancer through playwriting workshops with patients who were in remission (only two were still in treatment) and which was then continued by the staging of the texts produced by a director and professional actors. In this project, dramaturgical practice was at the centre of the process because the patients had to be introduced to playwriting, and it was precisely this practice of playwriting that allowed them to think about the addressed, polyphonic narrative of their illness and the possibility of del-egating their personal word to actors.

Finally, I will analyse the project *Si vous voulez de la lumière*. The director Florent Siaud and his Franco-Quebec company Les Songes Turbulents commissioned thirteen French-speaking authors to rewrite Goethe's *Faust*. This contemporary Faust, driven by the disorders of our time, is a haematologist to represent the figure of a scientist who feels powerless in the face of death and has the desire to push it away. His inability to accept the death of others leads him to a pact with a devil who is none other than a reciter in opera at the beginning of the show. Here, the dramaturgy is presented as the need to think of a narrative coherence around the complex and fragmentary journey of a haematologist and his confrontation with death and disease.

Composing human-scale dramas in simulated consultations

Medical role-play is practised in several university hospitals in France, with the use of simulated consultations developing gradually since the early 2000s. They were often the result of initiatives by individual teachers in conjunction with professional actors or patient-experts. The 2020 reform of health studies now requires all students in their final year of medical school to take Objective and Structured Clinical Examinations (OSCE). As part of these exams, students will be assessed on simulated consultations (general medicine interviews, diagnosis announcement), and the sys-tem we are running will therefore have to be expanded to prepare all future classes. The specificity of the CHUI project in Grenoble is that it calls on students from other disciplines (specifically the performing arts) to play the role of patients. The CHUI project sets itself objectives to be reached in two training courses which may seem totally different: the teaching of medicine and the teaching of the performing arts. The initiative for the University Hospital Improvisation Centre (CHUI) came from Philippe Chaffanjon, professor of anatomy at the Grenoble Faculty of Medicine, who contacted the Department of Performing Arts at Grenoble-Alpes University in 2015 with the desire to organise simulated consultations in order to give medical students a first experience in this field. During the last five years, we have been putting the two hundred fourth-year medical students through simulated consultations with twenty-five performing arts students who are enrolled in a twenty-four hour course in 'improvisation in the medical environment'. They work on theatrical improvisation and then learn ten scenarios and improvise with patient profiles (for example, the anxious patient, the talkative patient and the hyper-reflective patient). The simulated consultations are filmed, and then I evaluate the performing arts students on acting criteria and the medical students are also evaluated (without marks) on their listening skills.

Medical students are not assessed on their ability to make a diagnosis, as the frameworks distributed to the actors are mostly general and open to several possible interpretations. Instead, the medical student's ability to adapt their vocabulary to the interviewee, to produce a clear discourse, to show empathy and to listen to the interviewer is assessed. For the performing arts students, the aim is to develop their ability to interpret a role (that of the patient) and to improvise (as they interact live by bouncing off the questions asked by the medical student). They are evaluated on their ability to take on a predefined framework (a description of symptoms more or less directly related to a pathology) and to stick to it coherently. They have to improvise within this framework by inventing a social, family or psychological situation and as a particular character given to them a few minutes before coming to the consultation.

Simulated consultations make it possible to rethink the clinical interview as a stage with its own dramaturgy. Although one might have the impression that the link between the disciplines is a metaphor, one must on the contrary think that they develop a specific art of the gaze, because the stage direction and the psychological clinic were born at the same time in France:

> If, from one generation to the next, the medical disciplines of reference have changed, the same recourse to medicine persists, envisaged in its most innovative dimensions and serving to rethink, in a structuring and demanding way, the practice of staging. . . . One might see these statements as mere fashionable metaphors, which artists used and perhaps abused for a few decades. We believe, however, that the insistent reference to medicine, whose development and influence are major facts in the history of science in the nineteenth century, is worth more as a paradigm than as a metaphor. This paradigm underpins the affirmation, in modern staging, of a very particular visual regime, borrowed from the clinic.
>
> (Losco-Lena, 2016, p. 147)

Thus, in thinking up an interdisciplinary course, the medical trainers and I were able to see that we were trying to develop the same acuity of vision, the same attentive reading of the others, the same active listening, and we also understood that the practice of a body in play, in performance, was central to our two disciplines. But it was necessary to invent a common vocabulary and be able to understand each other's disciplinary culture, as Emma Brodzinski notes:

> Ideally, interdisciplinary endeavours involve artists and clinicians as equal partners in collaboration, who have a level of respect and understanding of each other's work to ask interrogative and apposite questions – as well as the ability to push for new questions and new

answers. Such a process, however, faces the problem of communication in that each party in such an encounter will have its own particular frame of reference and concordant professional language which may be a barrier to interaction.

(2010, p. 12)

The practice of dramaturgy is then embedded in the writing of the frameworks and patient profiles that prepares particular reactions for the medical students. The idea is to construct a fiction that meets a medical requirement but also triggers the need to listen, as Mermikides explains, 'the simulated scenarios . . . are understood as theatrical because they present human-scale dramas designed to change the way their audiences feel' (2020, pp. 56–57).

This writing of scenarios for simulated consultations pushes me to return to traditional dramaturgical forms (thinking about the psychology of the characters, constructing a linear narrative, inscribing oneself in a constrained space-time) and to abandon the post-dramatic forms to which I am accustomed in my discipline and in particular in the contemporary playwriting that I teach. In itself, the exercise of a simulated consultation is a fifteen-minute closed-door session, it has a beginning, a middle and an end, and the idea is that the audience (potentially the medical student but also the medical trainers who will watch the video) can identify with it as much as possible. This traditional dramatic form is also a privileged place of dialogue between the medical trainers, the patient-actors and me, and underpins the possibility of this interdisciplinary exercise, as Mermikides puts it very well:

Bringing together distinct disciplines invites unexpected innovation into the process as our assumptions are challenged by new knowledge, perspectives or representational strategies, thus drawing us to newer dramaturgical forms. At the same time, this interdisciplinarity can also provoke a simultaneous pull towards the familiar and the universal in search for common ground. While the latter statement might imply a degree of conservatism (and recourse to the established dramatic tradition), what can be more interesting is where the 'lowest common denominator' is found as a point of thematic intersection in terms of 'what is being presented'.

(2014, p. 139)

Here we find ourselves in a closed-door situation where the two actors do not experience the same level of reality. The medical student, even though they are playing the graduate doctor, is nevertheless experiencing an interview with a patient that is very close to their everyday life, and they are invited – even though this is ultimately impossible in the proposed context – to try to be themselves. In fact, they are supposed to be a better version, both by pretending to be a confirmed doctor and by trying to be as close as possible to an active and attentive listener, which they do not always manage to do in the reality of their externship.

The patient-actor, on the other hand, is aware at every moment that they are in a theatrical game. They have been prepared for several hours to take on the role of patients, different patients in the same evening, characters very different from them, with pathologies that they know absolutely nothing about. However, although they have been trained in improvisation, they do not know what's going to happen, and they therefore find themselves in a live writing situation which must aim for maximum credibility for the simulation to work. There is indeed a mimetic will which presides over the simulated consultation, as well as the search for real effects.

Thus, in the preparation of the actors, we utilise the Stanislavski method with the performing arts students. This method, which Constantin Stanislavski forged between 1898 and 1904 at the Moscow Art Theatre, consists of basing acting on the actors' interiority, notably around the technique of 'affective memory' (a concept borrowed from the French psychologist Théodule Ribot). The patient-actors must construct the thread of the consultation through the construction of a character whose motivations must be clear to them. To do this, I invite them to invent characters with past memories and stories and to invest in the character the emotional memory of each person. They can draw on themselves to bring a psychological truth to their character, and then they have to improvise from the medical framework and the psychological construction of a character in order to keep spontaneity in play with the doctor and create intimacy in the consultation space. This of course leads to fairly traditional forms of acting, within scenes corresponding to genres now shunned by contemporary directors, such as melodrama.

This course moved me. The challenge was not to become a service provider for the medical school, but to enter into a 'mutual recognition of disciplines' as Frédéric Worms suggested recently in the colloquium 'The indiscipline of medical humanities' organised by the University of Bordeaux in November 2020. It was a question of getting out of the usefulness of theatre. Yes, theatre can improve 'soft skills', but the aim is not to make doctors more human, because we can not make that claim. The idea is rather to build an interdisciplinary view of the medical interview as an intimate and social experience around the question of life stories, dialogue and polyphony of the disease. The medical or therapeutic interview summons dramaturgy as Maria Jesus Cabral notes:

> As an exercise in speech, the act of recounting in a therapeutic context remains an activity seen, perceived and heard in a situation of co-presence . . . from speech to silence, from speaking body language to its interstitial withdrawal. In this way, it summons the theatre, a social and communicative phenomenon as much as an artistic one, predisposed to link bodies and discourses.

> (2017: online)

And beyond this idea that the medical interview calls for theatre, I discovered to what extent dramaturgical skills prove to have mediating capacities in the interdisciplinary dialogue between the performing arts and medicine because they allow us to think about the construction of a common fiction.

Bringing the polyphonic story of illness to the stage: dramaturgy as mediation

In the course of clinical interviews with adult oncology patients (at the Grenoble University Hospital), a psychologist, Alexandra Dougnon-Denis, observed the extent to which all the representations (from the social environment, close relatives, the nursing staff or society in the broadest sense) of cancerous disease have an impact on the patients. Based on this observation, she was led to question the resilience of patients not in relation to the disease itself but to the representations of it and their traumatogenic potential. She then wanted to offer these patients playwriting workshops that would allow them to achieve 'assisted resilience' (Ionescu, 2011) by questioning the representations of the disease. The specific choice of playwriting, with its cathartic ideal, is at the heart of the project because this writing engaged the authors (the patients) in questioning the choice of words and the idea of incarnation but also what the idea of a spokesperson and the concrete representation (in a space, with bodies) of their illness meant. Eleven patients participated in the playwriting workshops which took place over five slots of three hours (fifteen hours of workshop). The patients were divided into two groups (one with me, another with Ariane Salignat), and each group worked on the same writing exercises.

It could be seen from the outset that there was a real resonance between this project on the representations of cancer and the characteristics of contemporary playwriting: the omnipresence of questions of life stories and the enunciative fragmentation that can result from this, beyond the sole patient-caregiver duo, to broaden the polyphony of the disease. Following these workshops, I played my role as mediator by linking these patients with a director and professional actors so that their texts could be performed. The work then continued with the stage dramaturgy.

At the end of the workshops, all the participants and their facilitators met with stage director Louise Bataillon, who was responsible for staging the texts in a practical workshop, in order to get to know one another and to start reading aloud some of the texts produced. While rehearsals were to begin with the two professional actors, Sarah Barrau and Geoffroy Pouchot-Rouge-Blanc, they could not take place due to the pandemic confinement. It was initially planned that the rewriting on the set would be done in the presence of the authors. As they were unable to carry out this rewriting work via rehearsals, Louise Bataillon and Stella Minichino, a student in the master's programme in artistic creation who was following my Arts and Health seminar, proposed distance writing sessions in order to think about the dramaturgy of the upcoming show. This could take into account all the texts produced in the writing workshop in order to think about a montage that would become the show. Seven of the eleven initial authors were fully committed to these six weeks of workshops to put together the show. New texts were written to fill in the gaps that Louise Bataillon had identified (texts on the announcement of the disease, or texts on the aftermath of treatment), then all the texts were sorted into five parts that would form the final text: 1) portraits; 2) the announcement of the disease; 3) the care, the changing body, the relatives; 4) the aftermath?; and 5) to you, the caregivers. Finally, it was a question of orchestrating each of the parts from the texts available, which were rearranged with each other and thus produced a certain chorality, allowing a new step in the distancing of each person's care path because it was no more a question of individuality but of collective speech.

At the end of September 2020, the whole team (writing workshop leaders, the psychologist behind the project, participants in the writing project, the director and professional actors) met for a reading of the entire text, the result of the dramaturgical work carried out during the 'lockdown' associated with the coronavirus (COVID-19) pandemic. Rehearsals then took place over a two-week period. During these rehearsals, the participants in the writing workshops were invited to come as often as they wanted to follow the rehearsals with the professional actors and share their feelings with us, a proposal which seven of them took up. After two weeks of rehearsal, the show was performed three times in October 2020 at the Maison de la Création et de l'Innovation on campus, in front of 150 spectators. Then the show was performed at the Autre Rive, a theatre in Grenoble, on 13 November 2021 and then at the Centre Hospitalier Universitaire in front of doctors on 15 November 2021.

This project allowed me to build my identity as a researcher in the medical humanities, specialising in dramaturgy. I had patients write a polyphonic and addressed account of the disease by listening to the wishes of the caregivers. I then accompanied the process of creating these texts for the stage while remaining outside the stage production. This project brought questions of dramaturgy around the work of writing from testimony and the construction of fiction but also around the theatrical representation of the disease and the world of health.

We built a dialogue with the patients, the caregivers and the artists around specific dramaturgical questions, such as the construction of a polyphonic narrative, the editing of texts from several workshops and the problems of enunciation. We introduced the patients to a collective thought about the dramaturgy of the text and of the stage, and it is through this dramaturgical thought that we were able to approach the story of the care path and the theatrical question of the representation of cancer. Indeed, we trained them in the entire dramaturgical process: first the playwriting, through exercises, then the composition of a theatrical text designed for the stage and finally the dramaturgy on stage with the actors.

Holding it all together to link narratives around the hypertextual figure of the Faust haematologist

In 2011, I co-founded the Franco-Quebec company Les Songes Turbulents with Florent Siaud who became the director. In 2021–2022, the company celebrated its tenth anniversary and its everlasting desire to bring together artists from different countries. To mark this anniversary, the company wanted to join forces with major theatres in different countries to create a rewriting of Goethe's *Faust I* and *II*, entrusted to thirteen authors from Quebec, the First Nations, Africa, the Caribbean and Europe. This vast rewriting is based on a collaborative utopia launched in 2017 and which was completed in 2021–2022. Since 2017, a three-stage writing structure has gradually emerged. Here, Faust becomes a renowned haematologist in a Parisian hospital where he falls in love with his patient Margot. Wanting to postpone death at all costs, he soon gives in to a futile pursuit of therapy, which raises the question of consent as much as that of the limits of science. On the run after using an illegal therapeutic technique, he and Mephisto reach the United States. The two companions encounter crowds raging against finance on Wall Street, digital companies trying to paint themselves green, but also the world of Silicon Valley in which the haematologist falls in love with an avatar of Marilyn Monroe in augmented reality. In a third phase, Faust and Mephisto continue their exploration of the world in a third circle and find only uprisings, sea dams and climate collapse. Worn out by cancer, Faust abandons himself to death.

All authors have been writing in a shared knowledge of the project, and each of them is responsible for their own art in this polyphonic architecture. The result is a writing process that proceeds by 'pollination', as Florent Siaud says: accompanied by long dramaturgical exchanges and constantly updated intellectual nourishment, each writing impulse follows its own destiny, but authors feel free to enrich their own writing with the ideas that have germinated in the rest of the show. To this end, regular re-readings (by the authors themselves, by the artistic coordinator, by other playwrights, by experts and members of the cast or design team) allow each draft to evolve towards ever greater precision, singularity and mutual resonance.

The director and several of the authors of the project came to Grenoble-Alpes University in 2019 to do a workshop with my masters students on the Création Artistique programme. Following this workshop, a central idea emerged: to make this Faust a haematologist. Indeed, the difficulty was to invent a contemporary figure of Faust. What scientist today could be this Faust, ready to do anything to overcome death, to understand humanity and to accept making a pact with the devil to do so? The idea of a haematologist emerged because they are constantly confronted with the death of their patients, patients of all ages, of all social and physical conditions, and one can imagine the disarray that this can cause them. The writing continued with the authors, and in October 2021, we organised a workshop with the director Florent Siaud, students from the Grenoble Conservatory, students in performing arts, an oncologist and a general practitioner from the Centre Hospitalier Universitaire and professional actors to work on texts that stage the world of health and question the issue of death.

During this workshop, authors sent us versions sometimes the day before the work on stage, and we had three professional actors as well as students from the Arts and Health seminar to read the texts and to do 'dramaturgy at the table' in order to detect the sensitive points and the dramaturgical challenges to be accomplished. During this residency, we invited an oncologist, Dr Isabelle Flandin, and a general practitioner, Dr Lucie Bosmean, to come and listen to a reading of Guillaume Poix's text which opens the show and presents Faust in his life as a haematologist. In this text, the pact between Faust and Mephisto, which is the narrative engine of Goethe's entire work, crystallises around theatrical and cinematographic fiction. The haematologist Faust answers his intern's invitation to accompany him to the opera. There he meets the actor Mephisto, who offers to take him to a film shooting where he will be asked, in spite of himself, to play a dead man. It is around this experience of the doctor playing the dead body that the unbreakable pact between this alchemist-turned-haematologist and a devil from the world of live performance unfolds.

In this first part, the subject of medicine renews the dramaturgic form. For example, the text opens with a letter that Faust records on his dictaphone for a colleague and which renews the form of the monologue with great credibility:

FAUST: Dear
colleague I have
again in consultation
your patient
for further management of a
Waldenström disease
(Silence.)
. . .
The patient
had informed me
last week
that he did not wish to
for the time being
not
to start this treatment
despite
despite my explanations about the short-term risk of
of this Waldenström's disease
of this Waldenström disease
disease, we agreed to
meet again
after a week
to arbitrate.
The intern knocks and enters. He is pale and stands at the wall. Faust continues to dictate his report
Meanwhile
I have discussed this case in the multidisciplinary consultation meeting on haematology
the indication for treatment
of the RCD type

is validated
with no other possible alternative
The intern crouches down.
We also agreed that it is not possible to carry out
the first treatment of
RITUXIMAB:
in a day hospital
for safety reasons
(The intern collapses to the floor. Suspension. He recovers and signals that he is fine)
(Poix, 2021, pp. 1–2)

The oncologist who was present at the reading was particularly moved by the hyperrealism of this opening monologue and by the stylisation of an everyday medical act that she had never conceived as a monologue but which actually is. The dialogue then started again around dramaturgical questions: how to render an inner monologue in the doctor's office, how the theatre can stage the plurality of voices that inhabit the oncologist during a consultation, how the theatrical form by means of the address and the work of a stylised orality can make explicit the words that the doctors never pronounce aloud. Thus it was around the dramaturgical work of the text that the dialogue started with the two doctors. We worked on the relationship between doctor and intern and on the emotionally loaded question of the announcement of the diagnosis, thanks to a second excerpt from Guillaume Poix's text where Faust explains to his intern what he sees in the patient when he announces the diagnosis:

FAUST: In the small office
(Silence)
Sitting
sitting behind
your chair
like this
you will be
and in front of you
she
this
woman
42 years old
who will die
she will look at you
(Silence)
Will wait
(Silence)
And
you will not know where to place your eyes
where to put them
you
feel a tension in your
your jaw
and chin the

temples too
they will pulse
your eyes
will not
stop falling
fall towards
your papers your documents your analyses
figures and units of measurement
frightening
data
frightening
averages
exploded
thresholds
pulverized
there will also be
the screen
the screen in front of you
the screen that will
malicious pleasure to
in spite of you
backlight
your emptiness
your inability to face the person in front of you who will be waiting, who can't take it
anymore
will know without knowing
will want to
shit
in the screen you will plunge like a
disgusting
and
this woman will always look at you
always
she won't take her eyes off you
she will have
put
her right hand on the edge of the desk
because she
she will have straightened up
she will not be able to brace her back against the back of the chair
she will not be able to
will barely fit on the edge of the anthracite polymer chair seat which is not comfortable
for any human being from here or anywhere else on the planet
she will fall
this woman

(Poix, 2021, pp. 3–4)

Conclusion: dramaturgy practices as essential mediation tools in the construction of medical theatrical fictions

This chapter aims to show, through the analysis of three medical performances, that dramaturgy is a privileged mediation practice in interdisciplinary projects mixing performing arts and medicine. Indeed, this practice, which is sometimes presented as the art of moving from text to stage, sometimes as composition, and which is often carried out by an outside eye, a third person, seems to be the most suitable for bringing together doctors, patients, artists and an audience around the complex story of a disease. Dramaturgy means encouraging dialogue in order to construct common fictions.

Thus, in simulated consultations, dramaturgy takes on its oldest meaning around the writing of scenarios and returns to the composition of a dramatic form in the Aristotelian model which allows mimesis and identification and which is a privileged place for dialogue with the doctors. At the same time, the work of the simulated consultations is in line with Eugenio Barba's more open definition of dramaturgy as 'the arrangement of actions' (2008, p. 54). In the context of artistic work with patients, dramaturgy is the practice that allows us to reflect on a delegation of narratives of illness and to accept the fragmentation and polyphony inherent to any collection of narratives in order to invent a common fiction that leaves room for varied expressions while building a thread that the spectator can follow. Everyone in the process embraced the 'shared dramaturgical state of mind' (Dort, 1986, p. 8). Finally, in a fragmentary and monumental theatrical project such as *Faust Augmenté*, it is also a question of finding the place of a collective and common fiction and here again the desire to 'coordinate the whole' (Martinez, 2002, p. 20) allows for a dialogue with doctors and artists. When I started working with the medical community, I felt displaced in my discipline. I had to find the place for dialogue with another disciplinary culture; I even thought I had to embrace another discipline. But with the experience of the projects reported on here, I understand that it is the specific view of my original discipline, dramaturgy, that has given me the tools to construct fictions with the world of medicine and to allow dialogues between performing artists and doctors.

Notes

1 In *Poetics*, Aristotle defines tragedy as a dramatic mode, as opposed to the epic mode represented by Homer. The dramatic mode excludes narration. It is a matter of arranging facts around a story and making characters speak, all with a view to coherence.
2 The project is described as 'storytelling and playwriting: tools for expression and evolution of cancer representations and support for resilience process'.

Reference list

Barba, E. (2008) 'Actions au travail', in Barba, E. and Savarese, N. (eds.) *L'Énergie qui danse*. Montpellier: L'Entretemps.
Brodzinski, E. (2010) *Theatre in health and care*. Kindle edn. London: Palgrave Macmillan.
Cabral, M.J. (2017) 'La médecine narrative par le discours et le théâtre', *Voix et relation*, 15 February. Available at: https://ver.hypotheses.org/2388 (Accessed: 6 May 2022).
Danan, J. (2010) *Qu'est-ce que la dramaturgie?* Arles: Actes-Sud Papiers.
Dort, B. (1986) 'L'état d'esprit dramaturgique', *Théâtre/Public*, 67, pp. 8–12.
Ionescu, S. (2011) *Traité de résilience assistée*. Paris: PUF.
Lessing, G.E. (2010) *La Dramaturgie de Hambourg*. Paris: Klincksieck.
Losco-Lena, M. (2016) 'L'Œil clinique de la mise en scène moderne', *Études Théâtrales*, (65), pp. 147–158. https://doi.org/10.3917/etth.065.0147

Martin, B. (2001) 'Dramaturgie et analyse dramaturgique', *L'Annuaire théâtral*, 29, pp. 82–98. https://doi.org/10.7202/041457ar

Martinez, A. (2002) 'La dramaturgie du cirque contemporain français: quelques pistes théâtrales', *L'Annuaire théâtral*, 32, pp. 12–21. https://doi.org/10.7202/041501ar

Mermikides, A. (2014) 'The appliance of science: devising, dramaturgy and the alternative science play', in Trencsenyi, K. and Cochrane, B. (eds.) *New dramaturgy: international perspectives on theory and practice*. London: Bloomsbury Methuen Drama Publishing, pp. 125–142.

Mermikides, A. (2020) *Performance, medicine and the human*. Kindle edn. London: Bloomsbury Methuen Drama Publishing.

Pavis, P. (2002) *Dictionnaire du théâtre*. Paris: Armand Colin.

Poix, G. (2021) 'Text 2: the meeting of Faust and Mephisto', 6 October version, *Faust Augmenté/Si vous voulez de la lumière*. Unpublished playscript.

Stanislavski, C. (2001) *La Formation de l'acteur*. Paris: Payot & Rivages.

18

PERFORMING GRATITUDE

A case study of the clap-for-carers movement

Giskin Day

The displays of gratitude for health care professionals and other key workers that took place in the early parts of the coronavirus pandemic constituted, it could be argued, the world's largest ever series of collective performances. Inspired by similar scenes in Europe, a ten-week campaign to 'clap for our carers' encouraged people across the United Kingdom (UK) to take to their doorsteps, windows, balconies and streets to express their appreciation. On Thursdays at 8 pm during April and May 2020, millions of people participated in a synchronous display of gratitude-motivated affect. Amidst the disciplined commitment to strictures demanded by the UK government to control the spread of the virus, clap-for-carers allowed for a state-sanctioned interval of cathartic hubbub. The resulting street-side performances were simultaneously earnest and playful, with some morphing into elaborate spectacles that found appreciable audiences on social media.

The clap-for-carers initiative seemed at first to be an unambiguously positive counterpoint to the dawning reality of the disaster about to be wreaked by the pandemic. Yet, for all the apparent simplicity of its structure, clap-for-carers was a complex and polysemous phenomenon. Throughout its run in the British summer of 2020, and the failed attempt at its revival at the start of the third national lockdown in January 2021, participants morphed between roles of audience, performers and critics. As I will elaborate, these ideologies were enacted through competing discourses that swirled around the weekly event – discourses that were suffused with references to embodied, symbolic and imagined performances.

Performance and health care have a history of shared analogies. As well as a mutual preoccupation with 'gazes and stages' (as discussed cogently by Mermikides, 2020), dramaturgical metaphors are prevalent in medical discourse. Operations are 'performed' in a 'theatre', medical professionals are defined by 'roles' and protocols are often developed as 'scripts'. Schechner draws attention to the carefully crafted codes of dress and behaviour in medicine that make it, along with professions such as law, a specific category of performance (2020). Imagining the health care worker as laudable for 'performing care' was already a plausibly available interpretation. This was all the more conceivable in the context of a pandemic in which expectations of roles deemed 'key', 'essential' and/or 'frontline', and concomitant risks, were a focus of acute attention.

The act of clapping as an expression of communal appreciation takes its cue from theatre, although its function is far from straightforward. Kershaw invokes a medical analogy when he suggests that applause might be an 'index to the health, or the disease, of a whole culture' (2001,

DOI: 10.4324/9781003036500-21

p. 134). He argues that the commercialisation of theatregoing has contributed to applause relinquishing its cultural power to judge the value of a performance. Instead, applause has become 'fatally tinged with a narcissistic self-regard' (ibid, p. 144) – an accusation that also came to be levelled at participants in clap-for-carers. The timing of applause is also significant. In the theatre, applause is usually a coda to a performance. Appreciation is expressed once a benefit has been realised. When gratitude is enacted in anticipation of a benefit, it runs the risk of being perceived as manipulative. Could the timing of the clapping – at the start of the pandemic – lend credence to the claim by Juri that clap-for-carers was a form of social distancing, separating those who 'do' on our behalf from those who merely 'watch' (2020: online)? Were we, Juri asks, applauding gladiators entering arenas to fight lions?

This chapter offers a case study of the clap-for-carers phenomenon. I draw on theories of affect and social practice to account for the emergence, flourishing and demise of the event. I trace its trajectory in public discourse from its inception as 'thick' civic engagement to its construction as an opportunistic political tactic and – ultimately – a dangerous distraction that authorised unrealistic expectations of health care workers. Although clap-for-carers as a synchronised communal practice was relatively short lived, I argue that it is likely to have a lasting legacy in the debates it spawned about the role of expressions of gratitude in collective life, particularly in the contexts of affectual authenticity and care justice.

Dramatic structure

Overture. Clapping for health care workers began in Italy, as an extension of impromptu balcony concerts, video footage of which started appearing on social media on 12 March 2020. From 14 March, people in Italy, Spain and Portugal took to their doorsteps and balconies – often timed to coincide with hospital workers changing shifts – in what the media often described as a 'standing ovation' for health care workers (Booth, Adam and Rolfe, 2020; Slisco, 2020). Other countries around Europe followed and, by the end of March, synchronised applause was being reported from cities across North America and some in Asia like Singapore and Mumbai.

Curtain Up. In the UK, the Clap for Our Carers campaign started with an Instagram post by Dutch Londoner, Annemarie Plas, who called on people to join in applause for the National Health Service (NHS) – the tax-payer–funded health care system that promises medical services, free at the point of care, for eligible residents of the UK. The first national clap-for-carers event took place on 26 March 2020. Its transmission was aided by the intensive involvement of mainstream and social media. A professional communications agency worked with Plas to promote the hashtag #clapforourcarers – although the 'our' was often dropped, probably for reasons of better scansion. Unlike some European cities where the applause took place every night until well into May when lockdown restrictions started easing, the UK's clap-for-carers became a weekly event held on Thursdays at 8 pm. In response to criticism that it was not just the NHS that deserved appreciation, the applause was extended from the NHS to all key workers from 2 April (Plas, 2020), although it never shook off the impression that it was primarily aimed at health care workers.

Rising Action. The simplicity of clapping – no special equipment required – encouraged mass participation, with many augmenting their noise-making by banging pots and pans, cheering, whistling and/or playing musical instruments. In some areas, the Thursday-night clapping morphed into impromptu concerts, perhaps causing the applause to be redirected to the performers rather than health care and key workers for whom it was originally intended. Although applause is primarily an audible phenomenon, the affordances of social media transformed it into a very visual one. Photographs and videos of people, including high-profile public figures and celebrities, participating in the applause flooded social media every Thursday night. The dramatic tension increased on 27 March when Prime Minister Boris Johnson and Health and Social Care Secretary Matt Hancock tested positive for COVID-19. The next day, Amged El-Hawrani became the first frontline NHS hospital worker to die from the disease amidst growing criticism of the government for failing to provide personal protective equipment (PPE) and testing for health care staff.

Climax. No official figures exist for how many people took part in clap-for-carers, but it was put at 'millions' by the BBC (BBC News, 2020b), and a YouGov poll of 1664 adults in June found that 69% of respondents said they had taken part at least once (Abraham, 2020). An analysis of tweets of gratitude to the NHS associated with clap-for-carers suggest that the event reached its apogee around the second week of April (Day *et al.*, 2021), bolstered by the discharge from hospital of Boris Johnson on 12 April after treatment in intensive care. Johnson issued an effusive statement expressing thanks to the NHS, and two nurses in particular, for saving his life. Later in April, a campaign to raise £1000 for the NHS Together Charities by 99-year-old Captain Tom Moore by walking 100 lengths of his garden gained momentum – it would eventually raise over £30 million. Around the same time, in an example of reproducing and repurposing creative action, numerous videos circulated on social media of health care staff applauding patients leaving hospital after recovering from COVID-19.

Conflict: A number of critical moments can be identified that started to erode the moral authority of the clap-for-carers initiative. Prominent from the start were accusations of hypocrisy aimed at Conservative government ministers who, when tweeting about taking part in clap-for-carers, were swiftly reminded of an incident in 2017 when Conservatives celebrated having voted against an amendment to end a public sector pay cap – widely paraphrased as voting against a pay rise for nurses. The clap-for-carers phenomenon also attracted criticism for attracting crowds outside hospitals in defiance of social distancing guidelines. Westminster Bridge, which affords a view of St Thomas' Hospital, was a particular focus for concern (Heren, 2020).

The release of a video, 'You clap for me now', on 14 April also proved divisive. It featured workers from Black and global majorities reading lines from a poem by Darren Smith, highlighting discrimination faced by immigrants working in key services (Smith, 2020). The video divided opinion, with many embracing its anti-racist message but others expressing outrage at the politicisation of the clap-for-carers event and describing it as 'petty moralising' (Gray, 2020). Yet another factor that destabilised the event was a widely shared article in *The Guardian* by an anonymous NHS doctor who decried the clapping as a 'sentimental distraction from the issues' and referred to 'creeping clapping fascism' (Anonymous, 2020).

Curtain Down. On 22 May, Annemarie Plas, the originator of the campaign in the UK, announced that 'Clap for Our Carers' should end, saying that it had 'become politicised' and that she did not want it to be perceived negatively. A third of respondents to a YouGov poll agreed that it had become politicised, with 63% approving of the decision to end the formal campaign (Abraham, 2020). The final organised clap-for-carers took place on 28 May. There was an attempt to organise a clap to commemorate the NHS's seventy-second anniversary on 5 July at 5 pm, but this had limited success.

No Second Run. On 6 January 2021, just as the third national lockdown got underway, Annemarie Plas announced that #clapforourcarers was being relaunched as #clapforheroes. It was patterned on #clapforourcarers with clapping called for at 8 pm. The proposed event generated a negative backlash on social media. Plas issued a statement saying she and her family had been targeted by abuse, and she was distancing herself from the applause and would no longer be promoting it. With the exception of a few corporate supporters, hardly anyone participated, and the event was not readvertised.

Gratitude as affect

Clap-for-carers is an example of socially synchronised affect. As a concept, affect is attributed to Spinoza whose argument in *Ethics* in 1677 took the form of a geometric proof written in Latin – a rhetorical tactic that, despite its formulation in logic, has led to much conceptual ambiguity (Robinson and Kutner, 2019). In the context of this case study, I take affect to be a dynamic capacity for embodied action that acknowledges the role of emotion – in this case, gratitude – in motivating, participating in and resulting from social encounters. Affect is often described as an 'energy' that characterises the structure of expression and connection, particularly with respect to rituals of public and private life (Papacharissi, 2015), or 'a force' that marks a body's belonging to a world of encounters (Seigworth and Gregg, 2010).

What is the value of taking the lens of affect theory to the clap-for-carers event? Perspectives incorporating affect aspire to explore, rather than explain, the mobilisation of people through connections and expressions oriented to other people via embodied thoughts and/or ideas. The emphasis on dynamism and networked flows, known as 'affective attunement' (Papacharissi, 2015), resonates with the clap-for-carers event that propelled people in lockdown to leave their sofas and engage in the rhythmic entrainment of applause for an audience imagined as health care and other key workers, but also for themselves, their neighbours and, for many, a virtual audience online.

Applause is a particular form of cultural patterning for, most often, the expression of appreciation. It is one of the principal means by which people share in collective emotions or emote together (Sullivan and Day, 2019). Drawing on a theory of affect advanced by the American psychologist Silvan Tomkins, Gibbs argues that mimetic communication, of which applause is typical, forms the affective basis for social processes and social bonding, fostering a 'sense of belonging' (2010). Clap-for-carers was both a response to and a reinforcement of the myth of social togetherness in the face of the prohibition of physical togetherness during the pandemic. Here I use 'myth' in the Barthesian sense as a culturally resonant, sense-generating narration of events rather than a falsehood (Barthes, 2000). Times of threat often fuel rhetoric around 'togetherness' which is harnessed to stoicism and resilience.

Jones has pointed out the parallels between responses to COVID-19 and the Blitz, arguing that the Blitz phrase, 'we are all in it together and we all need to come out of it together', was central to how people behaved in the first COVID-19 lockdown (2020). 'Blitz spirit' in Britain in the Second World War, as characterised by Kelsey, was a 'simple but powerful script' for ideological messaging (2013, p. 83). A survey of 1200 people on 21 April 2020 found that the belief that 'we are all in it together' was the most important factor driving self-reported lockdown compliance. Acting for the common good was found to be centred on sentiment supporting the NHS (Jackson *et al.*, 2020), suggesting that placing the slogan 'Protect the NHS' at the centre of the tricolon 'Stay at Home, Protect the NHS, Save Lives' was highly effective in mobilising public affect during the first national lockdown.

Gratitude and morale

Clap-for-carers arose out of an implicit but obvious anticipation of threats to the morale and wellbeing of health care workers posed by the pandemic. Morale in the NHS had been a matter for concern for decades before the pandemic. Constraints on funding and pay, increasing workloads, long waiting lists for procedures and insufficient bed capacity all contributed to a sense of impending crisis. Surveys found the majority of nursing staff felt overworked and underpaid (Marangozov *et al.*, 2017) and that a third of doctors were 'burned out' and suffering from secondary traumatic stress (McKinley *et al.*, 2020). The King's Fund, an influential charity with a focus on driving improvement in health care, has consistently highlighted that a major contributing factor to the erosion of morale is that staff feel undervalued (Finlayson, 2002; King's Fund, 2014; Burkitt *et al.*, 2018). Surveys of the public before the pandemic, however, consistently show a strong and appreciative relationship with the NHS (Burkitt *et al.*, 2018). It is perhaps the contrasting discourses of demoralisation amongst health care workers against overwhelmingly appreciative attitudes to the NHS that gave impetus to public support for clap-for-carers in its initial stages.

The relationship between receiving gratitude and raising morale is poorly theorised in the psychology literature, although some studies have implicated gratitude in increasing job satisfaction and protecting against burnout (Converso *et al.*, 2015; Starkey *et al.*, 2019; Aparicio *et al.*, 2019). However, we do not need theory to tell us that feeling appreciated is an integral part of morale, or to recognise that gratitude was deployed as a key morale-preserving strategy in government communications. Without exception, daily government press briefings during the first lockdown included expressions of thanks. This extract from Foreign Secretary Dominic Raab's statement on 9 April 2020, whilst Boris Johnson was being treated in intensive care for coronavirus, demonstrates the prominence of gratitude in government communiques:

> I want to say *a massive thank you* to everyone who has gone the extra mile during this very challenging period. *Thank you* to all of those who are looking after us in our time of need. The NHS workers on the front line who have treated the sick, saved lives and tended for those who, sadly, could not be saved. For the doctors and nurses who have died of coronavirus whilst caring for others, we will never forget their sacrifice, we will never forget their devotion to helping others. And I also want to say *a big thank you* to the carers, the charity workers, all those who are looking after, or even just keeping an eye on, those in their local neighbourhood. You are the lifeline to so many people in our communities. *Thank you* to the workers who keep the country running, the supermarket workers, the delivery drivers, the technicians, the cleaners, the public servants who just kept going, determined to keep providing the daily services we all rely on. I think you've certainly made us all think long and hard about who the 'key workers' are in our lives. *Thank you* to the volunteers who have stepped up across the country, whose big-hearted sense of responsibility defines British community spirit at its very best. And *a massive thank you* to every single person who has stayed home to stop this terrible virus from spreading, you have helped protect the NHS, and you have helped to save lives.
>
> (10 Downing Street, 2020: emphasis added)

Gratitude can be seen as fulfilling two main functions in this context. The first is the conferring of 'affective approval or encouragement', which the social philosopher Axel Honneth implicates in his account of recognition as central to social morality (Honneth, 1995, p. 95). Thanking phrases act symbolically here as insulation against criticism. Humility is signalled through repeated references to vulnerability by phrases like 'looking after' us. Blitz spirit is alluded to in the phrase 'British community spirit' and the emphasis on 'keeping going', with a sense of solidarity implicit in the use of collective first-person ('we' and 'us').

The second function of gratitude in this speech is to act as a political promissory note. Raab pledges to 'never forget' the sacrifices made by health care workers and to re-evaluate those in low-status, insecure employment on whom the nation now found itself utterly dependent. Clap-for-carers was directly referenced in the press questions that followed the briefing. Raab said,

'I'll be taking part in the clap for carers this evening. . . . And I'm sure, there'll be the, you know, appropriate level of recognition at the right moment once we're through the worst of it', implying that clap-for-carers was a placeholder for more substantial recognition to come. But, as Sorace has argued, gratitude is the 'ideology of sovereignty in a crisis', and it too easily slips from the recognition of individuals to an acceptance of the systems that reproduce their exploitation (2020: online). The problems besetting the provision of PPE and the roll-out of testing to health care professionals meant that the 'sacrifices' lauded by Raab and others in government briefings came to be seen not as unfortunate or inevitable but the result of incompetence.

Thanking allowed?

The prominence of gratitude in politicians' statements and the popularity of clap-for-carers in April fuelled a debate about what constitutes 'appropriate gratitude' and whose gratitude could be afforded credibility. Social media responses to clap-for-carers started to become more cynical, drawing attention to a perceived change in the primary audience for the event (Day *et al.*, 2021). Although the impetus was still gratitude to the NHS, it became, for many, a way to connect with neighbours and affirm a sense of community – sentiments that were both lauded and mocked on social media. The shift of focus to neighbours-as-audience played up to a long-standing trope of neighbourhood rivalry as a national characteristic. The stereotype, which references status aspiration, is a staple of comedy in British literature, particularly prominent in the novels of Jane Austen and forms the basis of many a sitcom – most notably the 1990s BBC series *Keeping Up Appearances*. It was not long before cartoonists and sketch-writers began satirising the event for its potential for one-upmanship. Comedian Will Hislop's parody of the event, for example, went viral on 9 May on Twitter. In the sketch, he mouths a conversation with his neighbour disparaging those who have not turned out to clap (O'Connor, 2020). Whereas previously, clap-for-carers could be seen as exemplary of Goffman's description of ceremony as a celebratory performance that highlights values of a society in 'an expressive rejuvenation and reaffirmation of the moral values of the community' (1969, p. 31), it began to be undone by associations with inauthenticity and accusations of 'virtue signalling'.

The expression 'virtue signalling' refers to behaving in a way designed to garner approval rather than acting from a place of conviction. When the phrase first proliferated on Twitter in 2016, writer David Shariatmadari, ironically with hindsight, reached for an epidemiological metaphor to decry virtue-signalling as an expression that had proliferated like a virus and 'against which quarantine measures now urgently need to be taken'. He argued that it was a lazy put-down and had become indistinguishable from the thing it was meant to call out: 'smug posturing from a position of self-appointed authority' (Shariatmadari, 2016: online). The shortcomings of the term notwithstanding, accusations of virtue signalling associated with clap-for-carers proliferated online. As a concept, virtue signalling is closely allied to 'slacktivism', a low-effort, low-engagement signal of support for a cause without actually effecting change in a meaningful way (Lodewijckx, 2020). Drawing on Goffman's conception of 'ritual equilibrium' (1967), Persson argues that the equilibrium of social interaction is vulnerable to sabotage, including by using humour or reframing the interaction order (2019, pp. 39–40). In the case of clap-for-carers, both apply: mocking the ritual and harnessing it to virtue signalling and slacktivism reframed the event as a performance primarily for impression management rather than gratitude.

Aspersions cast on authenticity are difficult to cast off – partly, perhaps, because Goffman's ideas are so pervasive about the inherently performative nature of social interaction, which he links to deception and illusion (1969). As Diski has pointed out, '[Goffman] presents a world where there is nowhere to run; a perpetual dinner party of status seeking, jockeying for position and saving face. Any idea of an authentic self becomes nonsense' (2004, p. 10). Of course, expressions of gratitude, whether enacted on the street as part of a social ritual or posted on social media, are not a guarantee of sincerity, but neither are they insincere by default: the point is that we do not have access to each other's underlying psychologies. Although clap-for-carers is a gratitude-motivated event, we cannot assume that participating individuals are experiencing the emotion in-the-moment of participation or when they tweet about it afterwards. What individuals say and do cannot be treated as a transparent window to their emotions and motivations. This does not prevent us investigating the 'display and management of subjectivity and attitude in talk' (Edwards, 2005, p. 19), but it shifts the focus to practices – collective, cultural and communal sense-making activities – rather than assuming individuals have coherent, distinct and articulatable emotions amenable to evaluations of authenticity.

Clap-for-carers as shared affective practice or 'group-thank'

How did clap-for-carers come to be conceivable as a collective practice? On the face of it, it seemed unlikely to catch on. Not only had the 2016 Brexit vote, narrowly in favour of UK leaving the European Union, caused deep social divisions that made ideologically aligned collective action improbable, but Britain ranks very highly on the 'individualism' scale, meaning that, unlike in 'collectivist' cultures, there is a highly developed focus on individual fulfilment and less emphasis on social interdependence (Hofstede Insights, 2020). However, research into 'display rules' – cultural norms for emotional displays in social contexts – suggests that, somewhat counterintuitively, individualistic societies are more likely to exhibit higher expressivity of positive emotions to those outside their immediate circles than those in collectivist societies (Matsumoto *et al.*, 2008). Display rules go some way to explaining why applauding health care and key workers seemed to be a more prominent responses to the early phase of the pandemic in Western European nations and in North America, although its conspicuousness may also be a function of the reach of reporting in the mainstream media and coverage on social media.

Durkheim coined an apt term to describe the emotionality of crowds: 'collective effervescence' (2012). The phrase refers to the idea that people in assembled social groups undergo an intensely affirmative experience that binds them to ideals valued by their social group, and are 'transformed through an emotional structuring of their sensory and sensual being' (Shilling and Mellor, 2016, p. 196), or what Sullivan and Day call 'phenomenological feel' (2019, p. 206). Hopkins *et al.* found that an important source of positive experiences in crowds was people's ability to realise the values associated with their social identities (2016). Although crowd studies have naturally focused on people in close physical proximity, clap-for-carers demonstrated that effervescence can still be generated when people are dispersed. Social media perhaps helped to generate the psychological effects of crowds when people participated regardless of whether they were in earshot of other participants.

Whilst clap-for-carers undoubtedly was fuelled by a celebratory atmosphere centred on the ethos and pathos of gratitude, there was always a potential for emotional dissonance between the group-based emotion in-the-moment and the contextual atmosphere of fear, anger, grief and shame engendered by the pandemic. In their study of national celebrations, Sullivan and Day showed that 'emotional enclaves' arise which challenge the credibility of a given celebration through questioning its inclusiveness, representativeness or appropriateness (2019, p. 212). The potential for calling out behaviours as hubristic and shameful exists alongside the celebratory activity. This is borne out in the context of clap-for-carers by the criticism of politicians as hypocritical for taking part (Wood and Skeggs, 2020) and also the condemnation of people perceived to be excessively revelling in the event, such as those gathering in a carnivalesque-like atmosphere on Westminster Bridge to applaud and cheer in sight of St Thomas's Hospital, London. The embodied connotations of carnival, already actuated by the street-lining nature of performances associated with clap-for-carers, here reached its apotheosis.

A Bakhtinian reading of clap-for-carers may illuminate why participation was so compelling. The pandemic foisted on us the suspension of free and familiar contact among people, yet, as Bakhtin argued, '[t]he category of familiar contact is always so responsible for the special way mass actions are organised' (1984, p. 123). Bakhtin juxtaposed carnivalisation with everyday life when he described carnival as bringing together 'all things that were once self-enclosed, disunified, distanced from one another' (1984, p. 123). Under pandemic restrictions, disunified physical distancing was massively amplified. This detachment set up an affectual flow of nostalgia for the possibilities of physical proximity permitted under non-pandemic life. Clap-for-carers, with its carnivalesque, ritual pageantry, gave those participating in a socially distanced manner the cathartic illusion of proximity.

Allied to the concept of carnival is that of the parade, particularly in a military context. It is this connotation, with the allied semiotics of 'heroism', that caused considerable disquiet amongst clap-for-carer's critics. Cox has pointed out that although valuable work performed by health care workers during the pandemic is worthy of recognition and appreciation, a narrative of heroism does not provide a firm basis on which to build a response to a pandemic (2020). The hero narrative is superficially fitting: the risks of continuing to work in a pandemic are appreciably greater than in usual times. But the hero narrative authorises the expectation of sacrifice and fails to acknowledge the limits of the duty to treat. Discomfort with the hero narrative as applied to health care workers perhaps helps account for the enthusiasm with which the public greeted Captain Tom's fundraising efforts (BBC News, 2020a). Here was a *bona fide* war hero willing – indeed delighted – to graciously accept deflected notions of heroism whilst acting as an honest broker for those eager to translate their gratitude to the NHS into charitable funding. Disquiet about hero rhetoric also heralded the entirely predictable backlash against the reshaping of #clapforourcarers as #clapforheroes in January 2021. The 'heroes' narrative had become – perhaps, in the context of the NHS, had always been – ideologically bankrupt.

'The loveliest cacophony in the world'

The legacy of clap-for-carers is likely to be evaluated, in the fullness of time, for its impact as a social movement. In their review of the literature in the context of implications for change in the NHS, Bate, Bevan and Robert point to the diagnostic characteristics of social movements (2004). They are radical or unconventional, political, transformative, collective and durable. People should join out of choice. Social movements come about spontaneously but require organisation to persist, and they are often characterised by conflicts with institutionalised systems of power.

Change wrought by clap-for-carers is difficult to disentangle from the totalising, transformative effects of the pandemic on society. Nevertheless, the magnitude of participation in the event itself, the debates it sparked and the social traces it left on balance qualify it as transformative, collective and durable. Can clap-for-carers be considered political? Although the originator of #clapforourcarers campaign, Annemarie Plas, called for it to end after ten weeks because it was 'becoming politicised' (SkyNews, 2020), in reality it was intensely political from the outset. 'When people come out *en masse* and cheer for the NHS', wrote Younge, 'it is, by definition, a political act' (2020: online). But, if we accept the event as intrinsically political, could it be said to have challenged institutional systems of power through conflict or resistance? Far from being subversive or unwelcome, clap-for-carers was characterised by consensual behaviour and initially, at least, as being in tune with power structures. However, there were identifiable points of conflict and resistance associated with the event that challenged systems of power, particularly in relation to care justice (Wood and Skeggs, 2020). At the very least, the event demonstrated a public appetite for challenging the limits of our imagination around care (Chatzidakis and Segal, 2020). Whilst it is easy to point to the hypocrisy of politicians who participated in clap-for-carers having equally enthusiastically cheered the maintaining of a public pay cap in 2017, all of us who joined in clap-for-carers are beholden to those working in health and social care not to be 'care-less' in the wake of the pandemic. To the roles of audience, performers and critics, we need to add 'script editor' to ensure that past injustices around care are remedied in post-pandemic society.

Clap-for-carers was associated both with activism, through the 'You Clap for Me Now' film that spotlighted contradictory attitudes to workers from global majorities, and ineffectual slacktivism. Musicologist Jutta Toelle pointed out in an interview for *Frankfurter Allgemeine* that there is an inverse relationship between audience participation in a performance and the role of applause (Hruza, 2020). If we are all players, to paraphrase Shakespeare, applause becomes less important. It is perhaps because we were *not* all players – some were required to step it up, while others were instructed to sit it out – that clap-for-carers became a guilty pleasure. Applauding health care workers afforded all the 'feels' of participation from the comparatively safe road-side vantage point of the spectator.

For all the criticism levelled at clap-for-carers, the intensity of emotions felt in-the-moment will be a lasting legacy of those summer evenings in 2020 when we were still flushed with optimism that the pandemic might be a short, sharp scratch rather than the deadly, deep wound it transpired to be. Rachel Clarke reflects on the impact of the applause in her description of the impact of clap-for-carers in her pandemic memoir:

> The idea of an impromptu ovation to express thanks to key workers has largely passed me by. But then, as I open the car door, applause begins to ripple and rise from my neighbours' doorsteps. . . . The entire village, it seems, is whooping and cheering, yelling 'N – H – S!' and letting rip this most thunderous of thank yous. . . . And, honestly, I could fall to my knees at the sound. Its kindness and sweetness and community spirit overwhelm me with raw gratitude of my own. I stand on the asphalt, open-mouthed, tears streaming. All these people, this passion, this trenchant solidarity. It is the loveliest cacophony in the world.
>
> (2021, pp. 160–161)

Shaw reminds us that moments of gratitude are valuable because they 'serve to enact assurances of our mattering, how they convey to us that others care about us and that we are worthy of their care' (2013, p. 423). Although clap-for-carers as an event is unlikely to be revived, as a social movement it continues to give impetus to and inform debates about how we value those who invest so much of themselves in caring for others. Of course, this appreciation must take a more sustained and material form than merely clapping if it is to serve care justice. Proper remuneration and safe working conditions are an entitlement rather than a reward. But we cannot value care only by the yardsticks of capitalist economies. Gratitude is the emollient of the social exchange upon which all care and caring relies. It requires frequent and generous application to soothe and lubricate relationships of mutual dependency, support and appreciation.

Acknowledgements

This work was supported by the Wellcome Trust [Grant no.212792/Z/18/Z].

Reference list

10 Downing Street (2020) *Coronavirus press conference*, 9 April. Available at: www.youtube.com/watch?v=18QhurjfnYs (Accessed: 26 July 2023).

Abraham, T. (2020) 'Third of Britons think clap for carers has been politicised', *YouGov*, 4 June. Available at: https://yougov.co.uk/topics/politics/articles-reports/2020/06/04/third-britons-think-clap-carers-has-been-politicis (Accessed: 26 July 2023).

Anonymous (2020) 'I'm an NHS doctor – and I've had enough of people clapping for me', *The Guardian*, 21 May.

Aparicio, M. *et al.* (2019) 'Gratitude from patients and relatives in palliative care – characteristics and impact: a national survey', *BMJ Supportive & Palliative Care*, 2(e4), pp. e562–e569. https://doi.org/10.1136/bmjspcare-2019-001858

Bakhtin, M.M. (1984) *Problems of Dostoevsky's poetics*. Edited by C. Emerson. Minneapolis: University of Minnesota Press.

Barthes, R. (2000) *Mythologies*. London: Vintage.

Bate, S.P., Bevan, H. and Robert, G. (2004) *Towards a million change agents: a review of the social movements literature: implications for large scale change in the NHS*. London: NHS Modernisation Agency. Available at: https://mahb.stanford.edu/wp-content/uploads/2012/08/rSUS-PEOPLE-SocialMovements-summary-NHS-copy.pdf (Accessed: 26 July 2023).

BBC News (2020a) 'Captain Tom Moore: NHS fundraiser "lifted lockdown blues"', 30 June. Available at: www.bbc.co.uk/news/uk-england-beds-bucks-herts-53178431?intlink_from_url=www.bbc.co.uk/news/topics/ckr483q4dwgt/captain-tom-moore&link_location=live-reporting-story (Accessed: 26 July 2023).

BBC News (2020b) 'Coronavirus: millions take part in weekly "clap for carers" tribute', April 23. Available at: www.bbc.co.uk/news/av/uk-52402181 (Accessed: 26 July 2023).

Booth, W., Adam, K. and Rolfe, P. (2020) 'In fight against coronavirus, the world gives medical heroes a standing ovation', *The Washington Post*, 26 March.

Burkitt, R. *et al.* (2018) *The public and the NHS: what's the deal?* London: The King's Fund. www.kingsfund.org.uk/publications/public-and-nhs-whats-the-deal (Accessed: 26 July 2023).

Chatzidakis, A. and Segal, L. (2020) 'Do we really "all care now"? Time to expand our caring imagination', *Red Pepper*, April. Available at: www.redpepper.org.uk/we-all-care-now-or-do-we-time-to-radically-expand-our-caring-imagination/ (Accessed: 26 July 2023).

Clarke, R. (2021) *Breath taking*. London: Little Brown.

Converso, D. *et al.* (2015, April) 'Do positive relations with patients play a protective role for healthcare employees? Effects of patients' gratitude and support on nurses' burnout', *Frontiers in Psychology*, 6, p. 21. https://doi.org/10.3389/fpsyg.2015.00470

Cox, C.L. (2020) '"Healthcare heroes": problems with media focus on heroism from healthcare workers during the COVID-19 pandemic', *Journal of Medical Ethics*, 46(8), pp. 510–513. https://doi.org/10.1136/medethics-2020-106398

Day, G. *et al.* (2021) 'An outbreak of appreciation: a discursive analysis of tweets of gratitude expressed to the national health service at the outset of the COVID-19 pandemic', *Health Expectations*, 25(1), pp. 149–162. https://doi.org/10.1111/hex.13359

Diski, J. (2004) 'Think of Mrs Darling', *London Review of Books*, 4 March.

Durkheim, É. (2012) *The elemental forms of the religious life*. Dover and London: George Allen and Unwin.

Edwards, D. (2005) 'Moaning, whinging and laughing: the subjective side of complaints', *Discourse Studies*, 7(1), pp. 5–29. https://doi.org/10.1177/1461445605048765

Finlayson, B. (2002) *Counting the smiles: morale and motivation in the NHS*. London: The King's Fund. Available at: www.kingsfund.org.uk/sites/default/files/field/field_publication_file/counting-smiles-morale-motivation-nhs-belinda-finlayson-kings-fund-1-march-2002.pdf (Accessed: 26 July 2023).

Gibbs, A. (2010) 'After affect: sympathy, synchrony, and mimetic communication', in Gregg, M. and Gregory, J.S. (eds.) *The affect theory reader*. Durham and London: Duke University Press, pp. 186–205.

Goffman, E. (1967) 'On face-work: an analysis of ritual elements in social interaction', in *Interactional ritual*. New York: Doubleday, pp. 5–45.

Goffman, E. (1969) *The presentation of self in everyday life*. London: Penguin Press.

Gray, F. (2020) 'Is the "clap for me now" video a wind-up?', *The Spectator*, 15 April.

Heren, K. (2020) 'Anger as people crowd together to clap NHS on Westminster Bridge for second week running', *The Evening Standard*, 24 April.

Hofstede Insights (2020) *What about the UK? Individualism*. Available at: www.hofstede-insights.com/country/the-uk/ (Accessed: 26 July 2023).

Honneth, A. (1995) *The struggle for recognition: the moral grammar of social conflicts*. Cambridge: Polity Press.

Hopkins, N. *et al.* (2016) 'Explaining effervescence: investigating the relationship between shared social identity and positive experience in crowds', *Cognition and Emotion*, 30(1), pp. 20–32. https://doi.org/10.1080/02699931.2015.1015969

Hruza, L. (2020) 'Und Jetzt Alle! [all together now!]', *Frankfurt Allgemeine*, 1 January. Available at: www.faz.net/aktuell/wissen/geist-soziales/klatschen-und-jetzt-alle-16556146.html (Accessed: 26 July 2023).

Jackson, J. *et al.* (2020) 'The lockdown and social norms: why the UK is complying by consent rather than compulsion', *British Politics and Policy Blog at LSE*, 27 April. Available at: https://blogs.lse.ac.uk/politicsandpolicy/lockdown-social-norms/ (Accessed: 26 July 2023).

Jones, E. (2020) 'The psychology of protecting the UK public against external threat: COVID-19 and the blitz compared', *The Lancet Psychiatry*, 7, pp. 991–996. https://doi.org/10.1016/S2215-0366(20)30342-4

Juri, C. (2020) 'Applause as a form of social distancing', *OpenDemocracy*, 1 May. Available at: www.opendemocracy.net/en/can-europe-make-it/applause-form-social-distancing/ (Accessed: 26 July 2023).

Kelsey, D. (2013) 'The myth of the "blitz spirit" in British newspaper responses to the July 7th bombings', *Social Semiotics*, 23(1), pp. 83–99. https://doi.org/doi.org/10.1080/10350330.2012.707034

Kershaw, B. (2001) 'Oh for unruly audiences! or, patterns of participation in twentieth-century theatre', *Modern Drama*, 44(2), pp. 133–154. https://doi.org/10.3138/md.44.2.133.

King's Fund (2014) *Growing concern about staff morale as NHS performance slips*, 30 October. Available at: www.kingsfund.org.uk/press/press-releases/growing-concern-about-staff-morale-nhs-performance-slips (Accessed: 26 July 2023).

Lodewijckx, I. (2020) ' "Slactivism": legitimate action or just lazy liking?', *CitizenLab*, 20 May.

Marangozov, R. *et al.* (2017) *Royal college of nursing employment survey 2017*. Available at: www.rcn.org.uk/professional-development/publications/pdf-007076 (Accessed: 26 July 2023).

Matsumoto, D. *et al.* (2008) 'Mapping expressive differences around the world: the relationship between emotional display rules and individualism versus collectivism', *Journal of Cross-Cultural Psychology*, 39(1), pp. 55–74. https://doi.org/10.1177/0022022107311854

McKinley, N. *et al.* (2020) 'Resilience, burnout and coping mechanisms in UK doctors: a cross-sectional study', *BMJ Open*, 10(1), p. e031765. https://doi.org/10.1136/bmjopen-2019-031765

Mermikides, A. (2020) *Performance, medicine and the human*. London: Bloomsbury Methuen Drama Publishing.

O'Connor, R. (2020) 'Comedian will Hislop goes viral for NHS clap for carers parody', *The Independent*, 9 May.

Papacharissi, Z. (2015) *Affective publics: sentiment, technology, and politics*. Oxford: Oxford University Press.

Persson, A. (2019) *Framing social interaction*. New York: Routledge.

Plas, A.M. (2020) *Clapforourcarers.com*. Available at: www.instagram.com/p/B-AJkisAhSF/ (Accessed: 26 July 2023).

Robinson, B. and Kutner, M. (2019) 'Spinoza and the affective turn: a return to the philosophical origins of affect', *Qualitative Inquiry*, 25(2), pp. 111–117. https://doi.org/10.1177/1077800418786312

Schechner, R. (2020) *Performance studies: an introduction*. 4th edn. Oxon and New York: Routledge.

Seigworth, G.J. and Gregg, M. (2010) 'An inventory of shimmers', in Seigworth, G.J. and Gregg, M. (eds.) *The affect theory reader*. Durham and London: Duke University Press, pp. 1–25.

Shariatmadari, D. (2016) ' "Virtue-signalling" – the putdown that has passed its sell-by date', *The Guardian*, 20 January.

Shaw, J. (2013) 'Gratitude, self-assessment, and moral community', *Journal of Value Inquiry*, 47, pp. 407–23. https://doi.org/10.1007/s10790-013-9396-7

Shilling, C. and Mellor, P.A. (2016) 'Durkheim, morality and modernity: collective effervescence, homo duplex and the sources of moral action', *British Journal of Sociology*, 49(2), pp. 193–209.

SkyNews (2020) *Coronavirus: founder wants 'politicised' clap for carers to end next week*, 22 May. Available at: https://news.sky.com/story/coronavirus-founder-wants-politicised-clap-for-carers-to-end-next-week-11992911 (Accessed: 26 July 2023).

Slisco, A. (2020) 'Netherlands coronavirus healthcare workers receive nationwide standing ovation for tackling pandemic', *Newsweek*, 17 March.

Smith, D. (2020) *You clap for me now: the coronavirus poem on racism and immigration in Britain*. Available at: www.youtube.com/watch?v=gXGIt_Y57tc (Accessed: 26 July 2023).

Sorace, C. (2020) 'Gratitude: the ideology of sovereignty in crisis', *Made in China Journal*, 18 May. Available at: https://madeinchinajournal.com/2020/05/18/gratitude-the-ideology-of-sovereignty-in-crisis/ (Accessed: 26 July 2023).

Starkey, A.R. *et al*. (2019) 'Gratitude reception and physical health: examining the mediating role of satisfaction with patient care in a sample of acute care nurses', *The Journal of Positive Psychology*, 14(6), pp. 779–788. https://doi.org/10.1080/17439760.2019.1579353

Sullivan, G.B. and Day, C.R. (2019) 'Collective emotions in celebratory, competitive, and conflictual contexts: exploring the dynamic relations between group-based and collective pride and shame', *Emotions: History, Culture, Society*, 3(2), pp. 202–222. https://doi.org/10.1163/2208522x-02010057

Wood, H. and Skeggs, B. (2020) 'Clap for carers? From care gratitude to care justice', *European Journal of Cultural Studies*, 23(4), pp. 641–647. https://doi.org/10.1177/1367549420928362

Younge, G. (2020) 'What, precisely, are we making noise for?', *Financial Times*, 5 May. Available at: www.ft.com/content/185dd664-83da-11ea-b6e9-a94cffd1d9bf (Accessed: 26 July 2023).

PART 3

Care and Cure

Introduction

The following chapters demonstrate the various ways in which performance, like medicine, can be used to make things better: serving to diagnose and, where possible, remediate human suffering. This 'therapeutic' agenda has been long imbricated in performance traditions across the globe. It is evident, for example, in the dramatic tradition of the western classical world and the Aristotelian paradigm in which a staged display of extreme distress leads to catharsis in the spectators as well the character (catharsis being a medical term). The projects and initiatives described in the following more purposely and tangibly pursue this therapeutic agenda, targeting specific health and social ills in individuals and communities, often in the hope of measurable benefits. We offer an array of case studies and vignettes, describing the aims, methods and outcomes of these projects, including insider accounts of the sort of performance practices that they involve. Apart from their shared mission to do good and to take care, however, our case studies operate within fields of practice – for example, public health; health promotion; theatre in development; arts and health; applied, community, socially engaged, activist and experimental performance; and more – that vary significantly. For example, they differ in terms of their alignment to the formal institutions of medicine and health care, the governmental policy of their specific locale and the different forms of performance – street clowning, one-to-one performances, catchy *sanedos*, gentle workshops and more – employed in their efforts to care and to cure. Our case studies also seek to address a wide range of health and social issues, criss-crossing across the Global North and Global South in response to areas of urgent, often overlooked, need. Despite their differences, two key themes thread through the projects and the discussion. First, the concept of care as a motivator and an ethical principle directed towards responsiveness and mutuality and, second, a desire to blur received distinctions between health care and the arts and the communities they serve, the merging of the social and artful. These themes are theorised and explicated further in the two final chapters of the part.

We begin in India: Shilpa Das describes a collaboration between the government of Gujarat, the Indian National Institute of Design and the international humanitarian organisation Humanity and Inclusion that sought to challenge the often extreme forms of stigma and marginalisation faced by people with disabilities in rural communities in Gujarat. A notable feature of this project is its basis

DOI: 10.4324/9781003036500-22

in the practitioners' deep understanding of the various communities they engaged with, including 'the visual language of the region, their symbolic systems, local art forms, preferred colours, colloquialisms, and local flavour in terms of the idiom'. As a result, the work involved the use of local performance traditions, notably the popular format of the *sanedo*, adapting this into 'forms of critique and resistance' that challenge 'dominant hegemonic (including medical) ontologies of disability and validating alternate epistemologies and practices'. We also see this adaptation to 'local' forms and practice to address issues of stigmatisation and marginalisation in Katharine E. Low's account of the 'quiet activism' practised by Positively UK, an HIV advocacy and peer support charity based in London. The focus here is on women living well with HIV, a community, Low argues, that is overlooked in the public imagination and in policy. While the HIV activism by gay and queer men is often 'spectacularly performative and blunt' – and rightly so – the small-scale participatory workshops delivered by Positively UK can make room for the 'softer, quieter voices' of 'those who are not used to taking up so much space', affording the possibility of enabling seemingly small but ultimately meaningful change.

From quiet activism, we turn to loud and colourful street clowning, as Sally Souraya offers an insider perspective of Rally Against Measles, a campaign delivered in a collaboration between UNICEF and Clown in Me, a clowning and street performance theatre company and non-governmental organisation based in Lebanon. Designed to raise awareness of the threat of measles and to advocate for uptake in vaccination programmes, the project involved the careful development of 'accessible, culturally acceptable, and compelling' events and activities, involving larger-than-life street performances of bouffon, clowning, puppetry and dance, as well as exciting opportunities for 'young and vibrant adults' to take part in competitive task and games. This, says Souraya, 'helped break down barriers that traditional, formal health promotion messages cannot and stimulated acceptance among the public'. This level of involvement and acceptance answers Jane Plastow's critique of the 'commonly accepted narrative' within theatre for development that the role of socially engaged theatre is 'artistically preaching development messages as designed by the rich and powerful to the poor – messages which often implicitly "blame" their ignorance and backwardness'. Her chapter describes Maternal Mortality in East Africa, a research project jointly funded by the UK Medical Research Council and the Arts and Humanities Research Council. By 'focusing on people rather than medical science', the project employed participatory workshops to capture people's experiences of maternity services in and around Ahero, a small market town in Kenya, leading to the creation of performance and film material that could be disseminated more widely. Plastow gives a striking account of the 'notable sense of panic' exhibited by a local minister for health in response to a documentary film that exposed how 'problems relating to maternal deaths stemmed from actions performed by the powerful and the state'.

'Applied theatre is, ultimately, concerned with power', state Andy Barratt, Chandradasan and Michael Wilson in their reflections on their Mental Health Literacy Project (MeHeLP) in Kerala, India. They ask: 'Who has the power to tell their stories; who has the resources, the space and the opportunity for their voices to be heard?' Their account of this project, designed to respond to high levels of mental illness in this relatively privileged area of India, demonstrates the potential for participatory and devised performance-making to unsettle hierarchies and give voice to marginalised communities, bringing together health professionals, patients and their families 'to create a genuinely democratic space in which experience, attitudes, and aspirations could be communicated freely'. We stay with the theme of mental health for the next two chapters. First, Yewande O. Addie, David O. Fakunle and Jeffrey Pufahl advocate for the use of performance storytelling as 'a viable form of care for mental and emotional health-related challenges, regardless of personal or societal cause'. Their three case studies, which all take place in the context of American universities, demonstrate the use of this adaptable format in relation to people recovering from substance use disorders, those living with obsessive compulsive disorder and those at risk of trauma caused by racism. Next, Cinira Magali Fortuna, Felipe Lima dos Santos, Jorge Antônio Nunes Bichuetti, Maria de Fátima Oliveira and Silvia Matumoto offer a rare insight into the use of schizodrama – a form of dramatherapy based on Deleuze and Guattari's philosophical concept of schizoanalysis – that has been integrated within the Brazilian psychiatric health care system. Accounts of three 'experiences' that took place in the Psychosocial Care Centre Maria Boneca reveal the improvisatory and responsive nature of this practice, its basis in the interactions amongst service users and therapists and the way in which 'the unprecedented and the uncertain' form part of the therapeutic process.

A similar level of responsiveness is evident in *Kicking Up Our Heels*, a playful project for the parents and carers of children being treated in Great Ormond Street Hospital, London. Brian Lobel and Emily Underwood-Lee describe how they drew on the practice of one-to-one performance, more commonly associated with alternative and experimental theatre than a hospital setting, in an effort to attend to the under-recognised needs of these carers. Donning eye-masks, bath robes and slippers, they engaged parents and carers in often brief but always 'care-filled and compassionate' interactions, 'intimate yet fleeting' and incongruously playful within the hospital setting. Their reflections on the ethical principles underpinning their own project, as well as the situation of their participants, brings them to the concept of care. Indeed, care is an important concept for understanding all the projects described in this part: care for others motivates the initiatives described in these case studies and characterises the ethos and ethics of the work. In particular, it becomes a way of digging into the paradoxical challenge baked into all forms of interaction in which one party attempts to remediate the suffering of another who is in some way vulnerable and in need.

All contributors to this section are engaged in relationships that require great responsibility and responsiveness but also great effort to avoid reinforcing the power differential inherent in any exchange based on the vulnerability of one party. Lobel and Underwood-Lee's description of the 'asymmetrical or unbalanced yet mutual encounter' between performer and audience in a one-to-one performance mirrors the 'reciprocal, asymmetric exchange' between applied performance practitioner and the community they choose to engage with. It also mirrors the 'asymmetrical or unbalanced' nature of the encounter between health or social care professional and patient, as explained in James Thompson's chapter on the art, ethics and performance of health care.

Care, then, is common to many if not all of the individuals who feature in these projects: health and social care professionals, including nurses, doctors and allied health workers; the researchers and theatre-makers and other artists delivering projects; the institutions supporting them; and the participants in those projects. Furthermore, Thompson's chapter reveals the practices of all these parties might be also productively thought of in terms of an aesthetic paradigm. It is not the case, he argues, that 'medicine' can be thought of as a form of care and 'performance' as an aesthetic practice. And he illustrates this by employing his concept of care aesthetics to explore sensory and crafted aspects of health and social care interaction, on the basis that 'medical practices and performance are understood to have a common concern with aesthetics: they both include relational, temporal, and affective practices'.

In the final chapter in this part, Simon Parry describes the work of Contact, a theatre and arts organisation based in Manchester, UK, notable for the active involvement of young people within the organisation and on its board, and its rich programme of theatre engaged with young people's understanding and experiences of health, medicine and biology. He describes how Contact's programming is situated within inter-sectoral and interdisciplinary networks and infrastructural frameworks, enabling a range of often novel partnerships among 'patients, broader publics, activists, health researchers, policymakers, clinicians, and other groups'. Through this, Contact usefully exemplifies Parry's conceptualisation of 'biosocial theatre', which he describes as 'a creative practice that thinks its artfulness and social function together' and that 'registers a relationship to the way the social is or has become entangled with the biological or biomedical'. The case studies and the theorisations offered in this part, then, enable us to also think 'artfulness' and 'social function' as complementary, indeed, as interrelated and mutual, and to see performance and medicine coming together in their shared commitment both craft and care.

19

PERFORMANCE, COMMUNITY AND DISABILITY IN GUJARAT

Reflections in hindsight

Shilpa Das

This chapter outlines a public health project which employed both participatory theatre techniques and local or folk performance forms in an effort to shift local understandings of and perspectives around disability in rural communities in Gujarat state in India. The project aimed to design, develop and deploy a strategic behaviour-change communication campaign to counter negative attitudes towards disability among rural communities in four districts of India. It also aimed to improve the competence and capacity of primary health care workers and engage with community-based organisations to increase their knowledge and awareness of disability and to transform the communication approaches of the government health department. In 2005, the NGO Humanity and Inclusion (HI) and the government of Gujarat invited the National Institute of Design (NID), Ahmedabad, to be a consultant on this project on the basis of NID's considerable media experience and resources.[1] The project continues to have currency and relevance in the state even today in terms of the lessons learned with respect to disability and medicine. The efficacy of project deliverables that pertain to theatre and performance, as exemplified in the use of a local folk form that coalesced song, dance, folklore and performance, the *sanedo*, to communicate key messages on disability, must be underscored.

In this project, everyday actions of the community around the disabled individual could be analysed through a performance vocabulary. A specific performance one night enabled looking anew at a life lived with disability and the phenomenon of disability at large. Metaphors are powerful in generating and giving life to community and have powerful narrational effects, and shared metaphors become part of how a community defines itself, how it talks to itself and how it produces and recognises both its positive and negative values. Performance was used as a productive metaphor for subjectivity, calling on the community in the village to conceive of nuanced ways of seeing disabled identity and other worldviews that elaborated on individual and environmental agency. An essentialised view of disability was counterproductive since subjectivity is not fixed but rather something that is produced through our interactions, and metaphors produced through our thinking often lie at its core. In this case, metaphors were offered through performance to layer people's perceptions of their own behaviour, attitudes and practices more complexly. They brought them up front in confrontation with their own social and cultural worlds, offering them other ways to understand society's interaction with disabled people.[2]

DOI: 10.4324/9781003036500-23

Contextualising disability

It is important to understand local perceptions of disability in order to appreciate the necessity and relevance of the project. Interviews in the field revealed that people in most villages, whether aware of medical causes of disability or not, attributed any kind of disability to cosmic factors such as fate, God's will and *karma*. The Hindu community tended to believe that disability results from the sins of the previous birth, evil doings of the parents in the previous birth, the wrath of God, black magic cast by a rival, excessive masturbation, sexual intercourse during pregnancy or soon after delivery, a pregnant woman watching television, intake of non-vegetarian food, excessive alcohol consumption and *mataji* (the mother goddess) possessing the body of a person, amongst others. The local Muslim community, by contrast, considered disability a blessing from God and people living with disabilities to be Allah's chosen few. Many people believed that vaccinations (injections) were a prime cause of disability (not improper administering of vaccines). Many others believed that any medical intervention in the case of disability would aggravate the disability and hence did not seek health care services for their disabled child. Due to issues such as poverty, inaccessibility of medical services, lack of education and certain embittered experiences of vaccinations administered by local doctors in the past, local mechanisms such as *bhuvas* or quasi-religious leaders were approached at the onset of disability or any health-related issue. Thus, medicine was not the dominant model of health care provision in some of the areas of these districts, and folk meanings and 'cures' for disability, rather than medical ones, guided those living with disability.

Most people were not aware of the medical assistance and care women need before and during pregnancy, during childbirth and after the delivery or of the developmental milestones of growth in a child. They were also unaware of the various types of disabilities and hence did not provide the early medical intervention to their children required in some disabilities. Most people were only aware of bus passes and disability certificates but not health services offered by the government to disabled people. Where there was awareness, there was a reluctance to avail themselves of these services because of poverty, lack of faith in government mechanisms or inaccessibility of those services. Surprisingly, most families of disabled persons were unaware of their psychosocial needs. Many parents of disabled children did not send their children to school for fear that they may be bullied in mainstream schools; sometimes they were seen to be ashamed to take their disabled children to social gatherings. Many parents felt that giving disabled children attention and special care would be a waste, since the other non-disabled children would eventually financially support the family in the future.

Objectives

With this background in mind, the objectives of the project were articulated as:

1. To understand the existing awareness levels, beliefs, attitudes and practices of the respondent groups on disability; the existing conceptions of disability likely to have a negative impact on those living with disability; awareness about the types and causes of disability, signs of early identification; relevance of good quality antenatal, intra-natal and post-natal care for the prevention of disabilities; the medical and rehabilitative referral services at local public health centre (PHC) level; and benefits available for disabled people.
2. To address negative attitudes which result in the marginalisation of disabled people.
3. To generate awareness of the problems faced by those with impairments.

4. To create desired social change through the campaign that would ensure the inclusion of disabled persons as full citizens with equal opportunities.
5. To sensitise government departments and public health workers to include disability information – prevention, early identification, treatment and referrals, if appropriate – leading to mainstreaming of disability in health care programmes.
6. To get the community to understand disability as a social issue and create behaviour change through communication design of posters, stickers, calendars, jingles, songs, audioplays, interviews and public service announcements, among others.

Aligning with the social model of disability, the project moved the lens of analysis from the disabled person to explore the role and liability of the family, community, medical establishment, society and other organisations at large in the construction of disability and its attendant oppression. The project proposed to keep the perspectives of disabled persons at the centre and create the desired social changes through a campaign that would create positive attitudes, health behaviours and practices both at the level of the general community and among village-level health workers.

Methodology

The project kicked off with the NID team conducting a review of existing disability-related communication materials such as posters, all of which turned out to follow the medical approach to disability. Second, a perspective building and sensitisation workshop on disability was organised with doctors, health workers, social scientists, media personnel and designers to understand the underpinning realities. The next stage entailed careful research of knowledge, attitudes and practices related to disability in the four districts. Intensive field research and interactive sessions followed over a couple of months, with a significant sample size of over 2000 respondents across different stakeholder groups: people living with a disability and their families, community members, Panchayat or village council members, *anganwadi* or rural childcare centre workers, NGO personnel, *bhuvas*, health service providers such as auxiliary nurse doctors, PHC, community health centre (CHC) staff, traditional birth attendants or midwives (ANMs) and other influential/opinion leaders. Different tools for data collection were used to gather information from each respondent group. For instance, in-depth interviews and focused group discussions were used with those with impairments, their families and the community, whereas in-depth interviews were conducted with government and non-government stakeholders. This gave an understanding of the way communities perceived disability and the disabled individual, the issues pertaining to disability and the core communication that needed to be disseminated.

Priority ranking of the essential messages that emerged from the fieldwork boiled down to four messages in the communication needs assessment: awareness building about disability: types and causes, prevention of some disabilities (e.g. polio) through vaccination and staying alert to signs of onset of disability, medical care and emotional support and benefits and services available. The last group of messages, especially, was a pitfall for us, as we were aware that ideas for prevention and cure posed ethical problems when seen through the lens of the social model and various empowerment models of disability. This was because we would be playing into the stigmatising medical model in which disability has an uncomfortable association with concepts such as illness, disease, congenital difference, dependency, lack, loss, tragedy and victimhood. But these messages could not be discarded, according to the government officials, doctors and the local NGOs, as the uptake for vaccination could not be jeopardised nor the availing of medical or rehabilitation facilities be lessened in a developing nation like India.

Communication need assessment

Each of these messages was broken down into several key sub-messages. Clarity emerged in terms of the precise communication need for each stakeholder group. For instance, with respect to government and private doctors, local communities often expressed that they did not want to seek medical assistance at the onset of disability in a child because of the insensitive behaviour of doctors and medical staff. Issues of perceived negligence on the part of doctors also emerged, which led the communities to resort to trusted local people named *bhuvas*, *ojhas* or *badwas* (who use a blend of medicinal and shamanic treatment and folk remedies to cure people in villages). So the communication need for medical personnel included making them aware of the repercussions of faulty prescriptions and wrong injections administered to patients; making them accountable and morally responsible; urging them to communicate to local communities about spacing between pregnancies, family planning, pre-, ante- and post-natal care and the benefits and services available to disabled persons and their families; and asking them to behave sensitively towards the local communities to encourage people to freely approach medical personnel for information on aspects including vaccination, rehabilitation and care.

In the villages of these districts, local CHC and PHC officials told us that *bhuvas* and *ojhas* were exercising their powers for their own advantage – for money or clout. For instance, they promoted practices such as sacrificing animals and birds to 'cure' a person of their disability or offering a silver tongue to *mataji* (goddess) to cure a person with a speech impairment. There were several instances where *bhuvas* indulged in harmful practices which caused a disability or worsened it, such as tying heavy stones to the leg of a child with polio or isolating a disabled child in a room for a month to effect a 'cure'. We aimed at getting the *bhuvas* to disseminate information on disability that the CHCs and PHCs recommended. We also aimed to make them feel morally responsible enough to urge people to consult doctors at the onset of disability so that timely measures for care and rehabilitation may be taken. Similarly, *dais* or midwives known to conduct most of the deliveries among low-income groups and who have a close interaction with pregnant women and young mothers also needed to be addressed by the campaign with respect to the ante-, neo- and post-natal care to be taken by pregnant women and their families that could sometimes prevent certain disabilities in the neonates, as well as the messages on disability.

Such findings were discussed in depth, after two months, in a perspective sharing workshop with representatives of the state government (the public health system), representatives from the district rehabilitation centres and representatives of civil society.[3] It became clear that the major change needed was to make communication strategies, implementation and action plans specific to the districts in a multi-pronged manner (keeping cultural and social aspects in mind) with respect to their needs, existing awareness levels, behaviour, social set-ups, cultural environment and local knowledge and practices.

Creative media strategy and communication development phases

Now the project entered the creative phase important to this chapter, not a mere creation of awareness material but developing a sustainable communication and dissemination strategy while exploring the possibilities of the various media that could be used. The field research gave satisfactory signals in this direction. For instance, in Hirapur village in Sabarkantha district, *bhavais* (a form of folk theatre) and street plays are quite popular. People said that messages delivered through them would be more effective in terms of understanding the key messages of the communications campaign and would have a marked effect on the viewers' minds. In another village, people said that if actors of Gujarati films were to deliver such messages, it would carry greater credibility. In a third village, they said *dohas* (a local form of poetry) or use of popular fictional or folk characters familiar to the local population would lead to greater impact on the local community. They said that involving an influential personality of the village or an opinion leader would also work well.

The media strategy and communication development phase ensued, emerging from the expressed needs of local people to meet very specific grassroots needs. The appropriate way was not to persuade people to adopt the new ideas or messages or pre-design communication campaign deliverables because this normally does not interest or influence local people and fails to make any impact. It was important to deploy a range of participatory methods and communication tools that emanated from the community itself. In order to do this, we would need to better understand local social set-ups, systems, cultural environment, knowledge and practices, as well as the visual language of the region, their symbolic systems, local art forms, preferred colours, colloquialisms and local flavour in terms of the idiom. The use of these aspects, we felt, would have a greater immediacy, would not seem alien to them and would be more readily accepted. After this, the knowledge of different stakeholders could be addressed, and their active involvement in the communication development initiative as active partners in the diagnosis, discussion and problem-solving process could be facilitated. Doing this through proper communication planning, multi-stakeholder dialogue and collaboration would systematically guide towards identifying the when, where and how of accomplishing the projected goals. The aspiration was to create a long-term impact on the community that would, eventually, become part of its folklore.

Finalising media tools

The next phase involved finalising appropriate media tools for the campaign to disseminate the messages and the communication strategy in terms of the content, time and manner of circulating the communication on disability. The tools finally selected comprised audio jingles and slogans, audio skits, audio plays, docudramas, public service announcements and documentary films, interview-based programmes and various kinds of print material. These were not seen as media products in themselves but as elements in a larger social and developmental process. Among these, the audio skits and plays and the docudramas to be aired on radio were envisaged as having high potential for performance aspects. But, as things would turn out, their thunder would be stolen by live folk theatre, as we will see later in this chapter.

A two-day creative workshop was organised in which the participants were visual artists, writers, playwrights, stage directors, musicians, film makers and radio programmers with experience in the sector of rural and social communication, disabled persons and eminent experts from different NGOs who had worked extensively in the field of behaviour change on various issues. The first day of the workshop was spent in acquiring a perspective on the issue of disability and in sharing the findings from the field along with the communication needs assessment and the media tools and types that the core team had determined. The participants were grouped into three: visual arts, audio-visual and theatre. In groups, the participants explored the scope that their medium allowed for creative ideas and their dissemination by way of slogans, jingles, radio programmes, flip books, interactive performance and other communication materials. Those in the theatre group had to focus on developing narratives, especially short skits and long plays, to generate awareness among and sensitise the community on the key messages pertaining to disability mentioned earlier.

On the second day, the team travelled to Samarkha, a village in the district of Anand where the participants of the creative workshop spent an entire day in refining and creating ideas along with people from the village, including teachers, disabled persons, members of the *panchayat*, women, youth and children. This proved invaluable in terms of getting an insight on the use of local material, readily identifiable characters and the local culture and idioms, all of which were incorporated in the communication material. For instance, the visual arts group created several posters and flip books along with disabled persons from Samarkha. The theatre group wrote and performed a street play with the youth from Samarkha, based on Bhikhabhai, a person with a learning disability, who was the target of much ridicule in the village. In the course of acting out Bhikhabhai's daily experiences and mannerisms through the play, some of the youth expressed that they now compassionately viewed his daily life experiences and realised what role they had themselves played in the collective opprobrium heaped on him.

But it is the work of the audio-visual group and the performances that followed that need special mention and detailed reflection here. Along with women from the village, the group created a new *bhajan* (devotional song) talking about the importance of ante-, neo- and post-natal care in the prevention of disability. More importantly, the group created short radio plays and programmes on public responses to health, wellbeing and disability. Among the most successful outcomes were their deployment of folk media and especially, folk song and dance performances at the research locations. These interrogated the social construction of normalcy and disability and yielded rich insights on the role culture plays in creating stigma about the disabled body and constructing categories that lead to the marginalisation of people with disabilities. Disability was the subject of these performances and was experienced in and through performance, and these performances proved to be forms of critique and resistance, challenging dominant hegemonic (including medical) ontologies of disability and validating alternate epistemologies and practices.

The power of folk media

Folk media are varied local media with limited geographical coverage, traditional to a particular community and intimate to it. They are relished in the form of theatre, puppetry, skits, songs, music, sayings, poetry and storytelling. They are orally handed down from one generation to the next and are moulded by the artists or performers to suit the times and the changing concerns, aspirations, hopes and fears, joys and sorrows, triumphs and defeats of a community. As they reveal the social and psychological attributes, the customs and conventions and living traditions of the community they originate in, they are a good means to know more about the life of rural people and of understanding their social behaviour and ways of living. They use familiar dialects for the most intimate expression and have a personal appeal that makes them readily understood and accepted.

Those in the social development sector are aware of the power of such media and strive to contemporise forms of folk media to reflect the changing preoccupations of the people. This requires skilled crafting of development messages into the fabric of the folk media. They are easily available at low cost, are relished by different age groups and genders and have greater potential than print media or even digital media for face-to-face communication and instant feedback. Most importantly, they are egalitarian, belong to the community and not to individuals or the state and hence are especially relevant for behavioural change. As Ranganath affirms, 'acceptability, cultural relevance, entertainment value, localised language, legitimacy, flexibility, message repetition ability, instant two-way communication, and so on are among their virtues' (1976, p. 25).

Often made successful or unsuccessful vehicles of social messages to change people's thinking by the government of India since Independence, folk forms performed *for* the folk and *by* the folk include *Nautanki* (a form of folk theatre in North India); *kathas* (a traditional mode of storytelling); *Yellamma* songs (in praise of Goddess Yellamma); *Yakshagana* (a traditional dance-drama of Karnataka); *Tamasha* (folk theatre of Maharashtra), which employs a harmonious blend of music, dance and drama; *Bhavai* (folk drama in Gujarat); *Pala* and *Daskathia* (folk drama in Odisha); and *Burrakatha* (ballad singing of Andhra Pradesh), among several others. They have conveyed messages on a range of subjects such as family planning, vaccination, sanitation, clean water, cooperative effort and rural development, most of which often have a direct or indirect connection with disability and the medical sector.

The efficacy of the *sanedo*

In this project, the audio-visual group made ample use of the popular and time-tested *sanedo*, a folk theatre form in Gujarat. The word has its origin in the Gujarati word *snehdo* or *sneh*, meaning love. A s*anedo* contains couplets of four lines and is usually played either during the Navratri festival where people dance to celebrate the Goddess Amba or the musical night attached to weddings: in short, any occasion for revelry. A *sanedo* can express romance or satire, poetry or beauty and dreams or cultural anxieties. The music played in the background during a *sanedo* recital is from a percussion instrument called *daklu*. The song is very relatable and the rhythmic foot-tapping, making it lively, joyful and interactive with its heady mix of gesture, mime, music, poetry and limited dialogue. Thus, the non-verbal aspect of purposeful communication is equally vital and leads to its dynamic nature. Though its current use is mainly for entertainment, ritual or aesthetic purposes, this traditional theatre form has great credibility to communicate messages with development content to rural audiences that may be illiterate or unable to interpret symbols, metaphors and messages from other types of media. There is a sense of legitimate ownership and pride that is associated with such media. They are decentralised, with each person who receives the message being a potential transmitter of the message and creating further interpretations of it. They are highly effective in mobilising the masses as they are collectively produced.

The performers are oral communication experts skilled at delivering messages. Typically, they are born in families that have traditionally been performing for generations, so they learn from early childhood by observation of the elders in the family. They are also experienced at creatively and innovatively capturing the attention of rural audiences with little formal education within the familiarity of the setting. Topics that may not be easily palatable are often strategically addressed and made more legitimate by putting the messages in the mouth of mythological, legendary or folk characters in a narrative framework. In Gujarat, the traditional jesters in folklore, and *bhavai* performances called *ranglo* and *rangli* may also be deployed to communicate sensitive messages such as family planning, for instance, with a dash of tomfoolery or rustic humour. Audiences easily relate to these characters through the shared understanding of the performative or theatrical conventions within which such characters operate. Most importantly, *sanedo* performances throw wide open the possibility of audience interaction in a participatory manner devoid of any hierarchies of artist and audience, where the performers seek the audience's response and validation from time to time in a recursive and repetitive manner. Thus, the meaning of the message to be delivered is continually created and re-created through the lively exchange between them. The audience breaks out into frenzy, singing and dancing into the night (when such performances are usually scheduled). The immense human resource thus created when deployed with familiar cultural heritage such as folk forms takes on a life of its own; mnemonic chains and opportunities for positive dialogue are spontaneously created and give the messages a lease of life long after a specific performance may be over.

The performance of *sanedo*

We witnessed first-hand how deploying the *sanedo* as a communication tool to convey the behavioural change messages on disability connected to the audience and galvanised an entire village. When the audio-visual team was scripting the *sanedo* lyrics, they integrated various important themes about the importance of vaccination, the benefits and health referrals available to disabled people, phenomenological aspects or lived experience of disability, the various stigma attached to disabled identity, the need for psychosocial care of a disabled person in one's family, different myths about disability and also how the medical establishment identifies it as a problem. In the evening, a show was organised for the village. This was an unexpected but pleasant development. News spread by word of mouth, which still seems to be an effective medium of communication in rural areas. By about eight o'clock in the evening, more than 200 people (out of which more than eighty were women) had gathered to watch the show. Posters were put up on an improvised rickety wooden stage; locally sourced lights, mics and speakers were arranged. The show began with a small audio skit. Surprisingly, the crowd listened to the audio skit silently and patiently. But the catchy *sanedo* was an immense hit. As the music was played and the singer sang, several young men started spiritedly dancing to the *sanedo* rhythm. Women were shy at first but kept pulling each other to their feet until some of them started dancing, demurely pulling the veils of their polyester and nylon sarees over their faces. The less shy ones danced merrily to the doting eyes of the village elders sitting in the *otlas* (the plinths bordering the street and forming the threshold space around the doorways of the houses). Children added to the performance by prancing around in paper masks and cloth capes. Someone pulled Bhikhabhai, the person with a learning disability mentioned earlier, into the fray. He happily clapped and swayed to the music, a performance that broke out of its allocated spaces in a way that Petra Kuppers would have termed 'characterized by a flow of energy, and a way of being alive, that negates fixity' (Kuppers, 2003, p. 1). A D/deaf girl danced with her friends, matching her steps to theirs in a watchful manner. A person who had polio in both his legs and who used crutches to walk created a moment of rupture by joining in the fray, asserting his individuality and creativity in terms of dance steps, claiming an unchartered space in the open by subverting the typical dance steps of the *sanedo* and what Kuppers (2003, p. 2) might have called 'sedimented certainties' of the *sanedo* for disabled and non-disabled people, modifying conventions to enable a different form of embodiment to emerge. People repeated the lyrics of the *sanedo* after the singer, gradually internalising the messages related to disability. Since the lyrics repetitively used the words, '*sanedo sanedo*', everyone chanted it in unison, which became a crescendo at the end of the evening's performance. The project team members were singing along too, taking photographs, delighted to see and feel the incredible pulsating energy in that village square. It was a night to remember.

Reflections

Reflections upon that evening and performance in hindsight today provide several valuable lessons for development communication. First, in the field, we must be mindful of ensuring sensitivity in community relationships and issues and the fact that we are always outsiders in the community. Second, we must play the role of an equal as opposed to that of an expert. It is important to take care to have extensive discussions with the artists beforehand on the messages to be communicated. In this project, artists deftly wove these into their existing tapestry by a turn of hand and the team mediated, facilitated and cross-checked the technical correctness as well as the adherence to a socio-cultural model of disability and rights-based approach to disability. Third, we need to understand that performance or participatory theatre is made for and by the community because it shuns top-down or one way communication. If it is entertaining, people want to actively engage with it; it strengthens community cohesion; it builds community, and in turn, community builds performance. A focus on process over product can pay rich dividends if it is not rushed. The *sanedo* was essentially to play the role of participatory performance. Fourth, we need to ensure that we do not establish new hegemonic systems of communication that would negatively disrupt the local cultural communication channels, reduce the form to a showpiece by ripping out its aesthetic totality, alter the moral equilibrium of the village or make culture a commodity to be consumed. Balancing all this out by keeping performance dialogic, making for new knowledges and very much a collective ritual, and not a mere set of movements and lyrics, is vital to make it all inclusive and accessible.

We learnt that we need to consider the audience and participants people with an autonomous and critical conscience capable of contributing to social change in line with what Brazilian educator Paulo Freire called a 'pedagogy of the oppressed' (1968). This means that disabled performers are capable of reinscribing their bodies through performance, tendering resistance and wresting agency by destabilising traditional social framings in a way that Kuppers would call 'a historical moment where a culture is examining its bodies, sorts and counts its differences, allocates new quarters and reinvents itself' (2003, p. 3). The performing of disability by the person with polio was, to my mind, a glimpse into disability culture that vanished soon after it emerged, but not before it fractured the old meanings and stereotypes of disability as locally understood. Similarly, this means reposing faith in the community's ability to learn through intense scrutiny and change by confronting the social reality of disability and by engaging in free dialogue and liberating action, that is, becoming change agents. It is, after all, up to the people in the community who form the audience to wrest the prerogative and use their indigenous ways of communication and decision-making to shape their own development through social change. With respect to disability, communication could not be a quick fix but rather an enabler that sustained a long process of behaviour change.

Spatially speaking, the fact that social hierarchies and patriarchal ideologies at the village level can be broken by folk media was brought home to us. The *sanedos*, even as they rang out in the entire village on loudspeakers, gave voice to those who may typically lack confidence. In fact, they participated equally and pushed through with a strength of their own, breaking the silence which tends to marginalise them. The *sanedos* conveyed a sense and knowledge of the age-old self as well, handed down by generations, and the modified lyrics of the songs made for a novelty and introspective awareness of the subject of disability. There was an irrepressible energy among people as they opened their hearts out to sing along with the singers about hospitals and doctors, immunisation, prevention of disability, caring for disabled people and shunning social prejudice about them. Thus, a complex structure was generated – the theme of disability, the *sanedo* and its rhythm, regional history, folklore and so on. This communication in a very broad sense had a role to play in mediating between opposing power groups and shifting paradigms in the social development process. It was able to give a voice to the marginalised, challenge and transform relationships of power and oppression and be a powerful tool for advocacy.

Other lessons we learnt were that folk media can engage locals to identify issues of concern, analyse and then together think about how change can happen. Further, deployment of folk media can help foster stakeholder empathy, trust and campaign 'ownership' in the communication because it incorporates and reconciles a variety of views from community members. In the project, these were local leaders like the village Sarpanch, the Anganwadi workers, the village *dai*, rural NGOs, local media and the team. It was in essence, 'done not only for the people but with the people' (Acunzo *et al.*, 2014). In this project, different stakeholders were inspired because they saw the messages regarding attitudes, behaviours and practices through a human lens, and this helped the team get insights about co-creation of some of the prototypes. This led to, in the short run, optimal acceptability, effectiveness and sustainability of the intervention. In the long run, this has led to positive effects and benefits for sustainable social change and people's empowerment. Finally, we realised that traditional media have the advantage of in-built instant feedback because of face-to-face interaction (Mathiyazhagan *et al.*, 2015). This helps assess the impact of the efforts. The positive feedback received went a long way in affirming the efforts that the team had put in over months and gave many insights and directions for further progress of the creative phase.

Epilogue

Even as the creative professionals were creating the content, we had to vet every outcome for ableist or disabling content. The drafts of all written content and rapid prototypes of all print, audio and video material were tested in the districts with the local communities and key stakeholders over days. Based on the insights obtained and meticulously recorded, the final concepts were developed, and material was refined content-wise and stylistically. The overriding learning was that no design outcome is right or wrong but is appropriate or otherwise for a given context. The project eventually concluded with production of all the design content, broadcast schedule finalisation for audio and video content, detailed documentation for each phase of the project and a report of detailed recommendations for dissemination of the tools designed.

Notes

1 The author was part of a team from NID comprising Tarun Deep Girdher as project head, Kavita Arvind and Snehal Rana, all of whom worked on designing the campaign in Mehsana, Sabarkantha, Surendranagar and Vadodara districts of Gujarat state. The four districts were selected based on diverse target profiles in terms of literacy levels, levels of awareness on the subject, socio-economic profile and exposure to communication material on health-related issues. About 1500 people were interviewed in all.
2 The project was also mindful about avoiding ableist metaphors in Gujarati such as '*andhlao na desh ma kano raja*' literally meaning 'the one-eyed rule the country of the blind'; '*gaando chhe*' or 'are you mad'?; '*akkal nathi*' or 'is your brain not working?'; and '*maari aankho ughdi gayee*' or 'my eyes were opened'.
3 Representatives of the state government included the chief district health officer, chief district medical officer, social defence officer, doctors and MPHWs (multi-purpose health workers). Representatives of civil society included NGOs and community members, especially disabled persons.

Reference list

Acunzo, M. *et al.* (2014) *Communication for rural development sourcebook*. Rome: Food and Agriculture Organization of the United Nations.
Freire, P. (1968) *The pedagogy of the oppressed*. London: Penguin Classics.
Kuppers, P. (2003) *Disability and contemporary performance: bodies on edge*. London: Routledge.
Mathiyazhagan, T. *et al.* (2015) 'Traditional media of communication', *International Journal of Social Science*, 4(1), pp. 159–169.
Ranganath, H.K. (1976) 'A probe into the traditional media: telling the people tell themselves', *Media Asia*, 3(1), p. 25.

20

QUIET ACTIVISM

A space to dare

Katharine E. Low

In the UK, women make up a third of the total HIV population (National AIDS Trust, 2022). Yet as highlighted by the HIV Commission, they 'do not experience the best HIV outcomes', and furthermore over 50% of women experience late diagnosis. Women are also not seeing the same decreases in HIV infection as is being experienced with other HIV groups (HIV Commission, 2020). It is thus unsurprising that a 2018 report by the Sophia Forum and the Terrance Higgins Trust found that women living with HIV reported often feeling 'invisible' or 'overlooked' by health care professionals (2018, p. 7). This is could also be understood as a moment of 'testimonial injustice', which Miranda Fricker describes as a form of epistemic injustice whereby 'someone is wronged in their capacity as a giver of knowledge' (2007, p. 7), fundamentally demonstrating the ongoing medical patriarchy experienced by many women living with HIV. This 'not counting' is replicated in a lack of attention paid to the female experience of living with HIV, particularly with regard to cultural reproduction and the artistic responses to what it means to live with HIV. This prevails despite the argument for the sustained relationship between performance and a demand for a cultural and governmental global response to addressing HIV being eloquently acknowledged and addressed in numerous accounts (see for example Campbell and Gindt, 2019; Kistenberg, 1995).

Thus, there exists an urgent need for more space and attention to be given to the female and non-binary experience of living with HIV. As the poet Bakita Kasada declared in her poem 'We Are', performed at the 'I Am Here, We Are Here' Conference in 2019:

Understanding our rights, in a way we didn't before
Realising our worth, when we previously didn't dare.

(Positively UK, 2019: online)

There is a need for places for women living with HIV to dare, and it is here that performance-making can become a site within which exploration, activism and daring can take place. This chapter addresses the need for quiet and subtle activism within the field of performance-making and HIV and considers the cultural representation of women living well with HIV.

Existing cultural performances and cultural responses that address the experience of living with HIV are often solely focused on the gay male experience (see Campbell, 2019; Schulman,

DOI: 10.4324/9781003036500-24

2022). Not dismissing the importance of these responses to the experience of living with HIV, this chapter suggests that other ways of making and forms of performance are required to capture and celebrate the female and non-binary experience of living with HIV. Specifically, in this chapter, I consider the role of small-scale, intimate moments of performance as a form of subtle activism and the impact it may have on challenging perceptions of what it means to live well with HIV if you identify as a woman. It is useful to unpack the concept of 'living well with HIV'. This term comes from my interactions with women at Positively UK and specifically with a poet and community facilitator, Mel Rattue. The term 'living well with HIV' is about acknowledging that living with HIV is no longer a death sentence and counters the idea that people are 'ill' or inca-pacitated by their HIV status so the phrase deliberately counteracts the stigma and assumptions associated that may be attached to the term 'living with HIV'.[1] 'Living well with HIV' is also a robust response to the frequent stigmatisation and lack of care experienced by women living well with HIV in a medical care setting (Namiba *et al.*, 2022). It is geared towards a targeted and joyful disruption of the disease – both psychological and medical – surrounding HIV and so becomes a reclaiming of space. This conscious disruption hopes to lay bare cultural misconcep-tions – as much for participants, who have a term that better represents their experiences, as for wider society.

Accordingly, this chapter contextualises the argument for women-focused performance in response to HIV against a background of existing and historical practice. It draws on my experi-ence of co-creating artistic work with women from Positively UK, a national peer-support and advocacy charity supporting individuals living with HIV. I consider three impacts which may occur in the performance of particular moments of quiet activism: the creation of new kinds of spaces; on peer support, leadership and learning; and finally, critiquing the values of the work. To begin, I turn to the experience of women living with HIV.

Women and HIV

Generally, women's experiences of health, from the reproductive cycle to responding to chronic health and mental health conditions, are often overlooked or forced into a medical system that has been predominantly designed for a male experience.[2] These oppressions are often exacerbated for women living with HIV, which speaks to a larger lack of attention paid to women's health. Women living with HIV encounter multiple oppressions through a patriarchal, stigmatised and medicalised lens, including an exclusion from a discussion of their health needs; they and their experiences are invisibilised, they are seen as a threat and are also vulnerabilised.

Beginning with exclusions, the multitude of times in which women have to renegotiate them-selves in order to be heard and believed is ever present and is particularly felt by women living with HIV (Namiba *et al.*, 2022). Women account for 53% of people living with HIV (UNAIDS, 2021) yet take up very little space in government cultural rhetoric. A 2020 UNAIDS review of the previous forty years of the HIV epidemic highlighted how AIDS remains 'the leading cause of death of women of reproductive age' globally and that the ongoing and blatant gender-based inequalities and inequities experienced by women and young girls continue to make these popula-tion groups significantly more vulnerable to HIV (UNAIDS, 2020, p. 2). This report was published before the real impact of coronavirus could be acknowledged for these population groups. Yet on the UNAIDS website in 2022 (UNAIDS, 2021), the key populations which are targeted for urgent action appear to overlook women, focusing instead on 'sex workers', 'men who have sex with men', 'people who inject drugs', 'transgender people', 'prisoners' and 'people living with HIV'.

While there is still a need for action within certain populations, this erasure of the female experience of living with HIV is deeply troubling.

This exclusion or invisibilisation is exacerbated for Black and Global Majority communities. Individuals living with chronic health conditions are often more likely to experience mental health issues, and COVID-19 has both replicated existing health inequities and compounded the existing racial inequalities in mental health care (Atayero, 2020). Recent studies have demonstrated that 'Black, Asian and minority ethnic (BAME) heterosexuals are disproportionately affected by HIV in the UK', accounting for 74% of heterosexual people living with HIV, with more than half of those individuals identifying as women (Dhairyawan *et al.*, 2021). As Dr Rageshri Dhairyawan has argued, health care is made 'hard to reach' for some populations due to lack of information in different languages, lack of culturally specific resources, lack of interpreters and hostile and racist immigration policies (2020). For women, this structural racism is future complicated; in addition to caring for themselves, they are also caring for their extended family and often for others within their communities, becoming the holders of significant information about their families and communities. They are aware of the potential social stigma of HIV, which can lead to further isolation and inequities in health. The result of this is that women living with HIV remain excluded, and this 'excluding' narrative means that, unsurprisingly, women keep their HIV status private. The lack of recognition and understanding of the impact the potential of your status being made public is often unacknowledged for women, which becomes another form of silencing and exclusion rather than being seen and heard as experts in their own lived experience. This feeds into an overall extension of the epistemic injustice experienced by women of colour with regard to their health. For example, in 2022 the Muslim Women's Network, in conjunction with the All-Party Parliamentary Group on Muslim Women, published a report on the Islamophobia in women's health and maternal care in which they found that women felt 'unheard and unseen' (Muslim Women's Network, 2022, p. 52). The invisibilisation is multi-faceted.

Alongside their exclusion and the invisibilising of their experience, when attention is given to women living with HIV, they are often vulnerabilised. For many women living well with HIV, they are both essentialised as vulnerable women and are dehumanised at the same time. This perspective is informed by Christina Clark-Kazak's work on age discrimination in migration and development policy (2022). Clark-Kazak has argued that the current 'categorical' approach to vulnerability is both dehumanising and essentialising to individuals. In her research she argues that migrants are regularly dehumanised as they are seen as being individual problems, rather than considering the wider, structural reason for their need to migrate, such as climate change or war. Within this dehumanising lens, those individuals are then essentialised and limited; if they are vulnerable because of who they are, they can never not be vulnerable. It becomes an inescapable perpetuating loop, because being vulnerable opens access, but this categorisation also confers a debilitating and limiting perception: the individuals are forever helpless and at risk. Fundamentally, Clark-Kazak argues that this all overlooks the power relations which render people vulnerable and the structural inequities which make individuals vulnerable to mistreatment in specific circumstances. Those individuals are seen within a 'deficit' model of being. Thus, if we consider Clark-Kazak's analysis, women living well with HIV are perceived as vulnerable because of their 'ill' bodies, but they are also stigmatised because of their illness due to the moral contagion (c.f. Low, 2020) which surrounds sexually transmitted illness. Clearly this categorical approach de-humanises these women while avoiding consideration of the structural inequities to the extent that no account of any facets to their lived lives like socio-economic positions (e.g. being a carer or a migrant, etc.) are taken into consideration or given space. Some of these women are vulnerable, others are vulnerabilised and are also perceived as a threat, which then leads to further stigmatisation (and thus made vulnerable again), thereby perpetuating a cycle of vulnerability.

For women living with HIV, this experience of being excluded, invisibilised and vulnerabilised forms part of a wider exclusion of women's bodies from society. The feminist geographer Leslie Kern researches and observes how women and women's bodies are viewed in urban settings, noting that on multiple occasions women's bodies are overlooked. She considers how women can reclaim spaces in these settings, acknowledging that:

> A geographic perspective on gender offers a way of understanding how feminism functions on the ground. Women's second-class status is enforced not just through the metaphorical notion of 'separate spheres', but through an actual, material geography of exclusion. Male power and privilege are upheld by keeping women's movements limited and their ability to access different spaces constrained.
>
> (2020, p. 13)

Outside the evident links to the experience of women living with HIV and having to negotiate their care within a patriarchal medical setting, this is an interesting conceptualising of the female body and how it is made to comply with a particular, often inherently patriarchal, structure. It is in rejection of such a structure that our practice of quiet activism is placed. Quiet activism is a means of reclaiming space. It is a taking up of and impregnating particular spaces with women's voices, histories and experiences in order to create a form of palimpsest in spaces, bodies and memories, which will continue to grow and spread. Thus, within our practice, we consider how women can reclaim spaces to be heard and to live in. Accordingly, as we place women living well with HIV at the centre of the work, from decision-making to implementation, it is pertinent to turn to the work of Positively UK, the charity with whom I co-collaborate.

Positively UK

Positively UK is a peer-led HIV advocacy and peer support charity based in London, with a national remit across England, networking and strategising with HIV charities across the UK. Today, Positively UK operates as an advocacy and support charity for anyone living with or affected by HIV and it was originally set up to support women living with HIV in the late 1980s who had little resource to information about HIV/AIDS. Positively Women was founded in 1987 by Sheila Gilchrist and Jayne[3] and later joined by Kate Thompson and Caroline Guinness. Sheila and Jayne came together to provide a weekly meeting space for women living with HIV, no matter how they had acquired the virus. As Gilchrist noted in 1988:

> although most women who knew they were HIV positive were or had been drug users, existing women's AIDS support groups excluded drug users. Most drug services were, and still are, male-orientated, and AIDS organisations ran groups consisting of mainly gay men. As a woman and an ex-drug user with HIV, I felt doubly isolated. Contacting other HIV positive people was invaluable, but to carry on living with the virus I and other woman in my position needed support which fulfilled our needs as women. This just did not exist – hence Positively Women.
>
> (Gilchrist, 1988)

Positively Women swiftly became an activating organisation, whose members went on to help found the International Community of Women Living with HIV (ICW) following a meeting in London in 1991. As an organisation, the ICW helped to support and advise similar organising structures to Positively Women in countries globally and was based in the Positively Women's offices (ICW Global, 2023).

Since its inception, Positively UK has been a peer-support charity, realising and valuing the value of peer-led support services, that is, people living with HIV supporting others recently diagnosed or encountering difficulties or new developments, such as pregnancy. Peer-led support and leadership is one of Positively UK's underlying principles, recognising the value of lived experience and knowledge informing HIV support and guidance; 85% of Positively UK's staff and 95% of its volunteers live with HIV, in keeping with Positively UK's principle that these individuals are 'best placed to support others, by using their personal and practical understanding of the health and social implications of living with a long-term condition that still carries stigma within society' (Positively UK, 2022).

Becoming Positively UK in 2010, due to a decision to not segregate the lived experience of HIV as being specific to one gender, the organisation offers a plethora of services, including: peer mentor training, clinical outreach, welfare rights advice, a women's space, a gay men's wellbeing space, an under 30's group and therapeutic gardening project. It is with the Women's space that we have most closely collaborated, co-delivering and co-creating a series of performance-based projects since 2016. In that period, we have explored topics from sexual pleasure to women who inspire us, women's rights and women's wellbeing and most recently the activist history of the organisation itself. In 2022, we co-created a series of exploratory workshops[4] using Positively Women's archives (based at the London Metropolitan Archives), taking time and space to reflect back on the past in order to consider what we can bring forward into the future. Part of this project also includes a public performance (a first for this group) and a series of historical podcasts.[5] The key focus is on creating a radically kind space that enables women to take up space and make use of it as they wish to (Low, 2021). It is part of a quiet performative activism, an idea that this chapter turns to next.

HIV and performance activism

HIV and performance activism have a long and rich history. In the early 1980s, the act of performing as a response and a call for action became a mainstay in the fight against the apathy that the AIDS pandemic provoked in governments and NGOs globally. The US saw the emergence of the work of ACT UP's performative demonstrations against the American Food and Drug Administration and the Federal Government. ACT UP's infamous 'die ins' at the headquarters of the FDA and the US Stock Exchange had significant political and social impact (Schulman, 2022). In South Africa and Uganda, there were community-led performances, giant puppets and theatre for development techniques were employed to raise awareness and share knowledge about symptoms and the potential impact of HIV and AIDS.[6] One example of activist performance which combined humour with basic safe sex facts is *For Fact's Sake*, a free educational performance that Pieter-Dirk Uys toured around South African schools. Renowned in South Africa for his satire and social activism in anti-apartheid politics and through his drag alter ego, the fabulous Evita Bezuidenhout, Uys directly drew attention to his positionality as an older, gay, white Afrikaans-Jewish man explaining to young people the importance of talking about and asking for help when engaging with sex. The performativity of Uys' practice broke down barriers in discussing sex for young people offering an 'honesty in the fact that sex can be funny, undignified and ridiculous' which offers 'an invitation into the performance and discussion around sexual health matters' (Low, 2017, p. 158).

The cultural space of what it means to live with HIV is often dominated by the male-identifying queer or LGBTQIA+ experience. This is understandably so, especially at the start of the emergence of AIDS, where men were disproportionately impacted and affected by HIV. This imbalance is evident in mainstream cinema, for example, in *Milk* (2008), *Philadelphia* (1993), *And The Band Played On* (1993) and *Longtime Companion* (1989), to television where HIV storylines were introduced into major British soaps such as EastEnders and Coronation Street and most recently Channel 4's *It's A Sin* (2020), which charts, for once, the British experience of the emergence of HIV (Wise, 2021). In this production, women were once again relegated to being carers, support workers, mothers and peripheral characters affected by the AIDS pandemic but not living with HIV themselves. On the stage, we have exceptional and historically important productions such as Larry Kramer's *A Normal Heart* (1985), Tony Kushner's *Angels in America* (1992) and Jonathan Larson's *RENT* (1993), as well as local UK-based productions such as Patrick Cash's *The Clinic* (2016), Outbox Theatre's *Affection* (2016) and Camden People's Theatre's intergenerational participatory *Kings Cross (REMIX)* (2017), all of which address the narratives of the local, queer community. The dominance of the male-identifying queer or LGBTQIA+ experience is not hard to find, but a woman's narrative – herstory – is notably absent.[7]

There is comprehensible significant public interest in considering and engaging with the experience of living with HIV and also in creating a space to comprehend, appreciate and recall the extremely difficult years of the 1980s and 1990s where friends, lovers, family members were dying and prioritising research for a cure. There is an essential and important need to memorialise and to remember what happened and to make space to hear these stories. We see this in the restaging of Kramer's *A Normal Heart* at the National Theatre in London in 2021, marking thirty-five years since its UK premiere, and with the restaging of Kushner's *Angels in America* in 2017 and 2018, which was a commercial success both on the West End and on Broadway.

Alongside more commercial performance-based responses, there have been striking forms of activism in response to HIV calling attention to the need for further support and awareness around what it means to live with HIV. ACT UP is one of the most famous examples of this, originating in the US but with branches emerging in other cities globally, including both London and Paris. The London branch of ACT UP is active and allied with key campaigns including PrEP[8] Health Promotion and Undetectable = Untransmittable (U=U),[9] (ACT UP London, 2022). Most recently, ACT UP London has engaged in a 'HIV/HEP Blind Date – World AIDS Day Special' in 2019, a World AIDS Day '#HIVisible ACTUP demo' and a Flash mob for the '#HIVisible 2gether' campaign in 2020. These are exciting and challenging performative responses. It is a very much a type of 'in-yer-face'[10] activism, flamboyantly loud, sensational and exhilarating. These performances take up space, demand responses from those witnessing them and, crucially, require significant emotional labour from those involved in the productions and the performative acts of activism.

Positively UK, performance and quiet activism

Whilst brilliant and provocative, these acts of activism are costly to those involved in terms of time and energy and but also in terms of personal investment and confidence. In my experience, many of the women who engage with our performance-based practice collaborations with Positively UK often lack time, space, energy and the desire to be so loud. Nor do some have the ability to be loud. Being outspoken may lead to community stigma and other potential dangers. There also exists an important need for quieter, reflective and potentially reparative space, a space for quietness, gentleness and subtlety. The noise can also drown out marginalised folx and voices. And within the existing, marginalised space of individuals living with HIV, where is the room for those softer, quieter voices? Those voices who do not necessarily have the capacity or the ability to commit to much larger acts of activism and performance, for those who are not used to taking up so much space?

HIV public activism is often spectacularly performative and blunt. While this is vital, the consequent space for activists or individuals who are not public with their diagnosis but who may like to consider where and how they might also share and extend their ideas and experiences are sidelined. Further, these public acts of activism often lead to a public disclosure of an individual's HIV status, not necessarily by directly pointing out someone's status; rather it becomes an assumed reveal through association in these acts of activism. The consequences of a public disclosure of an individual's HIV status are often both under-acknowledged and also complex for women living with HIV, not solely in terms of the practicalities (namely non-flexible working hours, childcare commitments) and structural racism (asylum and leave to applications pending) but also the social implications of a public disclosure, especially for women who may not necessarily be public with their diagnosis within their family and social circles.

The focus on the quotidian is significant for the argument in this chapter because it creates a space separate to HIV activism. What our work does is create a space in which other narratives of living with HIV can be explored and heard with a particular focus on the everyday because it is in the everyday that most of the felt experiences, structural oppression and racism occur. The quotidian is crucial because it is what the women experience in *their* every day and we do not usually hear this voice – a counterpoint to the single narrative currently dominating the HIV 'performance' space.[11] There is a need and a drive towards women who live with HIV reclaiming spaces in which their voices are heard, shared and listened to. A performance space that is quiet, gentle and subtle. It could be described as a domestic space, but doing so might taint the perceived value of such space, as the notion of domesticity contains the assumption that the work has less value. This is a fallacy. There is equal weight, action and affect that emerge from subtle and small forms of activism compared to larger, more 'in-yer-face' acts. Alongside this, the subtle, quiet space of making is also a curational space for individuals to hone and develop their leadership skills, to practice and explore ways of reclaiming spaces and holding leadership. It is key that we have more women living with HIV taking up spaces of leadership within the HIV field, where currently advocates and spokespeople predominantly reside in male hegemony.

I employ the concept of quiet activism as a means of drawing attention to the smaller, more subtle acts of rebellion, protest or dissent, which may not at first appear significant. For me, quiet activism is best understood through the lens of my concept 'apertures of possibility' (Low, 2020). Apertures of possibility offer an invitation to pause and look closely at the experiences that happen on the periphery of the main events in a workshop space. Apertures of possibility invite looking closely and with intent at small 'somethings' which appear in our practice; individually they may not appear significant, but when viewed collectively, their meaningfulness is quietly significant. An intentional part of this concept is the act of noticing. When these *noticings* are gathered together and considered, their import can reveal hidden subtle layers beyond the obvious action of the making or performance space. The noticing opens apertures of possibility, which are an invitation to reflect on the often ephemeral activities allowing different kinds of insights to be observed – and this practice, by nature, is gentle, kind and takes time.

So, in this context, considering quiet activism through a lens of apertures of possibility, I am drawing attention to several small moments in order to consider their potential effect. These moments could be overlooked or dismissed as insignificant, but I counter this perception. Rather, I invite a closer look at these moments as they offer an in-depth opportunity to look at another way of seeing something or recognising the value inherent in the work through observation, identifying their impact and effect. I have chosen an array of moments to illustrate how paying attention to a particular exchange, word choice or action allows for a deeper reading and recognition of the slight, almost insignificant moments that can, when experienced alongside other similar moments, exchanges and interactions have impact.

In the rest of this chapter, I consider three effects: first, what might occur when different kinds of spaces are created; second, how the discovery, peer learning and leadership that arise in these different spaces allows for a certain kind of reflection; and third, how this reflection prompts further questions around the values of this practice for both those involved in the actions taken in the workshop spaces and the wider field of applied theatre. Here the focus is placed on the principles of care and kindness where the needs of those attending are the peak of attention. Often a workshop will be held 'gently'. By this I mean a gentle, slow, warm and welcoming start, allowing the women to settle into the space. Directions of focus and intent for the activities are taken from cues provided by the women. There is no rigid workshop plan, for example; rather the space is set up with 'offerings' but the women participants choose what to engage with and also whether they engage in anything at all, so even the sharing of the space becomes a part of the quiet activism. Principally, the activities and the space are an offer of a joyous place where the women are the holders of power in the room.

Moment 1: a basket of joy => a different space created

By holding a quiet and kind workshop space, less extrovert members of the group can flex their use of the space. Take Abbo,[12] for example, a quiet woman from East Africa who now lives in London. She might often be overlooked in a crowd, but in the Positively UK workshops which she has attended over the past six years, she is seen and she takes up space. She is full of a quiet joy and care towards everyone in the space. In the small moments of performance, she radiates and demands attention, becoming a consummate storyteller, offering enticing titbits of knowledge (she speaks fluent Russian), weaving her audience into a tale of hilarity and mysterious improvised turns. On one occasion, in an exercise where we each offered another woman a metaphorical gift that we thought they might like, Abbo, considering my advanced stage of pregnancy at the time, offered me 'a pram for your bouncing baby and a basket of joy so you can continue to spread joy'. Although her comment was deeply pleasing to me personally, through the lens of an aperture of possibility, it is useful to consider the layers to such a casually spoken offering. She recognised the joy in the workshop space. There is an embedded recognition of the joy that is imbued within the space as well as an acknowledgement that there is potential for this joy to extend beyond the confines of this workshop, in this instance to my personal life. In our workshop space we have peer mentors, women living well with HIV from Positively UK, who in the room support newly diagnosed women navigate the space. But it is the gentle space that women like Abbo take up which has a significant effect – their acts of mentorship and modelling of quiet leadership linger. If we take a moment to consider the aperture of possibility, the lingering effect their presence and behaviour offer is quiet activism; their gentle extraordinariness is an alternative form of leadership and care, one which is a quiet and kind 'care-full' holding.[13]

This is a tiny moment, but it has had a great affective impact. Although it occurred in 2016, it continues to linger and have effect. It was noticed by others in the room, has been commented on by others (both at the time in the room and subsequently), and, on reflection, it has been the catalyst for my reconsideration of my style of facilitation, prompting a development into this mode of radically kind practice. This aperture invited me to further reflect on my practice, which ultimately further developed my facilitation approach.

Moment 2: Kasada's poem => a space for daring and reflection

But we also see this quiet activism in public events too. In 2019, Positively UK and Central joyfully co-hosted *I Am Here*, a two-day conference for International Women's Day, which also featured the Catwalk4Power.[14] As part of the event, leaders in the field of women living well with HIV spoke and offered workshops and creative activities for the attendees. In addition, the poet, HIV researcher and activist Bakita Kasada was invited to take part in the event and write a spoken word response to conclude the conference. The result was a public moment of performance, in which Kasada's poem summarised and performed back participants' ideas, responses and feelings in a manner that collectively held and heard those thoughts but which did not necessarily identify any particular person or space. Rather it spoke to the commonalities of experience. For example, Kasada acknowledges the road that many of women may have been on in their journey of diagnosis:

> Sometimes it's soft, bringing new friendships. Hope
> Sometimes it's clarity: hidden questions finally *providing relieving answers*
> Sometimes it's powerful; the thing that opens up doors to speak up (in our home, to ourselves, beyond)
>
> Understanding our rights, in a way we didn't before
> Realising our worth, when we previously didn't dare
>
> (Kasada, 2019)

In the act of writing and reading this poem, Kasada reclaims and holds a space of leadership and, in doing so, offers sisterhood and solidarity. Through her poem, Kasada invites others to consider what lies in the power to dare. It is an affective invitation to take up space, to work alongside in solidarity and sisterhood. Later on in the poem, Kasada offers:

> *There is enough power to share power*, share information
> of unknown lessons, from new perspectives
> *unlocking each other's potential*
>   messages from different tongues
> *speaking kinder to ourselves*
>   share that our treatment should empower us
> forgiving ourselves
>   amplify the voices of our sisters
> knowing we don't need to be forgiven – *this is not a moral issue*
> (Kasada, 2019)

These images from Kasada's poem are gentle, powerful and firm invitations to take up space and to speak up whenever you feel comfortable doing so. This affective invitation works because of the spatial setup or the 'event-ness' of the moment in which Kasada shared the poem: at the closing of a celebration of women living well with HIV. The ephemeral act of celebration is often overlooked. A celebratory event can lead to an affective atmosphere which begins to shift the microdynamics of the felt experiences and tensions in a particular site. The act of an open public event, a celebration and the sharing of the performance practice, has a profound effect on those involved and those who are audience members. It draws full attention onto a particular topic and may produce or provoke further reflection and thought. Fundamentally, it also reinforces an individual's personhood, where attention is given and framed with a particular gaze to the individuals' quotidian experience. For those present, the space becomes a space in which to dare or begin to consider daring in their quotidian. This begins to shift understandings and move away from that single narrative of what it is to live with a stigmatised chronic health condition as a woman in the UK. In this instance, the quiet activism is evident in the effect of Kasada's firm and gentle invitation to take up a different kind of space. By noticing this particular space, that aperture, we can see how a performative site and an invitation can set up an opportunity for daring, a space for participants to consider other possibilities while also being held and celebrated in their very being.

Moment 3: St Margaret's House => moving to leadership and daring

Continuing a deliberate looking through the lens of an *aperture of possibility*, it is important to consider the effect that small, delicate, subtle actions may have. If we recall the experience of women living with HIV having to negotiate their care within a patriarchal, medical setting, as described, it is possible to argue that many of the women's bodies and experiences have been forced to conform to a patriarchal structure in countless interactions their quotidian. So what happens when women chose not to conform, rather daring to take up space? How does this come about, and what can happen?

I propose this as a moment of quiet activism as a rejection of a 'conforming' or trope of a woman's body in a meeting space: Nobuhle's taking up of space in an unfamiliar site. Indeed, the manner in which Nobuhle, one of the service users at Positively UK, led and negotiated the discussions for our co-facilitated *Being Well and Wonderous* workshops as part of the Being Human Festival, which was hosted by St Margaret's House, is an example of quiet activism. In our meetings prior to the event,[15] we met with colleagues from St Margaret's House to plan how the day would unfold. As one of the group members, Nobuhle led our discussions, being very clear with our (delightful) male host from St Margaret's House what was required for the women who might be attending. Nobuhle underlined the importance of a crèche, delicious food and that the day should be structured and held by St Margaret's House to ensure that it was welcoming, joyful and easy to access for the people who were planning to attend. Nobuhle understood the basic needs and how the space needed to be different, what it needed to look like and, from an atmospheric point of view, the signals that were needed to communicate to the attendees that it was a welcoming space. On the day of the event, Nobuhle took up space: she arrived on time (early for her) and throughout the day encouraged and supported those around her. She participated fully in all the activities, making as many of the little booklets as she could while chatting with others around her. This suggests to me that she felt agency in the space, felt noticed and heard and that the space was her space. She was hugely comfortable in the space, and in her being so, she enabled others to experience similar relaxation and comfort, so much so that those individuals who had only booked in for the morning workshop extended their time with us, staying for the whole day and the afternoon workshop. By extending their engagement with the activities and discussions in the workshop space, the participants demonstrated how comfortable they felt in the room, recognising Nobhule's activism and working to support her vision. This underlines the success of Nobuhle's ownership and care-full setting up of the space from planning to delivery, a careful and quiet rejection of particular modes of behaviour. In doing this work, Nobhule took on the decision-making that usually lies with the community-arts facilitator.

Affective impacts

A final part of quiet activism is about also pausing and considering the impact and the perceived value of the work. One of the major complications around work in the field of sexual health or HIV-related performance is that, historically, funders often want to see quantifiable impacts for their funding, meaning that the funders may want to see changes in behaviour, often involving what is perceived as 'safe sexual conduct' or impact in terms of prevention (such as the adoption of PrEP) (cf. Low, 2020). Perhaps understandably, funders are after tangible, quantifiable outcomes. However, in reality, solely focusing on 'behaviour change' means more ephemeral aspects of sexual health are generally overlooked (c.f. Cáceres and Race, 2012; Kippax, 2012), and there is a need for more spaces in which to problematise ideas of health, questions of safety and ideas of sexuality all together. We need to work against the erasure of individuals' actual lived experience of HIV. Rather, in many of these positionings, the individuals in question have been 'vulnerabilised' and placed into a category of 'vulnerable', having neither a valued voice nor the ability to advocate for themselves. We refute this reading, rather arguing that in this moment of quiet activism, the participants are actually talking about what matters to them and not what matters to the funders. What happens in these moments is an opportunity for individuals to problematise ideas of health, questions of safety and ideas of sexuality on their own terms. It is not an externally driven agenda; rather it is a gently held space which is responsive to the 'wants' of the participants in the room.

These acts of quiet activism have such power because they are a rejection of the category of 'vulnerable' whereby their agency and being are reduced to a single narrative, a deficit model of being where there is little other explanation or experience in their lives. This is blatantly untrue, as we are all more than a mono-narrative (cf. Adichie, 2009). Too often women living with HIV are constricted, reduced to one particular narrative, and these quiet acts disrupt this narrative – they shift the deficit model of the vulnerability label to one where women are perceived as more than a single health status. These performative moments, Kasada's poem, Abbo's kindness in the space, Nobuhle's directness of what the other women needed in the meeting with St Margaret's House move their perceived ' "vulnerability" from a static statement of ontology to a state of being that can be shifted' (c.f. Feghali, 2022) – in the eyes of each other (peer learning), of other allies and of the general public they encounter. In this way the practice of quiet activism offers a space where there is a refusal to be 'vulnerabilised'. Rather it is a reclaiming of space as leaders, a reinforcement of individuals and their identities and the values they hold onto as being equally important and respected. These acts are a key moment in terms of leadership and development. As Kasada so eloquently says: '*There is enough power to share power*', if only we 'dare'. This is the invitation of quiet activism. What these women are doing is flexing the medical perception and reading of HIV. They bring into a public space their multiple selves and in doing so are disrupting a particular patriarchal and medicalised gaze.

To conclude, to dare. This chapter has addressed the overlooked and invisibilised nature of women living with HIV. It has put forward an argument for a space of quiet activism through which women's voices, histories and experiences can be ascribed into spaces, listened to and heard. It has argued how the performative, quiet moments of performance can offer a different type of value and effect for those who participate and those who witness these quiet acts. Within these acts there is a different kind of power in these moments, a different value – what those individuals are doing is a subversion of the idea that they are powerless and that their identities are solely their health status. Rather they dare – they take up space, take on leadership and offer peer support quietly, but with presence. There is an open invitation to others to continue to dare flexing and challenging.

Acknowledgements

None of this thinking or theorising would be possible without the work of Positively UK and the women who make use of its services. My thinking and my practice are intertwined with the model of leadership and advocacy that Positively UK offers. Their approach is fundamental to how I work and practice. To the women who have been part of one or all of the different activities and events we have co-run – thank you for your ideas, presence and daring. A final thanks to the wonderful Bakita Kasada for sharing her poetry with me.

Notes

1 I am acutely aware of the marginalisation which can occur within this statement, as there are those who are not living well with HIV. However by choosing 'living well with', I am challenging the stereotypes and shame associated with HIV, instead moving towards a recognition that – with access to the right healthcare and medication – HIV can be treated as a chronic health condition.
2 This 'overlooking' of women's health experiences has been observed in both the UK's House of Lords (2021) and the Department of Health and Social Care's policy paper on Women's Health Strategy for England (2022).
3 Jayne's surname is not shared at the request of her family.
4 For an account of these workshops, please see Positively UK (2022) *Positively past positively present*. Available at: https://positivelyuk.org/positively-past-positively-present/ (Accessed: 24 July 2023).
5 To listen to and subscribe to the podcasts, see Apple Podcasts Preview (2023) *Positively UK podcast*. Available at: https://podcasts.apple.com/us/podcast/positively-uk-podcast/id1558730896 (Accessed: 24 July 2023).
6 Here see the work of AREPP theatre for Life (Durden, 2011), Marion Frank's analysis of Uganda's response to HIV/AIDS (1995) and Thomas Riccio's analysis of puppetry in Kenya (2004). For a summary of this practice, see Chapter 2 in Low (2020).
7 In 2022, the Bearded and Flushed spoken word event indicates a shift in this. See Bearded and Flushed (2023) *Welcome to Bearded and Flushed*. Available at: https://beardedandflushed.com/.
8 PrEP is pre-exposure prophylaxis, the use of medications to prevent the spread of HIV before exposure to the virus.
9 U=U refers to the fact that a person with an undetectable viral load cannot transmit HIV through sex (it is untransmittable).
10 This term is taken from the 'in-yer-face theatre' genre, which describes a style of activist theatre-making that emerged in the UK during the 1990s (c.f. Aleks Sierz's *In-Yer-Face Theatre: British Drama Today*, 2001).
11 The publication of *Our Stories Told by Us: Celebrating the African Contribution to the UK HIV Response* in 2023 offers one counter to this narrative. See *Our Stories Told by Us*, available at: https://ourstoriestold byus.com/.
12 Individuals' names have been changed.
13 For a deeper discussion of the idea of 'care-full' holding in socially engaged theatre practice, please see Sue Mayo (2021).
14 See Positively UK (2020) *Catwalk4Power*. Available at: https://c4ptoolkit.positivelyuk.org/about.html.
15 The intention of the workshops was that it would be open to anyone who identified as a woman or as non-binary to gather together to talk about health and wellbeing and what makes us 'wondrous'. This was the first event that we (Positively UK and I) had ever facilitated which was open to the general public, culminating in a space where women living with HIV did not need to be identified with a label regarding their HIV status.

Reference list

ACT UP London (2022) *ACT UP London*. Available at: https://actuplondon.wordpress.com/ (Accessed: 18 April 2023).
Adichie, C.N. (2009) *The danger of a single story*. Available at: www.ted.com/talks/chimamanda_ngozi_ adichie_the_danger_of_a_single_story/c (Accessed: 18 April 2023).

Atayero, S. (2020) *Racial inequalities in mental health care*. A talk presented as part of the SWIFT symposia on race, ethnicity and health outcomes, 24 July, 2–4pm. Organised by The Supporting Women with HIV Information Network (SWIFT) [online, notes in possession of author].

Cáceres, C.F. and Race, K. (2012) 'Knowledge, power and HIV/AIDS: research and the global response', in Aggleton, P. and Parker, R. (eds.) *Routledge handbook of sexuality, health and rights*. Abingdon: Routledge, pp. 175–183.

Campbell, A. (2019) 'GL RY: A (w)hole lot of women trouble. HIV dramaturges and feral pedagogies', in Campbell, A. and Gindt, D. (eds.) *Viral dramaturgies: HIV and AIDS in performance in the twenty-first century*. London: Palgrave Macmillan, pp. 49–67.

Campbell, A. and Gindt, D. (2019) *Viral dramaturgies: HIV and AIDS in performance in the twenty-first century*. London: Palgrave Macmillan.

Clark-Kazak, C. (2022) *Age and vulnerability: from categories to an equity approach*. A talk presented as part of the vulnerability studies network, 15 March. Organised by the Vulnerability Studies Group at the University of Leicester. [online talk, notes in possession of author].

Department of Health and Social Care (2022) *Women's health strategy for England*, 30 August. Available at: www.gov.uk/government/publications/womens-health-strategy-for-england/womens-health-strategy-for-england#ministerial-foreword (Accessed: 18 April 2023).

Dhairyawan, R. (2020) *Racism and health outcomes: an overview*. A talk presented as part of the SWIFT symposia on race, ethnicity and health outcomes, 24 July, 2–4 pm. Organised by The Supporting Women with HIV Information Network (SWIFT) [online talk, notes in possession of author].

Dhairyawan, R. *et al.* (2021) 'Differences in HIV clinical outcomes amongst heterosexuals in the United Kingdom by ethnicity', *AIDS*, 35(11), pp. 1813–1821. https://doi.org/10.1097/QAD.0000000000002942

Durden, E. (2011) 'Participatory HIV/AIDS theatre in South Africa: a motivation to inspire practice', in Francis, D.A. (ed.) *Acting on HIV: using drama to create possibilities for change*. Rotterdam: Sense Publishers, pp. 1–14.

Feghali, Z. (2022) Personal correspondence with the author via email. June 16, 2022.

Frank, M. (1995) *AIDS education through theatre: case studies from Uganda*. Bayeruth: Eckhard Breitinger.

Fricker, M. (2007) *Epistemic injustice: power and the ethics of knowing*. Oxford: Oxford University Press.

Gilchrist, S. (1988, September/October) 'Positively women', in Nelles, B. (ed.) *Groups for HIV positive drug users' DRUGLINK*, pp. 9–11. Available at: www.drugwise.org.uk/wp-content/uploads/Groups-for-HIV-positive-drug-users-1.pdf (Accessed: 18 April 2023).

HIV Commission Equity (2020) *How England will end new cases of HIV: the HIV commission final report & recommendations*. Available at: www.hivcommission.org.uk/final-report-and-recommendations/equity/ (Accessed: 2 August 2023).

House of Lords and Winchester, N. (2021) *Women's health outcomes: is there a gender gap?* 1 July. Available at: https://lordslibrary.parliament.uk/womens-health-outcomes-is-there-a-gender-gap/ (Accessed: 18 April 2023).

ICW Global (2023) *History of international community of women living with HIV*. Available at: www.icwglobal.org/our-organization/history (Accessed: 18 April 2023).

Kasada, B. (2019) We Are. Poem Written by Kasada.

Kippax, S. (2012) 'Safe sex: it's not as simple as ABC', in Aggleton, P. and Parker, R. (eds.) *Routledge handbook of sexuality, health and rights*. Abingdon: Routledge, pp. 184–92.

Kistenberg, C.J. (1995) *Aids, social change & theater*. New York: Routledge.

Low, K.E. (2017) ' "It's difficult to talk about sex in a positive way": creating a space to breathe', in Baxter, V. and Low, K.E. (eds.) *Applied theatre: performing health and wellbeing*. London: Bloomsbury Methuen Drama Publishing, pp. 146–61.

Low, K.E. (2020) *Applied theatre and sexual health communication; apertures of possibility*. London: Palgrave Macmillan.

Low, K.E. (2021) 'The potential of radical kindness as a methodology in applied theatre in arts and health', *Performance Paradigm*, 16, pp. 164–182.

Mayo, S. (2021) ' "We know . . ." collective care in participatory arts', *Performance Paradigm*, 16, pp. 184–198.

Muslim Women's Network (2022) *Invisible: maternity experiences of Muslim women from racialised minority communities*. Available at: www.mwnuk.co.uk/INVISIBLE_Maternity_Experiences_of_Muslim_Women_FULL_REPORT_256_reportdownload.php (Accessed: 20 May 2023).

Namiba, A. *et al.* (2022) 'From presumptive exclusion towards fair inclusion: perspectives on the involvement of women living with HIV in clinical trials, including stakeholders' views', *Therapeutic Advances in Infectious Disease*, 9, pp. 1–17.

National AIDS Trust (2022) *HIV in the UK statistics*. Available at: www.nat.org.uk/about-hiv/hiv-statistics (Accessed: 2 August 2023).

Positively UK (2019) *We are*. Available at: https://c4ptoolkit.positivelyuk.org/poetry/weare.html (Accessed: 29 August 2023).

Positively UK (2022) *About us*. Available at: https://positivelyuk.org/about-us/ (Accessed: 18 April 2023).

Riccio, T. (2004) 'Kenya's community health awareness puppeteers', *PAJ: A Journal of Performance and Art*, 76(1), pp. 1–12.

Schulman, S. (2022) *Let the record show: a political history of act up New York, 1987–1993*. New York: St Martin's Press and Macmillan.

Sierz, A. (2001) *In-Yer-face theatre: British drama today*. London: Faber & Faber.

Sophia Forum and the Terrance Higgins Trust (2018) *Women and HIV: invisible no longer*. Available at: www.tht.org.uk/sites/default/files/2018-08/women-and-HIV_report_final_amended.pdf (Accessed: 2 August 2023).

UNAIDS (2020) *We've got the power: women, adolescent Girls and the HIV response*. Available at: https://www.unaids.org/sites/default/files/media_asset/2020_women-adolescent-girls-and-hiv_en.pdf (Accessed: April 18, 2023)

UNAIDS (2021) *Global HIV & AIDS statistics – fact sheet*. Available at: www.unaids.org/sites/default/files/media_asset/UNAIDS_FactSheet_en.pdf (Accessed: 18 April 2023).

Wise, L. (2021) *It's a sin: 'If Covid was an STD it would be hidden too'*. Available at: www.theguardian.com/tv-and-radio/2021/jan/09/its-a-sin-its-not-about-death-its-about-vibrant-beautiful-lives (Accessed: 24 July 2023).

21

RALLY AGAINST MEASLES

Performances for community mobilisation in Lebanon

Sally Souraya

'Children's lives are at risk', stated UNICEF Lebanon in 2018, raising the alarm to a measles outbreak declared in four areas of the country (UNICEF, 2018). With a 5.7% growth in the population by 2014 (according to the World Bank, 2020), a rise in poverty and the strain faced by Lebanon's health system, the 2018 measles outbreak constituted a very serious threat to children's lives compared to previous outbreaks. A key issue in this was the low vaccination coverage in several areas across the country. Whilst at least 90% of children in a given community need to be vaccinated to hinder the spread of measles, achieving this high level of population immunity remains especially challenging in Lebanon despite the availability of vaccines through routine vaccination services and mass vaccination campaigns (World Health Organisation, 2020). This is due to public mistrust in the vaccines and fundamental impediments, including erroneous beliefs, misinformation and misconceptions, leading to a false sense of safety and subsequent non-compliance to the full course of vaccines and boosters (El Zarif *et al.*, 2020; Mansour *et al.*, 2018). In addition, poverty and lack of legal paperwork among migrant and refugee communities constitute important factors that hinder vaccination in Lebanon.

For this reason, in 2019, a measles assessment mission recommended a national measles campaign targeting 1,170,000 children between the ages of six months and ten years of age (Reliefweb, 2019). This was part of a comprehensive integrated response by the Ministry of Public Health in coordination with the World Health Organisation and UNICEF. A key component of the response was social mobilisation and distribution of information, education, and communication materials across Lebanon and particularly to marginalised communities, which traditionally have lower rates of vaccinations among their children.

To support the national measles vaccination campaign, Clown Me In (CMI), a clowning and street performance theatre company and non-governmental organisation (NGO) based in Lebanon, collaborated with UNICEF Lebanon in 2019 and 2020 on a project to raise awareness of measles and advocate for vaccination through a street art intervention: Rally Against Measles (hereafter referred to as Rally) (CMI, 2020). Rally reached a total of 5945 people across six locations in Lebanon, far exceeding the initial target which was set at 1250 people. The Rally is an example of how arts-based approaches – and performance in particular – can be used as novel modes of large-scale community participation in health promotion initiatives, addressing serious health issues in a fun, educative and entertaining manner. This snapshot presents the Rally by describing the

DOI: 10.4324/9781003036500-25

performances and other activities that were included and providing insights on its creative process, development and implementation.

A partnership for mobilisation

CMI was initially founded in Mexico in 2009 and has been active in Lebanon since 2011. Our work introduces clowning to lay audiences as a comic and playful means to spread laughter and provide relief to disadvantaged communities while exploring human vulnerabilities and helping individuals to cope with them. Clowning is a familiar form of entertainment for Lebanese people, but the cornerstone of CMT's artistic mission and performance practice is to move beyond entertainment only, using clowning to raise awareness about social, environmental and health issues and advocating for the rights of citizens and refugees. Throughout the years, CMI has used clowning as their main methodology to connect with people and convey messages on important topics in a fun, engaging and memorable way, where people listen more attentively to education messages and understand them.

Despite theatre and performance not being used very often in health advocacy projects in Lebanon, CMI has experience of using these forms particularly in the streets and in public spaces to engage with local communities on health issues. In one of their projects 'The Caravan Series – Van12', CMI used storytelling and interactive performances to teach some fundamental protections from the United Nation's Convention on the Rights of the Child, including the rights to vaccination and the importance of breastfeeding. Building on this successful experience, the Rally represents another example of CMI efforts to use art-based participatory approaches to mobilise the public for a worthwhile and lifesaving cause: vaccination.

The Rally consisted of a one-day competition event happening across different towns and villages across Lebanon. In each location, five teams made up of local people competed in a series of games and activities (rather like a scavenger hunt) as they rotated through a series of 'stations'. Each of these stations featured a scene of up to five minutes (each performed in a different style), followed by a set of tasks and activities that would take between thirty and forty-five minutes, which the competing teams must complete successfully to win a monetary prize. The gamifications and prizes were integrated to bring more fun and provide an incentive for people to take part in the Rally, particularly given the difficult economic situation in Lebanon.

A total of thirty teams competed across the different regions. Each team consisted of five young and vibrant adults who lived in the targeted areas. The teams were formed locally in each community through a call for participation, looking for people who were excited to play and seek stimulating challenges, using their creativity on the streets to mobilise other people. The call focused on young adults rather than parents of young children (who would be responsible for decisions about vaccination) because parents are less likely to engage as participants for the whole day given their responsibilities. However, the Rally involved these parents as audiences and through direct and indirect interaction with the participants and the performers. This was not only a pragmatic way to ensure wider participation in the Rally, it also empowered young people to become local champions and take action to advocate for vaccination, in addition to their potential role as future parents in making decisions on vaccines.

The Rally was implemented in partnership with UNICEF with the aim to strengthen partnerships and community engagement to advocate for behavioural and social change, and demand essential health and educational services among the most disadvantaged. This is part of 'communication for development' (C4D), a cross-cutting programme strategy used and promoted by UNICEF to drive positive behavioural and social change for children and their families. C4D applies across a variety of sector-specific issues including overcoming barriers to vaccination. To achieve that, the Rally helped to build public trust in the measles vaccines, with performances, videos and activities set up to provide evidence-based information and address unhelpful beliefs, misinformation, and misconceptions about measles vaccination among the community. Throughout the process of conceptualising and developing the Rally, the CMI team worked closely with UNICEF zonal offices and health advocates on generating the key messages to be shared through the performances and stations by using easy to understand materials developed by UNICEF. They also collaborated on creating successful participatory methodologies and building robust models of partnerships. They reached out and engaged with municipalities, scouts' groups, and universities in the targeted areas in order to promote the Rally, recruit participants, and reach a wider audience, as well as facilitating the smooth implementation of the Rally on the ground through access to public space and organisational support.

Multiple stations and ways of engagement

A total of five stations were created for the Rally. Each station was dedicated to spread specific information about measles and vaccinations. The set, the costumes and the activities were carefully designed to suit the concept of each station as well as to deliver the key message. All stations included educational materials (for example, flyers and posters) and were placed in a way to be visible to passers-by and to facilitate social interactions. Adaptations to the stations and the performances were made to ensure a safe and socially distant environment for everyone. In addition, CMI produced six one- to two-minute-long videos before, during and after each Rally. The videos were posted on social media to promote the Rally, reach a wider audience and encourage people to get their children vaccinated.

Station one. The first station was focused on the main symptoms of measles, presented through a pair of twins infected with measles, depicted as bouffon characters. Their white stuffed, dotted costumes were designed specifically to make the measles' symptoms more visible to the public. Bouffon is a style of performance that focuses on the grotesque (for example, through exaggerated costume) and satire and was used to show the symptoms in a comic yet poignant and memorable way. The exaggerated elements of the bouffon's performance represented in both the costumes and the scene were purposefully used to alert the audience to the danger that measles symptoms represent and to reflect a sense of seriousness and laughter to address them. The scene was complemented by a backdrop of pictures of faces featured behind the performers to provide additional visual effects mirroring how the person feels while being sick with measles. The task which followed the performance required the contestants to knock on people's doors in the village, collecting data on those who were not vaccinated yet. Through this task, the contestants acted as health advocates trying to enrol people in the vaccination programme delivered by UNICEF and referring them to vaccination centres. The contestants informed people in the community about the context of the Rally and sought their consent when collecting their details. The bouffons accompanied the contestants throughout the task, adding an element of fun and supporting them in approaching families and children and in illustrating the information in a more accessible and comic way.

Station two. Station two introduced the concept of an outbreak and highlighted the highly contagious nature of measles. The performance featured an upper-class flamboyant lady responding to the news of a measles outbreak across the country. Using clowning techniques, the performer expressed her fears of the outbreak in a silly way by going from an extreme state of laughter to crying and vice versa. Accompanied by her bodyguard, whose sole role was to obey her orders, the lady demanded a solution and asked the contestants to organise a demonstration against measles.

Whilst the costumes and set design took the audience back in time to the sixteenth century with an extravagant bourgeois feel, the idea of a demonstration was more rooted in the current reality of protesting the political and economic situation in Lebanon. The contestants were asked to invent slogans and write banners on the spot and march in the neighbourhoods to raise awareness of measles and call other people to join them in their protest. Referring to practices and tools that people were familiar with made the task culturally viable and engaging both for the contestants and the public in the streets. The demonstrations created by the contestants across the different locations became themselves improvised performances. The contestants cleverly adapted slogans and songs from the Lebanese revolution in 2019 and 2020 to fit the task of protesting measles, presenting a memorable and accessible narrative which resonated with the audience. Proudly, the contestants enjoyed taking 'revolutionary' actions and hoped that 'their revolution on measles' would lead to better health outcomes.

Station three. This station consisted of a scene with two clown characters, arriving in an ambulance (a two-dimensional cut out). One character was a nurse wearing a costume with multiple fabric-made arms attached to it. The arms were designed to reflect the hard work and multi-tasking that nurses have to do whenever there is an outbreak and also to represent the multiple misconceptions associated with vaccinations, which were identified by UNICEF. The other character was acting as a medical mannequin on which the nurse demonstrated information related to measles, such as what measles is, how it manifests in the body, the symptoms, means of contamination and modes of prevention and treatment. Whilst this performance was very informative, the performers avoided jargon and only used simple and clear terms. Through their clowning characters and props, they turned the scene into a fun and engaging performance. To spread the information to a wider audience, the performers asked the contestants to make a short video in which they presented the information they had learned from the performance. After checking the content to

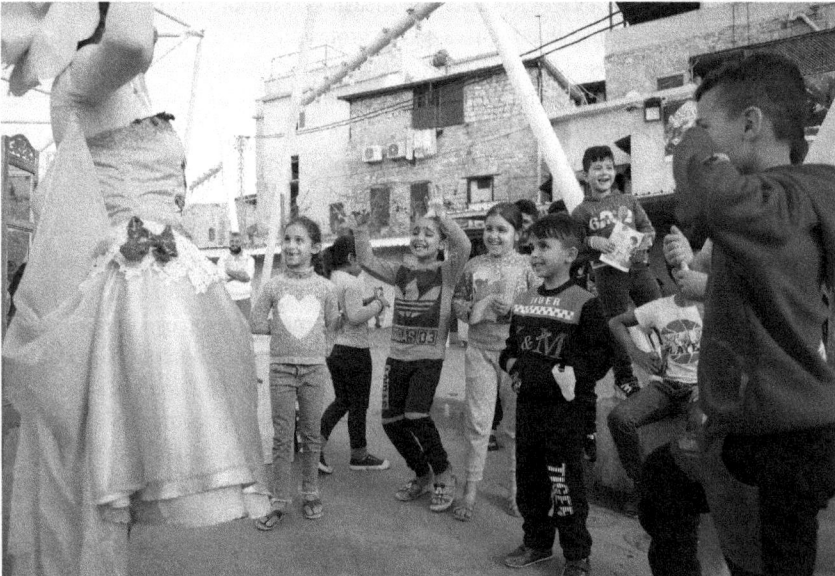

Figure 21.1 Children watching a performance as part of the *Rally Against Measles* with Clown Me In, 2019. Photograph by Wissam Andraos. Image Courtesy of Clown Me In.

ensure that all information in the videos was accurate, the videos were then immediately shared on social media. The number of views, comments and shares within an hour from posting the videos were then counted towards the final grade that each team received in the Rally. The performance at this station was a way to disseminate information and inspire the contestants to create their own awareness materials, not only that they were learning about measles, but they were also taking actions to raise awareness among their online communities.

Station four. With a touch of folklore and a mix of dancing and clowning, this station featured two men performing a comic classical dance while making a soup. The performers were dressed in *Abaya*, a traditional embroidered loose over-garment usually worn by women. With the set representing a Lebanese kitchen, the concept was to use the performance to provide the contestants and the public with nutritional tips to help strengthen the immune system in the case of measles. Initially, the idea was to ask the contestants to engage with their neighbours to collect ingredients and come together to prepare a soup or a healthy dish that would be helpful for someone who is ill with measles. However, due to the economic situation in Lebanon, which has put financial pressures on many families and left them without basic ingredients in their houses, the challenge was adapted, and instead the participants were provided with fresh ingredients to prepare their dish. Having male performers in this scene broke gender stereotypes that associated women with being the main carers whenever someone is sick.

Station five. This station introduced an old couple, represented by two human-size puppets, engaged in a familiar scene from Lebanese village life: drinking coffee and playing backgammon in front of their traditional house. The characters were both wise and witty, enjoying riddles and word games. They invited the contestants and passers-by for coffee and offered them a space for spontaneous interaction, conversations, games and laughter. In line with what they had learned about measles through the other stations, the performance ended with the puppets handing the contestants an envelope with five challenges and asking them to solve three of them. Examples of the challenges included teaching children a song about measles, taking a photo with as many people as possible holding the logo of the vaccination campaign and finding a couple who were about to get married and making them sign a vow to give the measles vaccine to their future children. Whilst the challenges revolved around simple social interactions, they represented powerful and meaningful actions, which sparked conversations around measles in the communities.

The process and beyond

As part of the creation process, the CMI team paid careful attention to cultural forms and their specificity in the context of the Rally. Through a back-and-forth process between the directors and the performers, the team discussed content-related challenges and how to respond to and address them. This included the risk of presenting narratives which failed to resonate with audiences or instil potential resistance to engagement with information. Thus, it was imperative to create a simple yet informative and engaging narrative that was accessible, culturally acceptable and compelling to the public.

Considering the content and the forms, the team reflected on how to bring both closer to the community using a language that echoed the 'streets' (from slogans of revolutions to daily life conversations) and roles that people could relate to. It was the responsibility of the performers to present these in a way that created a connection and initiated a dialogue between them and those who were participating in the Rally or watching it. Whilst the characters were perhaps amplified in their artistic and comic representation through bouffon and clowning, the narrative and scene remained accessible and reflected the subtlety and realism of local comic forms. The use of humour was carefully considered in this health-related context, where the characters were not in any way mocking measles as a sickness or sick people. Instead, they were finding and creating humour in situations that emphasised the importance of being vaccinated. In this instance, humour became an effective and ethical way for the performers to assume their responsibility to facilitate people's engagement with the theme and spread the message more clearly and widely.

In terms of its participatory approach, an emphasis was given to building the scenes and the actions around social interactions, which reflected and celebrated the values that these communities hold and their cohesive nature (for example, conversations over coffee and knocking on people's doors). In this context, 'word of mouth' was chosen as a performative act that tied all the Rally activities together and was an effective way of achieving its purpose in delivering health-promotion messages on measles. This participatory approach constituted a platform for the participants to act as performers and health activists, taking actions and raising awareness: this was a rewarding experience for them as they felt proud of making an impact on their communities. This highlights the value that the Rally had in creating both immediate and long-term results in the targeted communities.

The decision to incorporate a variety of performative styles and practices (bouffon, clowning, puppetry, dance) was made to ensure the Rally remained engaging through inciting curiosity and continual surprise for audiences but also operated as a strategy to anchor the educational elements and reinforce the messages through different mediums. The colourful costumes and set ultimately helped attract larger audiences and enhanced their engagement. They brought a different experience to the audience, which did not go unnoticed. The scenes performed at each station were all short and concise to hold the attention of the participants and the public focus on the key messages and to create a balance between the scene/content being treated as a spectacle versus being met with interaction and participation. Through their movements and voices, the performers tried to always capture the participants' attention while sensibly mixing entertainment and a sense of humour with the communication of measles messages to make them more memorable and effective.

One of the key insights gained along the way was the importance of simplicity and playfulness in engaging with the public. Even a simple question, such as asking people in the villages whether they have vaccinated their children or not, prompted a different reaction when presented in a playful way. Shifting such conversations from a formal health care setting to the Rally was a completely different experience for the community. Usually, people fear being accused of not taking care of their children and not taking the necessary measures to prevent them from being ill. The Rally's contexts helped break down barriers that traditional, formal health promotion messages cannot and stimulated acceptance among the public. Without shame or guilt, people felt more relaxed to share their experiences and were encouraged to come forward, ask questions openly and be referred to a vaccination centre.

'Where can we vaccinate our children?' became the mantra of success of the Rally, with many people repeatedly enquiring and expressing their willingness to take the step and vaccinate their children. For the performers and all those involved in the Rally, these were the most relevant moments, which made this whole experience an impactful one.

Reference list

CMI (2020) *6 Rallies against measles*. Available at: https://clownmein.com/performances/rally-paper-measles/ (Accessed: 28 March 2022).

El Zarif, T. *et al*. (2020) 'Challenges facing measles elimination: the Lebanese experience', *BMC Infectious Diseases*, 20(244). https://doi.org/10.1186/s12879-020-04956-1

Mansour, Z. *et al.* (2018) 'Factors affecting age-appropriate timeliness of vaccination coverage among children in Lebanon', *Gates Open Research*, 2, p. 71. https://doi.org/10.12688/gatesopenres.12898.1

Reliefweb (2019) *Measles – Lebanon | disease outbreak news*. Available at: https://reliefweb.int/report/lebanon/measles-lebanon-disease-outbreak-news-22-october-2019 (Accessed: 28 March 2022).

UNICEF (2018) *Measles outbreak in Lebanon: lack of funds hamper UNICEF's efforts*. Available at: www.unicef.org/lebanon/press-releases/unicef-lebanon-states-it-raises-alarm-it-targets-measles-response (Accessed: 28 March 2022).

World Bank (2020) *Population growth (annual%) – Lebanon 2000–2020*. Available at: https://data.worldbank.org/indicator/SP.POP.Grow?locations=LB (Accessed: 1 May 2022).

World Health Organisation (2020) *WHO UNICEF estimates time series for Lebanon (LBN)*, *WHO vaccine-preventable diseases: monitoring system. 2020 global summary*. Available at: https://apps.who.int/immunization_monitoring/globalsummary/estimates?c=LBN (Accessed: 28 March 2022).

22

SPEAKING TO POWER: SPEAKING TO PEOPLE

Responsive practice in relation to maternity issues in western Kenya

Jane Plastow

In 2018 a group of arts and social science researchers from Kenya, Uganda, Germany, Ireland and the UK came together in a project called simply Maternal Mortality in East Africa.[1] We were responding to a long-standing problem. One of the UN Sustainable Development goals is to reduce deaths in childbirth across the world to no more than seventy per 100,000. In the UK the current rate is seven. In the US, the worst-ranking country amongst industrialised nations, it is nineteen. In Kenya the figure is 342, and it is higher in the west of the country where we would be working. Of the thirty countries with the worst rates for maternal deaths, all but three are in sub-Saharan Africa. Many other causes of premature death have been relatively successfully addressed across the continent, but figures for death in childbirth have been coming down only slowly.[2] Numerous medical studies have been undertaken, but our research might be able to offer new and potentially useful insights by focusing on people rather than medical science. This article concerns the artworks that came out of the project.[3]

Most of the work discussed in the following comes under the heading of theatre for development (TfD). TfD is a term used to describe performance work in the political South that seeks to support development agenda. It is often seen as a branch of applied theatre but one used specifically in the poorer nations of the world. The term is contentious because it appears to imply both that the political North is 'developed' (hence indeed my preference for the term political South as opposed to the often-used 'developing world') and that all theatre here should have an ostensible 'development' agenda. Many other terms have been used: popular theatre, community-based theatre, campaign theatre and so on (Plastow, 2021). I simply use TfD here as a catch-all for theatre work that is community based and seeks to empower marginalised peoples in the South.

My mode of working in Kenya I call responsive practice. Originating in educational practice, the approach practice seeks to develop models that fit student needs as opposed to following predetermined rigid curricula.[4] More recently it has been adopted in relation to applied theatre (Hepplewhite, 2020; Elliott, 2020). I have been developing my interpretation of responsive practice in recent years on long term projects with multiple funders in both Kenya and Uganda (McQuaid and Plastow, 2017; Plastow and Elliott, 2020). For me the term links back to educationalist Paulo Freire's (1970) ideas of mutual learning between project facilitators and participants and of making that learning fit the needs, primarily, not of the facilitators or the funders but of participants.

DOI: 10.4324/9781003036500-26

This means that outputs cannot be pre-determined but will be decided as work progresses, always following an initial research process where participants are inscribed as co-researchers and their experiences and expressed needs drive all subsequent actions. The only activity that was planned in advance was a series of two-day arts-based research workshops, a tool which was used before each new phase of arts practice. From these, and from the data my fellow researchers were acquiring, we would plan the programme of activity.

The artistic outputs would face in two directions. The outward-facing work was to do with speaking to power. People living in poverty find it very difficult to get their voices heard in public or high-level fora; they lack agency, confidence and a platform. By making artistic works illustrating their experiences, the poor can begin to take power, crucially appealing to audiences simultaneously at both the intellectual and the emotional level. The inward-facing work would involve sharing information participants had decided would be relevant to affected communities. This would not mean message giving, as is so commonly practiced in TfD and indeed in behaviour change practices utilised across a wide range of disciplines from politics to health propaganda, but, building on the gaps in knowledge our research subjects identified and sharing the best relevant knowledge at our disposal, we would seek to overcome some of the poverty of information that is quite as crippling to many lives as is monetary impoverishment.

This article looks at four arts interventions carried out over two years in 2018 and 2019. These were, in order of execution: a series of two-day research workshops, a play made to show the perspectives of poor service users to senior medical personnel, a documentary film made for Kenyan television showing problems in accessing and delivering maternity care and a series of thirty workshops using sketches and interactive exercises conducted in a series of neighbouring rural hamlets focusing on the need for husbands and other community members to support pregnant women.

The research workshops

I began work with the research workshops. These utilised a format I have developed in recent years to seek to understand community perspectives on a range of specific issues. My collaborators in the workshops were local semi-professional theatre group, Lagnet Cric, based in the town of Ahero. Ahero is a market town some twenty kilometres from the main city in western Kenya, Kisumu, situated on the main international highway which runs into neighbouring Uganda. Crucial to our project was the fact that it contains a small state-run hospital where the majority of women in our study went for ante- and post-natal care and to deliver their babies.

Lagnet had been operating out of Ahero for some twenty years and had worked on a wide range of previous TfD projects with both local and international agencies. The group aspire to be full-time professional actors, though in practice this has never been possible. Theatre income is supplemented by a range of side-lines with members helping run market stalls, fishing (Ahero is near Lake Victoria, the largest body of fresh water on the continent), engaging in agriculture and running motor-bike taxis. Lagnet's local knowledge was enormously useful to the wider project beyond their acting skills, and they facilitated the research of all involved.

For my workshops I would run a session with Lagnet members themselves but would then ask them to find me groups of twenty women of child-bearing age from Ahero, twenty from a local village and twenty teenagers who had experienced pregnancy (teenage pregnancy rates are very high in this part of Kenya).[5] Participants would be paid only transport money to attend the workshops but would also be provided with lunch. Lagnet members were trained to help facilitate the workshops and to be note-takers, keeping track of the conversations held and issues raised to inform the research and subsequent practical work.

The central idea informing the workshops is to build a sense of relaxed community, as I have found that this enables participants to open up, share and discuss their experiences. The workshops only last four or five hours a day. This might seem a wasteful use of time, but that is not my experience. First, when working with mothers, many have family commitments that make a long research day impractical. Second, I have found that the coming together twice means that the sense of community, relaxation and openness is greatly enhanced on the second day. Participants have got over their nervousness and feel a growing sense of ownership of the workshop which tends to result in much richer and more nuanced information sharing. It is also important that participants be offered food. Most of the people I work with are notably poor, so to offer them a good lunch, which they have not had to prepare, was a significant luxury. Moreover, during lunch, conversations about the topics raised in the workshop continue. Lunch is a great informal research opportunity.

I always begin by explaining my reason for calling the workshop and that the participants are seen as co-researchers, sharing their knowledge but also helping sift what is being shared and identifying what they consider most significant and important. We sit in a circle, a configuration that is returned to at all discussion points, so that we are embodying the workshop principle of equality. In Ahero many people speak quite good English, but all information and discussion is always translated as we go along into the local language of Dhuluo and occasionally into Kiswahili, the more regional vernacular.

The secret weapon available to arts-based research workshops, and one I think social scientists often notably undervalue, is that however serious the subject matter of our investigations, we can make much of the process enjoyable, and fun is something many of my respondents do not have a super-abundance of. Fun relaxes people; it helps them buy into a process, and it helps them to open up far more than might a more formal interrogation. We begin always with games, games that introduce us to each other, games that enable us to know just a little about each other – What did we all have for breakfast? How did we each get to the workshop? – and then games that open up voices, singing maybe, and that get us physically moving, all tailored to the age, dignity and culture of the participants.

I have a number of possible exercises I use in these two-day workshops, but constant and central is the story-go-round. Many people have written about the power of story to validate, to support identity, to build community (Archibald, 2008; Frank, 2010), but my strategies have developed from some decades of experiential learning. In these first sessions in western Kenya I put people in groups of four and asked everyone to tell a short story about a problematic experience they had had with any aspect of their maternity care. I always emphasise when asking for these stories that people do not have to speak of matters that are traumatic; a simple problem with getting to an ante-natal appointment or an encounter with an unsympathetic health professional would be quite enough to build on. Asking for a 'big' story is in my view unethical, possibly traumatising for the teller and sensationalist.

The stories are exchanged (and recorded by the note-takers), and then three members of the group each join a different foursome. The other foursomes do likewise so that everyone now has a completely different group. The instruction this time is that everyone must tell not their own story but the story they think is most pertinent to the issue under discussion and would have most resonance among the wider community. Moreover, the story-teller must honour the confidence of the original tale-teller and tell the story as compellingly as they can. After this process, there is one more iteration of group change. This is the beginning of the development of critical thinking, requiring analysis and a move beyond the personal to begin thinking more widely about community. Again, everyone tells the story, other than their own, that they have heard in either of the preceding groups which they consider most powerful and representative. And then the groups vote on just one story of the four they have just heard that they will proceed to share with the whole group.

For this final stage, more time is given, and in this project, the Lagnet theatre members were to hand to help people realise their ideas performatively. Groups are encouraged to think about what might be the most appropriate and powerful way to tell their story. Many offer a fairly naturalistic theatrical presentation, but multiple narrators, mime, monologue and poetry may all play a part. The selected stories are shared with the whole group and can then be used in various ways. A particularly powerful tool I have found to be hot-seating: when characters are asked to remain in role and then anyone in the audience can ask them about their reasoning and motivation for particular actions. This enables the group to begin to analyse not just what goes on but why it happens, considering cultural and socio-political factors informing individual choices.

However the stories are presented, this activity leads into an extended discussion. People are asked what they saw in the stories and what had particular resonance for them. We discuss how representative particular tales may be. We also discuss how the process worked for all involved. Without exception, I have found that those whose stories are told are delighted to have their experiences validated in a public representation – even if sometimes elements of the story may have changed a little from their original telling. Often this is the first time people have shared their stories outside a very intimate circle, and this gives a feeling of being valued and heard. The displacing of stories from their original owners also prevents any element of blame or defensiveness. These are now the groups' stories in which all are invested.

Speaking to power

The stories I heard from women in and around Ahero had many common themes. The most striking was a perception that when poor, ill-educated women went to the hospital to give birth, they received a variety of abusive treatments, particularly from nursing staff. Much of this was verbal abuse: young girls would be berated for getting pregnant while they were still 'babies', while an older woman told of being abused for giving birth in her late forties, and very many spoke of being told off if they made any noise while in labour. There was also physical abuse. Women would be slapped if it was felt they were not making sufficient effort while in labour. There were many examples of neglect. Women would be sent away if they were not thought to be about to give birth, and several as a result bore their children away from any medical facility. Many women felt that nurses ignored their pleas for assistance at times in the process of birth, and most troubling of all were stories of women refused entry to facilities if it was thought that they might die, as this would reflect badly on the hospital.

While I was undertaking this preliminary research, our project leader, Shane Doyle, had been organising a meeting of senior local medical personnel and leading Kenyan professionals working on gynaecological matters. It had not been planned, but I was so struck by the recurrent themes – and the considerable horror I felt when being told many of the women's stories – that I decided, with the support of the research team, to make a play to show to the medics reflecting the women's experiences. At this point there was only about a week before the meeting.

I drafted an outline of a play that was based on the stories I had heard. It would centre round three women who had come to Ahero hospital to give birth: a teenage unmarried girl expecting her first child, an older woman coming for her fifth delivery and a woman who is initially sent away as she is told her labour is insufficiently advanced for her to be admitted. The delivery ward was staffed by two nurses more interested in chatting about their private lives than in their patients, while a lone doctor put in only very occasional appearances. The play would be performed by Lagnet, who, after the discussion of the scenario to confirm that they found it representative and credible, had just three days to rehearse.

Much was devised around the scenario. The company adapted a well-known tune to become a mourning song that framed the performance, and all the actors were given the opportunity to name someone they knew who had died in childbirth to whom they were dedicating their performance. The actors playing the part of the nurses managed to create an atmosphere that was simultane-ously hilarious and horrific as they discussed getting their nails painted while patients begged for assistance, and in a Brechtian adaptation, I got everyone to learn quotes from the Kenyan National Guidelines for Quality Obstetrics and Perinatal Care that spoke of compassion, respect and wom-en's rights and were painted on placards.[6] Only one woman died in the play but all were abused and ignored for much of their delivery, while the dead woman was smuggled out of the facility in an attempt to cover up what had happened to her.

My second speaking to power intervention I touch on only briefly here, as it was a documentary made for Kenyan TV and not a theatrical work. Following research into the understaffing of mater-nity services, and the frequent failure of on-call doctors to attend emergency calls, I, with an inter-national team of Kenyan, British and Austrian film-makers,[7] made a thirty minute film, *Sunset at Dawn*. This brought together observational techniques based in Ahero Hospital delivery ward with the partially re-enacted, partly described by family members and health staff, true story of a young woman, Judith Awino, who died in childbirth in 2017, having been denied entry to Ahero Hospital.

Speaking to communities

The major piece of community-facing work made for Maternal Mortality in East Africa was a series of thirty performance/workshops which took place in contiguous rural hamlets all around an hour's walk from a health facility. Again, production was preceded by two-day workshops with rural women. We already had much information on problems experienced by such women in rela-tion to pregnancy and childbirth, but we wanted to consult them on what they thought the most useful focus of these sessions would be. They asked that we emphasise the need for the support of husbands, who we were told often see pregnancy as purely a women's concern, and the problems many experienced with their mothers-in-law. Luo society is patrilineal, and in rural communi-ties when a man marries, he takes his wife to his parents' compound where a house is built for the couple. Mothers-in-law are in these circumstances ever present, and we were told they often have great influence over their sons and little interest in modern ideas about attending ante-natal services, vitamin-rich diets in pregnancy or going to a health facility to give birth. We also found there was much misinformation and many myths circulating about a whole range of issues relating to sexual and reproductive health, particularly when the topic of contraception arose, so we would also seek to engage with some of these. Theatre would be used as our primary tool of engage-ment not only because literacy is a problem for many older members of Luo rural communities but because it both engages interest through entertainment and allows a range of situations to be presented in a culturally nuanced manner that relates directly to local experience.

On the basis of our research, we created a two-hour performance/workshop. The devising pro-cess was led by Matthew Elliot, an experienced community arts facilitator, working with Lagnet, whose actors would be employed to conduct the series after Matthew and I had returned to the UK.[8] Rather than making a performance anyone could attend, we sought to recruit an average of forty adult participants in each hamlet, at least one third of whom would be male. This was done so that all involved had a measure of commitment to the work and so that we knew we could engage everyone in the participatory elements of the sessions. To achieve such attendance – and it is often difficult to secure the involvement of men who prioritise money-making activity and see pregnancy as 'women's business' – we employed Lagnet member Josephet 'Obul' Onyango, who in his work as both fixer and actor on *Sunset at Dawn* had illustrated not only his competence but his deep roots in the community, to visit communities in advance and mobilise our audiences. Notably he was much helped in this work by Denis, Judith Awino's husband, who had become a huge advocate for our work following his involvement in the documentary.

The sessions began with a series of sketches. We showed a husband and mother-in-law arguing over what to do with a young wife in labour as she sat voiceless between them, becoming ever more distressed. We showed a husband and wife embattled as she seeks to get him to understand that she needs to eat fresh vegetables in pregnancy and to take better care of herself while he worries about money and fears his authority is being eroded. We showed a pair of teenage lovers, with the girl abandoned by the boy as soon as she becomes pregnant, backed up by his mother even though she knows he is responsible. Five short sketches were linked by a chorus of doctors who, in white coats and big glasses, answered questions from patient-actors, dispelling some of the many misconceptions about the dangers of contraception.

Our performance was hugely serious in intent, but it included poetry and song, comedy and chorus, and was as slick, professional and entertaining as we could make it, as we were seeking to combat the making of formulaic, under-rehearsed, message-touting theatre that has been a feature of much theatre for development across the political South, The 'show' lasted some twenty minutes. The rest of the time was devoted to a series of participatory activities flowing from the performance. Audience members were invited to 'hot-seat' actors about their characters' thinking and motivations (the mothers-in-law were given a particularly hard time, including by older women). In small groups, participants were asked to discuss key questions that had often come up in our research: 'Is it OK for husbands to leave all aspects of pregnancy solely to their wives?' 'Should women give birth at home or in a health facility?' Discussion groups were facilitated by Lagnet, who also recorded key points in the debates, but the consensus of opinion was left entirely to villagers to come up with and report back to the wider group.

The final section of the workshops engaged with the highly controversial question of contraception. In many research workshops, women had told us they wanted to control the number of children they had, the average number desired being three. However, men almost universally wanted significantly more, the fathering of children being widely seen as a sign of virility. Religious factors also came into play, with many believing that it was a religious injunction to have many children and that contraception was divinely prohibited. Finally, there was much misinformation circulating about what is known across East Africa as family planning. The most widespread belief seemed to be that using contraception before having any children would imperil future fertility, and indeed concern that fertility would be damaged by any kind of contraception was widespread. Many also believed that intrauterine devices (IUDs) or long-term implants might move, get into the body and potentially kill the user.

Our doctor chorus had sought to dispel some of the most prevalent fears and myths, but the topic frequently led to both fierce debate and such a host of questions that the Lagnet actors were sometimes in danger of being overwhelmed. As Beatrice, one of the performers, recalled:

In those villages, there was no knowledge of Family Planning. So, when the actor began the discussion, there was a point where the community would ask her so many questions, she could not answer. We had to seek support from our chairman to control the debate.

It was important throughout that the performers tried never to cross the thin line between sharing information and promulgating messaging. Engagement in our sessions by community members was never a problem, and the information about pregnancy health and the importance of supporting pregnant women by the wider community was universally well received. On the matter of contraception, we often left communities with differing opinions. Indeed, I was at one workshop where a dominant man got everyone in his community to back up his strongly expressed view that contraception was not acceptable on religious grounds. Having shared our knowledge, we respected alternative views. It was crucial to our credibility and integrity that we remained peer-educators, not didactic preachers.

Analysing activity and impact: speaking to power

I am repeatedly somewhat surprised that so few applied or TfD arts events involve speaking to power. The commonly accepted narrative appears to be that artistically preaching development messages as designed by the rich and powerful to the poor – messages which often implicitly 'blame' their ignorance and backwardness – remains the only role for socially engaged theatre, at least in the political South.

One reason why so few of the development agencies which fund much of this work are interested in reversing the accepted order of messaging is that they do not wish to antagonise the powerful by critiquing them and imperilling either their funding or their permission to work in particular jurisdictions. Indeed, critique plays very little part in development arts agendas, vertically for fear of alienating the powerful and horizontally because opening up discussion involves risk that target communities may go off message, threatening the capacity of delivery organisations to succeed in achieving the aims of the often narrowly focused programmes for which they have received funding.[9]

Moreover, enabling the poor to speak to power is inherently political, and this runs counter to the behaviour change theories which have in recent years dominated international uses of the arts in the political South.[10] Behaviour change never means that the powerful should change their behaviour, only that the poor should do as they are told. Yet as I saw in Kenya, most of the problems relating to maternal deaths stemmed from actions performed by the powerful and the state – or more often from their inactions.

Pregnant women in Kenya are supposed to be given comprehensive information about ante- and post-natal care and about contraception, but most often this is given, if at all, in a very cursory manner. Nurses are not given decent conditions and are often over-worked and under-trained.[11] Doctors appear to be able to ignore their employment contracts at hospitals at will, frequently failing to carry out their duties,[12] and the state has significantly failed to deliver on its undertaking to provide free maternity services to all. In the face of all these issues, it appears quite as urgently significant to use the arts to ask these authority figures to engage in behaviour change as it is to empower the poor through increasing their knowledge of maternity-related issues.

My experience of trying to utilise the arts in Kenya to engage the powerful had mixed results. The play we made for the medical symposium organised by Shane Doyle was generally well received. It certainly made an emotional impact on some; both Shane and I recall a number of audience members crying at points in the play. Shane had been nervous that the critique embodied in the production might alienate his audience, but that does not appear to have been the case. He had several senior doctors tell him 'This is what it is like' (Pers. comm., 25 June 2021), and there was some discussion showing that the audience recognised the emotive power of the play and thought that this kind of methodology could be adapted to engage with a wider public.

The target of the play was primarily the behaviour of ordinary nursing staff, who were not present at the symposium, which perhaps explains why more senior medical professionals were relatively relaxed about the performance. The television documentary was another matter. Here critique was focused on medical officers (a group situated, skills wise, between doctors and nurses), doctors and the funding and organisation of state maternity services. The regional health minister sought to stop us filming, and senior medics then effectively prevented the programme being shown, even though it had been approved for transmission by the Kenyan Television Authority. There was a notable sense of panic among medics who saw the film, something I can only ascribe to a fear of what the public response to a screening might be. As I write, I have conducted further screenings for particular groups and occasions but have not found the best strategy for getting the film widely seen. In this instance political power prevented us sharing the film with the television-owning middle-class Kenyan community I had aimed to reach, who have little detailed understanding of the travails of the pregnant poor.

Speaking to people

I was, frankly, surprised at how positive the impact of the work was with communities in Nyanza. Many, myself included, have discussed the frequently limited value of one-off arts interventions (Odhiambo, 2008; Plastow, 2014). One-off performances and interactions may well be of only passing interest to communities, but this was not my experience here, and I was able to back up my impressions from workshops when I conducted evaluation focus group interviews in seven participating villages six months after the programme concluded. There are a few reasons why this may have been. First, the issue was one which resonated, particularly with women of child-bearing age, but also more widely within communities. Everyone knew someone who had either died in childbirth or lost a child at some point in pregnancy, and everyone had experienced problems in accessing the kind of maternity services that would make them feel relaxed and confident. Many were therefore willing to engage with our work and eager to both learn more about how to help themselves and to help us learn how they could better be supported.

The structures we used to research and inform communities seem to have been found accessible and relevant. The informal, playful, egalitarian atmosphere of the two-day research workshops, and the respect offered to contributors who understood that they were being valued as co-researchers whose knowledge and opinions would be fed into further concrete actions led to great openness in discussion, the sharing of a range of experiences and eagerness to suggest how community members wanted our work to move forward.

The workshop structure was an innovation for me, one that Matthew was happy to experiment with. My previous experience of taking plays into communities, even when they allowed for Boalian-style dialogic engagement, was that by no means everyone's voice could be heard and that the play limited the range of discussion to a particular topic or angle on an issue. A workshop gets round some of those problems but does not have either the aesthetic joy of a performance or so easily allow a culturally inflected framing of the topics under discussion The performance/workshop delivery was experienced very positively. In Ngere, I was told; 'It was real. In ordinary talks some go to sleep, but here all learnt'. In Bondo Kachola, one participant said that 'it gave room for all to contribute their ideas', while in Kakamu, a lady said simply, 'I liked the workshop because it was practical'.

Although our format only reached relatively small groups, we were working in small communities, adjacent to each other, and we thought this might promote meaningful discussion of the questions raised and information given after we had left. To a significant extent, this appears to have happened. In Ngere, I was told: 'The community is now talking freely about Family Planning and men's responsibility'. There were also specific stories of the beneficial effect of wider sharing of information. In Kagaga, a man told me; 'My neighbour is a drunk and he was careless of his wife. I went to see him and shared the information, and now he even went with his wife for the check-up', while in Kakamu, an elder reported: 'After the workshop I went to my house and talked to my daughters and said you must know this thing [contraception] and now they are using'.

For me these specific stories were the most powerful indication that our approach was seen as helpful. A couple of examples from many illustrate the kinds of changes people told me they had embraced. In Ngere Baptist, a man explained; 'Before I didn't listen about my wife's pregnancy. Now I went with her when she went to hospital for a check-up. My wife is happy'. In Kagaga, an older lady said 'To me as a grandma we used to go to the TBA, but now I know we need to send our daughters to the hospital'.[13]

Contraception was a more difficult area with a greater range of responses. In Kagaga, for instance I was told; 'Before there was a myth that FP (Family Planning) would give infection. Should you go before baby or after baby? Now more are going to the hospital for FP', though obviously the subject was still seen as delicate: 'Sometimes it is still difficult to speak, but we are seeing action with people going to hospital for FP'. In Koyare, one gentleman offered up a graphic picture 'Before women were like dogs, having babies all the time. So they had one on the back one in the hand and pregnant again. Now it can be different'. A woman explained, 'People are now using FP and seeing no bad effects. But people still do not discuss freely. But they go secretly. Like me'.

Conclusion

As I write in July 2021, I have just heard that I have been given funding to go and extend our village-based community information work in Kenya.[14] We will be building on the 2019 model and extending the work, at the frequently reiterated request of community members, to engage specifically with youth, discussing a range of issues around sexual and reproductive health while conducting more community workshops discussing contraceptive options. When I return I will also be strategising how we can best share our television documentary, probably via popular social media apps. Issues remain about the replicability of our information sharing; about how best to promote critical thinking, regarding the optimal model for development arts; about whether it is possible to work more closely with maternal health authorities and deliverers; and about how to make it possible to speak to power so that the voices of the poor may be heard and the excellent maternal health policies developed for use in Kenya may have a more realistic chance of implementation. As always, responsive practice-based research project work is an on-going, not a neatly compartmentalised, process.

Notes

1 The research team was composed of Shane Doyle, Paul Geissler, Benson Mulemi, Saudah Namyalo and myself.
2 Between 1990 and 2015, Kenya's MMR fell from 687 to 510, and progress has continued, but at nothing like the rate required. See Alkema, L. *et al*. (2016) 'Global, regional and national levels and trends in maternal mortality between 1990 and 2015', *The Lancet*, pp. 462–474.
3 Maternal Mortality in East Africa was funded by the Medical Research Council and the Arts and Humanities Research Council.
4 See www.responsiveclassroom.org/sites/default/files/pdf_files/RC_approach_White_paper.pdf.

5 Kenya has the highest teenage pregnancy rate in East Africa, estimated at 18–20% of girls. See www. thenewhumanitarian.org/news/2020/07/13/Kenya-teen-pregnancy-coronavirus.

6 Examples of quotes we painted on placards from the Guidelines included: 'Clients have a right to be treated with courtesy, consideration and attentiveness' (p. 21). 'When the mother comes into labour, the health service provider must provide a supportive, encouraging atmosphere for the birth' (p. 173).

7 The production team were myself, William Nyerere-Plastow, Dr Simon Peter Otieno and Tina Tschis- marov. The project was funded by HEFCE under the Global Challenges Research Fund.

8 For a more detailed analysis of the process and impact the community workshops, see Plastow, J. and Elli- ott, M. (2020) 'Translating "good" pregnancy in Rural Nyanza, Kenya', *Moving Worlds*, 20(1), pp. 83–96.

9 See Etherton, 2008, in *African Theatre: Youth*, where he discusses a programme working with young peo- ple that drew horrified responses from the INGO funder when the young people wanted to discuss matters beyond the remit of their programme because they feared this would alienate their funders.

10 See, for example, The Drum Beat Networks, www.comminit.com/health/content/drum-beat-networks, funded by USAID, which promotes a limited view of the social uses of arts for what it explicitly states is a 'behaviour change network'.

11 There are few specialist midwives in Kenya. Most of those working in delivery rooms are simply nurses who have been given limited training in midwifery as part of their general training.

12 Many doctors have private clinics, and it is widely felt that they neglect duties in state hospitals in fa- vour of these. Our documentary showed doctors failing to attend urgent on-call requests. For more infor- mation, see Research Journal of Finance and Accounting www.iiste.org ISSN 2222–1697 (Paper) ISSN 2222–2847 (Online) Vol 2, No 3, 2011 121 Ethical Issues in Health Care in Kenya. A Critical Analysis of Healthcare Stakeholders.

13 This comment brings up the difficult issue of recommending people to attend formal clinics when we know they are not well resourced. It appears that there are fewer dangers, limitations notwithstanding, to women if they give birth in the hospital compared to births which are TBA supported, though this knowl- edge is anecdotal.

14 I am grateful to the AHRC for funding further work with adult and youth groups on SRH in 2021–22.

Reference list

Alkema, L. *et al.* (2016) 'Global, regional and national levels and trends in maternal mortality between 1990 and 2015', *The Lancet*, pp. 462–474.
Archibald, J. (2008) *Storywork: educating the heart, mind, and spirit.* Toronto: University of British Colum- bia Press.
Elliott, M. (2020) 'We play as we mean to resist – theatre games as political participation', in Prentki, T. and Breed, A. (eds.) *Companion to applied performance.* London: Routledge.
Etherton, M. (2008) 'West African child rights theatre for development: stories as theatre; theatre as a strategy for change', in *African theatre: youth.* Oxford: James Currey, pp. 97–120.
Frank, A.W. (2010) *Letting stories breathe: a socio-narratology.* Chicago: The University of Chicago Press.
Freire, P. (1970) *Pedagogy of the oppressed.* New York: Herder & Herder.
Hepplewhite, K. (2020) *The applied theatre artist: responsivity and expertise in practice.* London: Palgrave.
McQuaid, K. and Plastow, J. (2017) 'Ethnography, applied theatre and Stiwanism: creative methods in search of praxis amongst men and women in Jinja, Uganda', *Journal of International Development*, pp. 961–980.
Odhiambo, C. (2008) *Theatre for development in Kenya: in search of appropriate procedure and methodol- ogy.* Bayreuth: Bayreuth African Studies.
Plastow, J. (2014) 'Domestication or transformation? The ideology of theatre for development in Africa', *Ap- plied Theatre Research*, 2(2), pp. 107–118.
Plastow, J. (2021) *A history of East African theatre.* Vol. 2. London: Palgrave Macmillan.
Plastow, J. and Elliott, M. (2020) 'Translating "good" pregnancy in rural Nyanza, Kenya', *Moving Worlds*, 20(1), pp. 83–96.

23

MAKING A DRAMA OUT OF A CRISIS

Using theatre to co-research mental health literacy in Kerala

Andy Barrett, Chandradasan and Michael Wilson

In 2019 a group of UK and Indian academic and health service delivery organisations met in Kochi to begin work investigating the experiences and understandings of mental health in Kerala. This thirty-month project, MeHeLP (Mental Health Literacy Project), had been funded by the Economic and Social Research Council (ESRC) and the Arts and Humanities Research Council (AHRC) under the Global Challenges Research Fund (GCRF) to explore how theatre and storytelling might be used as a method for increasing levels of mental health literacy in a relatively wealthy area of India that was experiencing high levels of mental illness. As a tool and language of research, such work has much to offer in a context where the arts are seen more broadly as tools of health promotion and education. This was a challenging proposition that moved away from the more traditional practice of theatre in health settings in India, exacerbated by the heavy bias towards health-based practitioners on the project and the wide geographical area in which the work was to take place. It also found itself having to adapt to cope with the coronavirus (COVID-19) pandemic, which accelerated public debate in India (as elsewhere) about mental health.

The project involved working alongside people accessing mental health care, their families and local communities to explore and re-present their stories and understandings of living with mental ill-health. It is important to note that our work was not designed as an intervention (in the sense of how the term is commonly used in health care settings) but as a feasibility study. Given the importance of cultural beliefs around this issue, our research aimed to examine how we could best promote socially and culturally appropriate mental health literacy (MHL) using participatory approaches. The changes that were made in response to the COVID-19 pandemic moved the storytelling work from a live, co-present encounter to a fully online space, which fundamentally changed the purpose of the artistic work, shifting it away from discursive intent towards more traditional understandings of health promotion. It also reinforced boundaries between health-based understandings and forms of artistic expression that our interdisciplinary work had sought so hard to break down.

Mental health in Kerala

The World Health Organisation (WHO) estimates there are over 450 million people suffering from mental disorders, accounting for around 12% of the global burden of diseases, a figure that is likely to grow over the following decade (WHO, 2001, 2010). Around 80% of these are located

DOI: 10.4324/9781003036500-27

in low- and middle-income countries (LMICs), with Rathod *et al.* suggesting 'Social factors, such as poverty, urbanisation, internal migration, and lifestyle changes' are key moderators of a high burden of mental illness, with subsequent economic consequences on individual and community development (Rathod *et al.*, 2017, p. 1; Semrau *et al.*, 2015). MHL is defined as the ability to recognise different types of psychological distress and disorder, a knowledge of risk factors and potential causes for these and an awareness of how to mitigate these through self-help or professional services which can develop mental health and well-being and is of huge importance in these contexts (Jorm *et al.*, 1997). Attitudes and behaviours around mental ill health in LMICs can often differ substantially from those in the Global North so that, for example, 'the cultural views and institutional biases against women and certain sections of communities (e.g., religious, certain castes) increase the burden of illness in these population subgroups' (Rathod *et al.*, 2017, p. 1). The National Mental Health survey of India has drawn attention to an urgent need for MHL, recommending the development of awareness and literacy programmes to strengthen early recognition of mental health concerns, to advocate for patients' rights and to enhance tolerance and de-stigmatise.[1]

The MeHeLP project was based in the southern state of Kerala, whose 35.5 million people account for around 3% of India's population. Kerala has a Human Development Index (HDI) of 0.79, the highest of any state in India, with its literacy rates (98.9%) and life expectancy of seventy-four years representing 'the direction in which other regions in India desire to travel'.[2] However, around 15% of the adult population experience mental ill-health at some stage in their lives, with 12.5% of individuals at risk of suicide, the highest in India and almost twice the national rate of 6.4% (Bal, 2016). These figures coincide with a rapid socioeconomic transformation that has been occurring across the country, with a decline of the joint family system, internal migration, a developing gap between high standards of education and low employment and pressure exerted on children within the school system to ensure success in this changing world. Kerala is also home to the 'gulf depression' of migrants and families that are left behind as work is sought in the Gulf States, a potentially contributory factor to a heavy consumption of alcohol within the state.

Kerala is tackling this situation through a range of community-based mental health models and the wide range of psychiatric, biomedical, ayurvedic and religious healing practices that people seek has been documented (Chua, 2009). However, MHL is still in need of development, as widespread stigma about mental illness remains, creating real challenges for marriage and economic prospects that impact on people's willingness to approach mental health facilities (Celine and Antony, 2014). The project partnered with two prominent mental health NGOs – Mental Health Action Trust (MHAT)[3] and MEHAC Foundation[4] – whose work and practice in their community mental health clinics are at the sharp end of the challenges Kerala faces. Their embrace of a wide range of strategies meant they were highly supportive of our theatrical experiments. Just as importantly this relationship allowed us to work across a very wide geographical spread, encompassing both urban and rural populations with different socio-economic challenges and local factors that impacted community mental health.

Before exploring our applied theatre and storytelling work, it must be stated that the majority of those working on the project came from the health field, which impacted the specific research aims of the project, namely:

- How is MHL shaped by economic, social and cultural contexts in Kerala?
- How do urban and rural communities construct a culturally and socially appropriate meaning for MHL?
- How can we best engage with urban and rural communities in Kerala to discuss mental ill-health?

- How might we use a participatory theatre model as an intervention for developing MHL?
- How can we best engage with communities, professionals, services, policy-makers and govern-mental agencies in promoting MHL?

The challenge of positioning the theatre and storytelling work as a central research tool and language must be understood in the context of an ongoing relationship in India between theatre and health, a relationship that our project was hoping to reset in some way.

Theatre and health/theatre as research

The traditions of community-based and street theatre in India stretch back to pre-independence, when from 1941 the Indian People's Theatre Association (IPTA) used 'street corner' theatre as a form of anti-colonial protest and propaganda (see Srampickal, 1994), in much the same way as agit-prop theatre groups of the political left in Europe had done following the end of the First World War. By the 1970s new forms of 'applied' theatre had begun to emerge in India, utilising other kinds of non-theatre public spaces. The principles and techniques of Augusto Boal's Theatre of the Oppressed, and Forum Theatre, gained popularity as a form of intervention (Van de Water, 2011; Ganguly, 2016; Ghoshal and Manna, 2017), and the Indian Theatre-in-Education movement evolved with theatre companies playing not only in schools but also with the purpose of educating the broader public, especially in marginalised communities. For example, Jana Sanskriti Theatre Company,[5] based in West Bengal, has worked nationally on projects related to child health, alcoholism and domestic violence, 'staunchly putting marginalised perspectives into dialogue with official governmental directives' (Chou, Gagnon and Pruitt, 2015, p. 614). Other companies with avowedly socially activist agendas include pandies theatre[6] and the Aagaaz Theatre[7] Trust, both operating out of Delhi.

Theatre for development initiatives, which align themselves to what Prentki describes as 'the goals of self-development and an improved quality of life of all people whose material conditions leave them vulnerable to hostile, predatory forces, both natural and human', have grown in prominence (1998, p. 419). Such work has commonly been adopted by NGOs and larger health campaigns in the service of the 'dissemination of information and awareness of health problems and other social issues to low-income, low-literacy populations' and is typified by the use of professional theatre companies in HIV/AIDS public health education programmes and prevention campaigns in the 1990s and beyond (Pelto and Singh, 2010, p. 147). Such work has not been without its critics, due to the role of external agencies in determining its direction. In reference to Theatre for Development work in Bangladesh, for example, Ahmed (2002) argues that such initiatives run the risk of prioritising the agendas of NGOs, wealthy donors and Western notions of development and need. Consequently, they may ultimately underperform when they fail to properly engage with the very communities they purport to help and empower.

In the UK, 'theatre and health' has become a growing field of practice interested in developing new vocabularies and re-conceptualising attitudes and approaches, whereas the situation in India is more commonly based on the conveying of officially sanctioned public health messages. Much of the interest in using theatre, particularly in rural areas, is driven by the vibrancy of traditional and vernacular forms of performance which, in creating strong bonds between performers and audience, make it highly effective as a medium of mass communication. This is particularly the case for clear health education messages, such as that used in the Kalajatha programme in Karnataka in 2001, where it 'was found to be a very effective medium in promoting health education and possibly behavioural changes' (Ghosh *et al.*, 2006, p. 6). Similarly the 2017 Actor–Doctor project in Ahmedabad explored the impact of twenty street theatre performances on five public health themes with the findings that 'Members of the audience, after watching the respective street theatre performances, were significantly more favourable towards . . . environmental health' (Sharma *et al.*, 2021, p. 89).

Dramatherapy is a slowly emerging practice in India, as indicated by the foundation, in 2019, of the Drama Therapy India collective which is beginning to 'explore training programmes, professional associations and research to grow, regulate and streamline the field' (Gopalakrishna, 2021, p. 147). There are also many Playback theatre companies creating improvisational performances in which individuals explore their own life stories. The recent *Even Mists Have Silver Linings* project, an example of the developing interest in using theatre to develop conversations around questions of identity, social acceptance and stigma, suggested that '[c]ommunity-based theatre is highly acceptable and effective as a medium for informing positive attitudes, improving knowledge, and promoting acceptance of and prosocial behaviours towards LGBTQ+ communities' (Pufahl *et al.*, 2021, p. 257).

Whilst the use of theatre as a tool for addressing a range of issues with marginalised communities and, as Jacob Srampickal would say, giving voice to the voiceless (1994), is part of a tradition stretching back over eighty years, its 'use in health research is more recent' (Fraser and al Sayah, 2011, p. 111). In particular, the use of theatre to address issues related to cognition and mental health has seen a significant growth in recent years, primarily in response to increased refugee and work-oriented migration on a large scale (Balfour *et al.*, 2015). Nevertheless, the application of theatre as a research method in health contexts, rather than simply as a tool for communication, has been less common. As Crossley *et al.* state, 'drama's potential to address issues of mental health and resilience in India . . . has not been comprehensively pursued as a methodology or, at the very least, not mapped and documented coherently' (2019, p. 222).

This understanding of theatre's engagement with health promotion as being a matter of message-giving is one that was made evident to the authors during work on a previous project.[8] In this case a community play had been made with the residents of a *basti* (slum) in the city of Pune, during which the experiences and challenges of internal migration; the impact of these on mental health; and the way these were addressed and ameliorated by individuals, families and the wider community were explored and shared. Swatantra, our partner theatre company in Pune, came to the project with a simple question: What is the message that we are telling the audience? The idea that the project was aiming to use theatre to find ways for people to tell their *own* stories, so the researchers could learn from this experience, was one they found challenging. Similarly, when the company went into the *basti* to ask what kind of street plays they should make and perform there, they were asked to create plays that called for better toilet facilities. Theatre, or at least the kind of theatre that was available to them, was understood by the *basti* community as highly instrumental, a promotional tool, albeit one that could also be used to their advantage to advocate for better resources. Indeed, when the final play was presented, in which people saw their own lives represented, this came as something of a shock to many. As one of the audience members told us: 'Nothing like this has happened before . . . this is the first time that someone has come here, talked to us, asked us'.[9]

Making the clinic plays

With the project team largely consisting of health-based academics and professionals, the applied theatre practitioners wanted to ensure that theatre did not simply become a mechanism for communicating the research outputs but an essential part of the research language, central to unlocking new forms of knowledge, through co-creating new forms of communication and conversation. The UK practitioners had many years' experience of community-based theatre work, and Lokadharmi, the Keralan theatre company partnering on the project, had a history of practice that ranged from classic plays of India, Greece and Shakespeare alongside street theatre and theatre for community education and engagement informed by Boalian practice.

The first stage of the work was the interviewing of patients, family members and health professionals identified from the clinic locations, run by MEHAC and MHAT. Both organisations collaborate with local communities and train health professionals and volunteers to deliver mental health services free of cost to people living with mental health issues from the lower socio-economic strata. MHAT has 56 clinics, some of which are locally owned and operated voluntarily, with those from non-professional backgrounds being trained to deliver mental health care to around ten to fifteen people a day. Day-care sessions are also run incorporating elements of vocational and psychosocial training. MEHAC has established a sizeable network of outpatient clinics across various districts in Kerala, providing assessment, clinical management, medication, therapy, rehabilitation and counselling. Each patient receives support from a volunteer whose role is to implement individual treatment plans, conduct home care services on a regular basis and to support their recovery, which may involve directing them to vocational training services. Their team includes psychiatrists, psychologists and social workers, most operating in paid roles and some volunteers who reside in the local area.[10]

This was a major undertaking that, from May 2019 to February 2020, resulted in 192 interviews with service users, caregivers and community members, with ninety-six from rural sites, seventy-two from urban sites and twenty-four from tribal sites. Such an extensive body of research had the potential to immediately impact the perception of the theatre work, to see it as something that should happen in response to these interviews. To counteract this, and to ensure that theatre's specific language register was fused into the fabric of the research from the very beginning, we asked those conducting the interviews to engage in 'theatrical reconnaissance', gathering images of artefacts that interviewees may have that might connect to the stories they were telling and paying attention to the way that interviewees used metaphors in their responses. Alongside this, Chandradasan, artistic director of Lokadharmi and director of the clinic plays, visited the clinics with the researchers to meet service users and the staff and examine the spaces in which the first shows were to take place, so that the physical environment and rituals of these spaces might inform the construction of the theatrical encounter. These were a combination of larger halls that held around 100 people, smaller buildings and open spaces.

For Sanjana Kumar, one of the researchers carrying out the interviews, this represented a new way of working. Whilst the documentation of artefacts was difficult to undertake, the focus on metaphor became transformational. When the team began to dig into the transcripts of the first interviews, the search for metaphors meant that 'they started looking at the data in a new way'. Instead of seeing them as collections of material to be coded, they 'started reading these narratives as stories', and those interviews without metaphor 'seemed to be lacking in some way'. Kumar now would 'look for the metaphors even as (she) was interviewing', aware that at these points the interviewees were moving beyond their explanation of a situation to reveal how they understood this situation and how it had felt to them. They were, in the language of theatre, showing, not telling. For Kumar this created a stark difference in how these encounters were understood and experienced; there was a beauty to the process that excited her, with the material being gathered having an additional layer, even though she knew that within the data analysis and subsequent coding the metaphors would be unimportant. Indeed, when Kumar and the other researchers returned to their data analysis after working in the rehearsal room with the theatre team, 'there was a shift, a switch; then the metaphors didn't matter as much, it had to fit into these boxes' (Sanjana Kumar, interview with the author, 6 January 2020).

The devising period took place over two weeks, during which six performers worked with the research team to create shows of around forty minutes in length, working location by location. Kumar talks of this period being 'emotionally charged, supercharged', with much of the early work spent reading a collection of narratives from each location to dig into key themes and issues. A generic framework was created, that of a problem play in which a character, family and wider social circle grappled with the challenges of facing some form of mental illness, with a seven-scene structure being created that was replicated for each location (Introduction/The Inciting Incident/ The Characters' Understandings/The Intervention/Response (Stigma)/The Question/The Resolution). So, for example, in Vailathur and Ponnani, predominantly Islamic communities with at least one family member working in the Middle East, the play focused on a character with post-partum depression exacerbated by her husband's work-enforced absence. As family members begin to voice criticism of her behaviour, her husband struggles to balance his need to earn an income and support his wife. After visiting a temple, faith healer and a doctor who prescribes medication, she appears to be recovering. Yet her ostracism from the local community, which comes to a head at a neighbour's wedding, causes her recovery to stall, and at this point the audience are asked by the characters how they may best move forward to break through this impasse.

The interview transcripts were a continual source of inspiration, specific lines being dispersed amongst representative characters who faced situations synthesised from the narrative material. More importantly, the metaphors that had been sought in the theatrical reconnaissance stage were given space to develop into stage pictures and choreographed routines. For example, in one scene, several masked characters surround a young woman who finds the demands of her family becoming impossible to bear; a rainstorm became a scene of social isolation; grotesque characters offered a kaleidoscope of quick-fix cures to desperate families; a busy office turned into an arena of physical competition. Themes of family stigma, social pressure, traditional and medicalised interventions were explored through characters suffering from a range of conditions that were most pertinent to their specific context and location (post-partum depression, psychosis caused by drugs and alcohol abuse, work-related stress).

The actors at the Lokadharmi Theatre Centre in Kochi used their skills in the devising process to quickly evoke a range of worlds and locations and move swiftly across time and space. For Chandradasan, this improvisatory working model, embraced by the company, was key in allowing the actors to escape from the parameters of many traditional Indian performance forms as well as connecting to indigenous traditions (often performed in similarly non-conventional spaces) where a set narrative may be interrupted and reshaped by the performers to respond to the immediate social, political and cultural realities of the day. The researchers were thrilled to see issues they had been told about coming alive in the space and became more confident in making suggestions as the actors looked for more nuanced understandings of the situations they were improvising. The text was co-created through this exchange, with the directors shaping and editing the material to provide clarity.

The first theatrical performances were hosted in the clinics for an invited audience of staff, service users and their families and were designed to provoke debate amongst those with lived experience of the issues we were addressing. Through providing a space for dialogue and conversation in a public space, it moved the conversations that had been recorded up to this point from a one-to-one situation to a social and collective one, as Jerome Bruner says, transforming 'private trouble into public plight' (2003, p. 35). This allowed us to discover ways in which, through responding to and building on each other's experience, mental health literacy was understood and practised. It was essential therefore that the audience were positioned not as passive observers of stories but as experts in a dynamic process that would initiate further debate and discussion both within and after the performance and could show the research team where they might need to move next. The plays then were a moment to share research but also to test and drive the research forward, an iterative process with the techniques of theatre being the tools that allowed this to happen in a specific way.

The nature of the venues demanded very simple theatre, with the actors using their voices and bodies to create landscape and atmosphere, resulting in an energetic and non-naturalistic aesthetic. Yet it was also important that there were moments when characters could simply explain directly to the audience how they were interpreting what was taking place in their lives, and this scene (The Characters' Understandings) was always the longest in the show, a moment of stillness that became a form of confessional from those who were facing mental distress, their families, friends and work colleagues. Most importantly, they signified to the audience that this was a shared space where they were able to communicate feelings directly, so that when the characters on stage asked them for their help to finally find a way to move forward, they might also speak openly and freely, which they did.

The creation of a participative environment encouraging mutual care was fostered in other ways. By sharing snacks with the audience, by having moments when the audience made sounds to create a storm or threw confetti at a wedding, by performing traditional songs or dances rooted in the location and inviting audience members to join in, the clinic setting was reinvented and re-purposed to become a playful space where all were invited to contribute and interact. By the time the characters asked for advice any barriers between performers and audience members, between health professionals and service users had been broken down, and a lively dialogue ensued that continued long after the play had ended. It was clear that the audience had recognised themselves and their situation, that they wanted to talk about what they had seen and what could be done and felt they had the space in which to do so. In the post-show discussions, audience members spoke freely of their lived experience of mental illness, elaborating on the crippling nature of stigma and isolation and the need for grassroots changes to counter this, a desire to see mental health education in schools and the importance of finding ways to address the issue of unattended mental illness. In Elapully and Attapadi, they spoke of rampant alcohol and drug abuse in their community, one woman telling of her abusive spouse and how she identified with the protagonist of the play. In Vailathur, a largely orthodox Muslim area, the company were told by the hosts to keep their distance from the women in the audience, who were expected to watch silently but who instead joined in with the singing of songs, participated in the discussion and got up on 'stage' to dance with the actors, to the astonishment of all present. Similarly in Malappuram, with its large Muslim community where women are less likely to speak out in public, Kumar was surprised at how willing the female members of the audience had been to 'voice their opinions, being very open'.[11]

These responses corroborated the findings from the field research whilst providing key insights into how challenges and issues might begin to be addressed, supplying new questions for the next stage of the research and design of the work. Yet there was one unexpected impact: post-performance follow-up with the host clinicians revealed an improvement in adherence to the treatment they had been prescribing. The plays, through being designed not as intervention but as discussion, had appeared to result in members of the audience taking certain courses of action in response to a genuinely collaborative and collective understanding of their situation. The siting of the plays within and around the clinics, and the anecdotal evidence of improved engagement with patients, has potentially important ramifications in shifting the perception of medical spaces. If the performances engaged with mental health in a collaborative manner, then the clinics this process was attached to might also be seen not simply as sites of medical intervention but of dialogue and social encounter, where a person's health is something to be responded to, rather than acted upon.

The clinic plays were to be followed with the creation of a single touring play that built on the responses to this work, this time for a wider, more public audience. This presented a new set of challenges, with the performance in all likelihood being less adaptable to local context and focusing on specific questions and key attitudes that had been uncovered. However, we had learnt the importance of the plays being able to communicate a diversity of experience that allowed audiences to draw their own conclusions and make their own sense of what they had seen. What had become clear from our work, and the responses to the shows, was the need to think about multiple mental health literacies which people deploy in different circumstances. Even those sceptical of traditional and spiritual approaches are knowledgeable about them, and the traditional practices themselves often involve detailed regimes of activities aimed at effecting an improvement in the person's mood or condition. Therefore, it is appropriate to consider mental health literacy not as a unitary universal phenomenon but instead as a mosaic of different literacies which may be deployed in different settings and in line with different experiences and which may operate in cooperation with each other to enable treatment but also facilitate a sense of meaning and purpose in life.

Unfortunately, before we were able to move into rehearsal, the COVID-19 pandemic meant that any possibility of creating a public interaction had to be abandoned. As a result, the next stage of the work was reconfigured into the creation of a series of short films, based on some of the storylines that had been created for the public plays. This resulted in a number of new partnerships being created with different film makers, each of whom responded to this material in very different ways. This process also drew attention to the potential dangers of artists and theatre-makers engaging in health-based projects as communicators of message rather than as co-researchers.

The theatre-makers had been clear about the importance of bringing the language and sensibility of theatre to the health research at the beginning of the project, to ensure that the discursive potential of theatre and its understanding of the affective power of narrative was utilised from the outset. The handing over of material, on the other hand, to film makers who had not been part of many months' worth of conversations, in which an understanding of the value of a heterogeneity of practices in response to mental health had mirrored the understanding of the value of different research approaches to the subject, was problematic. Left to their own devices, and without the researchers being able to provide constant insight and reflection, several of the films ended up creating messages that veered away from the understandings we had learnt. Rather than exploring how people deploy multiple mental health literacies according to different circumstances, this work tended towards placing emphasis on the importance of the clinical expert's role in prescribing medical amelioration. We had returned to the tendency within health-based arts work in India of a top-down message giving imperative; of taking information from 'experts' out to the population so that they can learn the 'right' course of action to be taken, and through doing so had shifted away from grounded cultural understandings towards a medicalisation of mental illness.

Reflection and evaluation

Throughout this project we sought to embrace a holistic understanding of how people address challenges to their mental health and, rather than extolling any kind of hierarchy of interventions, were more interested in how these might work together. Engagement with more traditional forms of help should not be seen as unhelpful or old fashioned but as a sign that people want to address these issues and are looking for ways for their needs to be supported. The creation of plays that were connected to specific cultural forms and invited the audience to join in with the performance (not just as those with lived experience of mental illness but as people who wanted to dance or to sing) amplified this purpose and was highly successful.

Whilst it is too early to understand the impact of the short films, it is clear they will have a longer life than the clinic plays and will reach a wider audience through social media and other platforms than the singular encounters of theatrical events in specific locations for small groups of people. Yet the very publicness of the latter, creating discursive spaces that had been lacking up to this point, created an open-ended narrative that drew the audience into conversation and democratised the very question of mental health literacies. If we were asking the audience to tell us what the characters should do to help them through a situation, then our job was simply to show the many ways in which this experience was currently being responded to and let them weave a path between these that would allow us to construct a wider understanding of how cultural and contextual factors impact on understandings of mental health.

The short films will largely be accessed individually, probably framed within wider messages around the importance of looking after one's mental health, and will therefore more likely be used as a more traditional form of health promotion.[12] While they will contribute to a wider discussion around mental health, they lack the discursive potential of the clinic plays. They may be shown in public as a tool of wider discussion, and this is already planned to happen. Yet this will still offer a fundamentally different experience and lack the more general participative impulse of the plays. The audience will not be offering advice to embodied characters who are representative of themselves but as a group of people asked for their reflections in response to something in which the potential for genuine reciprocity between the imagined space and the lived reality has vanished. In one of the clinic plays, a woman stood up from the audience in the middle of a show to console a character and offer advice. The imaginative space and the narrative that was being shared gave her the confidence not only to communicate her understanding and experience but to act on it by carrying out her own intervention. This move from individual recognition to public action is an incredibly radical and potent one that demands a particular form of narrative to help activate it, one that theatre has the potential to provide.

Concluding thoughts

Applied theatre is, ultimately, concerned with power. Who has the power to tell their stories; who has the resources, the space and the opportunity for their voices to be heard? As theatre practitioners, it was this focus on the idea of story rather than data that was central to our work, and to our research language, a language that, as Kumar indicated, complemented and developed the research whilst sitting outside the parameters of other aspects of the work. The levels of discussion and dialogue that resulted from the plays, and the uptake in clinic provision, shows that when people can see their experiences shared and explored in a collaborative way, allowing them agency over their own story, traditional doctor–patient understandings may be unsettled and create the kind of collaborative partnerships that are essential in dealing with mental health.

Applied theatre-makers understand the need for people to participate in the telling of their own truths and the potential of this to lead to the discovery of new truths and new ways of doing things. Story is a vehicle in which people explore their experience, and storytelling demands that there is somebody who is ready to listen. The clinic plays brought together health professionals, patients and their families and used the tools and processes of theatre to create a genuinely democratic space in which experience, attitudes and aspirations could be communicated freely. As Kumar observed of the audience: 'It was as though they were waiting for a chance to come and talk, and they were given this opportunity and space. So, I guess that's all everybody needs; if you give them a space the people will talk'.

Notes

1 National Mental Health Survey of India, 2015–2016. Prevalence patterns and outcomes. National Institute of Mental Health & Neurosciences, Bangalore, India, 2017. Available at: http://indianmhs.nimhans.ac.in/#.
2 MeHelp project website: www.mehelp.in/.
3 Mental Health Action Trust (MHAT). Available at: https://mhatkerala.org/.
4 MEHAC Foundation. Available at: www.mehacfoundation.org/.
5 https://janasanskriti.org/.
6 www.pandiestheatre.com/p/about-us.html.
7 www.aagaaztheatre.org/.
8 http://mhri-project.org/.
9 http://mhri-project.org/wp-content/uploads/2020/02/Pune-Report-v05.01-20190827.pdf.
10 The authors would particularly like to thank to Dr. Sanjana Ravi Kumar for providing this information.
11 A series of short films documenting the creation and production of the plays can be seen at www.youtube.com/playlist?list=PLcyav8zQAsKhLD8oLrrtp6RfyW9raIGeN.
12 The films are available at: www.moviezone.mehelp.in/.

Reference list

Ahmed, S.J. (2002) 'Wishing for a world without "theatre for development": demystifying the case of Bangladesh', *Research in Drama Education*, 7, pp. 207–209.
Bal, R. (2016) 'Prevalence of alcohol dependence among males in Thiruvanandapuram district, Kerala', *Research and Reviews: Journal of Social Sciences*, 2(1), pp. 1–7.
Balfour, M. *et al.* (2015) *Applied theatre: resettlement: drama, refugees and resilience*. Sydney: Bloomsbury Methuen Drama Publishing.
Bruner, J. (2003) *Making stories*. Cambridge, MA: Harvard University Press.
Celine, T.M. and Antony, J. (2014) 'A study of mental disorders: 5-year retrospective study', *Journal of Family Medicine and Primary Care*, 3(1), pp. 12–16.
Chou, M., Gagnon, J.-P. and Pruitt, L. (2015) 'Putting participation on stage: examining participatory theatre as an alternative site for political participation', *Policy Studies*, 36(6), pp. 607–622. https://doi.org/10.1080/01442872.2015.1095281
Chua, J.L. (2009) *The productivity of death: the social and political life of suicide in Kerala, south India*. Redwood City, CA: Stanford University Press.
Crossley, M. *et al.* (2019) 'Systematic review of applied theatre practice in the Indian context of mental health, resilience and well-being', *Applied Theatre Research*, 7(2), pp. 211–232. https://doi.org/10.1386/atr_00017_1
Fraser, K.D. and al Sayah, F. (2011) 'Arts-based methods in health research: a systematic review of the literature', *Arts & Health: International Journal for Research, Policy & Practice*, 3, pp. 110–145.
Ganguly, S. (2016) *From Boal to Jana Sanskriti: practice and principles*. London: Routledge.
Ghosh, S.K. *et al.* (2006) 'A community-based health education programme for bio-environmental control of malaria through folk theatre (Kalajatha) in rural India', *Malaria Journal*, 5(123), pp. 1–7. https://doi.org/10.1186/1475-2875-5-123
Ghoshal, S. and Manna, N. (2017) 'Boal's reception in India: dialogism of Jana Sanskriti's theatre of the oppressed', *Journal of Dharma*, 42, pp. 201–218.
Gopalakrishna, M. (2021) 'Drama therapy and psychiatric care in India: practice and potential', *Arts Therapies in Psychiatric Rehabilitation*, pp. 147–150. Springer. https://doi.org/10.1007/978-3-030-76208-7_19
Jorm, A.F. *et al.* (1997) ' "Mental health literacy": a survey of the public's ability to recognise mental disorders and their beliefs about the effectiveness of treatment', *Medical Journal of Australia*, 166(4): pp. 182–186. https://doi.org/10.5694/j.1326-5377.1997.tb140071.x

National Institute of Mental Health & Neurosciences (2017) *National mental health survey of India, 2015–2016: prevalence patterns and outcomes*. Bangalore, India: National Institute of Mental Health & Neurosciences.

Pelto, P.J. and Singh, R. (2010) 'Community street theatre as a tool for interventions on alcohol use and other behaviors related to HIV risks', *Aids and Behavior*, 14, pp. 147–157.

Prentki, T. (1998) 'Must the show go on? The case for theatre for development', *Development in Practice*, 8(4), pp. 419–429. https://doi.org/10.1080/09614529853440

Pufahl, J. *et al.* (2021) 'Even mists have silver linings: promoting LGBTQ+ acceptance and solidarity through community-based theatre in India', *Public Health*, (194), pp. 252–259.

Rathod, S. *et al.* (2017) 'Mental health service provision in low- and middle-income countries', *Health Service Insights*, 10, pp. 1–7. https://doi.org/10.1177/1178632917694350

Semrau, M. *et al.* (2015) 'Strengthening mental health systems in low- and middle-income countries: the Emerald programme', *BMC Medicine*, 13, p. 79. https://doi.org/10.1186/s12916-015-0309-4

Sharma, K. *et al.* (2021) 'Actor – doctor partnership for theatre-based public health education', *Health Education Journal*, 80(1), pp. 81–94.

Srampickal, J. (1994) *Voice to the voiceless: power of people's theatre in India*. London: C. Hurst & Co.

Van de Water, M. (2011) 'Jana Sanskriti: center for theatre of the oppressed', *Incite/Insight*, 3, pp. 7–10.

World Health Organization (2001) *The world health report mental health: new understanding, new hope*. Geneva: World Health Organization.

World Health Organization (2010) *Mental health and development: targeting people with mental health conditions as a vulnerable group*. Geneva: World Health Organization. Available at: www.who.int/publications-detail-redirect/9789241563949 (Accessed: 14 August 2023).

24

NARRATIVE RX

Storytelling's healing capacities in public health

Yewande O. Addie, David O. Fakunle and Jeffrey Pufahl[1]

This chapter presents three case studies as examples of how storytelling can be utilised in public health contexts, specifically to cultivate spaces for people to navigate personal experiences and embolden them to proclaim their truth for the sake of their mental health and emotional wellbeing. These US-based case studies focus on three different spheres of mental and emotional health: obsessive compulsive disorder (OCD), trauma from multifaceted determinants manifested through alcohol and substance use disorders and psychological distress caused by anti-Blackness. OCD is a mental condition that causes a person to experience distress from unwanted obsessive triggers; substance use disorders are diseases that impact one's mental state of being; and with the US declaration of racism as a threat to public health, health practitioners are now more openly addressing the relationship between anti-Black racism and psychological distress that manifests via anxiety and depressive symptoms (Devakumar *et al.*, 2020; Williams, 2018). In this context and others, storytelling offers mutually beneficial outcomes for both the narrator/writer of the story and the listener/audience. For the narrator it can be a cathartic, imaginative expression of self, and for the listener it can trigger deep introspection, empathy and reflective action (Addie and Pufahl, 2021).

We propose that performance storytelling is a viable form of care for mental and emotional health-related challenges, regardless of personal or societal cause, and should be utilised widely at the community level. To elucidate, we conceptualise storytelling as a practice and performance artform that can be usefully applied in public health for research and dissemination, and as a vehicle to promote social connection and healthy behaviors. We continue with a breakdown of each case study and a concluding section on potential future directions.

The value of storytelling

Stories help humans understand who we are in relation to ourselves, others and the world (Young and Saver, 2001). We tell stories to define who we are and to assign and construct meaning at every intersection of our lives, from small interactions to significant and tragic events (Bruner, 1990). Patrick J. Lewis, a Canadian narrative identity scholar, said 'we use the story form and the story forms us' (2009, p. 22). In the ongoing formation of self and story, our memories and identities are packaged into recognisable archetypes that we repeat and cognitively use to make sense of the world (Lewis, 2011). In this way, we make sense of life through stories on a metaphorical stage,

DOI: 10.4324/9781003036500-28

by performing layered versions of self through our social roles. We place our most intimate and authentic portrayals 'backstage', while using the 'frontstage' for public portrayals of self that are societally approved (Goffman, 1978; Sharma and Grant, 2011).

Beyond its individual, self-definitional qualities, storytelling is a tool for communal preservation through cultural dissemination. Our understanding of humanity stems from recorded pasts because stories are used to explain the mythology of who we are and where we come from. Yilmaz and Ciğerci (2019) maintain that presentation of narratives occurred in prehistoric and ancient civilisations, whether through cave-dweller paintings or oral tradition. Similar forms of storytelling practice endure in diverse ways; for example, ethnic groups in Senegal and Mali still maintain oral storytelling traditions through designated *griots*, professional storytellers and cultural historians that maintain the integrity of sacred information. Some stories that have been told and retold across time and cultures are immortalised in folktales, often with the social purpose of relaying wisdom through didactic messages and reoccurring character tropes (Lwin, 2009). Through such mechanisms, storytelling is ritualised to 'transmit histories, values, beliefs, cultures, and ideas about the social world' (Addie, 2019, p. 56). In the contemporary moment too, the process of relaying information from storyteller to audience, regardless of timing (that is, live rather than pre-recorded) or format (for example, in-person, virtual, and so on) creates a shared experience of social connectedness, whereby a community of listeners are engaged in co-constructing the reality of what is being shared. Jack Mezirow (2009) places stories at the heart of personal transformation; stories that contradict a listener's world view can force the listener to self-reflect and reevaluate their beliefs, assumptions and processes of meaning making. Through this process, both storyteller and audience can enter a collective experience of examining their lives and perspectives.

The National Storytelling Network (NSN) defines storytelling as 'the interactive art of using words and actions to reveal the elements and images of a story while encouraging the imagination of the listener' (2022). Because we live in a performative social world (Wulf *et al.*, 2010), the advent of communication technologies has expanded the storyteller–listener relationship to include imagined audiences, otherwise defined as the 'mental conceptualization of the people with whom we are communicating' (Litt, 2012, p. 331). Building on NSN's definition, we conceive performance storytelling as a process of meaning making that can take place between two individuals, in small groups of people known to each other, before a live public audience or imagined audience. Regarding our specific case studies, we present scenarios where storytelling is performed in intimate small group settings, on a theatrical stage and pre-recorded for imagined audiences.

Public health and storytelling

According to the American Public Health Association, the field of public health's mission is to 'promote and protect the health of people and the communities where they live, learn, work and play' (2022). Public health research and practice, like many intellectual endeavours, are extensions of inherent human curiosity about us and the world in which we live. The ingenuity that is generated by people engaged in public health work, such as vaccine intervention programmes and jurisdictional policies, is strongly aided by its multidisciplinary underpinning and the fluid relationships between people and their health. Similarly, ingenuity generated by storytelling is aided by its multidisciplinary nature and ability to reflect the fluidity of human experiences; the transfer of information between people is elemental to understanding life and how people navigate it. However, the extent to which creativity is allowed to manifest within public health has historically been structurally stifled, and the consequences of that deprivation have brought the field to a critical juncture.

The transition to the 'fifth wave' of public health – a focus on the influence and impact of cultural determinants – coincides with growing movements for epistemic justice and the need for more bases of knowledge to be recognised and utilised within science (Fricker, 2007; Davies *et al*., 2014). Public health's ongoing reckoning results from overdue acceptance that the field's epistemological and pedagogical foundations were dictated overwhelmingly by privileged White men and that their contextual disregard for any other viewpoint was often intentional.

What has become clearer is that the implementation of 'equitable' public health through research, policy and practice, among other manifestations, is ineffective if the approaches are crafted in disregard of the context of the people to be helped, willingly or unwillingly (Fakunle *et al*., 2021). Long acknowledged by the field, the navigation of racial, socioeconomic, educational, locational, personal, familial, historical and cultural contexts, all of which continuously interact with each other, are significant drivers of health and wellbeing. However, further translation of these contexts into public health work on all levels (i.e., local, state/provincial, national, global) is critical to reducing health disparities. As a universal practice evolved through cultural methodologies, storytelling is equipped to encompass the full spectrum of wisdom, knowledge, understanding, intuition and perspective by empowering human beings to willingly express their complete personhood. This is a relatively novel concept in public health, but not as novel in medical and therapeutic spaces. Rita Charon recognised this value and importance in her 2001 article, which introduced the term 'narrative medicine', and several institutions such as Columbia University, have a department or division dedicated to its practice (Charon, 2001). Preceding narrative medicine, psychotherapists used storytelling – in the form of 'the talking cure' – with people with mental and emotional health challenges (Marx, Benecke and Gumz, 2017). Both group and dramatherapy rely on storytelling to help treat unresolved trauma in a variety of populations such as veterans suffering from post-traumatic stress disorder.

To situate the practice of storytelling as an essential tool for healing, it is important to explain how we are using the term 'healing' and to differentiate it from 'therapy'. Here, 'therapy' refers to the treatment of mental and behavioural challenges by individuals with specialised training in disciplines like psychology, psychiatry and social work. Such training usually includes development of clinical expertise and is based on curricula determined by institutions and regulatory bodies. This includes all creative arts therapies, practitioners of which must adhere to qualifications and certification requirements (American Art Therapy Association, 2017). In therapy, an individual enters a therapeutic relationship with an accredited practitioner and specific goals are set and progression tracked. The individual often experiences 'healing' – improved mental and emotional wellness – through therapy. Conversely, an individual may experience 'healing' without engaging in therapy. We intentionally use the term 'healing' to encompass a wide range of practices, typically operating outside the Western scope of professionalisation (e.g., no explicit degree or certification), that seek to positively address intrapersonal, interpersonal, cultural, structural or systemic challenges, from which emotional, mental, behavioural or organisational consequences may result.

The following three case studies explore three different approaches to group storytelling. We acknowledge there is no 'one size fits all' approach to storytelling performance and hope to articulate through these examples how story performance can be beneficial to participants and audiences both in traditional performance settings (such as in a theatre) and non-traditional settings (in small groups and online).

Case study 1: storytelling in group settings

DiscoverME/RecoverME began as *Project Tell-a-Tale*, a practicum led by David O. Fakunle, then a first-year doctoral student at the Johns Hopkins' Bloomberg School of Public Health, with the aim of teaching individuals in recovery from substance use disorders (SUDs) storytelling for support and advocacy. In partnership with a local inpatient/outpatient recovery centre, the project provided instruction to individuals furthest along the centre's process for achieving sobriety, which allowed for programmatic flexibility and was the best assurance of participant retention. In designing the project, Fakunle was conscious that it was taking place at an institution notorious for historical medical exploitation of the local Black population – most famously the case of Henrietta Lacks (Skloot, 2010). Every effort was made to engage project participants as equal partners rather than the objects of research. To round out the facilitation team, Fakunle partnered with a fellow storyteller and educator, as well as a SUD recovery advocate.

The initial storytelling sessions were held during the participants' weekly support meeting and lasted between sixty and ninety minutes. Sessions consisted of one or two storytellers facilitating a group of around ten to fifteen participants. Participation was primarily self-selected, but for some participants attendance was mandatory due to legal obligations. Participants were primarily Black, between forty and sixty-five years old and residents of the Baltimore metropolitan area. Additionally, sessions were usually attended by the clinical director of the recovery centre who would listen and provide contextual clarity for facilitators and participants when warranted.

A constant in *DiscoverME/RecoverME's* approach was utilisation of traditional folktales to serve as primers for reflection and discussion. Narratives across various oral traditions in Africa, Asia and North America were chosen by facilitators for their abilities to solicit and elicit thoughtful insight. Stories such as *The Precious Stone*,[2] *The Healing Tongue*[3] and *The Real Meaning of Peace*[4] were successful in helping participants explore connections between the stories and their personal experiences, some of which related to challenges they were aiming to address. Early in the programme, the telling/performance of a folktale was used as an example for teaching basic narrative components such as structure (beginning, middle, end), characters, settings and themes for the clients to practice and then utilise within their own stories. Designed as a sixteen-week programme, that approach was quickly abandoned when faced with consistent turnover of meeting attendees. Methods were revised to focus on the use of folktales as a catalyst for collective sharing of personal perspectives, thus maximising empowerment in whatever amount of time facilitators had with participants. Thus, the project pivoted toward utilising techniques that reinforced storytelling's critical components in a simple, replicable manner and leveraging the group's core participants as peer leaders to orient new attendees. Additionally, sessions were altered from a rigid educational structure with a finite end to a more fluid, group conversation-style structure without a finite end.

Sessions revealed that vulnerability and connection were essential components of storytelling's potential for healing. Facilitators' willingness to share their personal narratives as part of the discussion process served as encouragement for participants to reciprocate, and vocalising appreciation to participants for listening to each other's stories reinforced the importance of receiving a person's truth. The main 'takeaway' finding was that facilitators modeling the behaviour of telling stories about difficult life experiences was the most effective approach for establishing collective trust (Ten Have and Jean, 2009).

Principles from the Virtues Project,[5] a global mental/emotional health initiative based in positive psychology, were incorporated to enhance participants' awareness of positive intrinsic qualities such as understanding, honesty, discipline and love. Facilitators identified moments in stories when participants demonstrated virtues and provided both appreciation for the qualities participants exuded and encouragement to continue doing so as part of their recovery. Recognition was most significant in stories of participants' active substance use, conveying that their past behaviours did not result from 'moral failure'. With heightened recognition of their fundamentally positive nature, participants were empowered to use past and current moments as emotional foundations for healing. What resulted were participants reorienting their shared narrative towards positive aspects of their character regardless of perceived or actual negative circumstances.

The developing partnership with the recovery centre's clinical director utilised insights from their observations of the project's impact outside of sessions. This included the frequency of participants' references to folktales shared, improvements in recalling past stories related to their use and greater willingness to explore life experiences more deeply in formal therapy sessions. Currently, approaches developed through *DiscoverME/RecoverME* have been utilised to explore other public health issues, such as community-driven asset mapping and understanding COVID-19 vaccine hesitancy, further exemplifying storytelling's value and potential (Fakunle *et al.*, 2021).

Case study 2: storytelling in group settings for a public audience

The University of Florida's (UF) Center for Arts in Medicine (CAM) has piloted several storytelling programmes and advanced research on the benefits of storytelling for patient populations, including Pufahl and colleagues' 2021 project with ten individuals with an OCD diagnosis and two caregivers. OCD is a complex and often invisible mental health disorder that can severely reduce social and work functioning as well as increase feelings of isolation and self-stigma in individuals in treatment or post-treatment (Weingarden and Renshaw, 2015). The programme facilitators wanted to investigate how storytelling might improve social cohesion and wellbeing among participants and support group members both in and out of therapy.

Participants were recruited in partnership with clinicians in the UF Center for OCD and Related Disorders to ensure they were psychologically able to participate. For added participant safety, the group was joined by a psychiatric resident physician who told stories from the clinical perspective and provided mental health support when necessary. The programme lasted ten weeks and culminated in a public performance at UF and subsequent performances at the International OCD Foundation and American Psychological Association Conferences. Selected stories were videotaped and installed on the Centre for OCD and Related Disorders website for ongoing public use.[6]

The group was led by Pufahl, a theatre practitioner and research assistant professor in CAM, and engaged in a structured programme focusing on how to craft and perform a story. Each week, group members built trust through improvisational exercises and games and then shared stories about their OCD with each other in a relaxed setting. Weekly stories were improvised around themes and prompts suggested by the facilitation team such as *At My Best*, *Aha Moments* and *At My Worst*. The sessions were recorded and transcribed and then emailed to participants to revise and memorise. The following week, group members would perform their stories from memory for each other. Participants then collaborated in pairs and small groups to improve each other's stories – working to shape narrative elements such as good beginnings, hooks, tangents and endings that contained a realisation from the narrator's current perspective. With Pufahl's assistance, the group collectively suggested staging and movement ideas to help the storytellers physicalise their stories and connect with an audience. After rehearsing the stories, the group engaged in collective reflection where they discussed connections and resonances. During this time, more memories were shared and often stories were changed or developed further to include more details and personal aspects.

As the stories were refined, group members engaged in a process of collective dramaturgy to create the performance. Each participant selected two stories they wanted to share, which were distilled onto colour-coded notecards, with each colour representing a previously explored story theme. Next, the cards were organised on a table and the group collectively decided the order of the stories, allowing control over the show's content and structure (Pufahl *et al.*, 2021, p. 3). The storytellers were asked to provide images that would be projected on a screen behind them to accompany their stories. These images included collages of artwork (both personal and found), personal photographs and geographical destinations. Finally, Pufahl staged the show by placing the storytellers in a semi-circle on stage and having them come forward to tell their stories.

The resulting play, *Inside OCD: I Am Not My Illness*, was advertised to the public through the UF Performing Arts and CAM websites and by word of mouth. Approximately two hundred people attended the performance, and most of the audience stayed for an in-depth post-show discussion with the storytellers. The audience and storytellers discussed the process of making the show as well as reactions to the stories and insights into living with OCD or living with individuals with OCD. Although the audience was not surveyed on their impressions of the show, a theme of enhanced understanding of the condition among audience members emerged in the discussion, and a feeling of greater solidarity towards the storytellers was felt by the participants.

Following the programme, participants engaged in an online survey and in-person focus group to evaluate programme impact. Feelings of increased social connection and self-confidence were reported by most participants, and more than half reported they felt more control over their OCD symptoms at the end of the process (Pufahl *et al.*, 2021, p. 6). Focus group responses were grouped into four key themes: understanding and acceptance, connection and self-disclosure, creativity and confidence and vulnerability.

Pufahl and colleagues' report that participants 'endorsed a better understanding of their OCD and increased confidence about sharing their 'OCD stories', gaining acceptance from family and friends and feeling less shame and guilt related to their OCD diagnoses (ibid, p. 7). Participants reported an increased ability to laugh and to put their OCD symptoms in perspective, both in terms of their own life stories and in terms of the larger lived experience of others (ibid, p. 7). The overall benefits of the programme included improvements in participants' social support structures, relationships and feelings of wellbeing, as well as increased feelings of confidence and social connectedness and decreased feelings of social isolation (ibid, p. 8). Some participants expressed relief in 'getting their story out' and sharing previously undisclosed details of their OCD experience with family and friends (ibid, p. 8). The authors note that while the programme was not designed with therapeutic outcomes in mind, it did indeed have therapeutic value for most participants and could be considered a valuable part of a holistic care plan (ibid, p. 8).

While the performances were an integral part of this programme and helped drive the participants towards creating an audience-ready product, Pufahl did note that some participants felt anxiety around the performances. Achieving a performance was offered as an option for the group, and Pufahl made it clear performances could be cancelled. By going ahead with the performances, the group was able to feel the accomplishment that comes with a public showing of work, but the true benefits of the programme happened in the small group sessions when the participants were able to form connections and lasting bonds with each other.

Case study 3: storytelling for online audiences

In the aftermath of George Floyd's murder by a Minneapolis police officer[7] and subsequent global protests,[8] in 2021 CDC declared racism a public health crisis in the US (Wamsley, 2021). Following this, many US institutions began to more critically focus on inequities and impacts related to anti-Blackness. Some of those efforts included earmarking funding for relevant scholarship. Based at the University of Florida (UF), a predominantly white university institution (PWI) in the South-eastern US, the *Black Student Storytelling Project* (BSSP) was developed in response to a call for projects that support research aimed at better understanding the Black experience, racial justice, diversity and inclusion on campus and beyond. The project sought to collect storied vignettes of experiences from enrolled Black students on the following topics: anti-Black racism, social support and racial representation within the student body, faculty and administration. According to UF enrolment data, Black students represent less than six percent of the entire student body, a marginal swathe of the overall student population. For those interested and willing to participate, this was an opportunity to give voice to experiences that are in some ways undermined or unheard; a way to share the ways Black students have cultivated community, to call out instances they perceive as being anti-Black in nature and to propose solutions. Self-identified Black students aged eighteen years or older of all classifications, ethnicities, nationalities and majors were invited to participate, and seventy-two stories were collected.

Students were given a list of prompts to motivate thematic focus on the three topics. The prompts were written in a neutral format to encourage participants to share a range of experiences they felt most comfortable with, be they explicitly negative, positive, empowering, disempowering or otherwise. Participants were advised to meditate on the prompts to thoughtfully reflect on what they wanted to share before recording. When ready, they were given opportunities to record ten-minute first-person narratives on a personal device or book an in-studio appointment. Some students chose to script their stories in advance, while others improvised. Most students shared stories about past events, while others storified ongoing experiences in the present.

Because the project's impetus and inquiry engaged emotionally charged sense-making, the team was intentional about making sure students understood their right to withdraw from the study at any point. Additionally, participants were provided with campus resource lists, which included access to counselling services. Out of seventy-two participants, fifty agreed to publicly archive their audio, which has since been indexed in a digital collection through the university's library system and oral history programme.[9]

Midway through the project, the research team hosted a focus group. In the session, story audio was played for a live virtual audience of leaders from several Black student organisations. This was done as a reflective, confirmatory process and to further clarify connections between project themes and direct experiences they may have had with the students they serve. Student leaders were also able to be reflective about their lived experiences and transparent about the ways they plan to respond to the topics featured in the clips. Themes that emerged from the analysis of the focus groups were used to develop a report of suggestive actions to the university as a way of improving the campus environment for Black students.

BSSP is a commemorative point of documentation that reveals cultural beliefs, values, and experiences of Black students within a university community. While this programme did not engage people with a diagnosed mental disorder, it provided insights into some of the psychological distress experienced disproportionately by Black people in the US. The collected stories help listeners understand racism's crucial infringement on both the physical and mental health outcomes for those who experience it on both individual and systemic levels. Through digitisation efforts, BSSP remains a source for those interested in using the content in courses, conducting additional analyses or pursuing similar research. The audio packages, which contain individual narratives spliced together, show how first-person accounts overlap across narratives to coalesce common threads and reveal both individual and communal identities.

Research from BSSP serves several audiences, presenting various mental health-related processing experiences in response to anti-Black racist stressors. For participants, the recording process was a storytelling performance, and though it technically occurred 'backstage', the accessibility allows it to reach an audience without the performer experiencing the anxiety of a 'frontstage' performance. Many participants informally described the process as liberating, in part to the project offering a space for them to express their experiences as Black students in the aftermath of a racially polarising year. In member-checking focus groups with other Black student groups, students affirmed kinship connections they felt with fellow students while listening to their stories. The stories helped reify and identify commonality among Black student collegiate experiences.

Historically, institutions of higher learning in the US have practiced structural and cultural educational violence through anti-Black oppression (Mustaffa, 2017). This harm is especially noted at PWIs, as many have financially benefitted from historical inequalities (Von Robertson and Chaney, 2017), they currently acquire significant material wealth from Black student athletes (Bimper, 2015) and maintain memorialisation of racist iconography. Through systemic micro- and macro-aggressions, White supremacy thrives by producing a marginalising environment for US students of colour. Within such a climate, providing an opportunity for Black students to thoughtfully reflect on personal experiences that link to experiencing and/or overcoming anti-Black oppression at a PWI is both a self-definitional performance and a cathartic act of resilient resistance psychologically grounded in liberatory wellness (Collins, Kohfeldt and Kornbluh, 2020).

The collected stories represent a shared anthology of experiences among an intersectional swathe (that is, LGBTQ+, Caribbean, African and Black American and varied by gender) of Black students, and through the archival process they can exist in perpetuity without threat of an erasure that can suppress already marginal traces of Black student identity. For consumers of the stories, performative elements like pregnant pauses, voiced inflections, certain language choices and the emotional recall present in the recorded stories represent a specific moment in culture and time; an overarching goal of the project is to establish some sense of kinship among those relating to the stories and/or empathetic reflective action that leads to personal transformation. Additionally, the archive serves as an educational balm for any problematic wounds of misinformation specific to anti-Blackness and to yield insights for university administrators as they craft policies that cultivate more inviting, equitable environments for Black students who traditionally experience deep feelings of cultural and social exclusion (Huelsman, 2018).

How this story concludes

The value of storytelling in public health becomes more evident by its continued inclusion in community settings for public education, stigma reduction, reducing feelings of isolation and increasing feelings of connectedness (McCall *et al.*, 2019; Tsui and Starecheski, 2018). Additionally, storytelling has forged more inroads in public health by incorporating oral histories and digital practices (Patel and Patel, 2017). The COVID-19 global pandemic is a uniquely relevant example of pathography at play, whereby historians are contextualising societal responses to previous pandemics like the 1918 Spanish Flu, journalists are writing about infection experiences, and health communicators are coalescing with both groups to disseminate protective information on digital platforms.

However, as we deal with fallout from public health disasters both preventable and unexpected, we must more intentionally utilise the healing capacities of storytelling. Performance storytelling can elucidate upstream drivers of health disparities and can help us understand deeply rooted cultural behaviours intrinsically linked to community health. For example, COVID-19 narratives and storytelling have remained pivotal among populations managing related ailments. In online communities, COVID long-haulers engage in collective storytelling about coping with long-term symptoms (Rushforth *et al.*, 2021; Teh, 2021) and storytelling has been a resource for helping children process pandemic-related grief while confined at home (Pascal and Bertram, 2021; Sullivan and Paccione-Dyszlewski, 2020). Older adults have relied on storytelling as they deal with loneliness (Kim *et al.*, 2021), and through stories the public gained a deeper appreciation for essential workers' perseverance in service and health industries (Pangborn *et al.*, 2022).

Beyond COVID-19, the cases studies exemplify capabilities of storytelling in addressing several aspects of public health. We envision a future where broad recognition of storytelling catalyses movement towards more social prescribing[10] in tandem with, or in lieu of, pharmaceutical remedies, and the empowerment of collaborative relationships between researchers and practitioners within health, health care and the arts and humanities.

Notes

1 Each of the authors, listed here alphabetically, contributed to this article equally and share first authorship. The 'Rx' in the title refers to a common abbreviation for a medical prescription (derived from the Latin recipe, to prescribe).
2 https://alltimeshortstories.com/the-precious-stone/.
3 www.oklahoman.com/story/news/1998/12/21/the-healing-tongue/62258414007/.
4 https://alltimeshortstories.com/meaning-of-peace/.
5 www.virtuesproject.com/.
6 https://coard.psychiatry.ufl.edu/find-treatment/disorders-treatment/inside-ocd-i-am-not-my-illness/.
7 www.nytimes.com/2020/05/31/us/george-floyd-investigation.html.
8 www.nytimes.com/article/george-floyd-protests-timeline.html.
9 www.jou.ufl.edu/black-storytelling-project/.
10 www.who.int/publications/i/item/9789290619765.

Reference list

Addie, Y.O. (2019) 'African story time: an exploratory study of narrative as a reporting technique in US news coverage of Nigeria's missing girls', *The Journal of Public Interest Communications*, 3(2). https://doi.org/10.32473/jpic.v3.i2.p53

Addie, Y.O. and Pufahl, J. (2021) 'From colored to black: a narrative medicine approach to theatre and community reconciliation', *Public Health*, 197, pp. 36–38. https://doi.org/10.1016/j.puhe.2021.06.005

American Art Therapy Association (2017) *American art therapy association*. Available at: https://arttherapy.org/ (Accessed: 14 January 2022).

American Public Health Association (2022) *What is public health?* Available at: www.apha.org/what-is-public-health (Accessed: 11 August 2022).

Bimper Jr., A.Y. (2015) 'Lifting the veil: exploring colorblind racism in black student athlete experiences', *Journal of Sport and Social Issues*, 39(3). https://doi.org/10.1177/0193723513520013

Bruner, J.S. (1990) *Acts of meaning*. Cambridge, MA: Harvard University Press. https://doi.org/10.1017/s0033291700030555

Charon, R. (2001) 'Narrative medicine: a model for empathy, reflection, profession, and trust', *Journal of the American Medical Association*, 286(15), pp. 1897–1902.

Collins, C.R., Kohfeldt, D. and Kornbluh, M. (2020) 'Psychological and political liberation: strategies to promote power, wellness, and liberation among anti-racist activists', *Journal of Community Psychology*, 48(2). https://doi.org/10.1002/jcop.22259

Davies, S.C. *et al.* (2014) 'For debate: a new wave in public health improvement', *The Lancet*, 384(9957). https://doi.org/10.1016/S0140-6736(13)62341-7

Devakumar, D. *et al.* (2020) 'Racism, the public health crisis we can no longer ignore', *The Lancet*, 395(10242), pp. e112–e113.

Fakunle, D.O. *et al.* (2021) 'What Anansi did for us: storytelling's value in equitably exploring public health', *Health Education and Behavior*, 48(3). https://doi.org/10.1177/10901981211009741

Fricker, M. (2007) *Epistemic injustice: power and the ethics of knowing*. Oxford, UK: Oxford University Press.

Goffman, E. (1978) *The presentation of self in everyday life*. London: Harmondsworth.

Huelsman, M. (2018) *Social exclusion: the state of state U for black students*. Available at: www.demos.org/sites/default/files/publications/SocialExclusion_StateOf.pdf (Accessed: 14 January 2022).

Kim, J.E. *et al.* (2021) 'Effects of social prescribing pilot project for the elderly in rural area of South Korea during COVID-19 pandemic', *Health Science Reports*, 4(3), p. e320. https://doi.org/10.1002/hsr2.320

Lewis, P.J. (2009) 'Who in this culture speaks for children and youth?', in Lewis, P.J. and Tupper, J. (eds.) *Challenges bequeathed: taking up the challenges of Dwayne Huebner*. Rotterdam, NL: Sense, pp. 13–24. https://doi.org/10.1177/1077800411409883

Lewis, P.J. (2011) 'Storytelling as research/research as storytelling', *Qualitative Inquiry*, 17(6), pp. 505–510. https://doi.org/10.1177/1077800411409883

Litt, E. (2012) 'Knock, knock: who's there? The imagined audience', *Journal of Broadcasting & Electronic Media*, 56(3), pp. 330–345.

Lwin, S.M. (2009) 'Revisiting a structural analysis of folktales: a means to an end', *The Buckingham Journal of Language and Linguistics*, 2(1). https://doi.org/10.5750/bjll.v2i0.16

Marx, C., Benecke, C. and Gumz, A. (2017) 'Talking cure models: a framework of analysis', *Frontiers in Psychology*, 8, p. 1589. https://doi.org/10.3389/fpsyg.2017.01589

McCall, B. *et al.* (2019) 'Storytelling as a research tool and intervention around public health perceptions and behaviour: a protocol for a systematic narrative review', *BMJ Open*, 9(12), p. e030597. https://doi.org/10.1136/bmjopen-2019-030597

Mezirow, J. (2009) 'An overview on transformative learning', in Knud, I. (ed.) *Contemporary theories of learning: learning theorists – in their own words*. London and New York: Routledge.

Mustaffa, J.B. (2017) 'Mapping violence, naming life: a history of anti-black oppression in the higher education system', *International Journal of Qualitative Studies in Education*, 30(8). https://doi.org/10.1080/09518398.2017.1350299

National Storytelling Network (2022) *What is storytelling?* Available at: https://storynet.org/what-is-storytelling/ (Accessed: 11 August 2022).

Pangborn, S.M., Boatwright, M., Miller, C. and Velting, M. (2022) '"I don't feel like a hero": frontline healthcare providers' social media storytelling during COVID-19', *Health Communication*, 38, pp. 1508–1518. doi.org/10.1080/10410236.2021.2017108

Pascal, C. and Bertram, T. (2021) 'What do young children have to say? Recognizing their voices, wisdom, agency and need for companionship during the COVID pandemic', *European Early Childhood Education Research Journal*, 29(1). https://doi.org/10.1080/1350293X.2021.1872676

Patel, N. and Patel, N. (2017) 'Modern technology and its use as storytelling communication strategy in public health', *MOJ Public Health*, 6(3), 00171. https://doi.org/10.15406/mojph.2017.06.00171

Pufahl, J., Nainaparampil, J. and Mathews, C.A. (2021) 'Inside OCD: perspectives on the value of storytelling with individuals with OCD and family members', *Healthcare*, 9(8), p. 920. https://doi.org/10.3390/healthcare9080920

Rushforth, A. *et al.* (2021) 'Long COVID – the illness narratives', *Social Science and Medicine*, 286, p. 114326. https://doi.org/10.1016/j.socscimed.2021.114326

Sharma, A. and Grant, D. (2011) 'Narrative, drama and charismatic leadership: the case of Apple's Steve jobs', *Leadership*, 7(1). https://doi.org/10.1177/1742715010386777

Skloot, R. (2010) *The immortal life of Henrietta lacks*. New York: Crown.

Sullivan, M.A. and Paccione-Dyszlewski, M. (2020) 'Consider storytelling to help children cope during COVID-19', *The Brown University Child and Adolescent Behavior Letter*, 36(11). https://doi.org/10.1002/cbl.30503

Teh, C. (2021) *When medical diagnoses miss the mark and their families don't believe them, some COVID long-haulers turn to online groups for help*. Available at: www.insider.com/covid-long-haulers-are-turning-to-online-groups-for-help-2021-4 (Accessed: 11 January 2022).

Ten Have, H. and Jean, M. (eds.) (2009) *The UNESCO universal declaration on bioethics and human rights: background, principles and application*. Paris: UNESCO.

Tsui, E.K. and Starecheski, A. (2018) 'Uses of oral history and digital storytelling in public health research and practice', *Public Health*, 154. https://doi.org/10.1016/j.puhe.2017.10.008

Von Robertson, R. and Chaney, C. (2017) ' "I know it [racism] still exists here": African American males at a predominantly white institution', *Humboldt Journal of Social Relations*, 39. Available at: https://digital-commons.humboldt.edu/cgi/viewcontent.cgi?article=1015andcontext=hjsr (Accessed: 14 January 2022).

Wamsley, L. (2021) 'Derek Chauvin found guilty of George Floyd's murder', *Kera News*, 20 April. Available at: www.keranews.org/news/2021-04-20/derek-chauvin-found-guilty-of-george-floyds-murder (Accessed: 2 August 2023).

Weingarden, H. and Renshaw, K.D. (2015) 'Shame in the obsessive-compulsive related disorders: a conceptual review', *Journal of Affective Disorders*, 171, pp. 74–84.

Williams, D.R. (2018) 'Stress and the mental health of populations of color: advancing our understanding of race-related stressors', *Journal of Health and Social Behavior*, 59(4), pp. 466–485. https://doi.org/10.1177/0022146518814251

Yilmaz, R. and Ciğerci, F.M. (2019) 'A brief history of storytelling: from primitive dance to digital narration', in Recep Yılmaz, et al. (ed.) *Handbook of research on transmedia storytelling and narrative strategies*. Hershey, PA: IGI Global. https://doi.org/10.4018/978-1-5225-5357-1.ch001

Young, K. and Saver, J.L. (2001) 'The neurology of narrative', *Substance*, 30(94/95). https://doi.org/10.2307/3685505

25

DRAMA IN MENTAL HEALTH CARE

The development and use of schizodrama in the Brazilian psychiatric support service

Cinira Magali Fortuna, Felipe Lima dos Santos, Jorge Antônio Nunes Bichuetti, Maria de Fátima Oliveira and Silvia Matumoto

This chapter introduces a novel form of psychotherapeutic practice called 'schizodrama'. Developed in the 1970s by analyst and activist Gregorio Baremblitt, schizodrama involves participants and therapists creating dramatic performances as a way of addressing a wide range of mental health conditions. Its development has also been strongly influenced by a number of diverse theatre traditions. Schizodrama offers a radical alternative to predominant ways of understanding and addressing mental ill health and its psychosocial and political impacts. Above all, it engages participants in dramatic or drama-like activities so as to produce ways of being and becoming other than the hegemonic ways of thinking, feeling, acting and accumulating (Bichuetti, Oliveira and Amorin, 2004). This chapter also pays tribute to one of its proponents, Jorge Antônio Nunes Bichuetti, who shares its authorship. Bichuetti passed away during the production and publication of this chapter but will always remain present, illuminating and inspiring new becomings in our lives.

Schizodrama as inventive and caring art

Schizodrama was created by psychoanalyst Gregório Franklin Baremblitt in the 1970s in Argentina. Since then, it has spread and developed in Latin American and European countries, with Brazil forming an important centre. The Gregório Baremblitt Foundation (founded in 1991) and the Félix Guattari Institute (founded in 1996) are both located in the state of Mina Gerais (in the cities of Uberaba and Belo Horizonte, respectively) (Amorim and Querrien, 2013; Amorim *et al.*, 2021).

Schizodrama dramatises the philosophical concept of schizoanalysis, which was developed by Deleuze and Guattari in their works, originally published in English in 1977 and 1980, respectively, *Anti-Oedipus* (2013a) and *A Thousand Plateaus* (2013b). In these works, they respond to psychoanalyst Wilhelm Reich's exploration of how oppressive regimes – his study is of the mass psychology of fascism (2019) – are made possible by our psychological and psychosomatic states. Deleuze and Guattari propose schizoanalysis as a process of exploring and countering internalised capitalist regimes, in part through an engagement with irrationality.

In keeping with this, schizodrama starts from the premise that hegemonic social relations and capitalist modes of production lead to the mass production of subjugated subjectivities. In this way

DOI: 10.4324/9781003036500-29

of functioning, the consumption of objects and the 'objectualization' of the human itself as a commodity to be sold and consumed produces devitalised existences. Schizodrama is used in 'klinics' (the termed coined by Baremblitt to indicate care work informed by schizoanalysis) with the aim of exposing and breaking stereotypes through individual or collective experiences. By doing this, schizodrama can renew life and creative potential and, to use the term developed by Deleuze and Guattari, produce subjectivities in 'becoming' (Baremblitt, 2013). It is a clinical intervention tool designed to enable an experimental deconstruction of one's 'sick' ways of functioning and the experience of inventing new ways of existing, new life trajectories (Baremblitt, 2019).

As will become clear in the accounts that follow, a schizodramatic session will typically be led by one or more therapists (psychodramatists) working with an individual or a group. It does not have a fixed number of participants, and the setting is freely assembled: it can happen in the frame of the room or in the free space of the street. The participants will be led through what we call an 'experience'. Each experience will be assembled in a unique way in response to the particular situation of pain or difficulty experienced by those being cared for. Therapists will draw from their own 'toolbox' of approaches, for example, using psychodrama, street theatre, performance, gestalt, bioenergetics, tribal and folk ritual, yoga and children's games and dances (including the Brazilian version of 'ring around the roses', called cirandas) (Hur, 2020). Baremblitt himself referred to a range of theatre practitioners as influences, including Artaud, Brecht, Boal, Beckett, Ionesco, Pavlovsky, Gó, Kabuki and more (2014). Baremblitt was not particularly concerned with the differences and tensions between some of these authors' productions or affiliations but focused instead on using any tools these authors' work could provide in the construction of schizodrama and its experiences.

In responding to the individual needs of participants, the therapist uses their body as an instrument of work, attentive to the emotions that they propose to the group and experiencing the group's scenes – stories not told with words and that are not concerned with logic – with participants. An experience does not obey a normalising script, though it will often move participants from the enactment of a dreaded scene, moving through painful repetition, to the explorative search for a way out from new departure points created in the process. The invented scenes are often guided by the possibility of becoming another through the playing of archetypes such as animals, children; warriors; 'mad people' (the 'louco/a' cultural stereotype); or forces of nature such as winds, tides, tsunamis, lightning, storms, breezes, light waves and waterfalls (Baremblitt, 2014). Music and props may also be used (Bichuetti, Oliveira and Amorin, 2004).

Schizodrama in the clinic provides care for someone's pain and allows everyone to review an issue and their own wounds through resonance. It also provides care by foregrounding a particular theme, allowing the participants to discover and reinvent themselves in the collective, therapeutic work. It explores the lived body on the limit, through intensification and experiment, dramatisation, with the opportunity of flight, of the jump, of the bridge, of the anchor, whilst avoiding the whirlpools and the abyss, with the production of new senses and new existential horizons (Hur, 2020).

Schizodrama is used in a wide range of settings and communities across health, education, the arts and prisons. In this chapter we describe its use in the field of mental health in a psychosocial care centre (CAPS) that dedicates its existence to the care of people in psychological distress. Before that, we provide some background on the development of the CAPS in Brazil.

The Psychosocial Care Centres

The psychiatric reforms emerged from a period of reform dating from the 1970s influenced by community psychiatry in the United States of America and specially in Europe. In February 1963, the Community Mental Health Center Act was decreed by President John F. Kennedy, redirecting the efforts of psychiatry towards prevention through paying attention to mental health in the community rather than the medicalisation and, at times, incarceration of those living with poor mental health (Paulin and Turato, 2004). In Brazil, this attention to preventative measures led to opposition to the established model of psychiatric care through private 'asylums' (Paulin and Turato, 2004). A series of national conferences in the 1980s and 1990s led to the emergences of new community-based services and programmes. A historic milestone for the mental health sector was the Regional Conference for the Restructuring of Psychiatric Assistance, held in Caracas in 1990, which led to changes at the level of the Ministry of Health. At this meeting, Brazil signed on to a final document entitled 'Declaration of Caracas' in which Latin American countries undertook to promote the restructuring of psychiatric care; critically review the hegemonic and centralising role of the psychiatric hospital; safeguard civil rights, personal dignity and human rights of users; and provide alternative services in their community environment (Hirdes, 2009).

Psychiatric reform is a complex political and social process, composed of actors, institutions and forces from different origins, which affects different territories, in the federal, state and municipal governments; in universities; in the health services; in professional councils; in the associations of people with mental disorders and their families; in social movements; and in the territories of the social imagination and public opinion. Understood as a set of transformations of practices, knowledge, cultural and social values, it is in the daily life of institutions, services and interpersonal relationships that the process of psychiatric reform advances, marked by impasses, tensions, conflicts and challenges (Brasil, 2005).

The psychosocial care centres in their different modalities are strategic points of attention for the Brazilian Psychosocial Care Network: these are open community health services constituted by multi-professional teams that work from an interdisciplinary perspective and primarily provide care to people with disabilities and mental ill health, including those with needs arising from the use of alcohol and other drugs, in their local area, whether in crisis situations or in psychosocial rehabilitation processes, and are substitutes for the asylum model (Brasil, 2022). The activities developed in these spaces are quite diversified, offering group and individual care, therapeutic and creative workshops, physical activities, recreational activities and art therapy, in addition to medication, which was previously considered the main form of treatment. In this service, the family is considered a fundamental part of the treatment process, accessing specific care (group or individual) and free access to the service whenever necessary (Brasil, 2022).

The CAPS Maria Boneca is a service associated with the Brazilian Unified Health System (SUS) through its sponsor, the Gregorio Franklin Baremblitt Foundation. This allied service has been in operation since 1991, having entered into an agreement with the SUS in 1994 (Baremblitt, 2013). In what follows, we describe three schizodramatic experiences that took place in Psychosocial Care Centre Maria Boneca CAPS. Each of these was witnessed by two of the authors of this paper. The aim of describing these experiences is to demonstrate the variety of ways schizodrama is used as well as exemplifying its extraordinary capacity to generate change.

Schizodramatic experience 01 – danced mourning, the angel becomings and (en)chants

3 March 1996: it was a sober day and everyone in the centre was sad, crestfallen, afraid: on the previous day, a plane carrying the rock band Mamonas Assassinas had crashed into the Cantareira mountains, killing all its members. The young musicians were famous for their comic satirising

of bourgeois life and for challenging politically correct standards of language and dance. Their sudden death at the height of the band's success produced feelings of grief and loss throughout the country, and at CAPS it was no different.

We felt that the sad occasion needed to be marked, so the usual schedule of activities at the centre was cancelled and, instead, all forty patients and six therapists came together to listen to the news and share memories. We decided to perform a schizodrama on the theme of pain, mourning, the accident and the band. It began with a warm-up, designed to make us present to each other and start to release the emotions – to 'deterritorialize'. We all came together in a circle in the garden of the Centre, in an area demarcated by the shade of the jabuticaba trees. The warm-up also involved walking around the space, following our gaze, until, on the lead therapist's demand, we expressed our grief: some broke into a waltz, others spun their bodies on the spot, sang, sighed or practiced holotropic breathing techniques. We then fell into silence, eyes closed, observing our physical sensations and emotions.

After a minute, the scene unfroze with one of the band's songs, 'Pelados em Santos' (Naked in Santos). The song is about a young man attempting a seduce a woman – he compliments her and invites her to the beach. But he is turned down because she thinks his car is too tacky. The rhythm of the song is infectious and soon we were dancing and singing. The therapist leading the session then invited each of us to 'connect' with an emotion we were feeling in that moment and express it through performance. A gesture. A bodily scream.

We were then divided into four groups, each group tasked to improvise a scene. Guided by the feelings expressed earlier in the session, these are the scenes that emerged:

Scene 1: The plane and its crash. Fatal shock.
Scene 2: Everyone standing around a body on the ground. Cries, a cry mixed with a painful prayer.
Scene 3: Boys play and then, scared by an angry dog, run away.
Scene 4: The band members arrive in heaven and perform a concert with the angels.

All seated in a circle, we took it in turns to reflect on the scenes. We also talked about what the band meant to each of us, its association with the joy and lightness of childhood. Given the significance of 'becoming child' in the work of Deleuze and Guattari, this theme of childhood was taken up in another set of scenes that the groups were then asked to improvise. This time, each improvisation was followed by discussion or exercises, chosen by the lead therapist in response to the scene.

Scene 5: Children fly kites and blow soap bubbles, and in a joyful ritual they move in a circle interpreting the band members as superheroes, flying and reaching the sky.

After this scene, the group applauded and hugged each other. A young woman started weeping and spoke of her loneliness. Making a swing with their crossed arms, other group members gathered her up and rocked her, soothing her with a lullaby. Later, she thanked the group, imitating the lead singer by saying she had found a 'madly loving family'.

Scene 6: The group has a picnic on the mountain and sings, playing in circles. They call everyone and they thank the joy of the art of the band through song.

This time, the therapist suggested a 'conversation circle' (a technique for structuring dialogue originally developed by Freire, 1970) that enables everyone to express their responses. Sensing the fragility and shyness of the group, the therapist then performed an energising rain dance, encouraging the group to join in. The shift of mood led to the spontaneous expression of gratitude, affection and farewell to the band.

Scene 7: Children play and night falls. Frightened, they experience the despair and terror of a severe panic attack.

In response to the sense of despair expressed in this scene, the therapist set up an exercise drawn from transpersonal psychology (Davis, 2010). Modelled on the principle of ego death and rebirth, the exercise supports participants' ability to cope with depressive experiences and psychological challenges. In the conversation after this, there was a comment expressing surprise: how the body discovers its own vitality.

Scene 8: The children fly flowers over the mountain.

The discussion after this last scene turned to the pain of losing people we love and people who are heroes to us. Someone suggested conducting a goodbye ceremony and the group accepted. There was singing: songs by Mamonas Assasinas, and also the hymn sung at the CAPS assemblies, 'O canto dos pescadores' by Dorival Caymmi, a song about the risks and joys of sea fishing on a raft. Standing in a circle holding hands, we recited the Lord's Prayer, which was followed by a group hug.

To close, a therapist suggested another conversation circle, in which we were asked to say a word to the Mamonas Assassinas and state what we would take away from the meeting and from the band. These are some of the things that were said:

'I felt stronger; it hurts a lot when we suffer alone'
'By playing we discover that we are strong and united!'
'I understood that the Mamonas are also the children that we have repressed and shut up
    inside our chest'
'I saw that playing relieves pain'

The experiment made CAPS more CAPS, a collective with body and movement, resistant, inventive, supportive, a society of friends. It involved us in becoming – becoming a child, an angel and a warrior. It exorcised the pent-up pains. It allowed the invention of a collective ideal.

Schizodramatic experience 02 – deserts, oases: the journey and the return

We present in the following a schizodramatic session involving a forty-year-old female patient, Sarah,[1] who was welcomed and cared for at the Psychosocial Care Centre Maria Boneca while she was going through a psychotic episode. The account is drawn from her medical records and as recollected by the psychotherapist, Luna.

When Luna first met Sarah, at 8 am one morning in 1993, she was crouched in a cardboard box in the stairwell of the reception area at the Centre. She was terrified, and it was only after long negotiation that she was persuaded to leave her hiding place. Once out of the box, Luna stayed with her but was not able to communicate, as Sarah's medication made her inarticulate. Sarah sat, making unintelligible sounds, until lunchtime, when she accepted a plate of pasta. It was only after this that Sarah agreed to accompany Luna to one of the therapy rooms.

For the first quarter of an hour in the room, Sarah sat up, making very loud noises. Then she announced that she was lost in the middle of the desert. Luna asked if she wanted company and

Sarah said yes. So began what would become a three-hour psychodramatic 'journey across the desert'. During this time Luna followed Sarah's cues as she described the various landscapes and encounters involved. Luna's role was to actively listen, fully alert and sharply perceptive, affecting and being affected, but not to try to understand or interpret the dizzying episodes that Sarah narrated. Her main technique for engaging with Sarah was to hand her objects that supported the imaginative journey: they hunted for gourds, wove objects into garments, built huts. Entire scenes were narrated, involving sand settlements, encounters with nomads, struggles with hostile people, kidnapping, rescue. An abrupt stop at an oasis, fresh water to drink and bathe in.

At the end of the afternoon, the patient announced that she did not want to leave the desert. At this point Luna felt it was important to convince her of the need to come back; that she could enjoy the trip, return when she wanted to, but not to become trapped in the 'desert'. At long last, Sarah returned from her crisis, exhausted and very calm. She was amused by all the paraphernalia she found as she came to: both patient and psychotherapist were wearing blankets.

A few weeks of daily treatment followed, involving intensive psychotherapy (workshops, group and individual therapy), nursing and medical care and engaging with the communal life of the Centre. It was only after this that Sarah reported the episode that had brought her to the clinic: a horrific hallucination of bloody slaughter which struck her while she was at a bus station on her way to hospital. When she started screaming, the police were called. They, in turn, had called the fire department, who took her to an emergency care unit, from where she was referred to a psychiatric hospital. It was her father who had taken her from the hospital to CAPS Maria Boneca.

It should be reported that Sarah has not had another mental health crisis since the schizodramatic session, despite concerns that the hallucinations might return.

Schizodramatic experience 03 – psychiatric reform fight in the bodies and in the streets: the broken-winged birds that fly

In the 'individual patient care programme' (Programa Terapêutico Singular) at CAPS Maria Boneca, a schizodrama is produced weekly, on Tuesdays from 1 pm to 2:30 pm. It is an activity open to everyone who wants to participate: patients, therapists, interns, visitors and academics from other municipalities who visit the CAPS. This programme has been in existence since the Centre was founded over thirty years ago, coordinated by the schizodramatist Maria de Fátima Oliveira, who has been joined more recently by Raquel Bessa, Camila Bahia and Lillian Naves. Ordinarily, it is the patients themselves who propose the themes of the schizodramas. The theme of the schizodrama described here was the campaign for psychiatric reform and the demonstrations that regularly took place during the annual Carnival in the streets of Uberaba (for the past eighteen years, CAPS Maria Boneca has had its own carnival block).

On an April afternoon around six years ago, a group of patients and four professionals and interns got together to work on a schizodrama that they wanted to perform on May 18, the National Anti-Asylum Fight Day in Brazil. Once the proposal was announced, an improvisation began to the sound of a drum, involving whole movement, dancing, inventing capoeira games, intensifying breathing, inventing songs, sounds. In the midst of all this noise, one of the patients who regularly participated in the schizodramas abruptly walked away, went to a spot on the balcony, bent down, picked something up and came back to the group crying. Gradually everyone stopped and surrounded this woman. She held out the palm of her hand and there was a bird with a damaged wing. She said she had noticed the bird while she was dancing and realised that it was not able to fly.

The group jumped into action: a cardboard box was found, food brought from the kitchen, the bird was carefully wrapped, the whole group surrounding and protecting it. The patient who found the bird stopped crying; she looked at everyone and said very seriously: 'Until I arrived at CAPS to be treated, I was just like this little bird. The crises, my depression left me unable to fly. Now I have an injured wing, I don't care, I fly anyway'. As she spoke, she moved her right shoulder in a gesture that suggested a broken wing, and there, sitting on the ground, many people imitated her gesture. A therapist repeated the movement. The group invented a dance, which entered CAPS history as the dance of the bird with a broken wing.

Later, the group discussed the intensity of the moment and decided to embody the metaphor of the bird with the broken wing as part of the schizodrama for the Anti-Asylum event: 'We the mentally ill, the "crazy" (loucos/as), are birds with broken wings, but we learned how to fly, a little crooked, a little unbalanced, we fly different from the others, but we fly'. After delicate debate among the group, it was decided that they would take many birds to the demonstration. One of the nursing technicians was talented at making origami and that day taught the group how to make birds. Soon, this practice flooded the Centre so that wherever you went, people were making these paper birds. The birds were shaped and painted to depict a species of stork native to Brazilian wetland areas called Tuiuiú. Some choose to write notes and attach them to the paper birds, in the manner of carrier pigeons – 'We are mentally ill. We are birds with broken wings, but we learned how to fly', one read. Other Maria Boneca patients expressed themselves after the schizodrama session, as follows:

'Don't lock up, life sweats. Help a broken-winged bird fly'
'Madness is the loneliness of those who love, let the birds fly'.
'Freedom even if you are crazy, don't lock the birds too'.
'A caress for you, a bird with a broken wing, take care of him'.

The tuiuiús appeared all over the CAPS, they attended the Carnival, flying through the city squares, handed out to passersby, 'forgotten' in the trees and delivered to schools. In fact, they lasted long after the Anti-Asylum demonstration, appearing as birthday gifts, in Christmas trees and around the building. They made further public appearances, for example, after environmental accidents at the ore damns in Mariana and Brumadinho, both in the Minas Gerais area. They composed with the rivers, houses and bodies that were covered in mud, transmuted in the schizodramas into green rivers, blue rivers, with macaws, rufous-bellied thrush and kiskadee. They featured in further Anti-Asylum demonstrations and on banners sent to the city of Brumandinho, as gifts made to the fire service and the psychology council there.

Mementos remain into the present day at CAPS Maria Boneca, where sooner or later one bumps into a tuiuiú that detaches from some object and enters the scene in these pandemic times, with so many broken wings that ask for shelter and care. As for the original bird with an injured wing, it was cared for in the house, attended to until one day it was not found.

Conclusion

The three schizodramatic experiences reported here took very different forms in response to the participant groups and their needs. This draws attention to a key feature of the experiences employed in schizodrama: its improvisatory nature. Rather than having a drama thought out *a priori*, the experiences emerge from the need for care, from the here and now connected to the local context and guided by principles such as the universal right to all forms of life.

The experiments depend on the skills of the therapists who draw on their knowledge and skill in crisis management and their many years 'klinical' experience through which they have developed therapeutic work (Bichuetti, 2000; Bichuetti *et al.*, 2013). This enables the therapists to accompany a process that emerges in the encounter with patients, maintaining the spontaneity that is an important resource in schizodrama. The therapist places themself as a radar, sensitive to movements and affections. They improvise and propose ideas for the scenes to be experienced, paying close attention to the effects produced in action then and there. There is no advanced planning about where the scenes will arrive, and it is not even known what will happen, so the unprecedented and the uncertain are part of the therapeutic process. In this sense, the unprecedented and the improvised are the result of interactions between patients with other patients and between patients and therapists and make up the power of care and the production of multiple meanings for experiences and suffering.

As these accounts illustrate, schizodrama works as a set of strategies, tactics and techniques that seek to act on the subjective, social, physical aspects of participants. In the language of Deleuze and Guattari, it provides experience of 'deterritorialization' rather than necessarily seeking what would conventionally be called a 'cure'. Nevertheless, Baremblitt reports a range of positive effects: the formation of a proactive attitude; greater lightness and softness in everyday life; decrease and/or disappearance of symptoms, repetitions, blocks and complexes; ability to combine delusions with reality, expanding the world view; creative becomings; containment of aggressive impulses; production of new meanings and outlining of novel directions of life project construction; and a greater capacity to love, work, play and dream (Baremblitt, 2013). Rather than seeing these effects as a cure for ill health, in the modus operandi of this clinic, a more modest claim is made: that participants manage to produce more meanings, allowing life with all its vicissitudes to move forward. According to Bichuetti, who passed away during the writing of this chapter and debuted on the path of the stars, leaving nostalgia, affections, encounters and enchantments:

> The Schizodrama, drama of becoming, a creative, singular invention by Gregório Baremblitt. We can approach this work proposal, which is a possibility and a path, perceiving the leap, the rupture, the innovation. . . . The schizodrama is, essentially, the possibility and the nomadic adventure of the new that emerges from experimentation, from life unveiled in the exploration of what a body can do. . . . It experiments, invents new possibilities of life. It explores, beyond the ego, the territories of becoming, the I unborn.
>
> (2021, pp. 30–31)

Note

1 Pseudonyms are used for any individual patients and therapists named in these accounts in order to protect anonymity.

Reference list

Amorim, M. and Querrien, A. (2013) 'Vingt ans de squizodrame au Brésil', *Chimères*, 80(2), pp. 19–30. https://doi.org/10.3917/chime.080.0019

Amorim, M. *et al.* (2021) 'Gregório Franklin Baremblitt, o guerreiro do devir: cuidado, insurgências inventivas, utopias libertárias', *Memorandum: Memória e História em Psicologia*, 38, pp. 1–11. https://doi.org/10.35699/1676-1669.2021.36967

Baremblitt, G.F. (2013) *Dez proposições descartáveis acerca do esquizodrama*. Available at: https://institutogregoriobaremblitt.wordpress.com/2015/05/27/dez-proposicoes-descartaveis-acerca-do-esquizodrama/ (Accessed: 12 March 2022).

Baremblitt, G.F. (2014) 'Presentación del Esquizodrama', *Teoría y crítica de la psicología*, 4, pp. 17–23. Available at: http://teocripsi.com/ojs/index.php/TCP/article/view/54 (Accessed: 2 August 2023).

Baremblitt, G.F. (2019) *Esquizodrama: 10 proposições descartáveis*. Belo Horizonte: Instituto Gregorio Baremblitt.

Bichuetti, J.N. (2000) *Crisevida – Outras Lembranças*. Belo Horizonte: Instituto Feliz Guattari.

Bichuetti, J.N. (2021) *Grupo como engenhoca de produção de saúde e vida, cidadania e devir*. Uberaba: Jorge Nunes Bichuetti.

Bichuetti, J.N., Oliveira, M.F. and Amorin, M. (2004) 'Esquizoanálise e produção do conhecimento: o uso do esquizodrama na pesquisa', in *Monografia (Curso de Especialização em Análise Institucional e Esquizoanálise)*. Belo Horizonte: Instituto Felix Guattari.

Bichuetti, J.N. *et al.* (2013) 'CAPS (Centre d'accueil psychosocial) Maria Boneca', *Chimères*, 80(2), pp. 42–51. https://doi.org/10.3917/chime.080.0042

Brasil (2005) *Reforma Psiquiátrica e política de Saúde Mental no Brasil: Conferência Regional de Reforma dos Serviços de Saúde Mental: 15 anos depois de Caracas*. Brasília: Ministério da Saúde. Secretaria de Atenção à Saúde. DAPE. Coordenação Geral de Saúde Mental, pp. 1–56.

Brasil (2022) *Centro de Atenção Psicossocial – CAPS*. Available at: www.gov.br/saude/pt-br/acesso-a-infor macao/acoes-e-programas/caps (Accessed: 10 March 2022).

Davis, J. (2010) 'An overview of transpersonal psychology', *The Humanistic Psycologist*, 31(2–3), pp. 6–21. https://doi.org/10.1080/08873267.2003.9986924

Deleuze, G. and Guattari, F. (2013a) *Anti-Oedipus: capitalism and Schizophenia*. London: Bloomsbury Methuen Drama Publishing.

Deleuze, G. and Guattari, F. (2013b) *A thousand plateaus: capitalism and Schizophenia*. London: Bloomsbury Methuen Drama Publishing.

Freire, P. (1970) *Pedagogia do oprimido*. Rio de Janeiro: Paz e Terra.

Hirdes, A. (2009) 'A reforma psiquiátrica no Brasil: uma (re) visão', *Ciência & Saúde Coletiva*, 14(1), pp. 297–305. https://doi.org/10.1590/S1413-81232009000100036

Hur, D. (2020) 'A Clínica do Corpo sem Órgãos: Esquizoanálise e Esquizodrama', *Porto Arte: Revista de Artes Visuais*, 25(44), pp. 1–17. https://doi.org/10.22456/2179-8001.110078

Paulin, L.F. and Turato, E.R. (2004) 'Antecedentes da reforma psiquiátrica no Brasil: as contradições dos anos 1970', *História, Ciências, Saúde-Manguinhos*, 11(2), pp. 241–258. https://doi.org/10.1590/S0104-597 02004000200002

Reich, W. (2019) *Psicologia de Massas do Fascismo*. São Paulo: Martins Fontes.

26

ILLNESS AND THE ONE-TO-ONE ENCOUNTER

Brian Lobel and Emily Underwood-Lee

We enter the room of a parent/carer and her 18-year-old child. Her child, who lives with complex medical needs, is about to transition to adult care after spending his whole life receiving paediatric care from Great Ormond Street Hospital. We are dressed in costumes related quite literally to self-care and relaxation: fuzzy slippers, colourful bathrobes, eye masks perched on our foreheads. We begin our performance/questionnaire which, despite our costumes, raises no red flags; this mother is used to being asked questions by medical staff she has never met and will sometimes never meet again. She slowly realises that the questionnaire is fun, funny, and art-y, and very quickly says 'I don't have very much to say . . .' about what it means to be a parent/carer of a child at Great Ormond Street, what it means to care for herself alongside caring for her child, what it means to relax, dream, and vision new futures.

'I don't have very much to say' she says . . . and then she speaks, uninterrupted, for forty-five minutes.

In this chapter we argue that there are useful parallels to be found between one-to-one performance and the medical encounter and that, by bringing this often avant-garde performance form to the hospital space, there is much to be gained for audiences/patients, institutions, and artists. Ultimately, we argue for a care-filled and compassionate ethical encounter that opens up new possibilities for one-to-one performance as part of the arts and health exchange. We consider the benefits of one-to-one arts encounters within the hospital space with particular reference to our *Kicking Up Our Heels* project – performed for parents/carers in 2018 and 2019 at Great Ormond Street Hospital, London (GOSH) – alongside *Footwashing for the Sole* (2009), a one-to-one performance by Adrian Howells. We have used the term parent/carer throughout to indicate the many routes by which we might come to be in a parental role for a child.

Kicking Up Our Heels was evaluated and reflected upon in 2020 by creative facilitator Anna Ledgard, who described the project formally as:

Artists Brian Lobel and Emily Underwood-Lee invited Parents & Carers to take part in a playful performative 'survey' about how they nurtured and looked after themselves whilst caring for a child in the hospital. In their responses parents were encouraged to get beyond the notion of the 'good parent' who subjugates their needs for those of their children. The responses were used by Emily Speed to design a permanent artwork, *Cocoon*, which was

DOI: 10.4324/9781003036500-30

installed at GOSH in February 2020 and was accompanied by a paper booklet *You are Doing a Great Job*, which incorporated ideas and activities offered by parents to improve their own and others' wellbeing.

(2020)

For our 'playful performative survey', dressed in colourful bathrobes and fuzzy slippers, we asked parents/carers survey-style multiple-choice questions about how much time they practiced self-care, walked in nature, slept, and so on, knowing that most answers to the questions would be 'Not at all!'. With a gentle wink and a shared understanding of how little they take care of themselves when their child is sick, we then asked them more open-ended questions about their own rituals, advice, and dreams of spaces that would enable more self-care. Ranging from five to forty-five minutes, the performances were attended by Brian and/or Emily, creative facilitator Anna, the parent/carer, and – more often than not – their child, either actively listening, contributing, or lying asleep. Though not always strictly 'one-to-one', the intimate interaction was much more akin to one-to-one performance than any traditional stage show, and it is through the lens of one-to-one performance that we examine the piece here.

Arts, health, and parents

The existing literature on the impact of parental mental health on the wellbeing of children is considerable (Barlow *et al.*, 2014), although there is less literature specifically engaging with the needs of parents/carers whose children are undergoing hospital treatment. In their review of the literature on psychological interventions for parents/carers of children with chronic illness, Christopher Eccleston *et al.* note that the data linking parental psychological health to paediatric patient outcomes is slight and has not been consistently replicated (2015, p. 26). Emily Law *et al.* note that, although difficult to prove causality, there is significant literature that demonstrates indirect links, specifically in relation to 'child mental health, behavior, and medical symptoms' and suggest that children's treatment should always be designed with a view of the needs of the whole family (2014, p. 880).

There is also a growing field of literature informing us that access to and participation in the arts is effective for improving wellbeing. Daisy Fancourt and Saoirse Finn conducted a review of over 900 articles examining the benefit of arts and health and found that engagement with the arts is effective for both prevention of ill-health as well as promotion of health-improving behaviours and for the management and treatment of health conditions. They identified claims for psychological, physiological, social, and behavioural benefit from engagement with the arts (2019, p. 3). In a modest study undertaken with participants in a ten-week arts on prescription programme, Anita Jensen and Wenche Torrissen found a specific link between aesthetic engagement and mental health improvement. Although the study only worked with seven participants, we are particularly interested to note that it considered the role of aesthetics where many other studies struggle to differentiate whether positive outcomes are a result of social engagement, movement, or community building which occur within an arts encounter but could also be found in many other community classes or social, physical, or cultural settings. Jensen and Torrissen state:

Although more research is needed to explore the complex connections between aesthetic engagement and wellbeing, this study has shown that aesthetic engagement can create deep emotional experiences that can change the distribution of the sensible in ways that have a significant impact on people's lives and wellbeing.

(2019, p. 246)

In the context of the United Kingdom, the 2017 report 'Creative Health: The Arts for Health and Wellbeing', commissioned by the All-Party Parliamentary Group on Arts, Health and Wellbeing, noted that there is inconsistent evidence linking the arts with health outcomes, and highlighted the research challenges of proving a causal relationship between arts participation and health and wellbeing benefits (2017, p. 11). However, with this caveat in mind, the 'Creative Health' publication still reports that participation and engagement with the arts can improve health and wellbeing significantly:

> [participation in the arts can] stimulate imagination and reflection; encourage dialogue with the deeper self and enable expression; change perspectives; contribute to the construction of identity; provoke cathartic release; provide a place of safety and freedom from judgement; yield opportunities for guided conversations; increase control over life circumstances; inspire change and growth; engender a sense of belonging; prompt collective working; and promote healing.
>
> (2017, p. 21)

We knew that parents' mental health was critical for enduring their own experience while parenting a child undergoing treatment at the hospital; we knew that, in turn, this would have a significant impact on the care they were able to provide to their child; we knew that parents' mental health and resilience could be improved by engaging in arts activities; and we knew that at the point that we entered the hospital, parents/carers were not attending arts events. These assertions provided the starting point for our *Kicking Up Our Heels* project created for GOSH Arts, the arts programme at Great Ormond Street Hospital. Though the GOSH Arts team, over the years, had repeatedly provided events specifically designed for parents/carers and also staged a range of events that parents/carers could participate in with their children or with staff from the hospital, we were told that parents/carers were very reluctant to attend anything that forced them to leave their child's room. Both the authors of this chapter, Brian and Emily, also had lived experience of hospital treatment for young people – Brian as a young adult cancer patient undergoing treatment for metastatic testicular cancer in the early 2000s (whilst living with his parents) and Emily as the mother of a child undergoing treatment for acute lymphoblastic leukaemia between 2011 and 2015. It was in 2018 that we, Brian and Emily, began conversations with Caroline Moore, then arts manager at GOSH Arts, in order to think about how we might be able to provide bespoke arts encounters for the parents/carers of children being treated at GOSH.

Parents

Influenced by Sara Ruddick's call to think of mothering not as a biological state but as a way of thinking and doing (1989), we define parenting as the work done by anyone in a position of care for a child, regardless of their route to nurturing. Ruddick, in her seminal book *Maternal Thinking*, asks us to imagine mothering not as the biological production of a child but as a way of thinking and acting that emerges from love. Ruddick is clear that, although this way of thinking maternally arises from biological mothering, it is not limited to biological mothers, or indeed to biological fathers, nor do all biological mothers feel love towards their child; instead, maternal thinking can be carried out by anyone, and maternal actions can be directed towards anyone (1989). In this way, maternal thinking can be extended not just to children by parents/carers but towards whomever needs our love and care. Virginia Held extends this thinking towards action and ethics, articulating that 'care is both a practice and a value' (2006, p. 42). It is not just in what we believe, but how this is enacted, that care is made manifest.

Rethinking parenting to extend beyond the biological acts of birth and caring for 'our own' children in this way is radical and political. It allows us to extend our thinking about parenting beyond the biological parent, and more usually the biological mother, to think of the wider relationships we might encounter and experience as family, and the infinite ways that family and community might be constructed and queered. In the UK, where the *Kicking Up Our Heels* project took place, we may come to be the primary care-giver for a child through legal, biological, or medical routes generally recognised by institutions, or we might come to be responsible for a child through our networks of care including chosen families, extended families, and infinite other constructions, or what bell hooks might term our 'kinship structures' (hooks, 2000, p. 37). At GOSH, we encountered people acting in parental roles who had come to that position in myriad diverse ways, including through friendships and through extended family relationships such as siblings, grandparents, aunts, uncles, and so forth. Further, when we begin to think about parenting as taking care and responsibility for another, we see many staff working within the hospital setting as in a parental role, including play workers, translators, porters, nurses, radiologists, and many more. Thinking of parenting in this way enabled us to work with anyone within the hospital who wanted to engage in an encounter with us. This meant that we initially worked with one hundred families or kin of young patients of GOSH but then extended the *Kicking Up Our Heels* project to provide a workshop at the annual GOSH staff conference in order to work with those staff members who also provide care and felt the desire for a space in which to reflect on their own needs.

Care

If we accept our proposal to redefine parental roles as being care-full of another, then we are required to consider exactly what is meant by care. Joan Tronto has made in-depth studies of what it means to care and how care is a political act. She helpfully articulates this: 'Care requires not only nurturing relationships, but also the physical and mental work of taking care of, cleaning up after, and maintaining bodies' (2013, p. 2). This definition of care is particularly helpful for our needs in this chapter as the parallels between caring as a parent/carer and caring as a member of staff within a hospital become immediately apparent. Tronto expands on her conception of care to note that it is a public value and that this is central to society (ibid, p. 18). Following Tronto, and in parallel with medical literature that notes that those whose wellbeing and mental health needs are not being met are less able to care for others (Cameron *et al*., 2020, p. 766), we can argue that without good care no-one can flourish, including those who are required to give care professionally or in parental roles. Here we are again reminded that if parents/carers and staff within the hospital are not cared for, they will be less able to care for their children/patients, and physical, psychological, and emotional outcomes will be worse for everyone.

Tronto notes several key aspects of care including: 'caring about', 'caring for' and 'receiving care' (2015, p. 7). 'Caring about' requires that we are attentive to the needs of others, be those others in our immediate circle, in our wider societies, or those other global citizens with whom we share the planet. 'Caring for' requires that we take responsibility for enacting care in whatever way we find it is required, and further requires us to be aware of the competencies and expertise that we may or may not have and that are needed for various caring roles. The consideration of caring competencies is particularly important when considering care for a child in hospital; for example, there are some acts that a parent/carer who is not trained in nursing will simply not be able to do. Erin A. Brown *et al*. note the centrality of caring for parents/carers in our attempts to provide better care to children in hospital in their review of 'parental moral distress'. In particular, they note that in hospitals parents/carers may feel unable to care or doubt their own ability to care for their children because they are unable to carry out some of the new tasks that are required in order for their child's needs to be met:

> parent moral distress may be one or more negative self-directed emotions or attitudes that arise in response to a situation in which important parental roles are perceived to be threatened or their ability to enact important roles is stymied.
>
> (2018, p. 828)

They note that '[w]hen we care about parents, we impact the children in their care' (ibid, p. 834). Tronto's final category of care is 'care receiving', which calls us to be responsive when we accept care and to identify and articulate our care needs. Tronto argues that caring for, caring about, and receiving care create an unending cycle where care is always circulating, repeating, and being reinvented (2015, p. 7). *Kicking Up Our Heels* adopted the philosophy that although the need to give care is infinite and can never fully be met, care is not finite or limited; instead, when we are all cared for, then our capacity to care also increases.

One-to-one performance

One-to-one performance, as we are exploring it here, relates to a form that has emerged from live art, fine art, and performance art traditions. In the one-to-one event, a performer and audience member have an intimate and interactive encounter designed by the performer for an audience of one. Rachel Zerihan usefully sums up one-to-one performance in her guide for the Live Art Development Agency: ' "One to One" or "One on One" or "Audience of One" are all terms used to describe a performance that invites one audience member to experience the piece on their own" (2009, p. 3). She then explores the dynamics of one-to-one performance, noting that it demands a rethinking of roles and power: 'questions around one's individual role in the performance's agency – in terms of cultural politics, erotic encounters, sacred moments, therapeutic interactions and risky opportunities – are brought to the foreground' (2009, p. 3).

Adrian Howells (1962–2014) was a one-to-one performance practitioner who brought major critical and popular attention to the artform. His body of work – which includes work as both himself and the alter ego Adrienne – often used quotidian scenarios to enable profound, unexpected, and revelatory encounters with audiences/strangers. These are described by Deirdre Heddon and Dominic Johnson:

> Whether spooning an audience-participant on a bed, or bathing, feeding, or holding one, washing one's hair or feet, Howells' encounters were rigorously planned and simultaneously, forcefully open to negotiation, challenge, and change.
>
> (2016, p. 9)

In *Footwashing for the Sole*, Howells, in his own words, 'simply washed, dried, anointed with oils, massaged and kissed the participant's feet', and the performance, including the conversation surrounding the act of footwashing, provides a useful parallel to the encounters we created within *Kicking Up Our Heels* (explored later) (2016, p. 189). In particular, Howells noted that *Footwashing* was designed to create and hold space for audience members:

> My intention was that during the foot washing and drying I would facilitate a minimal, spoken exchange. . . . This silent time was also intended to provide opportunity for internal contemplation and self-reflection. I sought to shift the focus and attention away from the experience being about me and my inclination.
>
> (Heddon and Howells, 2011, p. 7)

Using *Footwashing* as an example to think through care and the one-to-one encounter, there are a number of distinct elements of one-to-one that are worthy of critical attention:

- *Multiplicity of audience and audience experiences*: While in traditional theatre settings, we appreciate that every audience member has a subjective experience with a piece of art, with one-to-one performance, this is more true than ever. If Howells were performing *Footwashing* six to ten times a day, each of these performances, and each of these audience members' experiences, would be different.
- *Limited or expandable duration and quantity of performances*: If a one-to-one performance is twenty minutes or an hour for one person at a time, there will obviously be a limit to how often this work can be produced and how many people can see it. Because of the open-ended nature of our *Kicking Up Our Heels*, there is a natural emotional and physical limit to the amount of people we could perform with/to, just as with Howells. Thinking through emotional and physical capacity for holding space was critical.
- *It is not for everyone*: There are some elements of one-to-one performance that will intimidate or put-off audience members immediately upon hearing about them – particularly working and living in Britain, where a one-to-one interaction with a stranger is many Brits' worst nightmare. This will always be the case and is notable for when we think about whose voices are present, whose are absent, and who took themselves out of the performance/encounter of *Kicking Up Our Heels* before it even began.
- *Score and improvisation:* Most one-to-ones are built around the idea of a theatrical 'score', rather than a script. Because the audience will change, because the performer will get tired, because the day will get long, and so on, one-to-one performers often forego having absolute control over what happens or what is said, in favour of having an outline, both of texts and of actions, which provides touch points or milestones for the performance. Inside of this, audience responsiveness can guide the performance in one way or another, all of which contributes to the liveness and intimacy of the form.
- *Active participation of the audience:* Going hand-in-hand with a reflection on score/improvisation, the active and activated participation of the audience is often a critical feature of one-to-one performance.

And it is this final element, the activated participation of the audience enabling the show to exist, which is of particular interest in this study. Heddon, Iball, and Zerihan remark on activated participation: 'Crucial . . . , then, are the practices of exchange between selves enabled by One to One work' (2012, p. 121), while Kartsaki *et al.* posit 'the co-presence of performer and spectator . . . often refigures the 'audience' as participant or collaborator' (Kartsaki, Zerihan, and Lobel, 2014, p. 101).

The audience member must be prepared to offer themselves in a reciprocal encounter with the performer, some of which may provoke or challenge in unexpected ways (see Ursula Martinez's *Confront the Cunt* [2004] or Kira O'Reilly's *Untitled Action for Bombshelter* [2003] as two such examples).[1] Though not all one-to-one performances require the active and engaged participation of the audience member, most of these works place audiences in a position that often feels much more vulnerable than a traditional performance encounter, during which we can disappear within the crowd of the audience. But just like vulnerable audiences, the performer of one-to-ones must be willing to expose themselves to and be reliant upon the audience member in an utterly co-dependent encounter. This is not an equal encounter: the performer has designed the encounter, knows what to expect, is the 'professional' in the situation and in whom the audience member must trust. Instead, we might conceive of one-to-one performance as an asymmetrical or unbalanced yet mutual encounter. Adriana Cavarero discusses the option we all have when placed in a relationship of dependence to reach out to our other with the intent to either nurture or harm and positions care as a particular inclination towards a vulnerable other (2011, p. 202). Cavarero notes that, in a maternal encounter, the mother must literally lean over or reach out towards the defenceless, and often naked, infant child. Reaching out can be either benevolent or malicious and can be comforting or destructive; we can reach out to caress (as Howells does in *Footwashing*), or we can reach out to hit. Caring as an inclination towards a vulnerable other is inherent in both the one-to-one performance and the medical encounter.

Kicking Up Our Heels was a project for parents/carers by performers within the space of the hospital. All of these 'actors' (that is the parents/carers, the hospital as institution and the staff that make up that institution, and the performer working on the project) are in a relationship of both power and care. As outlined, care here is a complicated notion encompassing parental care for the child, the work of 'caring professionals', and the caring responsibility that must be taken on by a performer for the audience that they are engaging with. Each of these relationships requires us to put ourselves in a direct and unequal relationship with another – the parent/carer enacting power over the child, the hospital staff in a position of power over the patient and their family, and the performer asking an audience member to enter into an unusual encounter – one where the performer is in control and knows what to expect, while the audience member does not. When applied to both one-to-one performance and more traditional acts of care within the hospital setting, we must be particularly alert to the inequalities at play. As Tronto highlights, we must pay attention to the aligned but distinct aspects of caring about and caring for. In order to engage in caring encounters responsibly and productively within the hospital space, these encounters must be governed by an ethics of care. We perform our care in the actions we make (that is, the daily things we do) in the hospital space as well as performances (in the theatrical sense) that make up the principal method of the *Kicking Up Our Heels* project. When Nicholas Ridout proposes that the central question is 'how shall I act?' in his discussion on the ethics of performance, we see a double meaning – 'what actions shall I make?' and 'what theatrical performance shall I do?' (2009, p. 63).

To make performance that is ethical, we must consider the audience member someone for whom the performer has a responsibility and who should be taken care of, just as the hospital professional must be governed by robust ethical thinking in their own encounters within their working lives. Amanda Stuart Fisher highlights the potential synergy between ethical performance and ethical care, arguing that an analysis of care is essential to understand performance and also that an analysis rooted in performance studies can be a means of understanding the 'artful, aesthetic, rehearsed and performative' elements of performing care, enacted by those in social and medical settings (2020, p. 3). Elsewhere, James Thompson has noted that both care giving and socially engaged performance are aesthetic encounters that require attentiveness and craft (2020, p. 44). Through performance, we were able to offer an opportunity for both parents/carers themselves, and for all those individuals that make up the institution of GOSH, to pay careful attention and to reflect upon the parents' need for care within the hospital space.

One-to-one medical encounters

Victoria Bates and Sam Goodman discuss the history of the medical humanities, particularly noting that the evolution of medicine and the arts are inextricably interlinked. The result of this interwoven development, they conclude, is the 'socially contingent nature of both the arts/medicine relationship' (2013, p. 6), the need to take a 'broad approach' when we think about what might be considered for inclusion in a discussion of the arts and medicine (ibid, p. 5), and that 'the relationship between medicine, arts and humanities should be conceptualized in terms of reciprocity and exchange' (ibid, p. 5). This is particularly pertinent for us when considering performance. The well-rehearsed arguments of performance studies, which enable us to examine actions and language as a series of performed encounters, lend themselves particularly well to the hospital setting, with its history of the operating theatre as a site of spectacular revelations.[2] Similarly, every medical encounter requires a series of performances from the medic who must act out their reassuring expertise, the nurse who demonstrates compassion and professionalism, the radiographer who is a model of technical competence, and the patient who performs stoicism or humility. These performances of reassuring expertise, compassion, and so on, are in fact so embedded inside the medical encounter that they are formalised in medical education via objective structured clinical examinations (OCSEs). The OSCE (created in 1975 and developed upon in the last forty-five years) tests medical students on skills related to medical care (drawing blood, reading results, and so on) while also testing them on communication, breaking bad news, taking a history, and the like. Drawing on their learning, students navigate these 'scripts' and are assessed according to how they hit appropriate milestones during the encounter and acting with courtesy and professionalism (see also chapters by Bleakley and Marshall and Dalton and Hooker on medical education and performance in this volume). These examinations, and their stature inside medical education and thus medical practice, ensure a level of consistency inside health care, and without this series of performances the one-to-one medical encounter would collapse, just as the one-to-one performance encounter could not happen if the performer and audience member did not performatively signal their roles.

Care in performance – *Kicking Up Our Heels*

In the *Kicking Up Our Heels* project, parents/carers were asked to make actions with us through simple drama exercises and imagination activities, including those examples that we have shared in the following, that allowed them to make visible both the care they give and the care they receive while also taking time to reflect on the care they might need.

Care towards the other was evident in all aspects of the thinking, action, and values that informed the work we witnessed at GOSH, including the care shown by professional and administrative staff, support and clinical staff, allied health professionals, parents/carers, artists, and others. To act with care is clearly not an alien concept within the hospital, and yet, to show care to the parents/carers within the space was an area that we found to be overlooked, both within the processes and practices of the hospital and by the parents/carers themselves.

Ruddick asserts that, when we act with love, we are rewarded by seeing our child flourish (1989). Conversely, we can act with love and yet the child still succumbs to illness or to social or political events which prevent them reaching their full potential. When this happens, Ruddick notes, we are left with 'anguish . . . helplessness and guilt' (1989, p. 30). The parents/carers we encountered in GOSH were asked if they wanted to engage in a short performance encounter led by either one or the other of this chapter's authors to creatively imagine a space where they could be free from any anguish, helplessness, or guilt. We asked them to imagine that we had a magic wand that could ensure they could travel anywhere they wanted, real or imaginary, while knowing that everyone that might need them was safe and happy and that there would be no urgent calls from hospital staff or distressed children. The spaces that parents/carers imagined included:

- It would be a beach, white sand, clear sky, just the noise of the water and maybe family nearby. Cold drink like a Sprite or 7up. I don't want any music, just sea and birds.
- A proper bed, a separate room for the patient and family with a nice view.
- A holiday, with the kids. Big villa. Swimming pool. Infinity pool. Peaceful so you can hear the birds. Soothing. No phone charger. Archers & Lemonade. All the alcohol.
- Technology is an escape – I can keep in touch with friends, without having to talk about what's going on here. Normal life is an escape.
- Home. Most of his life was here in hospital.
- America, for treatment, anywhere for her.

These responses reveal not just what these parents/carers want but also what they are lacking: normality, care, sleep, and peace came out very strongly on the list of the kinds of care that parents/carers need but do not have access to when their child is resident in hospital. In articulating these things, which many take for granted, we are shown a vision of what is denied when caring for a child who is undergoing serious medical treatment. Parents/carers are able to speak from a position of authority about their own needs when sharing these images through engaging in a short interaction – they are treated as the expert on what it is that they desire, and power dynamics are momentarily reversed. We also worked to publicly acknowledge parents' own expertise by asking them to share advice that they would offer to another parent/carer coming into the space. When parents/carers shared this wisdom with us, we wrote it on an eye mask and offered it back to them; this gifting back of their own advice enabled parents/carers to recognise their own knowledge and also reminded them to show the levels of compassion towards themselves that they might show to someone else. The final 'You're Doing a Great Job' leaflet that was produced as part of the *Kicking Up Our Heels* project was subtitled 'advice from parents for parents'; again, this was an attempt to acknowledge the parents/carers themselves as experts in their own needs and situation and to attend to the inequalities of power found within the theatrical performance and hospital space.

What we learned from one-to-one bedside performances at GOSH

The nature of one-to-one performance makes it a challenging artform to document (lest you interrupt the one-to-one-ness) and evaluate (unless you capture and quantify each possibility for interaction), but over many performances, patterns and learnings begin to emerge. The learning we have drawn from our series of one-to-one performances, therefore, coalesces around some themes, while other details remain in orbit. The patterns and the outliers are, of course, both interesting to performance studies and health care practices. For example, we learned that the ubiquity of hospital surveys, which meant that parents/carers were used to sharing information, made it easier for us as artist/researchers to approach parents/carers. Parents/carers do surveys constantly and feel a drive to contribute to knowledge towards the betterment of the hospital and the affirmation of good practice; because of this comfort, we were probably successful (if we measure success by a parent/carer choosing to engage in an encounter with us) with 80% of the parents/carers that we approached, as reported in Anna Ledgard's final evaluation of the project (2020). Though the pull of the survey was a gentle way to begin a performance, some parents/carers still chose not to engage with us. Reasons for not participating cited by parents/carers were often related to their child's needs (or the child's needs being a convenient excuse when they just did not want to be bothered), exhaustion, not being the central caregiver so they would not want to speak on the subject, personal business, or a desire for rest. We also had to end a number of encounters soon after beginning them, and before the parent/carer was ready to finish, because of medical priorities; for example, when a child was called away for an x-ray or a doctor came for a consultation. The external evaluator noted in her final report:

> There was a high take up of parental involvement (80% of those who were approached took part). Most of those who declined did so for understandable reasons (clinical procedures/ other visitors etc.). When compared with the uptake of other parental surveys the artistic approach had a considerably higher uptake.
>
> (Ledgard, 2020)

We leave *Kicking Up Our Heels* with the knowledge that the survey technique is useful and worthy of more attention. Parents/carers desperately want to give feedback to the hospital but are often afraid to be critical or 'too difficult' lest it impact on their child's care. A performance survey might enable a moment to hear this feedback in order that the service can improve for all concerned. A notable example of this is that the findings from the *Kicking Up Our Heels* project were used to inform the development of the physical spaces of the new children's cancer centre at GOSH. Bringing performance, research, and other engagements to the bedside makes it easier for parents/ carers to fit them into their demanding, and often chaotic, days in the hospital, and allows participation where they might not be able to otherwise engage in any arts activity or in the feedback to the hospital that they are so committed to improving and supporting.

Another aspect of our performances that may account for our success in engaging with parents/ carers was the role of costume and status. We learned that ridiculous bathrobes and colourful shoes are a way to seem non-threatening and approachable to parents/carers and their children. Further, we found that being honest about our own position in the hospital as people who have a history of receiving care as patients and as a parent/carer of a patient enabled us to demonstrate that our knowledge was, at least in part, gained from personal experiences and to recognise that parents/ carers also have a level of expertise that they can share. Of course, there was not a parity between the parents/carers and us; we were presenting as artists employed by the hospital, which brings in a complex power dynamic around roles as well as serving to reassure the parents/carers that we had the necessary level of expertise to manage the performance encounter. Nonetheless, we wonder if these practices around status might also impact hospitals or health care practices in some way. To seem lower status, or clown-like, was helpful to break the ice, bring a smile, and get the conversation started in our performance, to bring our own history to the conversation broke down hierarchies of expertise, acknowledging that parents/carers within the hospital bring an expertise drawn from their own experiences.

From *Kicking Up Our Heels* we also learned (or were reminded) that people (parents/carers and children) love receiving a gift as part of the work; our inexpensive customised sleep-masks worked a treat. We learned (or were reminded) that language is always an issue in hospitals – particularly in an international space such as GOSH – but does not affect the ability to communicate about feelings well. We learned (or were reminded) that nearly none of these parents/carers had their first names used in the hospital. They entered the hospital with a sick child and instantly became just 'Mum' or 'Dad' to professionals and to other parents/carers. And we learned (or relearned) how parents/carers support each other in hospital settings in the smallest of ways that often feel unremarkable in retrospect ('I poured her a cup of tea') but life-altering and huge in the moment ('I will never forget that person who poured me a cup of tea just when I needed it'). All four of these lessons we might have predicted, but we hadn't, and the one-to-one form of work reminds us of small, individual stories and encounters and to consistently take in many different people's journeys in empathic ways.

And finally, we learned and felt deeply reminded that the length of the encounter is not an indication of the quality or depth of the exchange. Some of our sessions with parents/carers lasted well over an hour, some only a couple of minutes, but all parents/carers responded to say they had enjoyed the exchange and had a moment to reflect on their own needs. We are particularly grateful to Anna Ledgard, the external evaluator for the *Kicking Up Our Heels* project, who observed many of the encounters we undertook and was able to follow up with parents/carers about their experiences.

Final words

We are standing in the corridor after a long day of encounters with parents/carers. Our feet are tired from walking in slippers all day. We are introduced to a parent/carer who has expressed an interest in receiving a one-to-one encounter with us, but we have caught her at a bad time. Her child has just fallen asleep, so we cannot go into the room for fear of disturbing them. This is the parent's only chance to run out and get food. She chats to us for a moment and tells us she has to rush but would like to know more. We briefly explain the project and start a truncated encounter. We ask: 'Where do you find space for yourself in the hospital?' She replies: 'I hide in the bathtub. It is child sized so I have to curl up'. The whole event takes less than five minutes. Then she leaves to go on with her day.

The one-to-one encounter, either performance or medical, is defined in the moment by the people who are engaged in it; both are active participants, and, for the encounter to be successful, both must enter into a reciprocal, asymmetric exchange, with vulnerability and care. A successful one-to-one engagement in a hospital setting can enable us to find out much about what is needed, what the experience so far has been, to develop an intimate yet fleeting relationship, and to dream together.

Notes

1 *Confront the Cunt* is discussed in Lobel, B., Zerihan, R. and Kartsaki, E. (eds.) (2014) 'Performing ethos: ethics of one-to-one performance', *A Special Issue of Performing Ethos Journal*, 3(2); and *Untitled Action for Bombshelter* is documented in O'Reilly, K. (2018) *Untitled (bodies)*. London: Live Art Development Agency.
2 See Michel Foucault's *The Birth of the Clinic* (1973) for a discussion of the hospital as the site of spectacular revelations.

Reference list

All-Party Parliamentary Group on Arts, Health and Wellbeing (2017) *Creative health: the arts for health and wellbeing*.
All-Party Parliamentary Group on Arts, Health and Wellbeing (2017) *Creative health: the arts for health and wellbeing*. Available at: https://www.culturehealthandwellbeing.org.uk/appg-inquiry/Publications/Creative_Health_Inquiry_Report_2017_-_Second_Edition.pdf (Accessed : 1 December 2023).

Barlow, J., Smailagic, N., Huband, N., Roloff, V. and Bennett, C. (2014) 'Group-based parent training programmes for improving parental psychosocial health', *Cochrane Database of Systematic Reviews*, (5). Art. No.: CD002020.pub4

Bates, V. and Goodman, S. (2013) 'Critical conversations', in Bates, V. and Bleakley, A. (eds.) *Medicine, health and the arts*. London and New York: Routledge, pp. 3–15.

Brown, E.A. *et al*. (2018) 'Review of a parent's influence on pediatric procedural distress and recovery', *Clinical Child and Family Psychology Review*, 21(2), pp. 224–245.

Cameron, E.E. *et al*. (2020) 'Maternal psychological distress & mental health service use during the COVID-19 pandemic', *Journal of Affective Disorders*, 276, pp. 765–774.

Cavarero, A. (2011) 'Inclining the subject', in Elliott, J. and Attridge, D. (eds.) *Theory after 'theory'*. London and New York: Routledge, pp. 194–204.

Fancourt, D. and Finn, S. (2019) *What is the evidence on the role of the arts in improving health and well-being? A scoping review*. Copenhagen: WHO Regional Office for Europe. Available at: www.euro.who. int/en/publications/abstracts/what-is-the-evidence-on-the-role-of-the-arts-in-improving-health-and-well-being-a-scoping-review-2019 (Accessed: 13 January 2022).

Foucault, M. (1973) *The birth of the clinic*. Abingdon: Routledge.

Heddon, D. and Howells, A. (2011) 'From talking to silence: a confessional journey', *PAJ: A Journal of Performance and Art*, 33(1), pp. 1–12.

Heddon, D., Iball, H. and Zerihan, R. (2012) 'Come closer: confessions of intimate spectators in one to one performance', *Contemporary Theatre Review*, 22(1), pp. 120–133.

Heddon, D. and Johnson, D. (2016) *It's all allowed: the performance of Adrian Howells*. London: Live Art Development Agency.

Held, V. (2006) *The ethics of care: personal, political, and global*. Oxford: Oxford University.

hooks, b. (2000) *Feminist theory: from margin to center*. London: Pluto Press.

Jensen, A. and Torrissen, W. (2019) 'Aesthetic engagement as health and wellbeing promotion', *Journal of Public Mental Health*, 18(4), pp. 240–247.

Kartsaki, E., Zerihan, R. and Lobel, B. (eds.) (2014) 'Ethics of one-to-one performance', *Performing Ethos*, 3(2).

Law, E.F. *et al*. (2014) 'Systematic review and meta-analysis of parent and family-based interventions for children and adolescents with chronic medical conditions', *Journal of Pediatric Psychology*, 39(8), pp. 866–886.

Ledgard, A. (2020) *Kicking up our heels final report*. London: Great Ormond Street. Available at: https://storytelling.research.southwales.ac.uk/documents/2779/WEB_Evaluation_Report_KICKING_UP_OUR_HEELSFINALWEB.pdf (Accessed: 5 May 2022).

O'Reilly, K. (2018) *Untitled (bodies)*. London: Live Art Development Agency.

Ridout, N. (2009) *Theatre and ethics*. London: Macmillan International Higher Education.

Ruddick, S. (1989) *Maternal thinking: toward a politics of peace*. Boston: Beacon Press.

Stuart Fisher, A. (2020) 'Introduction: caring performance, performing care', in Fisher, S., Thompson, A. and Thompson, J. (eds.) *Performing care: new perspectives on socially engaged performance*. Manchester: Manchester University Press, pp. 1–18.

Thompson, J. (2020) 'Towards and aesthetics of care', in Fisher, S., Thompson, A. and Thompson, J. (eds.) *Performing care: new perspectives on socially engaged performance*. Manchester: Manchester University Press, pp. 36–48.

Tronto, J.C. (2013) *Caring democracy: markets, equality, and justice*. New York: NYU Press.

Tronto, J.C. (2015) *Who cares? How to reshape a democratic politics*. New York: Cornell University Press.

Zerihan, R. (2009) *One to one performance: a study room guide on works devised for an audience of one*. London: Live Art Development Agency. Available at www.thisisliveart.co.uk/wp-content/uploads/2020/02/OnetoOne_Final-copy.pdf [accessed 2 November 2023]

27

CARE AESTHETICS

The art, aesthetics and performance of health care

James Thompson

The concept of *care aesthetics* makes the claim that the caring relations between people can be understood for their aesthetics. This requires that human-to-human care experiences can be labelled aesthetic – and of course many traditions of aesthetics would not accept this – and simultaneously that care, more usually understood as a source for ethics, can also be understood for the craft and embodied sensory aspects of its practice. I have outlined this argument more broadly elsewhere (Thompson, 2015; Thompson, 2020) so the focus here will be more specific, examining the links between care aesthetics and health care, particularly in relation to its position in a collection exploring performance and medicine. This returns to the origins of my interest in this area which came from witnessing the extraordinary health care offered to my colleague, Antoine Muvunyi, from the Democratic Republic of the Congo (DRC), during his hospital treatment in the UK for a bullet injury. I worked with Antoine on a theatre programme on women and girls' rights in eastern DRC, where he was shot in an incident in which several other colleagues were killed. This event is documented in my article 'To applied theatre, with love' (Thompson, 2021) as part of a broader exploration of how we might find new registers for discussing socially engaged performance that do not rely only on the language of suffering. In terms of Antoine, I understood the health care relationship between him and his physiotherapist as an aesthetic encounter, but at the time I was unsure why I thought it so and certainly was unclear as to the implications for framing it in this way. There was something of the skill of the physiotherapist, in her embodied touch and manipulation of Antoine's fingers and palm, but also in his response as he held her in his eyes and expressed to me his trust in the relationship that made the process possible, and bearable. Their relationship was also composed of quiet conversations, gentle humour and shared stories. There was something *beautiful* in this act of care, and while fully aware of the difficulties of that adjective, it prompted a demand to know what the implications might be for an appreciation of care as an aesthetic practice.

Care aesthetics, medicine and health humanities

Here this initial inquiry is developed to explore how the practice of health professionals and other carers has been understood aesthetically. This draws on writing from my book *Care Aesthetics* (2022); however, for this edition, it will be connected to debates on the relation between

DOI: 10.4324/9781003036500-31

performance and medicine. At a simple level the phrase 'care aesthetics' neatly corresponds to the 'medicine' and 'performance' dyad examined in the book. Care operates as a subset of medicine broadly conceived, and aesthetics points to a sensory experience that exists as part of many performance practices. However, care and aesthetics are not intended to be synonymous or neatly contained within medicine and performance. Care is chosen to focus on those aspects of medicine that are connected to health care practices, whether in hospital or community settings, but specifically to point to those activities that have too often been delegated to the lowest paid members of staff. This is discussed later in the chapter in the difference between empirics and aesthetics in nursing 'knowledge'. Similarly, aesthetics is used to draw attention to those aspects of a performance that concern form, craft and embodied or sensory practices. It is also used to link performances of health care to the aesthetics of an environment, so that performance is not conceived as a response to the quality of that context but rather is considered for its own aesthetics, which is a constituent part of that wider environment. Aesthetics is used to designate a health care experience combining health performances and the environments in which they take place. Finally, as will be discussed in the pages that follow, aesthetics is used to examine how performance when applied to health care practices too often operates with an unacknowledged diminutive, whereby phrases such as *performing health care* struggle to avoid a sense that they signal a connection to fakery or pretence. Care aesthetics thus seeks to explore the hierarchies evident in medicine, between, for example, those that cure and those that care, and then the sensory and crafted aspects of performance practices. It will do so through accounts chosen from the health care literature where aesthetics is discussed, either explicitly or implicitly.

The writing here would fit within the field of the *health humanities* (see Crawford *et al.*, 2015; Crawford, Brown and Charise, 2020), which has documented the intersections between health broadly conceived and multiple disciplines within the arts and humanities. While in terms of the practice-based arts disciplines, this relationship is frequently about what the arts can offer health care, it is also a field that recognises an *art of* health as well as the *arts in* health. Crawford and colleagues mention a traditional approach to the relationship whereby the focus is on 'the potential for arts and humanities to make a real difference to the lived experience of informal carers' (2015, p. 146). The argument for care aesthetics extends this to formal health professional contexts but also seeks to move beyond this formula, to one which examines the aesthetics of health care practices, not what the arts, and theatre and performance, might bring to them. This is in fact part of the tradition documented by Crawford but often articulated as a form of minor key to more familiar preoccupations. So, for example, where there is the suggestion that the performing arts can be understood as health care practice, there is also the 'sub-argument that health practices can be understood as ways of being-in-relationship, aesthetically, in time' (ibid, p. 86). Similarly, rather than just a 'sub-argument', there is also the assertion in the same edition by Crawford that the two sides of the *health* and *humanities* relation, and that between medicine and performance here, might be explained under the one rubric where they are both 'relational-aesthetic-temporal phenomena' (ibid, p. 89). This is central to the claim of this chapter and aligns with the argument for care to be understood as a practical activity that has its own aesthetics alongside other arts and not as a sub-domain of them. Performance in this analysis is not offering medicine a way of understanding itself or of enhancing its delivery. Instead, medical practices and performance are understood to have a common concern with aesthetics: they both include relational, temporal and affective practices.

The claim that health care could be considered for its aesthetics is one that public health researcher Phil Hanlon has explained is not new but suffers from rarely being defined adequately (2012, p. 2946). The 'art of care', for example, is a phrase often endorsed but seldom defined with precision. The aim here is to discuss attempts to define what is often seen as an elusive quality in health care practice but also to offer a rationale for why *care aesthetics* might be a helpful framework for that process of definition. Where the 'art of care' should mean, in the words of nursing educators Peggy Chinn and Maeona Kramer, some property 'essential to the 'doing' of care work itself', it can frequently take on different and perhaps confusing connotations (2014, p. 234). Madeleine Bunting, in her book on the crisis of care, has argued that care is a 'close but poor relation of artistic creativity' and the approach here is to acknowledge the long history of aesthetic debate within health care research but also claim it deserves to be more than a poor relation (2020, p. 236).

Negative care aesthetics

The primary focus here is care aesthetic experiences that are positive contributions to health settings, but it is important to acknowledge that practices can be diminished in their sensory register or exhibit *negative* care aesthetics. Hilary Moss refers to this as an 'aesthetics of deprivation' that can be found both in the physical environments of, for example, hospitals and the practices within them (2014, p. 1032). She documents a hospital setting in which 'everything about the environment was professional, clean, and functional, but the effect was a sterile, clinical environment lacking warmth and humanity' (2020, p. 430). She is describing an aesthetic, the result of which was a sense of sterility and coldness. This, according to Moss, is counter to the needs of both staff and patients in these contexts and demonstrated the urgency of seeking out more 'aesthetically pleasing and supportive' ways of organising health care space (2014, p. 1032). Of course, there is a relation between the environment and the performances within it, and an austere context is likely to produce, and be the product of, a set of practices that have a particular diminished aesthetic. It is, therefore, not enough to discuss aesthetic deprivation in terms of the colour of walls, quality of light or other observable features of an external context; it must also be an analytic category for the practical interactions of people. Julia Twigg notes this when talking about the potential failures in care workers' practice. In a choice of words which is emphatically aesthetic, she argues that 'positive cruelty' is perhaps rare, but 'we can imagine rough handling, denigrating language, sneering or nasty words, a silent refusal to recognise the person, the demeaning exposure of the body, cold indifference to embarrassment or anxiety' (2002, p. 2). *Rough, cold* and *sneering* are exemplary words for an aesthetic of neglect, or 'negative' care aesthetics. They are clearly not synonymous with pleasure but with the sensations, feeling and forms of ugliness that can make health care unpleasant and of course abusive.

An examination of negative care aesthetics has been part of the critical work of both practitioners and researchers in health care, and it is notable that many of the challenges to the intolerable outcomes of poor health are presented in a language that might be referred to as *an aesthetic register*. However, in contrast to the 'ugliness' of poor care, there are numerous examples of *positive* care aesthetics documented in the health care literature. This is not therefore the performance of nurses or health care professionals struggling to manage their emotional labour, following the analysis of feminist sociologist Arlie Hochschild, which suggests the 'the induction or suppression of feeling' produces a sense in another person of being looked after (1983, p. 7). Hochschild's analysis operates in the diminutive register of performance mentioned previously, so that a health care professional is *merely* performing to 'sustain an outward appearance' (Ibid, p. 7). Care aesthetics is designed to be a critical concept and points to those instances when the care is wanting with limited bodily and sensory quality. However, it also seeks to validate the performance of health professionals for the aesthetics of their practice, in a way which avoids the implicit negative contained in Hochschild's presentation of emotional labour. Julia Twigg and colleagues note this when they explain that 'emotion can also make body work worthwhile, meaningful and rewarding' (2011, p. 462). This does not deny it can be tough, but that the performance of emotional work can also be a source of satisfaction. This frames the emphasis in the next section where examples of a positive care aesthetics are presented as a way of outlining what an enriched experience might be, rather than what it is not. Four examples are offered, taken from hospital settings and a care home hair salon, to raise some of the features that connect across the examples they illustrate. This intends to give a flavour of care aesthetics from the perspective of health care commentators and to demonstrate many of the themes that arise from an aesthetic focus. Quotations from the original sources will be given consecutively to help appreciate the patterns that repeat across them.

Positive care aesthetics

British author Marian Coutts wrote a memoir about her husband's illness and eventual death called 'The Iceberg' (2014) that is discussed by Bunting in her book *Labours of Love*. In her interview with Coutts, she quotes her as follows:

> When Tom was in hospital, I was aware of the charismatic power he had, even when he had no words. Once, I arrived early at the hospital to give him his clothes. The curtains were round his bed and three women were giving him a bed bath; they were talking in several languages. It was an amazing image to stumble on. Tom was totally relaxed. It was like a private party. I couldn't have arranged it better. I certainly couldn't have bought it. It was priceless. It was important, I felt, to bear witness to that kind of work, which is low paid and undervalued. It needs to be spoken about. . . . You could feel the levels of attentiveness in staff from the way they walked, their tone of voice, their touch. One consultant was under huge pressure, but she managed to keep that hidden from us. She made us feel like she had all the time in the world for us – to manage that professionally and personally is high art.
>
> (Bunting, 2020, p. 201)

From Chinn and Kramer, describing the work of a nurse in an outpatient clinic:

> Presley works in the orthopedic clinic of a large urban hospital and uses aesthetic know-ing with each young child who comes for cast removal. It is aesthetic knowing that helps him remove the cast in the least distressing way for the child. Presley understands that this child likely sees a large person approaching her leg with an electric cutter and other tools that resemble those in her father's woodworking shop. Presley might use a combination of distraction and humor as well as careful timing to move through the required procedure in an artful way.
>
> (2014, p. 33)

From Caroline Swarbrick, John Keady and Elizabeth Sampson in their account of a researcher's shift in role in her encounter with a distressed elderly patient who died soon after this account:

> I walk around the bed to the empty chair and pull it forwards and towards the bed so that Amy can see me and we make eye contact. I introduce myself by my first name and ask if she minds me sitting with her. She smiles at me. Amy immediately starts to shout loudly

for "Alice". I calmly ask who Alice is and she shouts "Mam, Mam". Amy starts crying and instinctively I reach out and stroke her hair and hold her hand, which she grips tightly. Amy stops crying and looks directly into my eyes. I ask her if she minds me stroking her hair, to which she replies "it's lovely". I carry on and Amy continues to shout for "Alice", whilst looking towards the corridor at the end of the bay. Suddenly, she stops, turns her head to me and says very matter-of-factly: "they tried to cut him out, but he wouldn't open his eyes" . . . She then starts to scream very loudly, shouting "Mam, Mam" at the top of her voice. . . . In a calm and soft voice, I continue to reassure Amy predominantly through physical touch, of which she is responsive. I am not sure how much she is aware of my presence. I stroke her hands and face. Amy looks at me and smiles.

(Swarbrick, Keady and Sampson, 2017, p. 204)

From Richard Ward, Keady and Campbell's study of hair care in an elderly care home salon:

Slow-motion video-analysis also helped to reveal the intricate nature of sink work. Thermal, haptic and multi-sensory experience is interlaced with apprehension and anxiety for many clients while the hairdresser combines touch and talk both to reassure and distract. Some clients were asked to count to ten, others strategically engaged in animated conversation and by taking advantage of her physical contact with clients the hairdresser could offer a reassuring back rub or accentuate the slow massaging of their scalp.

(Ward, Campbell and Keady, 2016, p. 1293)

One of the first things to note across these examples is that the phrases aesthetic knowing, fine art and art are used. The language of the arts is explicit, not in every example, but its use does illustrate immediately that the argument for care aesthetics is not something that comes to these practices from outside but is frequently articulated by those experiencing them. They are detailed accounts of performances, but it is the sensory and *haptic* nature of those performances that are highlighted rather than their artificiality or managed effort. The concept of aesthetic knowing, mentioned in the Chinn and Kramer quotation, originates in the work of nursing scholar Barbara Carper (1978). It is an important concept for understanding how aesthetics and art have been discussed in relation to nursing practice and will be discussed in more detail in the following. Besides these explicit art-related comments, each of the examples indicates a focus on the patient or client, a quality of attention and a sense of an engagement with a well-tuned insight to meet their different needs. The skills used to do this include touch and different ways of speaking, expressed in terms such as 'tone of voice' or humour. These encounters are explained as multi-sensory, combining handling, talking and crucially timing to ensure a considered process which creates a certain impression or ethos that is experienced bodily. Some of the interactions here are interpersonal, a relationship between a carer and a cared for, but some are concerned with more complex relational combinations, including those witnessing care or relying on care for one of their loved ones. While each of these quotations demonstrate an appreciation of the aesthetics within daily performances of care in an enriching, positive sense, they also express a sense of surprise that this quality of engagement is possible. There is an implicit awareness that normally constrained work schedules seem to dissolve or perhaps are jettisoned to ensure a practice that is truly attentive and appropriately caring of the patient. A beautifully executed health care performance, therefore, benefits from a sense of presence, its own expanded notion of time, a relational range of sensory and embodied skills and a close connection with another.

The aesthetic pattern of knowing

Barbara Carper wrote her seminal article 'Fundamental Patterns of Knowing in Nursing' in 1978, and it has produced substantial debate across nursing scholarship and nursing practice since then. Its basic premise was that the knowledge that nurses drew on in their practice included four main patterns of knowing. These were *empirics*, that is scientific understanding, *ethics* as the moral grounding of knowledge, *personal knowledge* of the self and others and finally *aesthetics* or what has been labelled the art of nursing. While the intention of delineating the different patterns was to name the different resources that a nurse might draw on to develop her or his practice in a holistic way, of course, in creating different categories, there is also the danger that they would be compared or set in opposition to each other. This is most acute in the tendency to set aesthetic knowing against empiric knowing, so that technical and scientific skills of nurses are positioned as a natural opposite of aesthetic-based skills. In the broader concept of medicine employed in this edition, this sets those that are involved in the technical work of curing, against those delegated to the embodied work of caring.

Gosia Brykczynska, in her work on nursing 'wisdom', has noted that 'of all the aspects of nursing, the artistic and aesthetic ones are the least commented and understood' (1997, p. 45). While this is true to an extent, there has, in fact, been substantial debate on and development of the concept of aesthetic knowing and the 'art of care' (see Chinn and Watson, 1994; Contreras Ibacache, 2013; Rovithis, 2002; Siles-González and Solano-Ruiz, 2016; Wainwright, 2000). Some of this work has sought to centre nursing studies and training within Carper's patterns of knowing (notably the work of Chinn and colleagues), and some has attempted to question its continued purchase, suggesting instead a move away from the boundaries it creates (notable in the work of Julie Duff Cloutier, Duncan and Hill Bailey, 2007). The argument here will explore the definition of 'aesthetic knowing' and its corollary the 'art of nursing' and then suggest some of the problems that emerge from both that definition and the extensive debates prompted by Carper's original work.

The first point to note about the aesthetic pattern of knowing is that it is used as a phrase almost interchangeably with 'the art' of nursing. Art and aesthetics are thus somewhat indistinguishable, so that Chinn and Watson might refer to the 'art and aesthetics of caring and healing' without automatically noting whether the use of the word 'art' signifies a nurse's practice as an art or if it is 'art-like' (1994, p. xiii). This is a corollary of the attempt here to distinguish between the performance of a health care professional and the aesthetics of the experience to which that performance contributes. The skill of nursing might be 'like an artist's brush', according to Karen Breunig in her account of how the absorption of an artist in their work is comparable to the feeling of absorption in a nurse-patient relation, but again it is unclear if 'the opportunity to be an artist' is the same as actually being one (Breunig, 1994, p. 201). Chinn and Watson in the following definition of the 'art of nursing' suggest the differences between art and aesthetic in a way that develops the distinction that I want to make here. For them:

> The art of nursing . . . includes intentional auditory, visual, sensory, olfactory, and tactile art or acts. . . . Among these are purposive movement, touch, sound, color, form, nature, and so on. Nursing as art is lived, expressed, and cocreated in the caring moment . . . the aesthetic character of the expressive form of caring, as revealed in the perception and action of the nurse, includes direction, force, balance, and rhythm.
>
> (Chinn and Watson, 1994, p. xvi)

This description links back to the previous examples that demonstrated the importance of multiple sensory practices. For me the 'art of nursing' here indicates the performance practice of this health professional. However, it is the phrase 'aesthetic character of the expressive form of caring' that is crucial because it asserts that caring as a form has an aesthetic. There is a problem, however, in that this is revealed in the perception and action of the nurse rather than as is suggested in the previous line as something co-created in a caring moment. Rather than these two terms – art (and for this edition *performance*) and aesthetics – being interchangeable, I want to insist on a distinction between them. The art or performance of care, therefore, refers to the activity of the nurse, located in their capacity realised in a moment. Aesthetics, on the other hand, is about the shape, form and feel of that moment as it is experienced between all those present. The first distinction to make from Carper's notion of an aesthetic pattern of knowing and the adoption of the art of nursing as its metonym is that by starting from the knowledge of a single person, there is a danger that the focus becomes about individual capacity rather than the shape of a moment created in the relation between at least two people. Contreras Ibacache repeats this when, in his work exploring the evidence for an art of nursing, he defines the art as a nurse's 'use of his or her internal creative resources to transform the experience of patients and co-workers' (2013, p. 333). Care aesthetics is used to avoid this focus on the performance of an individual and instead aims to examine the sensory and embodied experience of care between people. This, of course, might be instigated by the craft-like skills of a health practitioner, but it can also be an experience that emerges from the awareness and response of a patient, the interrelated actions of multiple workers, perhaps the family members visiting as in the previous example, and then the dynamics of a physical environment that shapes and prompts certain feelings and rhythms of engagement. When Mel Gray and Stephen Webb write about the history of social work being discussed as an art, in a parallel account to those that debate nursing, they complain 'the worker's talents are typically lumped together into something called "the art" of practice, but without clear definition about the meaning of the term' (2008, p. 183). The definition does need greater clarity, but I would add that the problem comes from starting from the 'worker's talents' and not how the real-time practice of workers with the people with whom they are in relation produces dynamic aesthetic experiences in which multiple factors play a role.

From the art of care to care aesthetics

Having a greater clarity about the difference between the performance of the nurse and the aesthetics of nursing indicates why care aesthetics is proposed as something distinct from the 'art of care'. The focus is on the sensory shape and feel of a caring encounter, not only the skills of one contributor. That said, drawing attention to the skills of the carer does help illuminate important contributing factors to care experiences. The positive element of Carper's framework is that it has enabled a focus on certain aspects of a health professional's work and in turn given it a value that is often elided. When Pam Smith notes a problem with a division between 'empirics' and 'aesthetics' by explaining how the more senior nurse does 'the "tricky dressings" and complicated medicines' where the untrained carers on the other hand just make 'people happy', her argument is that 'just' to make people happy is a combination of a set of complex 'caring gestures' that should be recognised (2012, p. 20). The hierarchy between the 'scientific' work of the cure and the 'softer' interpersonal effort of care should be challenged. While it is clear many health care settings have seen a gradual marginalisation and devaluing of the sensory skills of staff and a delegation of the more tactile and embodied practices to the lower paid, the emphasis here is that there should be no diminutive, no *just*, in the way these capacities are discussed. Caring gestures, in all their diversity and context-sensitive complexity, need attention and a commitment to their flourishing. *Performing care* must shake off this sense of the diminutive. 'Making people happy' is a vital part of nursing and many other health practices. Of course, even as we mention how they have often been separated from the more highly valued technical skills in nursing, Carper's differentiation of 'scientific' and 'aesthetic' patterns of nursing, and the distinction it seems to delineate, needs to be challenged by insisting that in fact they are often interwoven parts of the same practice. While warm words to a struggling patient might exist in a different register to fitting a canula, the argument here is that they both have a technique; there is a sensory, crafted element of each; and importantly they might co-exist as part of the successful completion of a single procedure. At best, there is an aesthetic knowing in the technical and a technical knowing in the aesthetic.

The focus in the 'art of care' literature on the specific skills of the health care practitioner has also led to a language that suggests there is something of an elusive nature to the practice. *Aesthetic* becomes not a descriptor of an experience brought about by identifiable actions but a signifier of a practice based upon almost mysterious and inexpressible intuition. Cloutier and colleagues have been particularly critical of this tendency as a response to the work of Carper, seeing her designation of empirics as that which is generalisable, and describable, and the aesthetic as 'beyond articulation' as an unfortunate starting point (Cloutier, Duncan and Hill Bailey, 2007, p. 2). They argue against *aesthetic* becoming a synonym for the unexplainable in nursing practice and insist instead that this trend is more an indication of the immaturity of qualitative enquiry, a feature of the time that Carper wrote her original article, than an accurate description of divisions in nursing practice. So rather than framing an aspect of caring practices as 'difficult to understand' or suffering from the dilemma that 'you know when you act artfully [but] you can never fully explain what you did', the argument here, in agreement with Cloutier, is that we should be finding a language and methodology for capturing this enduring part of health care practice and not giving it an analysis pass because it is 'art' and therefore enigmatic (Chinn and Kramer, 2014, p. 227, 236). This is not to deny the care experience as a situation-dependent moment that has particular rather than universal attributes. Alternatively, it seeks to meet the challenge of identifying the elements that are brought to a meaningful and 'positive' care aesthetic moment. In many ways, writers such as Chinn and Kramer who suggest the unobtainable or unrepresentable nature of the aesthetic knowing pattern of nurses' practice are also those who do articulate behaviours that are likely to craft powerful caring experiences. When they note that it is a practice 'expressed through the actions, bearing, conduct, attitudes, narrative, and interactions of the nurse in relation to others', they demonstrate that there are ways of explaining those capacities that make up this specific practice (ibid, p. 33). The challenge is to improve and expand the discursive register rather than rely on formulations that seem to endorse the 'art of nursing' as a quasi-mystical endeavour. In many ways the hard work of analysis in the chapters in this edition are testament to a desire to meet this challenge and move away from a sense that the arts and performance in health care are somehow based on something ineffable. Aesthetic experiences need a language, a way of capturing how they flow across time, and this makes Carper's categories useful in starting an exploration of those aspects of practice. However, the different patterns, empirical, ethical, personal and aesthetic, should be used in an integrative way to start describing and valuing the dynamics of nursing, and health care practices more broadly, where the aesthetic component is understood as a living part of a complete skill set rather than a particular term for all those parts that cannot be understood under the other forms of knowing.

The discourse of the 'art of care' being a zone of practice beyond categorisation produces two additional confusions about the use of the word art which have implications for the discussion of care aesthetics. The first is that commentators who might assert that 'no one, through pen or canvas, will ever be able to entirely capture the true art and the caring spirit of nursing' also argue that this inexpressible nature can be represented 'symbolically . . . as actions, sounds, or pictures, or in metaphoric language such as poetry or story' (Chinn and Watson, 1994, pp. xiv, 24). The art of nursing, therefore, as a practice beyond our ability to express it in ways that might be more familiar to the social sciences, leads to the necessity of an artistic treatment of that art form. Here we have an *art of* the art of nursing which shifts attention from the aesthetics of the care moment to a focus on attempts to portray that moment in a range of different expressive forms. Of course, this is not to deny that poetry or theatre which examines caring practices is of no value. The suggestion is that this demand for artistic representations of care practices confuses further the expression 'art of care'. It means there is a problematic lack of clarity as to whether the 'art of nursing' is a term referring to the art of the care experience itself or artistic work which is made in response to the practice of care. The purpose here is not to disparage artistic explorations of care, and in fact they might be ways of processing the care that is experienced. However, for care aesthetics, the 'art of care' does not need an art of 'the art of care' to make it have value or meaning as an aesthetic practice. Care aesthetics insists that, in the moment of its execution, care has an aesthetics – and an exploration of that moment, and the skills enacted in its realisation, are worthy of detailed attention.

If accounts of health care performances discuss artistic representations in a way that takes our attention from the caring moment to make the 'art made from care' a focus of analysis, there is a secondary problematic outcome. It leads to a tendency in training whereby developing aesthetic knowing can focus on artistic practices outside the care moment, encouraging students to represent care in different art forms, and then critique these representations, as a surrogate for developing their 'artful care' practice. While there is nothing wrong with health professional students being taught fine art or theatre as part of their courses, it is a confused notion of the 'art of care' or 'aesthetic knowing' that makes this the process by which they learn to bring a sense of well-honed performance skill to the caring moment. Judging the play a nurse writes about their experience as an attempt to assess their art of care draws attention away from care itself as an aesthetic practice. Care experiences need to be artful and life sustaining for those involved, and this demands that the practice be considered in its own right. The approach of care aesthetics is to insist that care involves an elegance and precision of touch, a deep understanding of presence, an awareness of body movement and a responsive verbal and embodied relational understanding of others and the space which they inhabit. These are capacities, skills and ultimately virtuosities that someone brings to a moment that are realisable by focusing on them and do not need alternative art forms to take their place. Of course, a care practitioner who develops a certain sensibility to others and their environment through an experience of other arts forms, might become a more sensorily aware human being, who may in turn be able to transfer their sensibility to the crafting of moments of care. However, the argument for *care aesthetics* is that the performance of care need not defer to other arts to make it valuable or successful.

From being there to being with

The distinction between the art and performance of care, which focuses on the skills of the practitioner, to care aesthetics, which attends to the sensory experience of care for all involved, is demonstrated in nursing scholar Fredriksson Lennart's work on caring conversations. At first his analysis offers an excellent account of the 'aesthetic knowing' of the nurse who must exhibit a sense of 'being there' with the patient. This involves:

Physically attending behaviour, sensitivity to body language, use of touch in a judicious way to comfort or express concern, making eye contact and leaning forward toward the other. Listening, comfortable silence, and communication of understanding of the patient's experience.

(1999, p. 1170)

However, a heightened capacity is then noted when the nurse demonstrates not just being there but 'being with' the other. At that moment there is a 'flow of feelings between two persons with different modes of being in a shared situation, in which the one caring is touched by the patient's feelings' (ibid, p. 1170). It is this *being with* in health care that care aesthetics is seeking to name and develop. It corresponds directly to the approach taken by Mel Gray and Stephen Webb in their discussion of the *art of social work*, where they are seeking to make the distinction between a focus on the virtuosity of the social worker and the more collective understanding of the aesthetics of a co-created moment. The 'art' in their words 'is immanent in the mutuality of the caring relationship and not merely in the qualities of the individuals doing the caring or being cared for' (2008, p. 183). It is not the 'interior aesthetic process of individual creativity' but a 'myriad of factors' such as 'the client – worker relationship, professional requirements, agency environment, social policy and so on' (ibid, p. 191, 183). This is precisely the differentiation that care aesthetics is seeking to make. It shifts attention to what Julia Twigg, in her account of bathing elders, refers to as 'the dynamics of the care encounter' where 'production and consumption collapse into one another' (2002, p. 1). An extension of this argument would be that *being with* is the exemplary condition of health care performance *and* the socially engaged arts, and that common concern indicates how they might learn from each other.

To conclude, care aesthetics is an approach to performance and medicine which locates the relation in these two areas not as one offering a service to the other but as an integrated proposal where practices of health care have an aesthetics which if properly noted and valued can improve the quality of the care experiences that are enacted in diverse health settings. It can highlight the performance of health care in all its rich complexity, avoiding a sense that performance is a diminutive or solely about the skills brought to an encounter by the one caring. Of course, while the focus here has been on care aesthetics applied to health, it is deliberately a concept that seeks to allow for the full range of caring practices, whether originating in the arts, in domestic care, in schools or many other social settings, to be explored for the dynamics of the caring relations that they perform. It is a concept that, I would argue, is inherent in much health and social care literature, and the ambition of naming it here is to provide a language for care and its aesthetics that values the too often ignored care experiences that are vital for people to live and thrive within the complex demands of our often care-diminished present.

Reference list

Breunig, K. (1994) 'The art of painting meets the art of nursing', in Chinn, P. and Watson, J. (eds.) *Art and aesthetics in nursing*. New York: National League for Nursing Press, pp. 191–201.

Brykczynska, G. (ed.) (1997) *Caring: the compassion and wisdom of nursing*. London: Arnold.

Bunting, M. (2020) *Labours of love: the crisis of care*. London: Granta Publications.

Carper, B. (1978) 'Fundamental patterns of knowing in nursing', *Advances in Nursing Science*, 1(1), pp. 13–24.

Chinn, P. and Kramer, M. (2014) *Knowledge development in nursing: theory and process*. Amsterdam: Elsevier Health Sciences.

Chinn, P. and Watson, J. (eds.) (1994) *Art and aesthetics in nursing*. New York: National League for Nursing Press.

Contreras Ibacache, V. (2013) 'Evidence of art in nursing', *Enfermería Global*, 30, pp. 333–338.

Coutts, M. (2014) *The iceberg: a memoir*. London: Atlantic Books.

Crawford, P., Brown, B. and Charise, A. (eds.) (2020) *The Routledge companion to health humanities*. London: Routledge.

Crawford, P. *et al.* (2015) *Health humanities*. London: Palgrave Macmillan.

Duff Cloutier, J., Duncan, C. and Hill Bailey, P. (2007) 'Locating Carper's aesthetic pattern of knowing within contemporary nursing evidence, praxis and theory', *International Journal of Nursing Education Scholarship*, 4(1), pp. 1–11.

Fredriksson, L. (1999) 'Modes of relating in a caring conversation: a research synthesis on presence, touch and listening', *Journal of Advanced Nursing*, 30(5), pp. 1167–1176.

Gray, M. and Webb, S. (2008) 'Social work as art revisited', *International Journal of Social Welfare*, 17(1), pp. 182–193.

Hanlon, P. *et al.* (2012) *The future public health*. London: Open University Press.

Hochschild, A. (1983) *The managed heart: the commercialization of human feeling*. Berkeley, CA: University of California Press.

Moss, H. (2020) 'Aesthetics of space', in Crawford, P., Brown, B. and Charise, A. (eds.) *The Routledge companion to health humanities*. London: Routledge, pp. 430–435.

Moss, H. and O'Neil, D. (2014) 'The art of medicine: aesthetic deprivation in clinical settings', *The Lancet*, 383, pp. 1032–1033.

Rovithis. M. (2002) 'Nursing as an art', *ICUs and Nursing Web Journal*, 9, pp. 1–14.

Siles-González, J. and Solano-Ruiz, C. (2016) 'Sublimity and beauty: a view from nursing aesthetics', *Nursing Ethics*, 23(2), pp. 154–166.

Smith, P. (2012) *The emotional labour of nursing revisited: can nurses still care?* Basingstoke: Palgrave MacMillan.

Swarbrick, C., Keady, J. and Sampson, E. (2017) 'Notes from the hospital bedside: reflections on researcher roles and responsibilities at the end of life in dementia', *Quality in Ageing and Older Adults*, 18(3), pp. 201–211.

Thompson, J. (2015) 'Towards an aesthetics of care', *RiDE: The Journal of Applied Theatre and Performance*, 20(4), pp. 1–12.

Thompson, J. (2020) 'Towards an aesthetics of care', in Stuart-Fisher, A. and Thompson, J. (eds.) *Performing care: new perspectives on socially engaged performance*. Manchester: Manchester University Press, pp. 36–48.

Thompson, J. (2021) 'To applied theatre, with love', *TDR: The Journal of Performance Studies*, 65(1), pp. 167–179.

Thompson, J. (2022) *Care aesthetics: for artful care and careful art*. London: Routledge.

Twigg, J. (2002) *Bathing – the body and community care*. London: Routledge.

Twigg, J. *et al.* (eds.) (2011) *Body work in health and social care: critical themes, new agendas*. London: Wiley.

Wainwright, P. (2000) 'Towards an aesthetics of nursing', *Journal of Advanced Nursing*, 32(3), pp. 750–756.

Ward, R., Campbell, S. and Keady, J. (2016) Assembling the salon: Learning from alternative forms of body work in dementia care. *Sociology of Health & Illness*, 38(8), pp. 1287–302.

28

AN ART OF CONTINGENCY

Producing biosocial theatre

Simon Parry

There is a diverse ecology of practices and organisations operating at the intersection of the biomedical, the artistic and the social. Such practices navigate the same ethical and political questions as those raised by socially engaged arts practice. They also face the complexity of biological, psychological and bio-psycho-social understandings of health. Artistic practices inevitably draw on and incorporate understandings of the body directly or indirectly derived from biomedicine when they respond to infectious disease or a health condition such as dementia. In her book *Social Works*, the theatre and performance scholar Shannon Jackson (2011) challenged any tendency to set the social function and aesthetic autonomy of an artwork in opposition. Rather she tries in her analysis to think both together, so see the artfulness in social practices and the sociability of arts practices. She pays attention to the ways creative practices, but also her own critique, illuminate or avow the supporting social structures that make them possible. However, social structures are themselves often entangled with ways of knowing. What happens, for instance, when the artistic practices or social structures also encounter medical practices or biological knowledge? Following Jackson, in this chapter, I am trying to pay attention to infrastructural or supportive practices that produce and are produced by what I am calling biosocial theatre. Biosocial theatre is a creative practice that thinks its artfulness and social function together. At the same time, it registers a relationship to the way the social is or has become entangled with the biological or biomedical.

In the first section of the chapter, I will develop the idea of biosocial theatre further as a critical framework and set of practices in a range of contexts including activist responses to HIV/AIDS in various parts of the world and in the work of particular artists in the UK. In the final section, I will focus on the work of Contact, a theatre in Manchester in the UK, and reflect on the way it is increasingly interpreting a long-standing social role in young people's performance culture to include a role responding reflexively to medicine and biology. Between 2011 and 2021, the theatre embedded a strand of health and science related programming within its core activities. It has also pioneered or developed innovative ways of working with health-related themes and within networks that cross over between different sectors (health/arts, public/private/voluntary) within the Greater Manchester city region and beyond. This engagement with medicine and biology through a programme of performance reflects a distinct reflexive or avowed attempt to constitute a biosocial theatre.

DOI: 10.4324/9781003036500-32

Biosociality and the biosocial

Biosocial theatre is more a proposed critical framework than a bounded set of practices. It sits at a confluence between sociological frameworks of biosociality or the biosocial (Rabinow, 2002; Youdell and Lindley, 2019) and theoretical frameworks derived from the study of arts practices. These discourses might include applied theatre, drama or performance (Shaughnessy, 2012; Nicholson, 2015), social theatre (Thompson and Schechner, 2004) and the kind of socially engaged arts practice discussed by Shannon Jackson, amongst others.

Biosociality was clearly articulated in the work of the anthropologist Paul Rabinow in the 1990s (2002), who identified social forms emerging from the practices and implications of bio-medicine, so for instance patient groups formed from those with direct experience of a health condition. Biosociality is built on Michel Foucault's critical account of biopolitics and the shifts in governmentality occasioned through the emergence of a range of technologies (2008). As such, much sociological work on biosociality is highly critical of the way biosocial forms are produced according to neoliberal regimes of biopower.

The sociologist Nikolas Rose (2007) has outlined a 'politics of life itself' that responds both to the emergence of the science and technologies of genetics, genomics and neuroscience and to the parallel and intertwined evolution of the global biotechnology industry, Big Pharma, private health care and a regulatory apparatus often set up at arm's length from national governments. The consequences of such shifts have been increasing demands for individuals to hold responsibility for their own health and to turn to the market to meet these demands. As Rose argues, such a 'complex of marketization, autonomization, and responsibilization gives a particular character to the contemporary politics of life in advanced liberal democracies' (2007, p. 4). Of course, such a complex gives rise to a pressure to perform and a wide range of different kinds of performance including ways patients perform their symptoms to gain access to treatments, modes of assessing the performance of health care or the promotional performances of new drugs or medical technologies. Such performances may also include apparently novel cultural forms. Rabinow refers to the use of fundraising téléthons by patient groups in what was, at the time, a new form of biosocial performance.

At the same time, researchers like Deborah Youdell argue for a biosocial approach to research that combines a critical, sociological engagement with concepts from the biosciences with a serious engagement with these concepts and indeed with bioscientists themselves. Working with the biologist Martin Lindley, for instance, she outlines a number of possible directions for a biosocial approach to the study of education. Attempting to allay the anxieties of fellow critical sociologists, which I think are probably shared by many socially engaged arts practitioners, Youdell rejects the idea that contemporary biology is necessarily deterministic, arguing that 'transdisciplinary' collaboration might support better understanding of 'multifactorial complex causality' (Youdell and Lindley, 2019, p. 11). So rather than the social and the biological set up in apparent perpetual (either/or) opposition, Youdell and Lindley propose programmes through which depression, stress and a range of other phenomena may be approached in a way that examines both their social *and* biological construction. They argue that emerging scientific work in areas such as epigenetics lends itself to such approaches better than sociology might have expected.

Building on Rabinow's analysis, I would argue that all cultural practices and therefore all theatre might be considered always already biosocial in the same way as all theatre is always already social. Rabinow's fundraising téléthons performed biosociality into being in certain ways, setting up particular kinds of relations between researchers, patient groups, clinicians, donors and broader publics. Patient advocacy groups developed new roles in the funding and governance of biomedical research partly through modes of performance. In this sense, performance became a key medium for the realisation of biomedical knowledge. However, the use of the idea of biosocial theatre prompts reflection on the extent to which biosocial theatres do or do not replicate the forms or functions of broader performances of biosociality occurring outside the structures of the arts or theatre. In the sections that follow I develop the idea of biosocial theatre as a framework for understanding a particular set of practices. These mostly emergent forms mediate biosociality through the spaces, cultural forms and social infrastructure of theatre, even if these may vary in relation to different contexts and conventions.

Biosocial theatre and performance

The framework of biosocial theatre as I use it in this chapter emerges from the study of practices where, to echo Jackson, the structures of biosociality are particularly clearly avowed. In these cases, theatres seem to be responding to, demonstrating and promoting certain kinds of biosocial consciousness. I suggest also that some forms of theatre have potential as sites of biosocial exploration and learning. This is partly because of their capacity to foster transdisciplinary collaboration. It is also to do with the potential for theatrical forms to allow for or even prompt what Lindley and Youdell, after Elizabeth Wilson, call the 'mutual rough and tumble' of such collaboration (Wilson, 2015; Youdell and Lindley, 2019, p. 15). Theatre contains but makes perceptible the mess and discomfort involved in encountering a phenomenon or experience from more than one disciplinary or epistemic standpoint. If performance can become implicated in the making real of biomedical knowledge, theatre can both illuminate the process and examine how the reality of this knowledge is incomplete. In her discussion of the relationship between performance studies and new materialism, the performance theorist Rebecca Schneider reminds us (as reader and audience) that '[t]heatricality, unlike performativity, makes sure we remember that not everything in the world is real – or not only real' (2015, p. 14).

Biosocial performance generally and biosocial theatres in particular operate in a variety of historical and geographical contexts establishing a range of different kinds of relations between patients, broader publics, activists, health researchers, policymakers, clinicians and other groups. The HIV/AIDS pandemic gave rise to a wide range of forms of theatre and performance responding to but also expressing and shaping forms of biosociality. Theatre played a key role in fundraising for AIDS research in the early days of the pandemic in the US in a way that perhaps mirrors the role of the téléthons (Roman, 1998). DramAIDe and Soul City in South Africa both emerged from health communication/education initiatives, as theatre and media companies, respectively, promoting drama as an approach to community consciousness-raising about HIV and AIDS (Chinyowa, 2009; Perlman, Usdin and Button, 2013). In Brazil, the Grupo Resistência Adquirida para Prevenção de AIDS com Arte na Rocinha (GRAPAAR) youth project in Rocinha, Rio de Janeiro and the Oficina de Teatro Expressionista para Homens que Fazem Sexo com Homens (OTE) functioned in a similar way to develop approaches to consciousness-raising from within communities affected (Albuquerque, 2004). Albuquerque shows how the work of OTE involved a bespoke training programme for performers that combined performance skills with understanding of the virus, sexual health and sexual practices. He also shows how the production of *Cabaret Prevenção*, which ran at Teatro Alaska for several months in 1995, involved the evolution of collective approaches to practices that included all elements of the production process (2004, p. 142).

These brief accounts show how cultural organisations in different countries changed and adapted social and aesthetic strategies in response to biosocial change. They also show how often new organisations have been created to provide the kinds of social and aesthetic forms to articulate the experiences of biosocially constituted groups and offer alternatives to patient organisations and/or even the activist groups that grew up in response to the biopolitics of HIV/AIDS. Contemporary accounts of collaboration between biomedical scientists and social theatre are often characterised in relation to discourses that might include arts-in-health, therapy, public understanding of science, public engagement with research, public or patient involvement in research and so on. However, these discourses often seem to understate the processes of biosocial knowledge production that might take place through the practice. The artistic/social practice is conceived as communicating, fostering engagement with, representing, consulting on, debating or even critiquing biomedical knowledge. However, it is less often conceived as a knowledge-making practice in itself and, where it is, there are distinct barriers between different kinds of expertise. This is despite the fact that many histories of activist interventions in the HIV/AIDS pandemic often do provide detailed accounts of knowledge (co)production (Epstein, 1996; Gould, 2009). This is an area for further creative and scholarly exploration.

Producing and programming biosocial theatre and performance

Outside the context of HIV/AIDS and within the UK, the work of Anna Ledgard and Mark Storor with individuals and communities alongside clinicians or health researchers constitutes a significant contribution to a practice of biosocial theatre that sits outside therapeutic, educational, commercial or purely aesthetic forms of theatre (Walsh and Ledgard, 2013). In a series of projects, Storor as artist and Ledgard as producer have worked with groups of people connected by a medical or medicalised experience from cystic fibrosis to testicular cancer and kidney dialysis. While Storor has worked with scientists and clinicians, he tends not to place scientific knowledge at the centre of the work. Similarly, while Storor involves patients, they are not positioned as patients in their relationships with him and often not positioned as patients within performance. In the case of his piece *Visiting Time* (2004), a performance by children in a hospital played with and disrupted any clarity about who was a patient, who was hospital staff, who was a visitor, who was an audience member and who was a performer. In other projects, he has involved a range of other people often without a clear differentiation say between professional performers, people with experience of illness, families and carers or clinical professionals. This playing with subject positions within modes of theatricality and the possibility, even if temporary, for individuals to break out of assigned modes of subjectivity begin to mark out the ways that biosocial theatres might constitute alternatives to dominant biosocial forms.

Storor makes performance work out of configurations of place, people, time and objects. The work often includes or emerges from narrative but is equally characterised by a vocabulary of rich symbolic imagery and atmospheric environments. It is creative of social forms as much as it is a creator of artistic forms within existing conventions. For instance, Storor has been working with Heart of Glass in St Helens in north-west England on a long-term project responding to health inequalities within the town. In 2015, Storor started what is planned as a twelve-year residency exploring life expectancy, suicide and other themes in response to specific health concerns of the town (Welsh, 2017). He also works in a variety of settings from a renal unit and a children's hospital to the former Admiralty Underwater Weapons Establishment on Portland, Dorset, UK. A concentration on the forms and politics of life itself perhaps leads to the need to imagine the timespans and spaces of practice as integral to its form. Storor's concern with the health of a town leads to a residency that plays out over a period that can shape and be shaped by a pattern or change in health of a town or community.

An artist's work over decades requires the development and evolution of structural or, as Jackson puts it, infrastructural relationships. These are developed and maintained by artists but also by networks of producers, programmers, commissioners and others. The role of the producer Anna Ledgard and now also the organisation Heart of Glass are integral to Storor's work as an artist. The producer supports the development of infrastructures and networks that make projects happen and coalesce them into programmes. Literature around theatre programming has tended to focus on debates about theatre's perceived elitism through reference to programming diversity or canons and the role that venue or festival programming might have in forming national or other identities (Harvie, 2005; Gilbert, 2007). What these sources recognise is the role of programming in constituting collectives whether across national or more local geographies. Biosocial theatres have the potential to constitute collectives that produce or shape a conception of health across a local, national or dispersed global community.

While there is research that looks at the role of the arts within health communication programmes (Sonke *et al.*, 2021), my interest is more on how programmes of artistic work might construct or reconstruct biosociality or the biosocial rather than communicate more or less predefined health messages, although there can of course be blurring across this apparent distinction. A number of organisations across the UK and beyond avow a commitment to doing this at a programme level in ways that, to greater or lesser extents, reflect similar political and aesthetic concerns to those of artists like Mark Storor. Heart of Glass has developed an extensive programme of biosocial arts practice over a number of years. The venue Summerhall in Edinburgh, UK, has run programmes of performance work setting medicine and theatre in relation as part of the annual Edinburgh Festival Fringe. Sick! Festival has programmed festivals in Brighton and Manchester, UK. Sick of the Fringe, an initiative developed by Brian Lobel and Tracey Gentles, assembled programmes for different venues between 2015 and 2019. Lobel has a track record as an artist and scholar working on a number of projects that together constitute a programme of creative responses to experiences of cancer (Lobel, 2019). Wellcome Collection in London has programmed performance alongside its biosocial exhibitions. The international network of science galleries promotes collaboration between biomedical science and artists including performers. Activist artists like Critical Art Ensemble have mobilised performance as critical response to biotechnology. An emerging literature tracks such practices within different critical frameworks (Shepherd-Barr, 2006; Da Costa and Philip, 2008; Mermikides and Bouchard, 2016; Parry, 2020).

These examples offer a collection of works that might support an understanding of biosocial theatre or investigations of relationships between theatres, publics and biomedicine. They also all institute, support and sustain such practices. Social theatres have often had to justify themselves to social institutions and the institutions of theatre. Similarly biosocial theatres sit between theatre as an institution and institutions that are often dominated by the structures of medicalised health care and biomedical research. There are many examples of plays or performances that might feature or draw on an individual doctor's, patient's or researcher's experience. Such examples may well have relied on the existing support infrastructures provided by their producing theatres or theatre companies. However, all the examples referred to previously have assembled programmes of biosocial performance and therefore encountered a consequent need for infrastructural or systemic support for such programmes that in most cases has meant a need for subtle or less subtle structural transformations.

The work of creating these programmes and indeed the associated social formations is institutional work. However, this work is not necessarily less artful or creative for all that. As Jackson points out, 'the de-autonomizing of the artistic event is itself an artful gesture, more and less self-consciously creating an intermedial form that subtly challenges the lines that would demarcate where an art object ends and the world begins. It is to make art from, not despite, contingency' (2011, p. 28). It is notable that both Theatre Rhinoceros in San Francisco and OTE in Rio de Janeiro chose the form of the cabaret for early theatrical responses to the biosociality of HIV/AIDS. Cabaret is a miniaturised programme that enables the assembly of diverse cultural forms with no requirement to account for their eclecticism or jarring transitions. In fact, it is often enhanced as aesthetic and social experience by the abrupt transition from one form to another. Many of Storor's performance works involve often physical journeys between different scenes or environments. Again the transit is a key feature of the aesthetic. These forms all constitute an art of contingency. Making biosocial theatre relies on structuring support for an art of contingency.

Structuring support for biosocial theatre: a case study of Contact, Manchester

The rest of this chapter focusses on the transformational work of one theatre in the production and programming of biosocial theatre. Many existing paradigms used to understand the relationship between theatres and biomedicine tend to frame any transformation in terms of the way biomedical knowledge may transform the practice of theatre or the way biomedical knowledge translates into theatrical form. I attempt here to register how the processes of transformation themselves involve work and that this work produces knowledge as much as it results from it. As the sociologist Sara Ahmed has put it in her work on institutional change, 'transformation as a form of practical labor leads to knowledge' (2012, p. 175). The labour lies in the creation/transformation of a theatrical infrastructure of time and space that allows for the emergence of novel social forms. At the same time, these social forms remain contingent on the different types of expertise that only become explicit (rather than tacit) through collective modes of theatrical production.

Contact is a theatre and arts organisation in Manchester, UK, founded in the 1960s. It is distinguished by its work by, with and for young people and has pioneered the involvement of young people in governance particularly since the 1990s. The organisation has been through a number of transformations in its history, which are partly reflected in its architecture. The redesign of the theatre building in 1999 prompted thinking about the mission of the organisation and planning the building crystallised thinking about the plan of the organisation. As the then–artistic director John McGrath commented in a conversation with James Thompson and Katharine E. Low, this plan was really a question: 'How would you put participation by young adults at the heart of the theatre?' (2010, p. 405). This ethical and political question still drives organisational practices at the theatre and again found new impetus in a major redevelopment in 2018–2021. The role of young people in governance and decision-making has played a significant role in the way (and the extent to which) the theatre understands itself as a theatre and interprets the implications of this for a programme of activity (Jancovich, 2015). Young people now make up half the board of trustees and are involved in running the theatre from programming and development through to different roles in production.

Since 2011, this programme has transformed, at least in part, into a programme of biosocial theatre as a direct consequence of the way the theatre has embedded in its constitution a reflexive approach to ethics and politics. Young people, unsurprisingly, express repeated concerns with 'the politics of life itself', to use Rose's phrase, in programming decisions, consultations and via creative contributions. There is an established and dynamic awareness in younger generations of the way, to paraphrase Rose, citizenship is interlinked with biological concepts (2007, p. 131). As an example, Contact's creative entrepreneurship programme, The Agency, which supports young people's creative responses to concerns in their local community, repeatedly produces projects with avowedly biosocial aims often responding to conceptions of mental health and illness ('Agency', n.d.). For instance, *Dawn to the Light* (2019/20) is a video game engaging with mental health and exploring interactive media as coping mechanisms. Other projects such as *Open Minds but Silent Sounds* (2016/17) and *Clay Help* (2018/19) explored different creative practices as responses to experiences of mental distress.

The agency also exemplifies the readiness of the organisation to think the social and the artistic together in that it employs a creative methodology derived from theatre to produce social outcomes that may have little resemblance to established or dominant forms of theatre. Contact's reputation and advocacy for including young people in decision-making has also clearly played a role in their developing relationships with key (bio)medical institutions, including Manchester University National Health Service (NHS) Foundation Trust, Vocal (a not for profit organisation supporting research involvement and engagement hosted by the NHS Trust), Greater Manchester Health and Social Care Partnership, University College London Hospitals NHS Foundation Trust and the Wellcome Trust. It has also underpinned the theatre's partnerships with biosocial organisations like the BHA for Equality in Health and Social Care, Brook Manchester and George House Trust.

Processes of infrastructural transformation that think the social and the artistic together necessarily encompass all the organisational functions of the theatre: executive, artistic, finance, communications and production. They emerge from activities of trustees, staff, artists, participants and audiences. Particularly since 2018, the changes have also incorporated the activities of architects, engineers, planners, public and charitable funders, as well as other stakeholders. A programme of biosocial theatre, as already outlined, is constituted by configurations of time and space. Producing biosocial theatre at Contact has involved making space for the programme inside and outside the theatre building and allocating time to it. Biosocial theatre also stakes out a position for theatre within the networks of biosociality and the associated networks of knowledge production.

Since 2018, the theatre has more explicitly marked out time in the programme for productions that respond to the biomedical in different ways through what they have referred to as a 'specific Health and Science strand of programming' ('Re:Con', no date). An examination of Contact's programming between 2011 and 2021, much of it from before this strand was explicitly identified, reveals repeated reference to medical or medicalised concepts: cholera, abortion, depression, trauma, female genital mutilation, radiotherapy, cancer, sexual health, HIV, endometriosis and fibromyalgia, amongst others. This approach, perhaps even before its explicit avowal, is distinct from the incidental and infrequent programming of theatre or performance dealing with health themes as with the vast majority of theatres. It is distinct from the way science festivals might programme theatre dealing with biomedical concepts. It is also somewhat distinct from but related to the advocacy and consciousness raising by theatres or other arts organisations in response to health crises notably in relation to the HIV/AIDS pandemic, as mentioned. These distinctions lie in evolving social/artistic processes but also in infrastructure even if this is often organic in form.

The programming strand is only lightly referred to within promotional materials. It reflects the increasing prominence of biosocial themes within the programme that emerge in different ways and date back much before 2018. It also registers the allocation of resources linked to but not wholly a consequence of a capital development grant from the health-focussed global research foundation the Wellcome Trust. The programming strand does not though correspond to an audience segment in any coherent sense. Contact does not seem to be looking for a health and science audience. Nor is the theatre setting up a health and science festival, although it has programmed collaboratively with Sick! Festival as part of the strand. Contact's health and science strand though is distinct from the festival as a programming construct perhaps specifically because it does not serve a major function in terms of marketing or production processes. It generates and is generated by communities of practice but does not attract a coherent audience group. Each of the projects construct a biosocial community of practice in tandem with reconstructing a theme as biosocial.

Contact's biosocial programming also cuts across its own programming framework that differentiates between different kinds of production which include 'professional theatre shows produced or commissioned by Contact; Contact Young Company shows, made by young people in collaboration with leading artists; visiting touring productions, selected by young people (Re:CON Young Programmers) and staff' ('Re:Con', no date). The first category might include *I Told My Mum I Was Going on an RE Trip* (2017) by Julia Samuels, a co-production with 20 Stories High dealing with abortion and reproductive health, or Amy Vreeke's *The year my vagina tried to kill me* (2018), reflecting on her experience of endometriosis. The second category includes *Under the Covers* (2015), engaging with young people's sexual health, and *There is a light* (2017), responding to the BRIGHTLIGHT study of young people's experiences of cancer. The third category would include work like *A Drunk Pandemic* (2019), inspired by the history of cholera, produced by the Japanese art collective Chim↑Pom. In this way, there is a continual innovation of social and artistic forms intertwined with the work on the theme. *RE Trip* was a recorded delivery verbatim theatre (and then television) play researched and written by Julia Samuels for a young professional cast and young audiences. Amy Vreeke's piece was a solo, autobiographical comedy performance by a young performer. *There is a light* was a collectively devised performance by Contact Young Company responding to a research study and young performers' personal experience. Contact's young curators programmed *A Drunk Pandemic* for the Manchester International Festival.

The performance programme also produces and is produced by different spaces in the building. The capital redevelopment (2018–2021), co-created by architects Sheppard Robson with Contact staff and young people, added a third main public event space called space 0 that works in parallel to the existing spaces 1 and 2 (Waite, 2020). The original 1960s design established Space 1 as a main stage with fixed audience seating and an end-on stage. The 1999 redesign by architect Alan Short added Space 2 as a smaller black box studio theatre. These spaces still retain this architecture and correspondent influence on production and programming. Space 0 is architecturally distinct from these spaces with a conceptual relationship to health and science programming and as a flexible events space. It can accommodate workshops, scratch performances, informal talks or cabaret. It is a space of/for contingency in the sense that it can be contingent on the theatrical or performative demands of disciplines other than theatre. At the same time, though, there is no sense that this space confines or circumscribes any biosocial programming, which continues to permeate the building in shows in Spaces 1 and 2 as well as in processes occupying office space and workshop/rehearsal space.

The health and science programming strand was given focus and added coherence when the Wellcome Trust award allowed for the appointment of a new role of Health and Science Producer (2018–2022). In this role, Chloe Courtney became a key figure in connecting collaborative networks around a number of different themes. This role is exemplary of the way biosocial theatres make use of and create different forms of expertise. Such producing and programming practice is of increasing importance and has a number of leading UK exponents like Anna Ledgard, Brian Lobel, Tracey Gentles and Jayne Compton (Switchflicker productions). Such producers are key to the development and curation of programmes and the formation of networks between creatives but also with health organisations and patient groups.

Sometimes the work of the biosocial theatre producer is about identifying and recruiting creatives with combinations of expertise derived from different sources. Lobel has developed a portfolio of work that originated with autobiographical performance about his own experience of cancer but then has produced, directed and advised on a number of projects that mix different forms of expertise in their creative processes. Cheryl Martin is an established artist who has regularly been produced or presented at Contact: *Alaska* (Flying Solo, 2016), *Who Wants to Live Forever* (2017), *I am because we are* (2018), and *One Woman* (2020). Martin's expertise, though, of particular relevance to *I am because we are* (2018), came both from her experience as a creative writer and performer but also her work as a biomedical research reporter in the 1980s working for the *Blue Sheet* – a publication that provided business and government news about health policy and bio-medical research. She specialised in AIDS and cancer and was working at the time when azidothy-midine (AZT) became the first drug approved by the US Food and Drug Administration (FDA) for treatment of AIDS. She also lived near Dupont Circle and had first-hand experience of how AIDS was affecting gay communities.

On the one hand, the practice of the creative producer requires a consciousness and recognition of the existence of different forms and sources of expertise but also the capacity to find processes and forms to accommodate them in productive relation. Sara Ahmed has talked about institutional work and specifically institutional change as 'an experience of encountering resistance and coun-tering that resistance' (2012, p. 175). Creative producers of biosocial theatre need to work with resistances to generate temporary communities of practice in ways that are generative rather than obstructive. Researchers reflecting on the process of making *There is a light* refer to 'potential tension between researcher and artistic team' (Taylor *et al.*, 2020, p. 11). While they frame their reflection in terms of knowledge dissemination rather than co-production, they acknowledge the way the theatrical (or dramaturgical) process moved control away from researchers and involved a multidirectional flow of different kinds of expertise.

The programme also evolves and develops its own forms of expertise associated with the pro-duction of biosocial theatre. It acts as a kind of creative biosocial laboratory. This laboratory is constituted from writers, performers and directors who include Cheryl Martin, Nathaniel Hall, Keisha Thompson, Yusra Warsama, Amy Vreeke, mandla rae, Ali Wilson, Mark Croasdale, Brian Lobel and Stacey Makishi. Artists have emerged through this period moving through different roles on different productions as a kind of biosocial training process. Yusra Warsama was an actor in *Crystal Kisses* (2010/11) and then moved on to co-write *Rites* (2015) with Cora Bissett. Nathan-iel Hall was assistant director to Stacey Makishi on *Under the Covers* (2015), directed *Not in my honour* (2016), worked as lead artist on *There is a light* (2017) and *Radiotherapy and Me* (2019) and has also presented his own show *First Time* (2021) at Contact. Amy Vreeke performed in *There is a light* before going on to make the solo show *The year my vagina tried to kill me*. The next generation of artists and producers emerging include mandla rae who has produced a series of projects about trauma and Ali Wilson who is establishing a programme of work dealing with neurodiversity.

This emergent expertise is somatic: it is expertise of and about the body (Rose, 2007, p. 74). It integrates and combines disciplinary biological knowledge derived from academic studies at school or in higher education; medical expertise acquired within health-related professions; and lived experience as survivor, patient, carer, friend or relative. The development, integration and learning of this expertise though is embedded within the social structures created by the cultural organisation. Such biosocial learning emerges through the creation of particular configurations of time and space and the convening of communities of practice that cut across categories of profes-sional/amateur, lay/expert, researcher/research subject and performer/participant. It also demands the creative use of different, sometimes novel cultural forms. The creativity relies on play between the realisation of projects and programmes and the un-realisation, to echo Schneider, demanded and enabled by theatrical form.

The institutionalisation of such processes often involves negotiating tensions between these kinds of expertise, for instance between medicalised knowledge and knowledge by experience. There is currently limited provision within higher education or elsewhere for formalised programmes that bring such forms of expertise together (Dewey Lambert and Sonke, 2019). Contact has a long-established capacity for supporting young artists and producers. However, in recent times, it has also shown the potential for its transformations to be led by these artists' and producers' creative practice. This capacity now offers an infrastructure for the emergence of a community of biosocial artists and producers, and through them approaches to the development of biosocial knowledge out of diverse artistic forms and types of expertise. The theatre's recent work opens up questions about the possible social, aesthetic and architectural forms appropriate to biosocial theatres. As a prototype of a kind of biosocial theatre, it also offers a site for the exploration of how the biological and the social might be held together by the theatrical in an art of contingency.

Reference list

'Agency' (n.d.) *Contact*. Available at: https://contactmcr.com/project/theagency/ (Accessed: 14 March 2022).

Ahmed, S. (2012) *On being included: racism and diversity in institutional life*. Durham: Duke University Press.

Albuquerque, S.J.M. (2004) *Tentative transgressions: homosexuality, AIDS, and the theater in Brazil*. Madison: University of Wisconsin Press.

Chinyowa, K.C. (2009) 'Theatrical performance as technology: the case of drama in AIDS education (DramAidE) in South Africa', *Studies in Theatre and Performance*, 29(1), pp. 33–52. https://doi.org/10.1386/stap.29.1.33_1

Da Costa, B. and Philip, K. (2008) *Tactical biopolitics: art, activism, and technoscience*. Cambridge: MIT (Leonardo).

Dewey Lambert, P. and Sonke, J. (2019) 'Professionalizing arts management in healthcare facilities', *The Journal of Arts Management, Law, and Society*, 49(3), pp. 155–170. https://doi.org/10.1080/10632921.2018.1559264

Epstein, S. (1996) *Impure science: AIDS, activism, and the politics of knowledge*. Berkeley: University of California Press.

Foucault, M. (2008) *The birth of biopolitics: lectures at the Collège de France, 1978–79*. Basingstoke: Palgrave Macmillan. https://doi.org/10.1057/9780230594180

Gilbert, H. (2007) *Performance and cosmopolitics: cross-cultural transactions in Australasia*. Basingstoke: Palgrave Macmillan.

Gould, D.B. (2009) *Moving politics: emotion and ACT UP's fight against AIDS*. Chicago: University of Chicago Press.

Harvie, J. (2005) *Staging the UK*. Manchester: University Press.

Jackson, S. (2011) *Social works: performing art, supporting publics*. 1st edn. New York: Routledge.

Jancovich, L. (2015) 'Breaking down the fourth wall in arts management: the implications of engaging users in decision-making', *International Journal of Arts Management*, 18(1), pp. 14–28.

Lobel, B. (2019) *Theatre and cancer*. London: Bloomsbury Methuen Drama Publishing.

Mermikides, A. and Bouchard, G. (eds.) (2016) *Performance and the medical body*. London: Bloomsbury Methuen Drama Publishing.

Nicholson, H. (2015) *Applied drama: the gift of theatre*. Basingstoke: Palgrave Macmillan.

Parry, S. (2020) *Science in performance: theatre and the politics of engagement*. Manchester: Manchester University Press. https://doi.org/10.7765/9781526150905

Perlman, H., Usdin, S. and Button, J. (2013) 'Using popular culture for social change: soul city videos and a mobile clip for adolescents in South Africa', *Reproductive Health Matters*, 21(41), pp. 31–34. https://doi.org/10.1016/S0968-8080(13)41707-X

Rabinow, P. (2002) *French DNA: trouble in purgatory*. Chicago: University of Chicago Press.

'Re:Con' (no date) *Contact*. Available at: https://contactmcr.com/about-us/programming/ (Accessed: 7 March 2022).

Roman, D. (1998) *Acts of intervention: performance, gay culture, and AIDS*. Bloomington: Indiana University Press.

Rose, N. (2007) *Politics of life itself: biomedicine, power and subjectivity in the twenty-first century*. Princeton: Princeton University Press. Available at: www.jstor.org/stable/10.2307/j.ctt7rqmf (Accessed: 17 August 2017).

Schneider, R. (2015) 'New materialisms and performance studies', *TDR: The Drama Review*, 59(4), pp. 7–17.

Shaughnessy, N. (2012) *Applying performance: live art, socially engaged theatre and affective practice*. Basingstoke: Palgrave Macmillan.

Shepherd-Barr, K. (2006) *Science on stage: from Doctor Faustus to Copenhagen*. Princeton: Princeton University Press.

Sonke, J. *et al.* (2021) 'Health communication and the arts in the United States: a scoping review', *American Journal of Health Promotion*, 35(1), pp. 106–115. https://doi.org/10.1177/0890117120931710

Taylor, R.M. *et al.* (2020) 'Brightlight researchers as "dramaturgs": creating there is a light from complex research data', *Research Involvement and Engagement*, 6, p. 48. https://doi.org/10.1186/s40900-020-00222-5

Thompson, J. and Low, K. (2010) 'John McGrath interview: contact theatre, buildings and young people's participation', *Research in Drama Education*, 15(3), pp. 403–411. https://doi.org/10.1080/13569783.2010.495274

Thompson, J. and Schechner, R. (2004) 'Why "social theatre"?', *TDR: The Drama Review*, 48(3), pp. 11–16.

Waite, R. (2020) 'Retrofirst stories: Sheppard Robson on overhauling Alan Short's quirky Manchester theatre', *The Architects' Journal*, 8 September. Available at: www.architectsjournal.co.uk/news/retrofirst-stories-sheppard-robson-on-overhauling-alan-short-designed-theatre (Accessed: 22 April 2022).

Walsh, A. and Ledgard, A. (2013) 'Re-viewing an arts-in-health process: for the best', *Research in Drama Education: The Journal of Applied Theatre and Performance*, 18(3), pp. 216–229. https://doi.org/10.1080/13569783.2013.810923

Welsh, J. (2017) ' "People congregate in shop fronts to catch a glimpse of the spectacle": Mark Storor's Baa Baa Baric', *The Double Negative*. Available at: www.thedoublenegative.co.uk/2017/10/people-congregate-in-shop-fronts-to-catch-a-glimpse-of-the-spectacle-mark-storors-baa-baa-baric/ (Accessed: 22 January 2022).

Wilson, E.A. (2015) *Gut feminism*. Durham: Duke University Press.

Youdell, D. and Lindley, M.R. (2019) *Biosocial education: the social and biological entanglements of learning*. Abingdon: Routledge.

PART 4

Side Effects

Introduction

The practice of medicine often throws up deeply ambivalent, uncertain or negative situations for individuals, for example, when disease or injury outwit our current capacity to cure; when treatment – or the withdrawal thereof – requires intolerable decisions; when human error, 'never events' or rare incidents of malpractice lead to devastating outcomes; or when clinical trials go beyond what is ethically acceptable. More broadly, the development of Western medicine asserts discourses about embodiment, normativity, productivity, responsibility, agency and criminality that reach far beyond the clinical situation. Medicine permeates our social, political, cultural, judicial, ideological systems and more, and historically, medicine has been used to legitimate and enact misogynist, racist, eugenic and genocidal programmes of horrific consequence. The capacity of medicine to do harm must not be overlooked. Performance can expose and critique the challenging and ambivalent personal and social consequences of medicine and medicalisation, and in this section our contributors examine performances that do just that.

We begin with the fraught topic of vaccination. This medical intervention has the power to eliminate horrific diseases but is also a prime target for public mistrust in biomedical research and of public health campaigns that involve coercion and abuse. As Stanton B. Garner Jr. states, vaccination raises a range of concerns in relation to 'bodily autonomy versus public health, the nature of immunity, social class, the aspirations and limits of scientific medicine, and the globalisation of health care'. His chapter describes three historically and geographically distinct case studies that illustrate how theatre engages with the controversies of a phenomenon that 'reaches from the global into the most intimate world of parenting and care'. George Bernard Shaw's anti-vaccination stance, as articulated in his preface to his 1906 play, *The Doctor's Dilemma*, as well as his letters, reveals that 'anti-vaxxer' standpoints are neither new nor as easily dismissed as some might believe. Garner turns next to the use of community theatre within vaccination campaigns in Africa and Bangladesh, suggesting that their participatory, interactive approach might go some way to remediating the harm caused by historic programmes of forced vaccination (another example of participatory performance within vaccination campaigns is provided by Sally Souraya in Part 3 of this volume). Garner concludes with Jonathan Spector's *Eureka Day* (2016), a play set in a progressive nursery school, which stages heated adversarial debates about vaccination in contemporary United States.

DOI: 10.4324/9781003036500-33

The Itch (2015) is a dystopian science-fiction play that uses a medical theme to examine 'oppressive state violence and resistance to it' in contemporary Turkey. Its creator, Deniz Başar, explains how the idea of a pandemic skin disease was inspired by the horrific effects caused by the tear gas used in the state-condoned police violence enacted on citizens during the Gezi protests in İstanbul, Turkey, in 2013 and how the play's setting – a fictional state hospital within a quarantined 'ghetto' – is located on the site of those protests. The main conflict within the play arises when two doctors charged with treating a journalist with a highly resistant case of 'the itch' clash over their 'different medical – and political – agendas in terms of his treatment'. Ironically, the planned production of this award-winning play was cancelled due to the COVID-19 pandemic, but subsequent staged readings in Canada prompt Başar to reflect on what happens when the metaphorical and allegorical references to disease and medicine are taken literally by a medical audience.

Traci Kelly's *Xenograftie (Artificial Sorrow)* (2013) is also inspired by real events. This site-specific performance is the artist's response to the shocking case of Kari Nielsdatter Spidsøen, a resident of a nineteenth-century leprosy asylum, who was pierced in the eye during an experiment conducted, without her prior knowledge or consent, by the hospital's director. Her name is known because she is a rare example of a marginalised person who challenged medical authority and was heard. Her story nevertheless exemplifies the 'asymmetrical power relations' within medicine, its potential to abuse and traumatise those supposedly in its care. Rather than dramatising these events, however, Kelly's performance, which took place in a museum on the site of a former leprosy hospital in Bergen, Norway, stages a ritual. At the heart of this is Kelly's gesture of gently tending to the body of a deceased rabbit, a proxy for all those bodies, human or otherwise, exploited for the 'extraction of knowledge'. The performance endeavours to form a 'new collective memory held by the audience as personal and historical trauma transitions into contemporary cultural currency'. The next chapter also engages with people, like Spidsøen, held in a closed medicalised institution. Clare Summerskill's *Hearing Voices* (2009) is a verbatim play drawn from the experiences of people committed to a locked psychiatric ward. Partly autobiographical, the play includes distressing testimonies from service users detailing failures of care, as well as insights into alternative provision for those suffering mental ill health. *Hearing Voices*, Summerskill tells us, 'presents the stories of people whose experiences and opinions are given scant attention' – indeed, whose experiences are at risk of being dismissed, following the argument that their mental health condition renders their evidence unreliable. Verbatim theatre, Summerskill argues, might offer a way of providing evidence of inadequate care, thereby offering 'valuable insight into the work and conduct of psychiatric professionals'.

The interrelationship between medicine and power is a consistent theme in the work of renowned UK-based playwright, Howard Barker. Alireza Fakhrkonandeh and Yiğit Sümbül offer a critical analysis of his 1998 play, *He Stumbled*, which they characterise as an 'implicit critique of medicine'. Barker, they suggest, uses 'the practice of anatomical dissection to evidence the objectifying and atomistic-analytical approach of medicine and how it diminishes and/or elides the holistic nature of human experience'. In the play, Doja, a famous anatomist, is called to a royal household to dissect and preserve the body of the recently deceased king. His 'detached and impersonal attitude . . . Doja's ingrained and customary temperament and professional stance' is eventually eroded, however, as he is seduced by the Queen and her son. When it is revealed that he has dissected a living person rather than a dead body, he turns the scalpel on himself.

Anatomical dissection and the medical gaze are further discussed in Laura Purcell-Gates chapter, which analyses two productions that employ puppetry to stage surprising medical case histories. Jane Taylor's *After Cardenio*, performed in the Anatomy Lecture Theatre at the University of Cape Town in 2011, is based on the case of Anne Greene, a woman hanged for infanticide, who revived on the anatomist's table just in time to avoid dissection. *The Depraved Appetite of Tarrare the Freak* (2017) is a puppet chamber opera by the company Wattle and Daub based on the case of polyphagist, Tarrare, as reported by his surgeon, Baron Percy, who dissects his body after death. Dated 1650 and 1804, respectively, these cases straddle the emergence of the shift, from "anatomical dissection (cutting open bodies in order to understand their interior structures) to pathology (cutting open the body to identify disease or disorder)". This shift in visuality and the gaze, argues Purcell-Gates, is manifested in the puppetry design of these two productions and in the way they represented acts of visual, legal and epistemological interrogation.

Next, Alex Mermikides and Katie Paterson discuss debates and controversies around hormonal contraception, within feminist 'fringe' performance, responding to the fact that between 2018 and 2023, no less than eight 'pill plays' were staged in small-scale and alternative venues across the UK. The chapter is based upon a roundtable discussion which brought together the creators of these performances, examining their motivations and the political stances they take in relation to a deeply contradictory and controversial medical intervention. The pill, argue Mermikides and Paterson, has been hailed as an 'unqualified good that can liberate women from childbearing and domestic servitude' but also maligned 'as a harmful imposition oppressively regulating women, alienating them from their own natural reproductive cycle and introducing toxic and carcinogenic substances into the body' and implicated in horrific eugenic programmes designed to control fertility in certain populations. The chapter reveals the capacity of performance to represent these ambiguities and draw attention to the way women's experience has been overlooked.

We close this part with Gianna Bouchard's lucid analysis of two plays, *Harvest* by Manjula Padmanabhan and *Made in India* by Satinder Kaur Chohan (first performed in 1999 and 2017 respectively), that interrogate racialised and exploitative practices involved in a global biocapitalist market that mines black and brown bodies for the benefit of those in the global north. Padmanabhan's *Harvest* is a dystopian vision of the future of organ transplantation. In it, a young man based in Mumbai contracts his body to a wealthy white client who systematically commandeers his family's privacy, autonomy, his brother's eyes and body for transplantation, and, prospectively, his wife's reproductive capacity. *Made in India* is concerned with the practice of surrogacy, a form of assisted fertility which involves a surrogate gestating a baby on behalf of another. While surrogacy, like organ donation, tends to be conceived of a 'gift' and a generous sacrifice, in cross-racial surrogacies operating between the global north and south, stark differentials in the economic status of surrogate (in the play, a widow living in Kerala for whom surrogacy is the only way of providing for her daughters) and prospective mother (a white, affluent English woman) render this discourse questionable. Indeed, in these plays, states Bouchard, the concept of the gift in such exchanges is thoroughly 'shredded'.

29

AT THE NEEDLE POINT

Theatre and vaccine scepticism

Stanton B. Garner Jr.

On 8 December 2020, William Shakespeare became the second person in Britain to receive the recently approved Pfizer-BioNTech vaccine for coronavirus at the start of the country's largest vaccination campaign in history. The 81-year-old Warwickshire man was injected at a hospital in Coventry, twenty miles north of the more famous Shakespeare's birthplace, by May Parsons, a nurse who emigrated from the Philippines seventeen years earlier. The happy coincidence of Shakespeare's name and the significance of the occasion triggered an avalanche of memes, jokes and puns ('The Two Gentlemen of Corona' and 'The Taming of the Flu' were popular). Several Twitter users remarked how well the patient looked given that he was 456 years old, while another posted, 'Actually I heard the second person to get the vaccine was Christopher Marlowe but William Shakespeare took all the credit'. For his part, the playwright's namesake focused on the significance of his injection: 'It could make a difference to our lives from now, couldn't it?' (Spearman, 2020).

The idea of vaccination, of course, would have been unfamiliar to the historical Shakespeare, whose career was interrupted by outbreaks of bubonic plague and who lived in an England where typhus, malaria and smallpox were regular threats. Although variolation – a method of inoculation in which healthy people were exposed to material from smallpox sores – was practised in China, India, Africa and the Ottoman Empire, it was not until the eighteenth century that this practice was adopted in Europe and North America. Vaccination, which involved the injection of a less risky substance, was introduced in 1796 when Edward Jenner scratched fluid from a cowpox blister onto the skin of James Phipps, an eight-year-old boy. After developing mild symptoms, Phipps demonstrated immunity when exposed to the deadlier disease. Smallpox vaccination quickly spread to other parts of the world and by the end of the nineteenth century additional vaccines were developed for rabies, anthrax, cholera, typhoid and plague.

From a public health standpoint, vaccination is one of the greatest triumphs of modern medicine. Smallpox has been eradicated, polio is no longer the scourge it once was, and worldwide deaths from measles declined 73% between 2000 and 2018 (World Health Organization, 2019b). Vaccination is responsible, in part, for decreased childhood mortality and increased life expectancy across the globe. Despite these advances, though, a significant percentage of the world's population does not participate in vaccination, and their passive or active opting out threatens to

DOI: 10.4324/9781003036500-34

limit or reverse the previously mentioned gains. The medical term for this phenomenon is 'vaccine hesitancy', which the World Health Organization defines as 'the reluctance or refusal to vaccinate despite the availability of vaccine' (2019c). This and other terms – anti-vaccinationism, vaccine refusal, vaccine scepticism – cover a range of individuals and social groups, including those who lack necessary information on vaccines, those who are uncomfortable with the growing reach of biomedicalisation and those who pursue conspiracy theories and partisan agendas. With the politicisation that surrounds COVID-19 vaccination in the United States in 2021, it would be easy for someone like me – who has received every recommended vaccine since childhood and believes in vaccination with the fervour of many people born in the shadow of polio in the 1950s – to reduce all vaccine sceptics to the latter category. In truth, though, the resistance to vaccination is as old as the practice itself, and it has manifested itself in a variety of forms and sociohistorical contexts. There is a reason for this continuity. Vaccination, after all, raises a number of personal, social and political issues: bodily autonomy versus public health, the nature of immunity, social class, the aspirations and limits of scientific medicine and the globalisation of health care. In the words of anthropologists Melissa Leach and James Fairhead, 'Vaccination reaches from the global into the most intimate world of parenting and care. At the needle point, the most global meets the most personal of worlds' (2007, p. 2). Understandably, the emotions occasioned by this practice are driven by a range of factors. As Eula Biss observes in her book *On Immunity: An Inoculation*, 'Our fears are informed by history and economics, by social power and stigma, by myths and nightmares' (2014, p. 37).

When the coronavirus pandemic surged in early 2020, theatres shut down in New York, Lagos, London, Sydney, Tehran and elsewhere in the world. Asked when they would feel safe returning to the theatre, a majority of New Yorkers responded at that time that they would do so only when those in attendance were vaccinated. Theatre, of course, is a contagious medium and amidst the most serious global pandemic in one hundred years, the performing arts depend on people being inoculated. But the connection between theatre and modern vaccination runs deeper than this. Not only has theatre served as a vehicle for the passionate debates that have surrounded vaccination since the late nineteenth century, it has also been deployed in global public health initiatives in vaccination campaigns. In both capacities, theatre has provided an instrument with which vaccine hesitancy has been acknowledged, explored and – in national and international educational programmes – countered through story-telling. The present chapter offers snapshots of this important, but understudied, interaction. The first section examines George Bernard Shaw's anti-vaccination writings and the origins of his position in the nineteenth-century anti-vaccination movement. The section that follows discusses the role of interactive community theatre in vaccination campaigns in Nigeria (1994) and Bangladesh (2019). And the final section looks at Jonathan Spector's 2016 play *Eureka Day*, which stages the controversies over vaccination in the contemporary U.S.

'A notorious and avowed anti-vaccinationist'

In 1881 the aspiring writer George Bernard Shaw contracted smallpox during an outbreak of the disease in London despite having been vaccinated as a child. 'I was a fully vaccinated person', he later wrote, 'guaranteed immune from smallpox for the whole of my natural life' (Shaw, 1932, pp. 102–103). His signature beard – so much a part of his celebrity later in life – obscured the pockmark scars on his face. This experience confirmed Shaw as a life-long anti-vaccinationist, a position he advanced in letters and published texts and in his 1906 play *The Doctor's Dilemma*.

Nine months before this play's premiere at London's Royal Court Theatre, Shaw wrote the following in a letter to Charles Gane, secretary of the National Anti-Vaccination League:

> [V]accination is nothing short of attempted murder. A skilled bacteriologist would as soon think of cutting his child's arm and rubbing the contents of the dustpan into the wound as vaccinating it in the official way. The results would be exactly the same. They *are* exactly the same.
>
> (quoted in Dukore, 2020, p. 289)

Shaw's opposition to vaccination was intensified by the fact that smallpox immunisation was compulsory in England and Wales as a result of the 1853 Vaccination Act. All infants were required to be vaccinated within three months after being born, and parents who did not comply with this law were subject to a fine. Subsequent acts in 1867 and 1871 extended compulsory vaccination to age fourteen, increased the penalties for parents who refused to vaccinate their children and established compliance officers to track down and prosecute those in violation of the law. Parents who refused or could not pay the fines and court costs, most of whom were working-class or poor, could have their possessions sold or be sent to prison. A law that had been irregularly applied was now heavily and consistently enforced.

Opposition to compulsory vaccination, which increased dramatically after 1867, manifested itself in a loosely coordinated network of national and local associations. Drawing Britons from all classes, the anti-vaccination movement was, as Nadja Durbach notes, not 'a fringe movement of eccentric Victorians but . . . a widespread popular phenomenon that was central to the problematics of both the body and the state in nineteenth- and early-twentieth-century England' (2005, p. 12). This movement asserted the rights of English citizenship against what it saw as an increasingly interventionist state, and it challenged the shift in public health policy from sanitation reform to a reliance on scientific medicine (Durbach, 2005, pp. 18–19). As the century progressed, anti-vaccinationists found allies with other Victorian dissenters: vegetarians, anti-vivisectionists, food reformers, trade unionists, factory reformers, alternative medicine practitioners, religious dissenters, spiritualists and proponents of women's suffrage. Like these other movements, anti-vaccinationism reflected nineteenth-century concerns about individual and parental rights, social class and equality, bodily integrity, medical professionalism, industrialisation and nationhood.

In its efforts to have compulsory vaccination repealed, the anti-vaccination movement skilfully exploited the resources of Victorian print and civic performance culture. In addition to three periodicals – *The Anti-Vaccinator*, the *National Anti-Compulsory Vaccination Reporter* and the *Vaccination Inquirer* – anti-vaccinationist societies produced books with titles like *The Dangers and Injustice of Compulsory Vaccination: or, The Great Medical Delusion of the Nineteenth Century*, which was published in 1873 by the Mothers' Anti-Compulsory Vaccination League. Supporters of this cause wrote letters to newspapers; distributed leaflets at meetings, debates and vaccination stations and mounted postcard campaigns to new parents hoping to dissuade them from complying with the law (Durbach, 2005, pp. 47–50). Propagandistic slogans were prominently displayed on banners and placards at protests and demonstrations. As the Leicester Demonstration of 1885 illustrated, these events could be highly theatrical affairs. Between 80,000 and 100,000 anti-vaccinationists converged that March for a mass procession through the city. Trolleys and carts displayed diseased cows and horses (the source of lymph, which was used in smallpox vaccination), furniture seized by vaccination enforcers and a gallows, on which a dummy of Edward

Jenner was hanged to the delight of onlookers. At an assembly after the procession in the market-place, this dummy was tossed around by the crowd until it lost its head. The day of the demonstration had been declared a holiday, and with '[f]lags everywhere; music everywhere; rosy faces everywhere; happy laughter everywhere', the carefully planned and orchestrated event resembled a civic festival (Biggs, 1912, p. 111).

Shaw did not attend the Leicester Demonstration – nor, as far as I have been able to determine, did he participate in any of the movement's other forms of public protest – but by the early twentieth century he had become one of the country's leading voices against vaccination. This stance formed part of his career-long campaign against the practices, scientific claims and institutions of modern medicine. His preface to *The Doctor's Dilemma*, which was included in the 1911 published edition of the play, includes a lengthy attack on vivisection and a critique of private medical practice in addition to its argument against vaccination. In this important text, which is almost as long as the play itself, Shaw combined the arguments of earlier anti-vaccinationists with his sometimes idiosyncratic beliefs and commitments.

Shaw's preface denounces vaccination as 'dirty, dangerous, and unscientific' (1911, p. 35). In the absence of sufficient controls, vaccination introduces pathogens other than the ones intended for immunisation and, hence, causes illness instead of preventing it. Moreover, the science with which the practice was currently supported – the germ theory of disease, which was developed in the latter decades of the nineteenth century and which Shaw criticised throughout his career – mistakenly identifies microbes as the cause of disease rather than one of its symptoms. One consequence of this mistaken belief, Shaw maintained, is the privileging of bacteriological over sanitary measures for disease. 'The simplest way to kill most microbes', Shaw writes, 'is to throw them into an open street and let the sun shine on them' (1911, p. 28). Like anti-vaccinationists before him, Shaw was a fervent believer in urban sanitary reform; as a member of London's St. Pancras Vestry, or parish council, he had urged the health and sanitary authorities to take measures to stave off the smallpox epidemic of 1901–02 (Dukore, 2020, pp. 290–291). In other writings, Shaw supported a robust policy of isolating those who were afflictèd with the disease. Importantly, he also advocated systemic solutions. As a committed socialist, Shaw attributed what he called the 'vaccination craze' to the economics of private medical practice. As long as underpaid doctors depended on paid procedures such as vaccination to earn a living, they would prolong the practice. If doctors' salaries were independent of the number of vaccinations performed in a system of socialised medicine, 'vaccination would be dead in two years' (1911, p. 77). Though Shaw was wrong about vaccination in important ways – stubbornly so – his objections to the practice were grounded in an expansive vision of public health and the institutions that supported it.

As those who have read them will attest, Shaw's prefaces often float free of the plays themselves, which counter the polemical voice of Shaw himself with the dialectic encounter of positions and ideas. To a degree, *The Doctor's Dilemma* is no exception. The play's medical figures debate the merits and proper procedures of vaccination in the play's opening act as they do other aspects of their profession and the treatment of illness. Unlike the preface, Shaw's play satirises the vaccinationist position through the flawed logic of all positions and the seeming nonchalance its participants display toward the consequences of their medical interventions. But Shaw and the anti-vaccination movement that informed his writing are reinforced through playfully metadramatic means. In Act 3 the artist Louis Dubedat, whose medical treatment constitutes the play's 'dilemma', declares himself to be 'a disciple of Bernard Shaw'. Sir Ralph Bloomfield Bonington, one of the doctors who considered his case, responds, 'Say no more, please. When a man pretends to discuss science, morals, and religion, and then avows himself to be a follower of a notorious and avowed anti-vaccinationist, there is nothing more to be said' (Shaw, 1911, p. 152).

Theatre and vaccine education

The refugee camps in Cox's Bazar, Bangladesh, house a million Rohingya refugees who were settled there after fleeing ethnic and religious persecution in neighbouring Myanmar. On a cloudy day in 2019 a large group of spectators watches actors perform in an open area in one of the camps. Three women performers carrying cloth bundles representing their babies discuss childhood vaccination. 'You are not going to vaccinate your child?' asks one of the mothers, to which the grandmother of the second replies, 'I have never been vaccinated, why should my grandchild be?' The first mother takes her child to be vaccinated and the injection process is mimed for the watching spectators. Later in the performance, the second baby gets sick. 'My baby's hands and feet are numb', his mother exclaims in desperation. 'He is not responding to me anymore' (World Health Organization, 2019a, online).

The community theatre project in Cox's Bazar, which was sponsored by the World Health Organization (WHO), reflects the globalisation of vaccination since its discovery by Jenner in 1796. In 1802 a Scottish physician named Helenus Scott vaccinated the first child in Bombay, and the following year Spanish physician Francisco Javier de Balmis embarked on a three-year expedition that brought smallpox vaccination to the Spanish Americas and the Philippines. Vaccination campaigns were conducted in Africa and Asia during the late nineteenth and early twentieth centuries by British, Belgian, French and Portuguese colonial medical authorities. Since then, international vaccination efforts have been conducted and supported by non-governmental organisations (NGOs) such as the WHO, the United Nations Children's Fund (UNICEF), the Red Cross and Red Crescent and the Global Alliance for Vaccines and Immunization, which was established in 1999.

Because contemporary global vaccination initiatives have concentrated on sub-Saharan Africa, south and southeast Asia, Oceania and the Caribbean, the vaccine hesitancy they provoke reflects the colonial and neocolonial histories of these regions in relation to public health practices. For all the gains that immunisation has brought to countries like Haiti, Senegal and Cambodia, the history of vaccination in the so-called 'developing world' was often marked by mistrust, cultural conflict and coercion. In colonial India the early practice of transferring lymph from one person to another threatened Hindu caste distinctions by introducing the bodily fluid of Untouchable children to those of high-caste parents. Replacing this practice with the use of calf lymph also encountered resistance, since cows are sacred animals in Hinduism. Because India had its own tradition of inoculation – variolation – that was embedded in ritual and religious practices, vaccination was seen as irreligious. As David Arnold notes, 'It treated smallpox purely as a disease, stripped of any religious significance – if indeed it was seen to have any connection with disease at all and not to be merely the 'mark' the colonial state made on its subjects' (1993, p. 143). The notion of subjection in Arnold's characterisation was evident in other beliefs that vaccine objectors held about the practice. Despite the fact that many Indians welcomed vaccination, its association with the imperial state apparatus added an element of coerciveness – implicit or explicit – to the practice. The experience of Indian bodies being subjected to and by scientific medicine continued beyond the end of British rule. During the final years of the WHO's global Smallpox Eradication Program, holdouts in rural villages in India and Bangladesh were forcefully vaccinated. In the words of one physician-epidemiologist who participated in this programme, 'We went from door to door and vaccinated. When they ran, we chased. When they locked their doors, we broke down their doors and vaccinated them' (quoted in Greenough, 1995, p. 636). Though abuses like this are prohibited in today's health campaigns, mistrust of outsiders remains a feature behind vaccine suspicion in many countries and communities. In the early 2000s, for instance, some parents in northern Nigeria refused to have their children vaccinated against polio because they believed the campaign was part of a global plot against Islamic Africa (Leach and Fairhead, 2007, p. 2).

What joins this belief with vaccine hesitancy elsewhere in the world is a disconnection between claims of science; the lived experiences of people's lives; and social, religious, familial and other worlds in which these lives find meaning. Overcoming this disconnection is one of the central challenges facing international, national and local vaccination campaigns. Educating people about the facts of vaccination is important, but this is often insufficient because facts are understood in personal and communal contexts. Bernice Hausman notes,

[W]hat counts as a fact leading parents and individuals toward particular health care decisions is not always, or even primarily, scientific facts. And if it is one, it may be a scientific fact calibrated for the circumstances of an individual's, or a family's, experience.

(2019, p. 120)

Over the last several decades theatre and the stories it tells have provided an effective way to achieve this calibration. That it did and continues to do so is no surprise. Theatre is a communal medium, and the stories it tells in the following examples are by, for and about the people who participate.

One of the earliest and most ambitious uses of theatre in vaccination education took place in Nigeria in the early 1990s as part of UNICEF's child immunisation campaign. Earlier efforts to educate Nigerians using television, radio and print media had had limited success in rural communities, where electricity was often unavailable and literacy rates low. In order to reach and engage these populations, those overseeing the campaign turned to popular theatre, which had demonstrated its effectiveness in addressing public health issues in other international settings. In 1990, the Nigerian actor, dramatist, singer and storyteller Jimi Solanke was invited to train community theatre groups as part of an initiative to bring the message of immunisation to villages in the southwestern states of Ondo and Oyo where vaccination rates were particularly low. Because the work of these groups was so successful, the initial project was expanded into a nationwide programme – the Network of Educational Theatre (NET) – that addressed additional public health issues such as maternal health, guinea worm eradication, food security, AIDS and malaria. As part of the continuing immunisation campaign, local groups around Nigeria performed *The Postman Calls*, one of twelve plays that Solanke wrote based on the 1989 UNICEF/WHO children's health publication *Facts for Life*.[1]

Central to this programme's success was its responsiveness to the individuals and communities it served. As Alfonso Gumucio Dagron suggests, 'The beauty of popular theatre in Nigeria is that it can be built on existing ritual manifestations, taking advantage of local culture to communicate new messages of benefit for the community' (2001, p. 115). When the actors arrived, drumming and singing, in a designated village, they gathered with community leaders to discuss recent events and personalities in the village so that they could incorporate this material in their performance. The performances themselves – which consisted of drama, songs (often local ones) and dialogue with the spectators – were engaging and participatory. During *The Postman Calls*, spectators were invited to ask questions, provide what information they knew about vaccination and the diseases they protected against and share personal experiences. Performances concluded with the actors and spectators dancing, singing, then sitting together to discuss the play and the issues it raised. Members of the local government health staff were available after every performance and they administered vaccinations to the large number of children who lined up with their mothers.

A similar integration of theatre and public health was employed twenty-five years later in the Cox Bazar Rohingya refugee camps. The WHO-funded educational theatre project there was part of an ongoing effort to combat the low immunisation rate in a highly vulnerable population surviving under poor living conditions. The goal of its organisers was to train young Rohingya and Bangladeshi performers to provide information to people in the camps and the adjoining host community who held misconceptions about vaccinations and what they do. Based on a survey they conducted in summer 2019 to understand the barriers to immunisation, they developed an interactive community performance about the consequence of non-vaccination and the benefits of vaccination to children, pregnant women and the community at large. During the performance actor-facilitators provided the spectators with information on such points as the number of recommended vaccinations, the importance of keeping vaccine cards and the locations where their children could be vaccinated. As in Nigeria, theatrical intervention was integrated with actual vaccine administration.

The specific performance referred to at the opening of this section, video segments of which can be viewed in a WHO feature article about the Cox Bazar project, demonstrates the project's strategies for addressing the beliefs, fears and misconception of its audience (*Community Theatre*, 2019a). As Munir (not his actual name), one of the actor-facilitators quoted in the WHO article, explains in translation, 'In the Rohingya community, most of the people believe that vaccination makes them sick because sometimes it causes fever, swelling and body pain' (World Health Organization, 2019a, online). Early in the performance Munir invites the spectators to share what they know about the symptoms of vaccination. When they shout out answers – boil on the arm, fever – actor-facilitators representing fathers step forward and insist that they will not allow their babies to be vaccinated because of these symptoms. Munir solicits applause for them as a way of acknowledging the fears they expressed. One of these fathers is important to the story that follows, in which two families debate the issue of whether to vaccinate their newborn infants. Their actions and interactions with each other reflect the kinship structure and religious beliefs of the production's Muslim audience.

When the drama concludes, the actor-facilitators and spectators applaud each other, and the latter depart with the knowledge they gained from the performance. Vaccination rates among children and pregnant women increased in Cox Bazar as a result of this project. The Rohingya and Bangladeshi young people who trained in order to perform in it also benefited from their work. 'Our parents and grandparents didn't receive vaccines, so we don't know much about it', says Rahema (also not her actual name) in translation. 'By taking part in this community theater, I learned about the importance of vaccination and shared this information with my family and community. I want to help Rohingya people understand the benefits of immunization' (*Community Theatre*, 2019a). Because a theatrical project like this educates its performers as well as its spectators – and because its intervention addresses the lives and concerns of the community – the vaccination advocacy it stages will likely continue.

Eureka day

In her recent book *Anti/Vax: Reframing the Vaccine Controversy* (2019), Bernice Hausman challenges the popular view held by pro-vaccinationists that vaccine sceptics are science deniers whose beliefs mirror those of climate change and Holocaust deniers. This view, she demonstrates, has become increasingly inflammatory in contemporary media and in books such as Paul A. Offit's *Deadly Choices: How the Anti-Vaccine Movement Threatens Us All* (2012). As long as the vaccination debate is framed in this way, attempts to communicate with vaccine resisters will fail, since the issues at stake are as much social and political as scientific: '[V]accine skepticism is linked to various beliefs and practices that are actually not unusual in American society, and . . . such skepticism is sustained by popular suspicions of government, sponsored scientific research, and pharmaceutical companies' (Hausman, 2019, p. 13). Instead of falling back on tropes of ignorance, gullibility and misinformation, Hausman proposes listening to vaccine sceptics and understanding the assumptions, concerns and decision-making process of those who choose not to vaccinate their children or themselves. As members of the Vaccine Research Group at Virginia Tech, US, Hausman and her collaborators conducted semi-structured interviews that allowed vaccine sceptics to tell their own stories. The reasons these interviewees offered were varied, complex and – in many cases – understandable. The concerns about vaccine safety that some expressed, for example, makes sense in view of the fact that Johnson & Johnson, a pharmaceutical company that produces one of the main COVID-19 vaccines currently in use in the United States, was fined in 2019 for its role in the country's prescription opioid crisis. Historically, moreover, some people have suffered adverse consequences from vaccination. The statistical chances of this happening are small, but this may not be sufficient assurance if you are deciding whether or not to have your own child vaccinated.

The controversy that Hausman analyses is at the centre of Jonathan Spector's *Eureka Day*, which premiered in 2016 at the Aurora Theatre in Berkeley, California, and enjoyed popular runs in Washington, DC, and New York in 2019. The play takes place in the library of a progressive private elementary school in Berkeley where Don, the school's head, and four parents who serve with him on the school's executive committee hold their meetings. Diversity, inclusiveness and social justice are the guiding principles at Eureka Day: the walls are adorned with posters that display slogans like 'Berkeley Stands United Against Hate' and 'We are the Resistance', and the banner welcoming students to the 2017–18 school year includes the equivalent dates in non-western calendars. When the play opens, the committee is attempting to navigate the demands and pitfalls of inclusiveness. Eli, a stay-at home multimillionaire who is having an extramarital affair with a bi-racial Japanese/White committee member named Meiko, supports the request submitted by one Eureka Day family that 'Transracial Adoptee' be added to the school's list of identity categories because 'everyone should Feel Seen by this community' (Spector, 2022, p. 9). Suzanne, one of the school's founders, argues against this by pointing out that 'adoptee' is not a racial category. Their discussions are comically fraught, with characters working carefully and often at odds with each other to ensure that they avoid saying or doing anything that could be construed as causing offence to anyone. Carina, a lesbian African American woman who recently enrolled her child in the school after moving to California from Maryland, watches the conversation with a mixture of bewilderment and bemusement.

What begins as a lighthearted satire on over earnestness and self-congratulatory political vigilance takes a more serious turn when one of the students in the school comes down with mumps. The committee convenes for an emergency meeting in response to a letter that the school received from the Alameda County Health Department requesting that students who cannot provide documentation of immunity to mumps be excluded from school until the danger of infection passes and that those parents who have delayed or refused having their children vaccinated do so. Their discussion centres on whether the school should include a statement with the letter acknowledging the diversity of opinions on vaccinations and the right of families to make their own choice without judgement. Carina, whose child is immunised, is shocked to learn that California allows personal exemptions to mandatory school vaccinations. Suzanne, who opposes vaccination, argues in favour of parental freedom. At issue in this scene and the ones that follow is whether the school's commitment to diversity of opinion can negotiate an issue this divisive.

Not surprisingly, it cannot. The committee holds a live-screen Facebook meeting – what Don refers to as a 'Community Activated Conversation' ('it's a bit like a Town Hall but more participatory') – with the rest of the school's parents to discuss the outbreak and the health department's mandate, which the school intends to follow (ibid: 47). The parents' comments, which are projected on stage so that the audience can view them, begin with the friendly chit-chat typical of such meetings, but when one parent expresses shock that half the school are 'anti-vaxxers', their exchange shifts to defensiveness and accusation. Those who oppose vaccination provide a range of justifications that characterise contemporary American anti-vaccinationism, and those who support it mount familiar arguments and lines of attack in its defence. One parent's suggestion that all children stay at home so that unvaccinated children do not fall behind is met with outrage by parents who refuse to have their children disadvantaged because other parents are willing to endanger theirs. As the conflict escalates, any pretence of civility gives way to personal attack, sarcasm and insult: 'Remember that time I got crippled from polio? Oh, no wait. I didn't. Cause I got FUCK-ING VACCINATED' (ibid: 76). Don, the only one who can follow the online comments on his computer screen, grows increasingly distraught as the acrimonious discussion spins out of his control, and his only recourse at the end of the scene is to slam his computer shut, cutting off the feed. So much, it seems, for inclusiveness and consensus.

With politically enlightened parents reverting to their worst selves, the Community Activated Conversation scene is wildly funny. The issues and emotions that underlie it, though, are real. Eli's son catches mumps from Meiko's daughter and becomes so sick that he has to be placed in a medically induced coma and sustains substantial hearing loss in one ear. A petition circulating among a group of fifty parents states that they will not return to Eureka Day unless they revise the school's immunisation policy to require vaccinations for every student. Carina and Suzanne continue their argument about vaccinations and personal belief. Carina, who signed the petition, upholds science as an arbiter of controversy, and her role as a newcomer to the world of Bay Area culture endows her position with a certain authority. Suzanne's defence of vaccine scepticism is undermined, in the audience's eyes, by the patrician condescension she exhibits toward Carina, which comes to the surface when she reveals her mistaken assumption that Carina, as an African American, required financial aid to attend the school. But her position and the concerns it reflects are by no means discounted. In an unexpected moment when the two are alone on stage, she tells Carina that shortly after her daughter received her one-year shots, she started wailing, eventually stopped babbling and sleeping through the night and died in her sleep one night. Her monologue is devastating, and though Carina will later point out that the two events are not necessarily connected, the evidence of science sits uncomfortably with the apparent, though no less real, evidence of experience.

In the end, the school adopts the vaccination requirement. Eli has offered to offset the financial losses suffered by the school on the condition that it do so, and he is supported in this position by Don, Carina and Meiko, who has been a vaccine sceptic up to this point. The play ends with the final minutes of a committee meeting to mark the start of a new year. The books Suzanne contributed to the library are gone, and her place on the committee has been taken by a new member. Don acknowledges that not everyone is continuing on the school's journey with those who remain but affirms 'how special a thing it is we have here because it's a thing we Make Together' (ibid: 147). In the absence of Suzanne and other parents who share her beliefs, however, what 'Together' means for a school founded on the principles of inclusiveness and consensus is not the same as it was at the start of the play. Some conflicts, it is clear, cannot be resolved.

By exploring the disagreements that led to this outcome and the lived realities they reflect, *Eureka Day* joins other theatrical attempts to advocate, analyse and intervene in the fraught relationship between vaccination and its sceptics. As we saw with Shaw's anti-vaccinationist writings, these relationships involve long standing issues concerning individual and parental rights, medical professionalism and the claims of collective responsibility. The continuing volatility of these issues in *Eureka Day* and the heated conflicts associated with COVID-19 indicates the persistence of anti-vaccinationist attitudes and beliefs despite the greater safety of vaccines in the early twenty-first century. At the same time – as the international vaccination campaigns in Nigeria and Bangladesh remind us – these attitudes and beliefs are conditioned and localised by history, culture and politics. Hence, this chapter has argued, the striking, if underappreciated, role of theatre in the history of vaccination debates. Because vaccination 'reaches from the global into the most intimate world of parenting and care', it finds a natural place in a medium – like theatre – that joins the social, the political and the personal.

Note

1 Information in this and the following paragraph is taken from Gumucio Dagron, 1994, 2001, 2008. Gumucio Dagron (1994) includes Solanke's training manual for actors who performed as part of the NET initiative.

Reference list

Arnold, D. (1993) *Colonizing the body: state medicine and epidemic disease in nineteenth-century India.* Berkeley: University of California Press.

Biggs, J.T. (1912) *Leicester: sanitation versus vaccination.* London: National Vaccination League. Available at: https://wellcomecollection.org/works/zkaqv9kh (Accessed: 26 May 2021).

Biss, E. (2014) *On immunity: an inoculation.* Minneapolis: Graywolf Press.

Dukore, B.F. (2020) 'Bernard Shaw and the smallpox epidemic of 1901–2', *SHAW: The Journal of Bernard Shaw Studies*, 40(2), pp. 285–297. Available at: www.jstor.org/stable/10.5325/shaw.40.2.0285 (Accessed: 17 May 2021).

Durbach, N. (2005) *Bodily matters: the anti-vaccination movement in England, 1853–1907.* Durham: Duke University Press.

Greenough, P. (1995) 'Intimidation, coercion, and resistance in the final stages of the South Asian smallpox eradication campaign, 1973–75', *Social Science and Medicine*, 41(5), pp. 633–645. Available at: https://www-sciencedirect-com.utk.idm.oclc.org/science/article/pii/0277953695000356 (Accessed: 31 May 2021).

Gumucio Dagron, A. (1994) *Popular theatre in Nigeria.* Ibadan: UNICEF.

Gumucio Dagron, A. (2001) *Making waves: participatory communication for social change.* New York: Rockefeller Foundation.

Gumucio Dagron, A. (2008) *Photo essay: developing locally relevant theatre in Nigeria.* Available at: http://archive.cfsc.org/photogallery.php%3Fid=371.html (Accessed: 7 June 2021).

Hausman, B. (2019) *Anti/Vax: reframing the vaccination controversy.* Ithaca: Cornell University Press.

Leach, M. and Fairhead, J. (2007) *Vaccine anxieties: global science, child health and society.* London: Earthscan.

Offit, P. (2012) *Deadly choices: how the anti-vaccine movement threatens us all.* New York: Basic Books.

Shaw, G.B. (1911) *The doctor's dilemma.* London: Penguin.

Shaw, G.B. (1932) *Doctors' delusions, crude criminology, and sham education.* 2nd edn. London: Constable.

Spearman, K. (2020) 'The wheel is come full circle: Shakespeare gets the COVID vaccine – and there are memes', *The Daily Dot*. Available at: www.dailydot.com/unclick/william-shakespeare-covid-vaccine-memes/ (Accessed: 18 May 2021).

Spector, J. (2022) *Eureka day*. New York: Dramatists Play Service.

World Health Organization (2019a) *Community theater – bridging the immunization gap in the Rohingya refugee camps*. World Health Organization South-East Asia Region. Available at: www.who.int/bangladesh/news/detail/15-12-2019-community-theater–bridging-the-immunization-gap-in-the-rohingya-refugee-camps (Accessed: 28 May 2012); www.youtube.com/watch?v=wKJtpDRadWk (Accessed: 8 June 2021).

World Health Organization (2019b) *Measles*. Available at: www.who.int/en/news-room/fact-sheets/detail/measles (Accessed: 20 May 2021).

World Health Organization (2019c) *Ten threats to global health in 2019*. Available at: www.who.int/news-room/spotlight/ten-threats-to-global-health-in-2019 (Accessed: 20 May 2021).

30

CONSTRUCTING A FICTIONAL SKIN DISEASE

Pandemic as a political allegory in *The Itch*

Deniz Başar

This chapter focuses on *The Itch*, a dystopian science fiction play I wrote in the close aftermath of the Gezi protests in İstanbul, Turkey, in 2013 (see Tanyıldız, 2017). Starting as a peaceful demonstration by environmentalists against the proposed redevelopment of Gezi Park into a shopping mall, these protests were met with large-scale state-condoned police violence, including excessive use of tear gas on civilians and other forms of physical violence, along with mistreatments in police stations. I had first-hand experience of the unrest, both as a protestor at the time of Gezi and later due to the MA research I was conducting on the independent theatres of the Beyoğlu distinct of İstanbul (Başar, 2014). Tear gas was the initial inspiration for the idea of an itching pandemic: when skin is exposed to too much tear gas, it creates allergic reactions such as rashes, itching, redness or dryness. Because, as writer Sergio Del Molino defines it in his meditative book, *Skin*, on the relation between skin and psyche: '[t]he metaphor is the epidermis: that is the place where we carry our dead friends with us' (Del Molino, 2021, p. 17). I finished the play in 2014, just a few days after the funeral of one of the victims of the police violence of Gezi, fourteen-year old Berkin Elvan (see Akıncı, 2018). In the writing phase of *The Itch*, I imagined it would be staged in one of the black box theatres located in the Beyoğlu district. If the play had been staged in such a venue, the audience would have been transported into the future of the exact same location that they were in at that moment. Influenced by these events, *The Itch* imagines a dystopian future in which the divisions exposed by the protests, between social justice-minded civilians and the far-right tendencies in political power, have taken an extreme form.

My focus here was my decision to explore this theme of oppressive state violence and resistance to it, through a play with a medical theme. Arguably, the central character in the play is the illness itself, which is partially embodied by all of the characters, either in their bodies or in their ideological blindspots. *The Itch* centres on the character of Toprak, a Kurdish man who is forcefully hospitalised because he is suffering from a particularly resistant case of 'the itch', a novel pandemic skin disease that is sweeping the globe. The main conflict within the play arises when the two doctors assigned to his case, İpek and Celal, have different medical – and political – agendas in terms of his treatment. Turkish names are generally derived from the in-use nouns in contemporary Turkish. Toprak means 'earth' or 'soil', İpek means 'silk', Celal means 'rage'. Toprak is a unisex name (the character is male), İpek is for women, Celal is for men. These names were chosen to immediately give an insight about these characters. The name of Toprak indicates the character's

DOI: 10.4324/9781003036500-35

suffering is related to the suffering of the earth, İpek's name highlights her elegance and softness along with her class background and Celal's name alludes to his alliance with the authorities.

The play takes place in a hospital room which we see over the course of a few days as the conflict between the two doctors and the patient unfolds. The two medical professionals, both specialists in 'the itch' (as it is now established as a separate branch of medicine), are on the opposite sides of the medical-ideological spectrum of how to deal with the pandemic, and Toprak is an unusually treatment-resistant patient. Cameroonian scholar Achille Mbembe notes that 'the primary function of the medical gesture was not the absolute eradication of illness or the suppression of death and the advent of immortality', in his contextualisation of this view it would make 'the ill human' as into someone with no 'possibility of an authentic encounter with other humans', which is exactly where the two doctor's ideological positions oppose each other (2019, p. 24). İpek believes in the totality of healing; she is against sacrificing the lives of the current patients by dehumanising them for their illness and therefore opposes ideological and medical paradigms that would eventually allow violent experimentations on patients for a 'greater good' such as a complete eradication of the disease. On the other hand, Celal is introduced as a doctor who seemingly wants to eradicate the illness and does not respect the itching patients' lives, as he is willing to treat them as livestock for experimentation. At the beginning of the play, İpek has just returned to İstanbul to take on this position; therefore she has not yet figured out all the corruption happening in the hospital, which she only begins to notice at the end of the play. In Celal and İpek's medical debate in the first scene, their alliances and privileges are demonstrated: İpek is an internationally successful doctor, whereas Celal is an institutional power holder domestically, with – as it is later revealed – strong alliances to the deep state; Celal has a superior position to İpek due to being a man in a patriarchal institution, whereas İpek has a superiority over Celal as a person a from higher class with better family connections and fluency in foreign languages. It is revealed at a certain point that Toprak is conscious, unexpectedly so since many patients as severe as he lose their mental capacities. This is why when he is introduced at the beginning, he is pretending to be unconscious so as not to reveal his agency, which would make things more dangerous for him in the institutional machinery – especially when Celal is in control. It is also suggested in the play that he got 'the itch' because he witnessed too much human pain as a journalist, which means his capacity of resilience is what made him ill. But unlike many others with the illness, Toprak does not die: he holds onto what he witnessed to be able to pass it on.

The setting alludes to the main theme of the play, which is how the state constructs spaces and institutions to ideologically and physically penetrate the body and how resistance can be possible under such intense attacks on the integrity of the body. In the play, all the action takes place in one hospital room. We learn that the hospital is located in what used to be Taksim Square/Gezi Park (site of the uprisings) in what has now been made into a quarantine zone by the state to segregate the ill. In the universe of the play, there are six degrees of 'the itch', the first degree being the lightest and the sixth degree being the severest. Starting from the fourth degree, 'the itch' patients are considered dangerous due to the loss of mental capacities and tendencies of violence and are segregated. This camp, which is referred to as 'the ghetto', is right in the centre of the city; it occupies the heart of the city. Philosopher Giorgio Agamben argues that '[t]he camp, which is now securely lodged within the city's interior, is the new biopolitical nomos of the planet' (2004, p. 179). This means that the realities such as spatial segregation, ghettoisation and apartheid not only directly inflict violence onto dissenters but also turn everyone into potential subjects of violence by normalising such socio-spatial organisation. Beyoğlu district is made into a quarantine zone, a ghetto for the ill, and the humans locked in the ghetto are stripped of their rights as citizens and reduced to the status of 'bare life' in Agamben's terms. None of these locations were chosen by coincidence: Beyoğlu has always been an anxiety-inducing space for conservative politicians due to its historical cosmopolitanism, and the Gezi Uprising was positioned against the neoliberal-conservative spatial plans of the government to reshape this symbolic space according to their agenda.

The camp has an even more sinister purpose. As we learn in the climactic dialogue between Celal and Toprak, the state hospital has been conducting secret experiments on the ill to create super-human soldiers immune to 'the itch'. We also learn from Toprak that refugee children are being brought into the ghetto illegally by the state to save the rich and powerful itching patients by transplanting children's skin onto them, since children do not get the itch until adolescence. This detail was inspired by the Syrian refugees who were visibly occupying urban spaces in İstanbul when the play was being written in 2014, raising questions of the precarity of the refugee children under these circumstances.

The ghetto in the play is constructed as the spatial manifestation of the phobia of touching the ill. The main character who has the itching illness, Toprak, is Kurdish: which suggests an overlapping pattern of stigmatisation. His ethnic background locates his pain in a geo-political context. Kurds are one of the most ethnically stigmatised and one of the largest minorities in Turkey. The undercurrent of the play is this landscape defined by colonialism, playing out at both national (against minorities) and global (against third world countries) levels. The world map of the play spirals out of İstanbul and Turkey through the character dialogues (as İpek tells of her time in Brazil as a doctor to Toprak) and relates to the experiences of the itching pandemic, particularly in Latin American countries. Suffering under similar colonial projects and military coups, these regions share similar histories and hold the potential to build healing practices in dialogue with each other for the itch. Through such dialogues, the play spirals out of the spatial limits of İstanbul and develops a more global understanding of interconnected networks of information, bodies and power structures.

The basis of this ideological and medical debate between these two doctors resides in the body of the patient: Toprak. Toprak is someone who is described in the play by the established medical discourse as 'someone who should have died long ago', due to the intensity of his unendurable pain and the incurability of his diseased body. He is someone who should 'not have stayed conscious' according to the same medical literature. There is a hint of a certain fear that the medical establishment has, particularly embodied in Celal's discourse: the medical establishment is uneasy with the conscious patient who can articulate their own pain in their own terms. Toprak is aware of this, which is why he reveals that he is conscious only when İpek appears within the institutional setting. The conscious mind of Toprak is a threat to the medical establishment represented by Celal, because it resists the abstraction of the illness, as a concept separate from the individual patients' bodies. This is why Celal, as an authoritarian figure who fails to produce any kind of compliance from Toprak, gets more and more aggressive towards 'the ill human' as the play progresses.

The central medical and ideological divide between İpek and Celal materialises not only in their verbal debates but in their ways of relating to Toprak. The moment that Toprak decides to trust İpek is when she touches him without wearing gloves:

Toprak: Won't you wear gloves?
İpek: The disease is not transmitted by touch. This is a well-known fact.
Toprak: It is not known how it is transmitted which means it can be by touch.
İpek: Yes, it is not known but we are close to sure that it is not due to touching.
Toprak: But it is not proven.
İpek: One out of a thousand is a negligible percentile.
Toprak: Why don't any doctors touch patients, then?

İpek: Fear. There are fears in people that the conscious mind cannot conquer. Like the fear of darkness. Maybe you know, one of the most feared illnesses in history was leprosy and it is not transmitted by touch either. But all the doctors used gloves. One of the deadliest epidemics of the last century was AIDS and it was the same case. The virus was not transmitted with touch but still many doctors wouldn't touch patients. The creature named human is full of unexpected fears.

(Başar, 2015, p. 256)

Here, the decision to touch is an ideological choice as much as a scientific one; İpek choses to show physical solidarity with Toprak by shouldering the institutional stigma she will receive due to her choice. The play ends with an unexpected twist, with a fragile alliance formed between İpek and Toprak to work together to understand the disease, which may or may not defy the larger system. Such a fragile alliance was also formed during the Gezi Park Uprising, where people from Western Turkey started to develop an embodied understanding of the Kurdish resistance and the meaning of positioning against the state.

The Itch won an important award in the 2014 Mitos-Boyut theatre publishing agency's annual contest, which is the largest playwriting competition in Turkey, and was published in a volume of plays that was granted the award in 2014 (Başar, 2015). The play was potentially going to be staged in the 2020–2021 season by the İstanbul Municipality Theatres, under the direction of Semah Tuğsel, but the season was cancelled, ironically, because of the coronavirus pandemic. Between 2018 and 2020, Dr. Art Babayants started to assign the play to his theatre students in the University of Regina, and later in the University of Ottawa, which triggered productive debates about biopolitics amongst students. During the summer of 2020, an interview about why I wrote the play was published in a prominent left-wing Turkish-language online newspaper (Başar, 2020), focusing on how many things in the play corresponded to the present realities of the pandemic as the fears of the pandemic triggered authoritarian tendencies in many states along with overt and visible racism, accompanied by anti-immigration rhetorics.

In the play, the hospital becomes a metaphor for the state, and the effects of state oppression and resistance to it are reimagined through the image of a contagious skin disease that each character seeks to address. But what happens when the medical metaphor is taken more literally? This is what happened when the play was performed as a staged reading for an audience of medical practitioners in Canada rather than its intended location in a theatre near the site of the Gezi Park protest where the play itself is set. In the relatively safe space of a medical humanities conference, far from the violence and unrest in which the play was developed, the play nevertheless revealed the potential violence inherent in medical practice. I remember the reaction that the play received when it was read in a room full of medical professionals and doctors with various specialisations and students of medicine, along with a few artists and scholars who were instructors in other workshops of the conference in 2016 in Hamilton, Ontario, Canada (Canadian Society for the History of Medicine, 2016). There was an intense silence at first, which then led to questions during the post-show discussion such as 'How did you understand the insider position of a healthcare worker?' or 'How did you get the scientific references right?'. While modern medicine is assumed to be objective and neutral for outsiders, insiders know the dirty history of the discipline, ranging from human experiments to the societal results of defining states of being that are not illnesses as disease (such as 'hysteria' or non-heteronormative desire) or the multiple cases of the medical status quo denying scientific facts due to ideological positionings.

It seemed that the majority of the audience members missed the nuances of the İstanbul-based references in the text and the integral ties of the allegory of the skin disease pandemic to what was happening in Turkey during the early 2010s, but the meaning was still clear, the moral questions that the text was engaging with communicated effectively to the audience, which allowed for a brief acknowledgement of the ideological position of medicine and its ties to state politics.

Especially in the post–COVID-19 world where 'the new biopolitical nomos of the planet' (Agamben, 2004, p. 179) is clearly divided on the line medically drawn between 'the ill human' and the healthy human, the 'possibility of an authentic encounter with *other* humans' (Mbembe, 2019, p. 24, emphasis added), becomes the only hope for a more just world. Such encounters can be sustained within the medium of theatre better than other artistic mediums due to the fragile dependency of theatre onto temporary communities constituted by its audiences in each performance event. Therefore, the fragile alliance between İpek and Toprak can be embodied best in theatre thanks to the medium's potential of contaminating bodies not just with diseases but also with critical thinking by physically confronting the audiences with the meaning of illness in relation to the state apparatus.

Reference list

Agamben, G. (2004) *Homo Sacer: sovereign power and bare life*. Reprint edn. Stanford: Stanford University Press.

Akıncı, E.F. (2018) 'Sacred children, accursed mothers: performativities of necropolitics and mourning in neoliberal Turkey', in Brady, S. and Mantoan, L. (eds.) *Performance in a militarized culture*. Abingdon: Routledge, an imprint of the Taylor & Francis Group.

Başar, D. (2014) *Performative publicness alternative theater in Turkey after 2000s*. M.A. thesis. Boğaziçi University.

Başar, D. (2015) 'Kaşıntı [The Itch]', *Mitos-Boyut 6. Oyun Yazma Yarışması*, 2014, Beyoğlu, Mitos Boyut, pp. 241–84.

Başar, D. (2020) *Derinin altı derinin üstü: Deniz Başar'la 'Kaşıntı' oyunu üzerine [Over the skin, under the skin: Interview about 'The Itch'with Deniz Başar]*. Interviewed by H. Aktürk for Gazete Karınca, 24 July. Available at: gazetekarinca.com/2020/07/derinin-alti-derinin-ustu-deniz-basarla-kasinti-oyunu-uzerine/ (Accessed: 1 August 2020).

Canadian Society for the History of Medicine (2016) *A palpable thrill: an introduction to medical humanities*. Available at: cshm-schm.ca/cfp-a-palpable-thrill-an-introduction-to-medical-humanities/ (Accessed: 1 November 2021).

Del Molino, S. (2021) *Skin*. Cambridge and New York: Polity Press.

Mbembe, A. (2019) *Necropolitics*. Translated by S. Corcoran. Durham: Duke University Press.

Tanyıldız, G.S. (2017) 'The Gezi protests: the making of the next left generation in Turkey', in Muhannad, M.A. and Hadj-Moussa, R. (eds.) *Protests and generations: legacies and emergences in the Middle East, North Africa and the Mediterranean*. Netherlands: Brill, pp. 143–167.

31

XENOGRAFTIE (ARTIFICIAL SORROW)

Traci Kelly

The following text contemplates a site-specific performance based on the medical history of Kari Nielsdatter Spidsøen, a woman with leprosy subjected to unethical experimentation in nineteenth-century Norway. The account of the performance interplays with the artist's own childhood experience of medical internment and utilises the presence of a rabbit as a surrogate for the medical subject. The performance was staged in St Jørgen's Lepramuseet (a museum on the site of a former leprosy hospital) in Bergen, Norway, in 2013.

The rabbit escapes (1963)

I am two years old and lying in an iron cot towards the end of a row of identical cots running down the middle of the ward. The nurses have just given me the spoonful of 'sweet' that puts us to sleep each evening. The little girl three cots away has just had a small piece of dead brown earlobe snipped away, as she does every evening. I am paralysed with fear that this may also be my fate. I am here to convalesce after dying twice during a surgical operation. My misery is full until three months later when my father, alarmed that I am 'looking like a skinned rabbit', discharges me against medical advice.

The rabbit fails (1879)

'. . . she stayed anxiously beside the door and started to weep'.[1]

The 'she' is Kari Nielsdatter Spidsøen, one of Bergen's many leprosy sufferers of the nineteenth century, whose body becomes colonised by a disease that will damage organs and limbs and cause chronic disfiguration. She is one of over eighty people with advanced leprosy interned in the Lungegaardshospitalet.[2] Kari was admitted when she was sixteen – she is now thirty-three. The doorway she stands beside is the medical office. She has been called there, and as doctors in white coats gather and Kari glimpses a sharp instrument, she knows that she is central to the proceedings. Unwilling and unknowing, Kari panics and is reduced to floods of tears. Afraid and pressured, she finds herself amongst ambitious men competing to discover the cause of leprosy. Daniel Cornelius Danielssen is convinced it is a hereditary blood disease. However, his son-in-law Gerhard Henrik Armauer Hansen, who is the resident physician, discovered six years earlier that it is caused by

DOI: 10.4324/9781003036500-36

what he called a 'bactillum' (a form of bacteria), though he has not been able to meet the scientific requirements needed to prove this. In order to evidence infectious transmission, he has previously made multiple attempts to inoculate rabbits. The disappointment and frustration born of repeated failure foments his gambit for human-to-human transmission. So, in the medical office and without consent or anaesthetic, Hansen uses a sharp implement to breach the conjunctiva of Kari's eye. It conveys 'bactillum' from a different type of leprosy to the tuberculoid one she is already suffering. Hansen is hoping to manifest a lepromatous-type nodule in Kari's eye, thereby gaining proof of transmission and cementing his place in medical history. There is no mention in the medical records of who the donor might be and whether their consent was sought. Kari's experience is recorded because the trauma of the action led her to report the incident to her pastor, who advanced the complaint to the hospital board. In turn, the board forwarded it to the legal authorities, and in an unlikely event, Hansen was charged with causing bodily harm to an innocent patient (Blom, 1973). His defence hinged on the scientific and national importance attached to the research which he proposed necessitates the act (Vogelsang, 1963). In an entwining of medical science and national value, Kari's subjectivity is undermined and obscured for a 'greater benefit'.

Untypically in a case involving a marginalised woman, a guilty verdict is returned of medical criminality, and Hansen is stripped of his resident position at the hospital.[3]

This event, along with my childhood experience of medical institutionalisation, informs my site-specific performance *Xenograftie (Artificial Sorrow)* at St Jørgen's Hospital. Built in the twelfth century, the site was established as a leprosarium in the fifteenth century to house the most advanced sufferers in a closed complex composed of hospital, chapel and small cobbled yard for air and exercise. Within the compound, patients were subjected to an imposed medical and religious regime where everyday autonomy and privacy were eroded. Married couples were separated, and two to three occupants shared a small bedroom (measuring three by four metres) along with a small, numbered cupboard next to the kitchen area to store meagre belongings.

The rabbit is the understudy (2013)

Xenograftie (Artificial Sorrow) involves a gesture of artificially inducing tears, creating a leakiness between ideas of the operating theatre, the courtroom theatre and the theatre of performance. A slaughtered rabbit takes the lead role. Like my childhood experience, in a certain way it has also endured two deaths combined in a single event. One death is metaphorical and arrives at the hands of capitalism – a result of being an unsold unit in the pet industry. Its surplus to requirement status means it must be culled to protect the profit margin. The second is literal and comes at the hands of a pet lover who purchases it at a discount to use for dog food; she stands beside the household door, holding the rabbit tightly under one arm. The rabbit glimpses a blunt instrument and, like Kari, intuits that it is central to the proceedings. In a unilateral transaction, it receives a hefty blow to the skull. The lights go out. Ahead of the blunt force trauma I have negotiated with the pet lover to borrow the rabbit from the food chain and return it two days later for its intended purpose. The dead rabbit arrives with me a day ahead of the performance so that we are able to become familiar with and adjust to each other. It now has an open wound running the length of its underbelly where the innards have been evacuated. Its lips are bloody. I cradle its soft fur, figuring out which way to hold it so that it offers the best fit for both of us– elongated, close to my warmth, held firmly and tenderly. I stroke the rabbit with my hair, its fur brushes my cheek and back of the hand in the softest of greetings. The rabbit's body unfolds to me inflections and possibilities – missing organs, violent ruptures and how to give rise to a voice. My place, the rabbit's place, our place in all of this.

The rabbit wears fur

The rabbit wears a coat of fur. I wear a white dress and silent-sole pumps. My attire is simple and unencumbered, somewhere between the medical and religious, reflecting the simultaneous occupations of the site as hospital and church. My head is surrounded by a protective guard normally used for sick animals. Like a clerical ruff it stiffens my posture, and the semi-opaque material makes my vision slightly milky. Across my chest are strips of double-sided tape which cling to my skin and are placed there ready to receive added material.

The rabbit plays dead

The performance begins when, wearing the post-operative cone for animals and carrying the slaughtered rabbit, I tentatively descend the staircase of the museum. The audience must part as I form a path through their midst. Unprompted, audience members gradually form a small cortege in my wake. No matter how carefully and lightly I step, each tread groans. One hand gently trails behind on the banister indicating a certain reluctance to arrive. I approach the ground floor central hall which, like the galleries above, is flanked by rows of empty rooms, each containing two single beds either side of a small devotional table. The old wooden architecture and furnishings are warmed by the sun and smell slightly sweet. The atmosphere is subdued and the smell reaches as far as my stomach and tightens invisible strings into knots. I lay the rabbit down gently on the large table where over centuries interns have shared meals and fates. Now it is laid with neat rows of sealed 8 × 8 zip-lock bags, each containing samples of my razored hair. To the left are equal rows of repurposed sardine tins. They recall Bergen's history as a former fish canning port and reflect that the museum is a site of cultural preservation. On the underside of the tins a sequential number is stencilled in the same manner as the occupant's cupboard doors. A single tear-shaped pearl-headed pin stands upright in each tin, held in place by a volume of salt. As in the bacillus transplant to Kari's eye, cultivated pearls are also formed around a foreign body introduced into the soft tissue of a living being. The other items on the table are a circular watch glass used as a resting place for a bottle of Hypromellose (more commonly called artificial tears), a kidney-shaped enamel dish holding a pair of snips and a small crucible to temporarily hold the displaced pins prior to relocation. Inside the drawer of the table close to my left hip there is a small gold-rimmed magnifying glass.

As I take a seat at the table the audience gathers silently in front of me and leans from the gallery above and I begin to enact a cycle of gestures. Reaching out to the rabbit I carefully shear a section of fur from the area around its open wound and place it upon my own chest. I mirror this action by taking a lock of my own razored hair from one of the sealed bags and place it along the rabbit's incised underbelly. After each transplant I spin the watch glass, making my decisions in the moment whether to let it cease its own momentum or whether to arrest it beforehand. When it stops or is stopped, I remove the bottle of artificial tears balanced finely in its centre. Raising my head and looking up, I drop tears from the bottle's pipette over the top of my head cone and into the corner of my eyes before returning it to place. I then upturn a tin of sea salt, either pouring it into the rabbit's cavity as a healing and preserving substance, or spilling it onto the table as an uncontainable excess. I think of lives that have expired in this place and how each new death necessitates the patient's cupboard being disembowelled of contents. The displaced pearl-headed pin from the volume of salt is used as a rudimentary suture to close the rabbit's wound. At the end of each cycle, I take the small gold-rimmed magnifying glass from the table drawer and hold it over my handiwork, checking for finer material through the increased scale. During a prior visit to the museum, I notice the scientific lens instruments that opened up the possibility of new discoveries and understandings and that were used so unswervingly on designated bodies. Towards the end of the 45-minute performance my eyes are sore and my vision marred, an irritation that focuses my attention. The cycles continue until the incision on the rabbit's underbelly is completely sutured with pins and dressed with my hair.

The reiteration of cycles is a device to allow the performance to gradually evolve into a denser realisation. The repetition slows down time as a strategy to create a thinking place for the audience and to grow a space of connectivity between myself and the rabbit. When all the cycles are complete, I signal the end of the performance by slowly rising from the table and exiting alone via another staircase to a private room. There I am confronted with a wave of loss and sorrow. I slowly remove the furry double-sided tape from my chest. Its pull is strong and also lifts my skin cells, raising a blush to the surface. The recto-verso tape-membrane samples both of our bodies but in the moment of separation is nothing more than bio-waste.

Years later, I process my decision to leave the performance space alone whilst the rabbit remained part of a brief installation. The intention behind leaving this trace of the event is to allow a space for processing and speculation, but with the passing of time I admonish myself for leaving the rabbit at risk to the care of others.

The rabbit is a 'she' (1879)

An ophthalmologist present at Kari's incision challenges her account in court of how painful the procedure and after-pain were. Although admitting that no prior check for sensation was made, he proposes that her tears were a hysterical outpouring caused purely by imagination. It is not considered that her anxious tears prior to the not-yet-revealed operation welled from an embodied archive of the self under pressure. The doctors gathering as they call her to the office was enough to bring that archive to the surface in a visceral response. Philosophically the female is aligned to the animal processed through terms of 'Can it think?' or 'Can it speak?' (Derrida, 2008). These questions are aimed towards determining a reasoning subject or, as in Kari's case, a non/hysterical subject. In the same year as Hansen's criminal experiment, Jeremy Bentham reframed and challenged the hierarchies and borders of human and animal subjectivity by shifting the prerequisites of thought and speech and positing the defining criteria as 'Can it feel pain?' (Burns, 2005). For Bentham, the benchmark of how we approach and interact with other beings is based upon the ability to suffer and not the ability to reason. This radically shifts the criteria from an intellectual premise based on reason to a phenomenological experience grounded in sensation. If we were to adopt the ophthalmologist's account of Kari's hysteria, in Bentham's terms she remains a validated subject.

In *Xenograftie (Artificial Sorrow)*, it is through an act of self-determination that I introduce a foreign substance to my own eyes. The intrusion bites the membranes and creates a tearful response. Through the distilled cyclic nature of the performance, I am repetitively moving material, building a located disturbance to form an inverted lens that places scrutiny back towards the wielder. The corporeal performance event forms a new collective memory held by the audience as personal and historical trauma transitions into contemporary cultural currency. In the act of introducing artificial tears to my eyes to produce the imagery of crying, one could quickly assume that fakery denotes inauthenticity – a presumption that can be challenged. In working with Kari's particular history of weeping, it seems disingenuous to appropriate her tears-as-voice, by reperforming crying as a seamless copy. In the performance it is vital that the teardrops are introduced as a foreign body and that the audience are fully aware of the artifice of the gesture. In mapping my performance ethics, I choose to work with the Hypromellose, but in a turn of events the artificial tears bite and real tears flow, creating a confluence.

The rabbit runs ahead (1879–2022 and onwards)

Kari's induced tears flow through time and representation accompanying multiple acts of corporeal usurpation. *Xenograftie (Artificial Sorrow)* is a performative response and a cultural enquiry into aspects of medical trauma coalescing around asymmetrical power relations. It points to the struggle that sick bodies experience when trying to instate or retain corporeal autonomy when medicalised. This is particularly vivid when they are designated automatic donors of scientific material under medical ownership (Robertson, 2011). Through his trial Hansen answered to established points of law covering medical conduct, but there is an absence of evidence to suggest he ever acknowledged, took moral responsibility for or grew into an understanding of his unethical conduct. Arguably, bodies have a tendency to run ahead of ethics, creating the conditions that belatedly stir ethics into consideration. As I treat the rabbit's corpse, my actions could also be read as a further mastering of a purloined body stripped of agency. In a sense the rabbit reveals something to me, which rather places me in the situation of Hansen, validating the treatment of Kari's body because it will offer something to him. The extraction of knowledge at the expense of another is a knotty matter requiring consent and perhaps mutuality. The performance and the rabbit unveil my cultural culpability and embroilment with the demise of other bodies, shattering the privileged illusion that I am sitting outside of or beyond the discourse.

Translations across bodies of knowledge, which are necessarily bodies of experience, sit complexly and may never meet a tidy resolve. Unethical medical explorations lie beneath the surface of many treatments that allow us to live extended disease-free or disease-controlled lives. Despite the disturbing aspects of Hansen's conduct that are entangled with my own performative actions, there is also another dynamic in play. The memorialisation inherent in an act of recalling extends the will to fix a narrative. In contrast, *Xenograftie (Artificial Sorrow)* fosters multiple simultaneous stances through engaging acting-out-memory. The acting-out is politically prolific and carries agency that continues to evolve. Performance as a transient form, and gesture approached as micro-culture, creates the space for multiplication and interconnected transmission.

Notes

1 Vogelsang, T.M. (1963) 'A serious sentence passed against the discoverer of the leprosy bacillus (Gerhard Armauer Hansen) in 1880', *Medical History*, 7(2), p. 184. https://doi.org/10.1017/s0025727300028210.
2 Pleiestiftelsen No.1 was one of Bergen's three leprosarium operating in the nineteenth century. It was the youngest site, in use from 1857. The oldest site was St. Jorgen's, utilised as a leprosium from the fifteenth century and in 1849 Lungegårdshospitalet was opened with space for 84 live-in patients. Hansen worked briefly at Pleiestiftelsen No.1 before moving to Lungegårdshospitalet. All three sites were within close walking distance of each other. This was probably instrumental in establishing a dynamic research community. The performance *Xenograftie (Artificial Sorrow)* takes place at St Jørgen's Hospital which is now a leprosy museum.
3 The consequences are somewhat mitigated as Hansen is supported by the director general of the Norwegian Health Directorate to keep his appointment as medical officer of health for leprosy in Norway until his death in 1912.

Reference list

Blom, K. (1973) 'Amauer Hansen and human leprosy transmission: medical ethics and legal rights', *International Journal of Leprosy*, 41(2).
Burns, J. (2005) *An introduction to the principles of morals and legislation*. Oxford: Clarendon Press.

Derrida, J. (2008) *The animal that therefore I am*. Translated by D. Wills, Edited by M.-L. Mallet. New York: Fordham University Press.

Robertson, J. (2011) 'The leprosy-affected body as a commodity: autonomy and compensation', in Ferber, S. and Wilde, S. (eds.) *The body divided: human beings and human 'material' in modern medical history*. Farnham, Surrey, United Kingdom: Ashgate Publishing.

Vogelsang, T.M. (1963) 'A serious sentence passed against the discoverer of the leprosy bacillus (Gerhard Armauer Hansen) in 1880', *Medical History*, 7(2).

32

HEARING VOICES

The creation and staging of a play based on interviews with psychiatric patients

Clare Summerskill

Hearing Voices is the title of a play that I wrote based on interviews with five mentally ill patients who I had met on a secure psychiatric ward where I, myself, had been hospitalised. The piece was initially presented as a rehearsed play reading at The Cochrane Theatre, London (on 10 January 2009) and was performed by members of my theatre company, Artemis. The script also includes accounts of my own hospitalisation and extracts from interviews with professionals who work in mental health. Directed by Lorae Parry and funded by Arts Council England, the play was performed in ten theatres in 2010 and, in the show, I acted 'myself'. The shows were well attended, and several sold out, reflecting the high degree of general interest in the subject matter addressed by the piece.

A few years prior to the production, I had suffered a breakdown triggered by the ending of a long-term relationship but ultimately the result of deep-rooted childhood trauma. In the two years that followed, I experienced severe depression and suicidal ideations, both symptoms of post-traumatic stress. Finally, I took an overdose and was admitted to a central London hospital. I stayed on a locked psychiatric ward for two months, and, during that time, I met other patients with whom I became close. I heard many of their stories and they heard mine, and we built friendships which sustained us during that difficult period. After I was discharged, I kept in touch with these friends and asked them if I could interview them about their own life experiences and their views about the psychiatric system. From those interviews, I created a verbatim play.

The rehearsed play reading of *Hearing Voices* at The Cochrane Theatre was free, and the audience numbered more than 250 attendees. A question and answer session was held after the performance. The feedback provided by audience members indicated a sharp divide between those who had, as psychiatric patients, experienced a poor standard of treatment and those who worked within that profession, some of whom claimed that the dramatised incidents they had just witnessed could not have possibly occurred. These scenes included patients being left on the floor calling out for help but receiving none, nurses treating emotionally distressed patients in an aggressive manner, medications being mixed up and given to the wrong people and ongoing chaos on the ward. This was exacerbated by daily thefts from bedrooms and illegal drug use by some of the patients which seemed to be ignored by staff, who rarely left their office.

DOI: 10.4324/9781003036500-37

The discussions that took place after the play reading were intense and, at times, conflictual. I had written the piece in order to reveal to a wider public some of the more shocking incidents I witnessed in hospital, but I had (perhaps naively) not realised beforehand that this subject matter would be so contentious. I suggest that two main factors fuelled the impassioned debates which occurred. First, in recent years, the practice of psychiatry in the UK has come under criticism as not necessarily providing the most effective treatment of those who suffer from mental illness, and, second, feedback in different forms provided by those who have experience of mental illness and the psychiatric system has often been dismissed as non-empirical and, at times, invalid because those sharing their stories have (or have had) diminished mental capacity.

The clinical psychologist Peter Kinderman, author of *A Manifesto for Mental Health: Why We Need a Revolution in Mental Health Care*, cites the findings of a report on schizophrenia, published in 2012 by the UK charity and pressure group, Rethink Mental Illness, who call for 'a radical overhaul of poor acute care units' (2019, p. 3). The chair of that report concluded that 'the message that comes through loud and clear is that people are being badly let down by the system in every area of their lives' (2019, p. 3). Kinderman states: 'we need to make residential mental health units places of safety' (2019, p. 4). Whilst some may automatically assume that any low standards of care in mental health care must be the result of underfunding, Kinderman notes that the UK spends a relatively high proportion of the overall health care budget on mental health, 'around 12% . . . compared to only 5.5% as the European average' (2019, p. 3). This statistic indicates that there are factors, other than financial restraints, which contribute towards the causes of poor treatment of patients within the psychiatric system.

Anna Harpin (now anna six), in *Madness, Art and Society*, argues that psychiatric professionals' lack of focus on talking therapy with those who are mentally ill and the reliance on prescription drugs to treat mental distress is a deliberate consequence of those in positions of power within society averting their responsibilities to face up to and treat deep-seated, underlying social problems (Harpin, 2018, p. 101). She also suggests that: 'chemicals are, in this sense, less volatile material than child abuse, domestic violence, racism, LGBTQ+ oppression, poverty and so on' (ibid: 101). Harpin states: 'if psychiatry can be experienced as brutal or brutalising for a sizeable group, then artistic practice may yield valuable insights for both care and personhood' (ibid: 101). The theatrical representation of those who are mentally ill and the kind of treatment they receive would therefore seem to be an effective way to convey patients' experiences and provide valuable insight for psychiatric professionals. But Harpin cautions that: 'creative practices are all too often marginalised as the soft distraction from hard science, overlooked as of anecdotal interest but of no real clinical value, or simply jettisoned entirely from the debating chamber' (ibid: 4).

Furthermore, historically, whether for theatre or other forms of research, when those who have suffered from mental illness have been interviewed, doubt has often been cast upon their experiential narratives. From the field of sociology, Angela Sweeney documents the ways in which testimonies of survivors of the mental health system have been invalidated. As a survivor herself, she observes how: 'historically, our experiences have been disbelieved or dismissed, while our distress has been reduced to symptoms of a psychiatric condition' (Sweeney, 2015, p. 5). Both during and after my hospitalisation, talking therapy was never offered. Therefore I decided I would call my play *Hearing Voices*, not because it focused on schizophrenia but because no-one working within the psychiatric services appeared to want to hear the 'voices' or the personal stories of the patients, and my intention was to somehow redress this imbalance.

The play and its contributors

The play opens with a scene showing how I came to be hospitalised, and then it moves to the setting of a locked psychiatric ward, where I am seen struggling to understand whether I was allowed out (*no*), when I could speak to a consultant about my treatment or medication (*once a week for a ten-minute session*), what the general rules were (*it was only after a month that a nurse explained to me where I could find clean linen and towels*) and why the nurses seemed so disinterested in the patients (*a question that was never answered!*). As the play progresses and I meet other patients, I inquire about their own mental struggles and personal histories. These scenes (scripted entirely from the content of interviews conducted with them after we were all discharged) include me (playing myself) asking the questions and them responding. Two of the friends I made in hospital were Alison and Mary, who had both been diagnosed with schizophrenia.[1] Neither of them had worked for many years, but they used to hold down full-time jobs in local government and teaching. I also met an Irish woman called Eilis who had been hospitalised more than twenty times over a five-year period after taking overdoses, and I became very close to a young Hindu man named Tony, who frequently self-harmed to the point of endangering his life. Another patient I met while I was in hospital was Debbie, a mother of five and a singer-songwriter, who had been diagnosed with bipolar affective illness.

I also secured interviews from four contributors whom I term 'alternative' professionals who worked in different areas of mental health in the UK, not necessarily within the psychiatric system, but in what I regard as a kinder and more humane way. One of them ran a sanctuary in London for those with suicidal ideation called Maytree, one was a psychiatrist in the NHS (the UK National Health Service) who worked with schizophrenic patients in non-medical ways, one had worked as operations manager for The Samaritans (a charity offering support to those who feel suicidal) and had been involved in writing reports about self-harm and the fourth was a doctor who suffered from bipolar affective illness and had been hospitalised many times herself on psychiatric wards. By including excerpts from their interviews, interspersed in the script at relevant moments, I intended to demonstrate that there are more effective ways of treating people in mental distress, other than those currently offered by the NHS.

Interviewing Debbie

A few months after we had both left the ward, I visited Debbie and told her about the work I did when I was not ill – writing verbatim plays from interviews with people about a particular subject or theme. I then explained that I wanted to create a piece based entirely on stories of people who had experience of psychiatric services, myself included. My interview had two key aims: to question Debbie about her mental illness, inquiring as to how she and her family dealt with her condition, and to ask her how she thought the psychiatric system had treated her over the many years she had been unwell. The questions I asked her regarding the first of these matters were 'open' questions, in that I had no idea how she would reply and I was not looking for any particular kinds of responses. Also, I had no previous knowledge of how Debbie had navigated life as someone with serious mental health issues. But as far as my questioning Debbie about her views on the psychiatric system in general, I am fully aware that her answers might partially have been informed by the fact that she already knew that I thought quite badly of the treatment I and other patients had received in hospital. An examination of the transcription of the interview I conducted with Debbie reveals that, at certain points, I did express my views on what I saw as the low level of care psychiatric nurses and consultants displayed towards their patients. In the interview, Debbie also expressed very strong opinions about what she had experienced as poor treatment not only during our shared hospital stay but at other times when she had been hospitalised, sometimes forcibly. This extract was included in the script:

Debbie: It seems to me the nurses aren't there to care for sick people, it's almost like they're there to punish you for having a few more screws loose than them. They've got all their marbles, they've got a good job and you're in there. It becomes almost like a prison situation. There's no caring.

(Summerskill, 2010, p. 36)

Debbie's comments helped to consolidate my own ideas about the general direction the final theatre piece was to take: to demonstrate, through personal narratives, that psychiatric patients in secure wards can sometimes be treated less as mentally frail people in need of help and more as prisoners who have, in some way, transgressed society's laws and moral codes and who should not expect to receive sympathy or solicitous forms of caring while they are hospitalised.

A difficult staging decision

During the week-long rehearsal period for the play-reading, which I directed, I made the choice to have the actress who played Debbie narrate certain excerpts from her interview in a way that appeared as if she was 'on an episode': quite loudly and with an intense fervour. This is one extract from the script where a manic style of acting was employed by the actress who delivered her lines:

Debbie: Before my last episode I'd just given up the Lithium, 'cos I thought I was going to have a baby and I didn't tell anyone I'd stopped taking it and then about ten days down the line I was just back into darkness. My mental state of perception and understanding goes like to other places, like when you're really enthusiastic about things as a kid. And my brain is taking me enthusiastically down a road or a path in my head, but I'll just be laying there, I can't move . . . I'm off, I'm gone. Ga-ga. And it's twenty-four hours. You don't sleep. It's terrible 'cos you're running around.

(Summerskill, 2010, p. 46)

At each performance, the way the actress who played Debbie presented her lines – in a loud and hastily-delivered manner – proved to be extremely dramatically powerful, but there were, of course, serious ethical implications in taking such a theatrical decision. Even though I had included in the script the exact words Debbie had spoken in her interview, I employed a large degree of dramatic licence by directing the actress who played her to perform as if she was *currently* experiencing a bipolar episode rather than discussing her experiences in a reflective, calmer state, which was the case when I interviewed her. The test of whether this proved to be dramatically effective and achieved in a way that still demonstrated respect for the contributor was by having Debbie come to the show and seeing this portrayal of herself. Fortunately, she seemed very pleased with the dramatic representation of her character, and, during a follow-up interview, she said: 'I am like that! I do recognise myself' (Debbie, 2012).

The positionality of the playwright

The playwright's positionality in verbatim theatre work is of particular concern in the creation of theatre based on interviews with members of marginalised communities. It is often the case that the agenda of the theatre-makers is one that reflects that of the contributors but it must also be noted that verbatim plays are frequently created by those who hold far more power in society than those whose stories they seek to present dramatically. Ethical concerns about exploitation are therefore pressing in these situations and most especially in works which draw their content from interviews with extremely vulnerable contributors, such as those who are mentally ill. In such situations, an even higher level of self-reflexivity and ethical vigilance by the theatre practitioners is required in order to mitigate charges of appropriation and exploitation.

In identifying my own positionality as the playwright in *Hearing Voices*, I see that I was in a highly unusual relationship to both the subject matter and to the contributors. I regard myself primarily as an 'insider' since I had shared the experiences of being on the same locked psychiatric ward as the other patients I later interviewed for the play. I also had a shared experience of being extremely mentally unwell, although we were not suffering from the same conditions. My understanding at the time that I scripted the play, and one that I still hold, is that these shared experiences gave me 'permission' as a writer to conduct interviews with people from an extremely marginalised and vulnerable sector of society, whom I would certainly otherwise never have approached. Although I was exceedingly ill at the point when I met the contributors, I later recovered sufficiently to interview them, secure funding for a tour of the show, write a script and, at a later stage, create a film version of the play[2] and also employ critical reflexivity upon some of the practical and ethical issues that arose during the production process. In short, I had sufficient mental health, clarity and capacity to achieve all these steps, which a long-term mental health sufferer might not possess.

Hearing Voices presents the stories of people whose experiences and opinions are given scant attention. It also sheds light on some of the poor practices displayed by psychiatric staff on a NHS ward that I and my friends had witnessed as patients, thereby employing theatre to expose an area of social and political concern. I could make no claim to objectivity when describing how we had been treated as patients – nor did I intend to. However, I hoped that my personal experience might prove to be a powerful way to expose what I and my friends had experienced as generally harsh and uncaring treatment offered by the National Health Service to those suffering severe mental distress. As my research indicates, creating verbatim theatre which employs exact word-for-word accounts from patients who have spent time on a secure psychiatric ward is arguably, as important as it is ethically problematic.

Notes

1 At their request, I have employed aliases for four of the patient interviewees, but Debbie wished her real name to be employed in the script.
2 Three films can be found at: https://www.youtube.com/watch?v=02hUsBm8ptQ (accessed 6 December 2023).

Reference list

Debbie (2012) Interviewed by C. Summerskill, 12 February. London.

Harpin, A. (2018) *Madness, art and society: beyond illness*. Abingdon: Routledge.

Kinderman, P. (2019) *A manifesto for mental health: why we need a revolution in mental health*. Care Cham, Switzerland: Springer.

Summerskill, C. (2010) *Hearing voices*. London: Tollington Press.

Sweeney, A. (2015) 'Sociology and survivor research: an introduction', in Staddon, P. (ed.) *Mental health service users in research: critical sociological perspectives*. Bristol: Policy Press, pp. 1–9.

33

DEPTH, INTIMACY, AND DISSECTION

Howard Barker's critique of medicine in *He Stumbled*

Alireza Fakhrkonandeh and Yiğit Sümbül

A sustained engagement with medicine constitutes one of the persistent preoccupations of playwright Howard Barker's work since the 1990s, reaching its full-fledged dramatic articulation in *He Stumbled* (published 1998, premiered 2000) and *Blok/Eko* (2011). In these plays, Barker critiques three central features of medical discourse and practice: the medical gaze, the biomedical treatment of pain, and the objectification of the patient as an embodied sentient being. By subjecting his characters to tragic experiences involving intense pain, transitivity of the flesh, transgressive desire, and crisis in (self-)knowledge, Barker throws into relief the aesthetics of subjectivity and ethics of relationality. This chapter, accordingly, will demonstrate how the dramatic method Barker employs in his critique of medicine can be characterised as at once phenomenological and evental.

More specifically, in Barker's work, there are two crucial phenomena, both featuring as evental moments, that substantiate these twofold characterisations of the body and embodied subjectivity in *phenomenological* and *evental* terms. These are the experience of extreme pain and of interpersonal proximity (or evental intimacy). It is on this premise that we find 'the chiasmatic' and 'proximity' accurate terms for capturing both the nature of the body and its mode of relationship with the Other in Barker. The chiasmatic – a term deployed and elaborated by both Merleau-Ponty and Derrida – designates a non-synthetic and non-sublational mode of relationship between two phenomena which is not amenable to unitary identification, binary opposition, or dialectical synthesis. In contrast, the chiasmatic involves a relationship informed with simultaneous infinite proximity and irreducible différance, the simultaneity of reversibility and divergence – akin to the relationship between the two hands of the same person or that between a person and their own image in the mirror (see Merleau-Ponty, 1968, pp. 130–155). Our conception of proximity derives from the philosophical insights purveyed primarily by Levinas, but also those proposed by Deleuze. First, proximity is neither a subjective nor an objective relation or communion. It is rather a contaminating communication of anarchic sensibility, involving the transitivity of the affects and the adoption of an abject or accusative position prior to assuming a subjective position or positing (or comprehending) the Other in a representational present (see Levinas, 2006, pp. 7, 9–10, 16, 100). Second, rather than designating a sense of adequation, proximity is informed with an obsessive urgency and repetition of a rapport with alterity (see Levinas, 2006, pp. xxv, xxxiv, 91, 197). Third, proximity is an intercorporeal co-implication and interlacement which is irreducible to manifestation. Fourth, in proximity subjective identity and autonomous agency of the self are rendered infinitely

DOI: 10.4324/9781003036500-38

passive in its exposition. Though, it is worth indicating that passivity, as intended here and elaborated by Levinas, is the ultimate state of passion for self-transcendence, openness towards alterity,
and carnal-spiritual closeness and affinity between two individuals or singularities. Fifth, in proximity a heteronomous, compelling excess persists in negation. This negation, nevertheless, should
not be interpreted as the counterforce to, or opposite of, affirmation, nor as being susceptible to the
Hegelian labour of the negative. It, contrarily, emanates from and is intimately bound up with the
notions/phenomena of pain (see Levinas, 2006, p. 88), traumatic affectivity, and persecution, in
addition to being beset/overcome by a sense of delay and guilt involved in the proximal relation.
Sixth, in terms of temporality, proximity occurs in a diachronic mode rather than a synchronic
one. Hence, precluding the possibility of synchrony (time of consciousness, intentionality, and
identity), present and representation – which are the conditions for and conducive to symmetry and
identity, adequation, and knowledge (in the form of thematisation and conceptualisation). Seventh,
as regards the spatiality of proximity, it should not be conflated with contiguity or conjunction.
Rather, it involves an immediacy closer than that of image and intuition (Levinas, 2006, pp. 97,
100, 127). Finally, proximity is an approach of an exteriority which itself holds no sway over self
but against which self has no power either (see Libertson, 1982, p. 208).

Accordingly, this chapter explores Barker's implicit critique of biomedicine – manifested in
his treatment of the body, relationality, self-knowledge, and desire – with a specific focus on *He
Stumbled*. As will be demonstrated, the play is informed with a critical consciousness of the history of medicine and its objectifying dualistic approach to the body, subjectivity, and mind-body
relationship. In *He Stumbled*, Barker uses the practice of anatomical dissection to evidence the
objectifying and atomistic-analytical approach of medicine and how it diminishes and/or elides
the holistic nature of human experience. Furthermore, dissection is used in this play to explore
questions of 'depth' and 'intimacy'. 'Depth' is depicted, in Barker's drama, as a critical site of
both embodied self-knowledge and evental relationship with the virtual (see Deleuze, 1990, pp. 8,
94–95, 150–152) and/or the other. Both of these dimensions are posited by Barker as essential and
yet missed or dissolved by the discourse of medicine and its valorisation of an atomised 'actual'
(part of the body) and its insistence on the necessity of transparency and visibility to the therapeutic medical gaze (see Fakhrkonandeh, 2021). Indeed, 'depth' in Barker, constitutes a space-site
where the chiasmatic (or relational) natures of the flesh, affectivity, and knowledge are manifested.
In other words, depth features as a site where the performative interplay between presence and
absence, between interior and exterior, and between visible and invisible – as productive dynamics
in the aesthetic, ethical, and hermeneutic dimensions of human experience – is thrown into relief.

On the other hand, 'intimacy' is where the aesthetic, ethical, and affective-cognitive subtleties
of depth evince themselves. The dramatic method Barker deploys to foreground this difference is
'performance'. More strictly, in the play's depiction of dissection, Barker stages medicine in its
most manifestly performative moment. Thus, the performance of medicine-as-dissection meto-
nymically stands for the biomedical approach to the embodied subjectivity where the 'quintessen-
tial' medical intervention into human/personal depth and privacy is shown to blatantly miss and
destroy them both. The play also illustrates, by way of irony, how medicine misses its infinite
interplay between the depth and surface as an aesthetic and ethical space for the re-fabrication of
the self and for relating to the beyond-the-self.

Dissection and medicine in *He Stumbled*

In the play, Doja, a renowned anatomist, is summoned by royalty upon the death of the King
(Tortman) to conduct the solemn, ritual-like ceremony of dissecting the King. There are two other
central characters in the play: Turner (the Queen) and Baldwin (her son). Doja becomes an object

of desire for both Turner and Baldwin. Baldwin, who harbours an intense desire for knowledge of the secrets of human life and relationships, becomes obsessed with both the mysteries surrounding his father's cadaver and with Doja, who, thanks to his knowledge of the human interior and his claims to healing and alleviating human pain, has assumed an aura of sacredness and awe. This leads Baldwin to anticipate Doja's assumption of his father's position both politically–symbolically and psychosomatically (that is, in his mother's affections).

As this brief outline suggests, the critique of medicine in *He Stumbled* is highly subtle: the dissection that takes place throughout the play is a ritualistic act rather than a medical one, meant to preserve the body of the recently deceased King Tortman for posterity, encasing and anointing the organs so they can be dispatched as relics to various regions in the realm. Its purpose is not to ascertain the cause of death (as in an autopsy), nor increase knowledge of anatomical structures (as in dissections that take place in the context of scientific discovery or medical education). Indeed, the historical period of the play's setting, though unspecified, seems to predate the advent of medicine in the early modern period. Rather, discussions between the characters as to the religious nature of dissection and the rarity of Doja's services, as well as the setting being the Kingdom of Sicily, suggest a late-Medieval or early Renaissance epoch.

Although the origins of the practice of dissection date back to Ancient Egyptian and Greek civilisations (more specifically to the Alexandria of the third century BC) where the human body was dissected for preservation and/or anatomical examination, the practice became popular in the early modern period when pathological anatomy was seen as a source of medical knowledge (see Foucault, 1973, p. 126). Then, the practice of dissection revolutionised the medical sciences by providing the clinician with the knowledge of the deepest secrets of human anatomy and the mysterious ways in which diseases manifested themselves in the organism. The late-Medieval or early Renaissance period in which Barker seems to set *He Stumbled* is a transitional moment in this history of dissection. Sawday describes this period as 'culture of dissection . . . devoted to the gathering of information and the dissemination of knowledge of the 'mystery' of the human body' (Sawday, 1995, p. 4). While dissections at this time were strictly exclusive to the ruling class for preservation or consecration purposes, the quest for knowledge prefigures the development of the secular scientific medicine in the Enlightenment period which would follow.

He Stumbled, then, offers an anachronistic critique of medical discourse and its cognate branches such as anatomy and dissection as an objectifying and allegedly objective approach to the body. This critique owes much to Foucault's account of the emergence of scientific medicine ('the clinic') and the way it reframed the status of both the dead and the living body. The structural opposition pervading *He Stumbled*, accordingly, is that between the (dead) body under anatomy's scrutiny and the lived, subjective body. This structural opposition is played out in tense situations where the body as the object of anatomical practice/gaze (anatomised, laid open, de-subjectified, and accessible human flesh) and the subjective body (disruptive, elusive, desirous, living) are juxtaposed to accentuate different aesthetic, ethical, and sensory-affective dynamics informing each mode.

The play opens with a corpse in the middle of the stage ready to go through a protracted process of dissection. *He Stumbled* is suffused with a morbid ambience and macabre mood where the sacral rituals of dissection of the 'holy' body of the king are conducted ceremonially upon the stage with clinical precision, whilst transgressive desire and the prospect of erotic jouissance – epitomised by the stark nakedness of female flesh and seductive manoeuvres of the Queen – erupt on the stage to subvert this clinical objectivity and affective detachment. This tension-laden dynamic does not cease at the table of dissection but rather advances to culminate in a bravado of self-dissection by the anatomist/lover himself.

Dissection as performance

What distinguishes dissection from other forms of medical practice is its performative nature. Dissection merges with the medical gaze, thereby being enhanced with the power of the touch-as-penetration, in an attempt to fathom 'the tangible space of the body, which at the same time is that opaque mass in which secrets, invisible lesions, and the very mystery of origins lie hidden' (Foucault, 1973, p. 122). It penetrates the human body by means of the incision of the skin, removal of the internal organs, and examination for pathologies. Various scholars have drawn attention to the inherent theatricality of the practice of dissection. Sawday, for instance, states how 'the body was produced (in a theatrical sense) as the flimsy vehicle for a complex ideological structure which stretched into every area of artistic and scientific endeavour in the early-modern period' (1995, p. 4). Ferrari, on the other hand, accentuates how 'the two kinds of architectural structure (the anatomy theatre and the theatre proper) for centuries led a parallel existence' (1987, p. 86).

By the same token, in *He Stumbled*, Doja, who has taught his assistants to have a 'character of spirituality [and] . . . reverence for the flesh' (Barker, 2012, p. 287), performs the dissection on King Tortman as if it were a religious ritual or a sacred art whose significance arises from his intimacy with the inner space of the body and its secrets: 'My arm aches and if I cannot exert the fullest concentration on my task the perfection for which I am renowned will certainly be compromised' (Barker, 2012, p. 258). The aura of artistic authority and sacredness is acutely registered in the language (Latin) Doja uses while conducting the ritual of dissection with his assistants, Pin and Suede:

Doja (To Pin):	Dextra . . ./Inflexit . . ./Contorturn./Occlusit . . ./In axio . . ./In axio . . ./Dixi . . .
Pin:	*(Working deep in the chest):*
	In axio . . .
	(An atmosphere of tranquillity surrounds the work of the clinicians, cutting and cleaning with a practised routine, hypnotic to BALDWIN, who sways on his stool . . .)
Doja:	Et implacit . . .
Pin:	Sub sternum . . .
Doja:	Implacit . . .
Pin:	Implacit . . .
Doja:	Testoria . . .
Pin:	Fluvio . . ./Fluvio . . .
	(SUEDE holds up a pan. DOJA lifts out the heart and suspends it in the manner of a priest raising the host. It leaks blood. BALDWIN is a miracle of balance as he inclines in fascination . . .).

(Barker, 2012, p. 259)

Doja's resort to Latin can be interpreted as his attempt to dispel the perceived taboo and evilness of the practice of dissection in the late-Middle Ages where human anatomy was considered God's perfect design and thus sacred. Sawday refers to human anatomy as it was perceived by mediaeval anatomists as 'a text written by God, comprised of all the different members, sections, subsections, and partitions revealed in dissection' and describes the task of the anatomist as 'to re-create, in order to read, the precise system of division by which the body-book had originally been composed by the divine author' (Sawday, 1995, p. 135). The Latin words Doja uses are expressive of a feeling of the sublime while he performs the ritual of dissection as an act of transcendence and of his occupation of a liminal-transcendental position between inside and outside, surface and depth, the physical and the metaphysical, intimacy and detachment, visible and invisible – Eros and Thanatos.

Distance and intimacy

Doja's attractiveness to Baldwin is enhanced not only by his use of Latin, with its religious and sacred overtones, but also by his access to the interior of Baldwin's father's body and the increasing erotic attraction and intimacy between Doja and Turner. Hence, Baldwin construes Doja's ability to penetrate the bodies of his parents as justification for his being intimate with Doja (see Rabey, 2009, p. 111). In the play, Baldwin tells Doja: 'You put your hands inside my father, Mr Doja . . . And you are now proposing [to my mother] . . . everything conspires to make me intimate with you' (Barker, 2012, p. 274). In fact, as it becomes apparent in the play, what Baldwin so feverishly pursues is the realisation and witnessing of an obscene primary scene (or Oedipal scenario, which is eventually realised), the spectacle of Doja having sex with his mother in the presence of the dissected body of his dead father.

In the first half of the play, Doja maintains a detached and impersonal attitude towards the dead body at hand, remaining unaffected by the horror and mortality, death and decay, an attitude which, as we gather, is Doja's ingrained and customary temperament and professional stance. Baldwin, perceptively seeing through Doja's cold aloofness, identifies a subjective desire for *jouissance* latent in the ostensibly clinical/objective mode of his intervention into the human body: 'With you, the knife is perhaps, the mirage that shimmers on the horizon of your life . . . the alibi for ecstasy never quite attempted' (Barker, 2012, pp. 296–297). Elsewhere the same stance in Doja is recognised by a courtier named Todd: 'How you have loved to be beyond . . . keeping your intimacy for the dead . . . and visiting, as it were . . . just visiting . . . the living' (Barker, 2012, p. 292). In the meantime, Turner spares no efforts to make a ravishing spectacle of herself in order to seduce and prise open Doja's clinical composure and also to confront him with mysteries and excesses of subjective and intersubjective flesh and spirit. Gradually, Doja is captivated by the queen, who is readily associated with a corpse, bereavement, death, nakedness, abject states, contamination and infective partaking of bodily fluids, and religious relics.

Self and other

In keeping with its critique of the objectifying treatment of the body in the biomedical paradigm (particularly in its earlier manifestations), *He Stumbled* is primarily preoccupied with the question of the locus of the essence of the embodied subjectivity/individuality (or singularity) and of carnal-spiritual desire between the self and the Other. The former is shown to be an embodied, relational, and integrated yet open phenomenon characterised by intentionality, integrity, and autonomy. The latter is demonstrated to involve a non-dualistic dynamic and thus defiant of the objectifying and reifying logics of the biomedical discourses. *He Stumbled* proceeds to reveal both the body and the mode of relationality between self and the other to be inherently non-dualistic (or chiasmatic) phenomena – hence amenable to an eventual dynamic and approachable through an eventual aesthetics. In accord with the epistemology of his objective-medical profession (anatomist), Doja initially embodies a dichotomous conception of the relation between flesh/body (which is deemed an inanimate, inert matter) and soul (which is considered the immaterial and eternal locus of man's essence). Doja's remarks about the king's corpse and his admonition to Baldwin about the necessity of adopting a dispassionate stance towards it attest to this point: 'It is the degenerate and spoiling prison of a dead man's soul. . . . But I must cut him all the same, . . . And you must watch without exclaiming' (Barker, 2012, p. 257). Confronted with Doja's Cartesian postulation of a dualism between body and mind – where the mind is accorded essential primacy as the ideal locus of rationality and authentic seat of selfhood, and body treated as an addendum, the material base of the mind – Baldwin protests:

Doja: The flesh is not the man . . . [. . .]
Baldwin: Stop . . . ! [. . .] The flesh is not the man . . . ? *(He looks at DOJA)*
The flesh is not the man? What is the flesh, then? Is the flesh not this man's and no other's? If the flesh is not the man, why are you here?

(Barker, 2012, pp. 256–257)

Their discussion captures the complexities surrounding the double-edged status of the human body in contemporary medical, socio-cultural, and philosophical (more specifically, phenomenological) discourses. The fact that the primary objective of dissections is either the determination of the cause/ manner of death or the examination of human anatomy (or, as in the case of Barker's play, consecration) reduces the human body to a site of disease or a scrapped machine, failing to account for the complexities of human body, its individual history, and the embodied nature of human subjectivity. In line with this, 'a dissection might denote not the delicate separation of constituent structures, but a more violent 'reduction' into parts: a brutal dismemberment of people, things, or ideas' (Sawday, 1995, p. 1). In this regard, *He Stumbled* can be argued to offer a phenomenological critique of the reductive and analytical approach of biomedicine and other contemporary approaches (in neuroscience and cognitive science) to the human body. More specifically, Barker's representation of the human body in the play through scenes of stark nakedness, extraction and ingestion of bodily fluids, and inter-corporeal proximity can be characterised as phenomenological and evental.

Earlier, Turner poses a provocative question to Doja which sets into motion the vexing concerns of the play. She articulates the opposing values and terms at stake throughout the play: the fraught relation between surface and depth, visibility/transparency and invisibility, scopophilic vision and tactility/olfaction, chiasmatic intimacy and penetrating knowledge, integrity and fragmentation:

It must be the same with character. We love what we see. But that is rather little of it. Really, life is solitude. We attach ourselves to surfaces. But what is intimacy, Mr Doja? A fiction, surely.

(Barker, 2012, p. 260)

Here Turner is as much non-committal as she is inviting; she gives as much as she withholds; she unfolds and instils as much as she elicits. *Prima facie*, she seems to be sceptical of the possibility (or even the necessity) of reaching the depth (as the site of truth, essence, or naked knowledge of the Other) by deeming the superficial contact of surfaces and a superficial or inauthentic knowledge or communication as the only available or ultimately attainable means and manner of contact. Highly revealing is that in response to Turner's query, Doja draws a blank and fails to provide a residual, let alone convincing, answer:

Doja: Intimacy I know rather little of.
Turner: Is that so? [. . .] Perhaps it frightens you. [. . .] Certainly it frightens me. [. . .] Knowing how little intimacy there is, we are correct to fear it, Mr Doja . . .

(Barker, 2012, p. 260)

Later, whilst Baldwin is bluntly endeavouring to draw Doja's attention to his mother's sexual appeal and profligacy, Turner lays bare the purpose underlying Doja's adoption of the posture of intellectual autonomy and clinical detachment. She avers that Doja's stance is nothing but an existential and psychological shield and shelter he has assumed to evade a heteronomous relationship or an emotive-affective involvement which might eject him from his egocentric solipsism and undermine the inveterate habits of his idealist-materialist mind. Turner suggestively interrogates Baldwin: 'What is the point of it, when what we require of Mr Doja is that he lays aside his cleverness, which he assures me –' and not lingering to add the thrust: 'Is nothing more than a means of fending off his fear of intimacy' (Barker, 2012, p. 272). Here the term 'intimacy' is conjured once more to express the space and mode of relationality and affectivity which stand in contradistinction to synthetic unity or detached identity. Doja, perplexed and missing the meaning of 'expression', says:

Doja: Did I say that . . . ?
Turner: Say . . . ? I don't know about say, you expressed it, and you express it now, Mr Doja . . .
           I am the same, which is why I am able to recognize in you the preposterous evasions we
           undertake in order not to –

(Barker, 2012, p. 272)

Intimacy/proximity features in Barker's theoretical and dramatic works as an interpersonal and chiasmatic space not only for the occurrence of evental relationships between the self and the other at aesthetic and ethical levels (see Levinas, 2006). It transpires as a space for socio-political and existential-psychological resistance to the functionalisation and objectification of the body, relationality, and embodied subjectivity by both the reifying logics of consumer capitalism and the medical-clinical discourse/paradigm.

As opposed to the ocularcentric strain informing the scientific paradigm, which he has hitherto been shown to embody, Doja experiences an encroaching tactile profusion combined with a corrosive sense of being enveloped with an uncanny smell. As he explains it bemusedly to Laybach, a priest, whilst groping for its cause, source, and meaning:

Doja: There is a smell on me . . ./A smell which nauseates me and yet . . ./A smell I –
Laybach: Death . . .
Doja: Is that what it is . . . ? It's from a woman's body . . .

(Barker, 2012, p. 277)

The second measure taken by Barker to foreground the chasm between body as an object and body as an (inter-)subjectively lived and libidinal space manifests itself in his according prominence to 'skin'. The significance and implications of Barker's subtle gesture come to the fore if we notice how skin not only serves as the paradigmatic figure for the chiasmatic state of flesh but also embodies ambiguity, intercorporeal proximity, and a Mobius-like two-foldness (simultaneously surface and depth, single sense and milieu of all the senses, that is, synaesthetic). Nevertheless, notwithstanding fulfilling such a vital function and serving so many purposes, skin is a highly fragile organ and hence the organ most intimately associated with abjectness and abjection (see Fakhrkonandeh, 2017). Skin, in the play, is persistently invoked as the primary organ and the trope/figure for the individual's psychosomatic boundaries, subjective sensibility, and interpersonal affectivity: 'Oh, how painful your life must be . . . *(The KING looks at DOJA . . .)* I have flayed kings . . . but in your case, there is no skin that I can see . . . the nerves are naked . . . and wind even, gives you agony' (Barker, 2012, p. 311). Elsewhere Baldwin evokes the figure/organ of skin in the same way designated previously: 'Nothing/Nothing/Is lost on me/I am/Oh, misery/Oh, melancholy/Intuitive to an inordinate degree/My skin/So thin/I feel a thought alight on me' (Barker, 2012, p. 273). Crucially, Doja's perception and description of Turner's skin corroborate and are consonant with the descriptions of the skin as a double-edged organ, simultaneously sublime and abject: 'Her skin [. . .] Has that peculiar [. . .] That simultaneously [. . .] I can only describe it as possessing the identical extreme of fecundity and death/associated with [. . .]/Compost./Manure/Ordure [. . .] Intoxicating/Nauseating' (Barker, 2012, pp. 289–290). Insofar as intimacy/proximity is concerned, this act of according primacy to (non-penetrative) touch and smell reveals an anti-idealist, anti-metaphysical, and phenomenologically inflected insight.

The interplay between surface and depth on the one hand, and the interior and exterior on the other, fosters an ironical situation in *He Stumbled*, where the medical profession, despite its unconditioned access to the interior of human body, attains a superficial understanding of ethical, existential, and psychological intricacies of the embodied subject. It thus illustrates how the clinical-medical knowledge falls short of accounting for the critical and vital dimensions of human life and interpersonal relationships, such as intimacy, mind-body integrity, intentionality, relationality, secret, and mystery (of desire and spirituality). In the play, the interpersonal relationship, in eventful moments of eroticism and proximity/intimacy, reaches a profound level of affective contagion and chiasmatic intertwinement. Turner states:

> You have kissed me where the daylight has not visited. [. . .]/Even so, one might, such intimacies, and still, the most profound, and then, next day, despite the, with a new sunrise, even/Everything that occurred was novel to/Me/Everything/The dress/The manner/ The conversation/Never/Never/Before/I was a stranger to myself
> (Pause . . . DOJA looks into her stricken face . . . he leans into her and breathes the odour of her body)
>
> (Barker, 2012, p. 284)

Gradually, by the incursions Turner, Baldwin, and the whole unnerving ambience of the play make into his sensibility, Doja becomes obsessed and carried away with Turner's insinuating conduct and mysterious smell which evoke the prospect of *jouissance* and transgressive eroticism with her. Seated at the luxurious table while Nixon, the Queen's servant, is serving various exotic delicacies, Doja advances towards Turner 'who is still, observing him, he extends a hand, stops . . . *(DOJA places himself behind TURNER, his hands spread on her torso. He kisses her neck)*' (Barker, 2012, p. 275). Doja's subsequent utterances are revealing: 'I – [. . .] DOM Manifestum . . ./et . . ./Mammarum . . ./Exposito . . ./*(He unhitches her dress . . . her breasts are exposed . . . she is immobile . . .)*/ I've no desire to . . ./I've no –' (Barker, 2012, p. 275). Doja's language and bodily actions are in a jarring juxtaposition. Here, Doja's attempt to maintain his distance and detachment by resorting to the use of Latin (both as an expression of an ecstasy and transcendence of common language and a token of entering a sacred space) is palpable in his utterances which are punctuated with the eruption of impulsive drives and semiotic flows, alternating between science of anatomy and non-knowledge of fascination and (inter-)affectivity.

Later in the play, Doja's contracted captivation with Turner's sacred secret and erotic spirituality coupled with his desire for intimacy with her manifests itself in terms of possessiveness and jealousy but also an interrogation of the source and limit of Turner's morbid love for her dead husband: 'Do you still love this *(Pause . . .)*/Man or memory do you still *(Pause . . .)*/Mess or monarch' (Barker, 2012, p. 304). This trend reaches a climactic point when Doja urges Turner to drink the blood and bodily fluids of her husband. The act of ingestion and (melancholy) incorporation (of the blood and bodily fluids), in addition to involving a reciprocal, transgressive initiation into a mutual obscene intimacy and a space of secret partaking, designates de-cathection and dissipation, that is, ingestion for the purpose of mnemonic-erotic-physical defecation and dissolution. Thus, the absorbing or partaking of the abject fluids by them in this instance is not primarily carried out with the intention of intensification of intercorporeal proximity, envelopment, and incorporation, and this strain specifically arises from Doja's mechanical and objective-analytical attitude towards the human flesh:

Doja: Drink your husband . . .
 (Pause . . . the tin roof rattles in the wind . . . TURNER is rigid with horror . . .)
Turner: Drink
Doja: I'm your physician, do take my advice . . . *(He holds her still . . .)*
Turner: Drink
Doja: I say advice, in cases of this gravity I think advice is not –
Turner: Drink
Doja: The word, advice, no, it's imperative –
Turner: Drink
Doja: Your health depends on it –
Turner: Drink my
Doja: And mine the surgeon's sickness also must be cured . . .
 (He continues to grip TURNER with one hand, and with the other lifts a beaker of fluid from the anatomy table to TURNER's lips . . . A long pause . . .)

(Barker, 2012, p. 304)

Perhaps no other scene so vividly illustrates the principal characteristics, in Barker, of the body and evental ethics of inter-personal proximity – including the fluidity of the flesh, the chiasmatic transcription of carnal-spiritual schemas, and inter-affective contagion. The concomitant crescendo of Eros (desire) and Thanatos (dead priests) – involving Doja's movement towards carnal-spiritual proximity with the Queen and the dead (where the threat of death or execution due to an adulterous relation with the Queen is looming near) – reveals not only Doja's experience of abjection but an evental moment here. As is evident, the modality of relationality between Doja and Turner – proximity/intimacy – primarily belongs to the order of the caress, haptic vision, and the imbibing of the fluid (flesh) of the dead. What the dynamics of intimacy/proximity reveals is an ontological and ethical principle in Barker's work: the invisible, death, Thanatos, and the other as the (inassimilable) lining of the mirror of the visible, life, Eros, and the self.

Towards the end of the play, we witness another moment of the ethics of the event – involving a process of self-overcoming and becoming-other in proximity with the Other – in two characters, Baldwin and Doja, who both undergo psychosomatic and existential-ethical upheaval. In Doja's case, this cataclysm is evidenced by his relinquishing of his career which has been an indispensable part of his character:

> Always I have preserved the most clinical and frozen distances between myself and the material remains of the – [. . .] nothing to me . . . ! [. . .] In this case however . . . a profound loathing for this degenerating flesh makes me recoil from the most mundane professional activity, I –

(Barker, 2012, p. 292)

One of the reasons he advances is the collapse of impersonal distance: 'The necessary reverence for the dead I found in this particular instance is rapidly diminishing [. . .] I experienced disgust –', which is, according to him, 'the nightmare of anatomy . . .' (Barker, 2012, p. 297). He adds:

Doja: I have abandoned my vocation.
Baldwin: Can you abandon a vocation, Mr Doja? Perhaps it has abandoned you?
Doja: It's fled, certainly . . .

(Barker, 2012, p. 228)

Similarly, Baldwin claims to have been initiated and in consequence undergone an upheaval, a reconfiguration of identity, sensibility, and perception by incorporating new affective states and knowledge: 'I talk of ecstasy/Me/Me Mr Doja/Ecstasy . . . ! [. . .] I am a changed man/No/Not changed/Oh, preposterous and incredible claim is anybody is anything changed no not changed merely reasserted/I am reassorted' (Barker, 2012, p. 296).

Doja's obsessive concern both with the 'clear and distinct' determination (at personal, interpersonal, and existential levels) and with his autonomy reaches its climax when he tries to conduct an act of vivisection on himself, an act verging on perversion, if not near psychosis, where the category of the Other seems to have been dismissed or dissolved. Sawday refers to pathological anatomy as an inherently ambiguous practice: 'the anatomist is . . . a self-reflexive figure – a dissector and a dissectee' (1995, p. 207). The act of self-dissection can also be considered an act of suicide impelled with the intention of utmost self-possession, self-affirmation of personal will and meaning. In this act, the subject-object dynamics of dissection is also subverted:

DOJA's hand is seen to make the movements of swift dissection, the other assisting it, nimbly, as if inspired, rapid as a concert pianist, an apotheosis of a skill. [. . .] the sound of instruments exchanged, the frantic activity of DOJA's hands . . . a spectacle of will, dexterity, endurance . . . of magic.

(Barker, 2012, p. 251)

The subversion of agency (the dissector taking himself as the object of dissection) transpires right at the moment when Doja realises the king has been alive all the time and he (Doja) has been a pawn in a game contrived by the queen. In a way, he and his psyche/soul have been the objects of dissection of the queen throughout, the objects of a subtle charade concocted by her (with the acquiescence of her husband the King/Tortman) to gratify her transgressive character and her pursuit of ecstasy. Doja's act of auto-dissection can be considered a symptomatic attempt at self-determination and affective-intellectual autonomy governed by a restricted economy of totality (self-totalisation). It thus reveals the extent to which he, as a sovereign clinical-medical mind, is intolerant of loss, the experience of the nonsense of the inter-corporeal sense, mere experience of exposure to the Other, and excess.

Doja's self-dissection can also be argued to illustrate a tragic/transgressive attempt at reaching a depth at the core of one's selfhood where not only the secret of desire (Eros) and death (Thanatos) but also the knowledge of their evental force and their intertwinement can allegedly be found. Such an approach to depth – as at once literal/physical and metaphorical/metaphysical – is highly consonant with the Calvinist doctrine of self-knowledge or self-examination. Sawday considers self-dissection not only within the context of the Socratic aphorism of 'Gnothi

Seauton' (Know Thyself), but also of the Christian doctrine of transparency, self-scrutiny, and self-exposure:

> What the device of self-demonstration guaranteed was a literal interpretation of the searching, inward gaze recommended by philosophical self-examination. But this inward gaze also gestured towards a tradition of representation which was to become familiar in later, Baroque, images: that of Christ in self-dissection, exposing his own sacred heart.
>
> (Sawday, 1995, p. 117)

Doja's self-dissection at the end of the play can thus be interpreted as a metaphor for his self-examination after realising his having been blinded by his passion and seduced into non-knowledge and loss by the Queen.

Conclusion

Barker's twofold – evental and phenomenological – critique of biomedicine finds its most reverberating articulation in the climactic scene of the play. Earlier in *He Stumbled*, Barker had posited the medical-anatomical discourse's objectifying-atomising epistemologies through the anatomist Doja's predilection to conceive of depth literally-physically – hence Doja's use of dissection as a means of disclosing the secret/cause of pain, sickness, and death. Barker's critique of this symptomatic approach to depth is, above all, attested by his decision to conclude the play with a stark act of tragic opening: self-scarring/wounding. In the throes of a crisis of knowledge and self-knowledge riven with loss between transgressive desire and death, Doja feels impelled to undertake an act of self-dissection in a bid not only to reach an insight into the secret of his own desire for Turner, but also to regain his medical-objectivist mastery lost in his erotic fascination with her. As he avers to Turner: 'It is not pleasure, is it . . . you two share . . . But terror . . . ? *(She remains motionless . . .)* What's common love alongside that . . . ?/Answer me . . ./ No/No/They all say that/They all/They all say that/Don't answer/No/I'll cut/I'll/I cut/The master me' (Barker, 2012, p. 315). Ironically, however, this literal perception of depth evidences yet another poignant moment of tragic blindness and failure on Doja's part notwithstanding the apparent heroism and authenticity of his endeavour. This blindness specifically stems from his literalist approach which is symptomatic of the persistence of his anatomical-medical attitude towards the embodied self.

In *He Stumbled*, scar marks the pain and violence of the evental experience of 'becoming-otherwise' undergone by Doja. As Kuppers explains,

> The scar is self and nonself: it implicates and questions the subject's agency and yet asserts the viability of the body/mind as a creative, adaptive, and plastic entity. The scar moves matter into a future of a new flesh: a different subject emerges, a re-creation of the old into the new, into a repetition that holds on to its history even as it projects itself into an unpredictable future.
>
> (Kuppers, 2007, p. 19)

This passage cogently captures the aporias of Doja's evental experience of becoming-other through self-vivisection, where the critique of medical discourse and practice is pushed to a self-reflexive extreme.

Reference list

Barker, H. (2012) *He stumbled. plays three*. London: Oberon Books.

Deleuze, G. (1990) *The logic of sense*. Translated by M. Lester. London: The Athlone Press.

Fakhrkonandeh, A. (2017) 'Noli Me Tangere: the efflorescence of the third skin in the torsions of pain in Howard Barker's *The Europeans*', *Textual Practice*, 33(1), pp. 99–133.

Fakhrkonandeh, A. (2021) 'Poetics of the event or evental poetics? Writing as becoming imperceptible in Howard Barker's *hurts given and received*', in Mukim, M. and Attridge, D. (eds.) *Literature and event twenty-first century reformulations*. London and New York: Routledge, pp. 93–114.

Ferrari, G. (1987) 'Public anatomy lessons and the carnival: the anatomy theatre of Bologna', *Past & Present*, 117, pp. 50–106.

Foucault, M. (1973) *The birth of the clinic*. Translated by A.M. Sheridan. London: Routledge.

Kuppers, P. (2007) *The scar of visibility: medical performances and contemporary art*. Minneapolis and London: The University of Minnesota Press.

Levinas, E. (2006) *Otherwise than being or beyond essence*. Translated by A. Lingis. Pittsburgh: Duquesne University Press.

Libertson, J. (1982) *Proximity: Levinas, Blanchot, Bataille and communication*. The Hague: Martinus Nijhoff Publishers.

Merleau-Ponty, M. (1968) *The visible and the invisible*. Edited by C. Lefort. Translated by A. Lingis. Evanston: Northwestern University Press.

Rabey, D.I. (2009) *Howard Barker: ecstasy and death: an expository study of his drama, theory and production work, 1988–2008*. London: Palgrave Macmillan.

Sawday, J. (1995) *The body emblazoned: dissection and the human body in Renaissance culture*. London and New York: Routledge.

34

STAGING CORPSES

Reanimating medical history through puppetry

Laura Purcell-Gates

At the beginning of Jane Taylor's play *After Cardenio*, performed in the Anatomy Lecture Theatre at the University of Cape Town in 2011, its stage walls covered with drawings by South African artist Penny Siopis, a puppet revives on the anatomy table. The moment stages the true event that occurred in Oxford in 1650, when Anne Greene, a woman who had been hanged for infanticide, revived just before her anatomical dissection (Watkins, 1651). Taylor came across the story of Anne during her research into Cardenio, a character in the Miguel de Cervantes novel *Don Quixote* (she had been commissioned by Stephen Greenblatt to explore the 'missing' Shakespeare play *Cardenio* as part of the Cardenio Project). In Taylor's play, Anne is represented by both a puppet – who begins the play lying on the anatomy table as anatomists circle around her, observing her body – and by a woman who begins the play lying beneath the table.

On another stage several years later, another puppet revives on an autopsy table. At the beginning of *The Depraved Appetite of Tarrare the Freak*, a puppet chamber opera by my company Wattle and Daub,[1] an eighteenth-century French surgeon, Baron Percy, autopsies Tarrare, the polyphagist (a person with excessive appetite) whom he had tried, and failed, to cure. Like *After Cardenio*, *Tarrare* tells a true story, though in this case the reanimation of the puppet is not drawn from historical records. Tarrare revives when Percy decides to tell his story and invites his medical assistants, two puppeteers and two singers, to assist him by bringing the corpses in the autopsy room to life. The stage is Percy's autopsy room, littered with corpses and body parts that are reanimated/puppeteered by the human performers to tell the story of medical 'monster' Tarrare, a man who could not stop eating but never gained weight.

Both shows explore true stories drawn from medical history. In the intervening years between the revival of Anne Greene and the autopsy of Tarrare, the European medical establishment's approach to cutting open bodies had shifted from an anatomical dissection model (cutting open bodies in order to understand their interior structures) to an emergent pathology, in which the autopsy was intended as a diagnostic tool (cutting open the body to identify disease or disorder). In *The Birth of the Clinic*, Michel Foucault argues for the emergence of the clinical or medical gaze in the late eighteenth century. He traces a shift in visuality from previous classificatory medical structures, in which the patient's body is rendered legible by viewing it through existing structures of medical spatialised knowledge, to the anatomo-clinical method, in which the patient's body and disease are produced through the clinician's gaze (2003, pp. 2–4).

DOI: 10.4324/9781003036500-39

This chapter analyses *After Cardenio* and *Tarrare* with a focus on this theme of medical visuality and the gaze, as reflected in the contrasting designs of the Anne Greene and Tarrare puppets in terms of their visual penetrability. In *After Cardenio*, Anne is represented by both a human actor and her puppet counterpoint, the only puppet on stage for the bulk of the play. This splitting of the figure of Anne into human and puppet allowed Taylor to explore Descartian questions of soul and body – though whether the human represented the soul and the puppet the body, or vice versa, was left intentionally ambiguous (Taylor, 2012). Just before Anne's revival on the anatomy table, we see her anatomists, Dr Petty and his assistant (played by human actors), peering into the dark space between her legs in an unsuccessful attempt to observe her womb. This moment of peering – craning the neck, narrowing the eyes, tilting the head, bodily adjustments intended to find just the right angle that will allow one to catch a glimpse of that which is hidden – recurs throughout the production, as attempts by medical and legal institutions to peer into Anne's life, to see the truth of her narrative and her body, never cease. In one scene, Dr Petty admits to the audience that while he does not wish Anne dead, he is disappointed that her revival has denied him possession of her womb, which he had been promised. The puppet that portrays Anne is life size and fully intact, her body appearing whole and sealed. Designed by South African sculptor Gavin Younge, she is covered in vellum. Taylor emphasises the aptness of using a material that is both skin and book for the puppet that embodies the subject of her literary-theatrical project (Taylor, 2019, 2012). Younge used actual medical prosthetic eyes as the puppet's eyes, and these seem to look outward from their sockets: 'when she looked at you, she *really* looked at you' (Taylor, 2012). The only portal into her body is the hole in her back that takes her puppeteer's hand. She can be puppeteered, but she cannot be seen into.

In *Tarrare*, the puppet design materialises the medical gaze. The characters from Tarrare's life, including himself and his doctor Percy, are all played by puppets, each of whom apart from Percy is designed to resemble a corpse. The show's conceit is that the six human performers on stage with Percy, who play his medical assistants, bring Tarrare's story to life in Percy's autopsy room through singing, playing musical instruments, and puppeteering the corpses. The titular puppet in *Tarrare* was constructed to look like a fragmented corpse. His torso ended at the sternum, leaving a gap where the belly would be. His skin was designed to look like wrinkled, decaying flesh. We made three different Tarrare puppets for the show, each of which could perform a particular function, like swallowing cats and snakes, grabbing his own ribcage to stretch it open, or vomiting a large satin sheet of 'blood'. Each of these puppets, in contrast to the Anne puppet in *After Cardenio*, is open and porous; the audience, and Percy, can always see into Tarrare's interior. In the autopsy scene that bookends the performance, Tarrare's body is ripped open, his guts spilling out. Unlike the Anne Greene puppet, whose interior is inaccessible both to the audience and to the anatomists, the interior of the Tarrare puppet is always accessible and visible.

The reanimation of corpses is used in *Tarrare* as a metaphor for the staging of a historical story. Corpses also played a key role in the history of medicine and the emergence of the medical gaze in the period between the two medical cases depicted in these productions. At the end of the eighteenth century in France, hospitals became centralised and institutionalised as medical treatment was increasingly governed by state oversight, and because ongoing revolutionary military action necessitated centralised medical treatment centres for wounded soldiers (Foucault, 2003). Foucault identifies this period with the emergence of the medical, or clinical, gaze, an epistemic shift in the organisation of medical knowledge. The new medical model replaced the holistic view of patient disease, which was based in part on the patient's own narrative of illness, with the doctor's authoritative ability to describe and diagnose disease based solely on his penetrating gaze onto the components of the patient's body. This is a body that is, in Foucault's words, 'entirely legible for the clinician's gaze: that is, recognisable by its signs, but also decipherable in the symptoms whose totality defined its essence without residue' (ibid: 159). Foucault links this shift with the 'minute but decisive change' in the doctor's first question to his patient from 'What is the matter with you?' to 'Where does it hurt?', a change that marks the decline of the patient narrative and the rise of the clinical model in which the patient's body is framed as legible object (ibid: xxi). Foucault's genealogical approach is set in contrast to a historical understanding of the development of modern medicine as simply the uncovering of transparent facts that had always been available to doctors. Foucault instead frames the birth of the clinical model of medicine as an epistemological rupture, allowing for an understanding of the resulting shifts in medical practice as both helpful and harmful to patients. This is a complexity that, as we dealt with the story of one particular patient from this time, we wished to maintain.

In the sections that follow, I further discuss visuality both in relation to puppet design in each of the two productions, and in relation to anatomical dissection in the mid-seventeenth century, and the late eighteenth-century emerging practice of pathological autopsy. I suggest that both productions use puppetry to make visible these respective medical epistemological paradigms. *After Cardenio* uses the puppet's interior inaccessibility to materialise the inaccessibilities of Anne's life and alleged crime of infanticide, and to explore the mid-seventeenth century English legal imperative to produce material objects as evidence for even invisible and intangible facts, in this case, Anne's intention that her child should live. *Tarrare* draws on the fragmentation of the body made possible through puppetry, including the incompleteness of Tarrare's body, the visual accessibility of his interior, and the actual pulling apart of his body into specimens, including in the production's final image of his head in a jar. These fragmentations allowed us to use puppetry to represent, explore and intervene in medical historical narrative through materialising the medical gaze.

Visibility and hiddenness in *After Cardenio*

In *After Cardenio*, Taylor explores the discursive intersections between seventeenth-century philosophical and religious thought and emergent neurology, which sought to understand the workings of consciousness across states of alertness, sleep, coma and death (Taylor, 2019, 2012). The piece begins in the anatomy theatre, when Anne Greene, who had been hanged for infanticide, revives on the anatomy table. The remainder of the piece follows the struggles of Anne to remember what happened to her, to explain to her anatomists what happened to her between death and revival and to prove to them her innocence of infanticide in an echo of her trial. A dream sequence later in the play sees Anne as puppet and Luscinda (the character name for Anne's puppeteer, who also plays Anne's human aspect) philosophising about issues raised by the play, including the inaccessibility of the female voice in the archive. It ends with an irruption of the Cervantes novel into the narrative, when Don Quixote, as a Sicilian marionette, appears to rescue Anne from the Oxford dons – though a final voiceover by the actor who plays Anne calls into question conventions of gendered narrative resolutions. Beginning with a thwarted dissection, the play can be read through the framing of anatomical dissection, a practice that is about revealing what is hidden, the interiority of the human body. *After Cardenio* engages with themes of hiddenness, and particularly inaccessibility, via intersecting medical, religious and legal discourses of the seventeenth century. At the core of these explorations is the figure of the puppet: the materiality that both promises and prevents access to the hidden.

The hidden, in *After Cardenio*, is multifaceted. The interior of Anne's body, rendered inaccessible through her unexpected revival of consciousness, is the first hidden and inaccessible space that the piece introduces. In a scene shortly after Anne revives, her anatomist William Petty, who at the beginning of the show was seen peering between the puppet's legs into the inaccessible dark space of the womb, laments to the audience the loss of the opportunity to examine this interior space of her body: 'I was sorry at first that she was so much alive/For I'd been promised her corpse so I could study her womb'. His regret at the lost opportunity reflects the status of the female body as only of value in relation to its reproductive organs. Petty's desire to possess Anne's womb reflects a male medical entitlement to the female reproductive system. His regret also reflects the shortage of corpses available for dissection at the time in England. The bodies of those sentenced to hanging were allowed to be dissected. In 1636, fourteen years before Anne's hanging, a charter of King Charles, in an attempt to address this, expanded the hanged criminals eligible for dissection at Oxford University from the city limits to within twenty-one miles of the city, but in practice this still did not produce enough cadavers to meet the demand (Mitchell *et al.*, 2011).

The unexpected inaccessibility of Anne's womb to her anatomists serves as a starting point for a layering of inaccessibility in the piece, much of which is linked to themes of the womb: birth and child rearing. Anatomy here intersects with seventeenth-century legal discourses, as the anatomists attempt to uncover the truth of what happened to Anne's child. Anne maintains that the infant was born dead, and that she is therefore innocent of her accused crime of infanticide. The fact of the birth – what Petty calls 'the fact of the matter' – is inaccessible to her interlocutors, as there were no outside witnesses to it. Anne responds to Petty with 'I am the matter of fact. But fact is dead. So matter stands accused'. This line foregrounds the materiality of Anne's body, the only remaining trace of the death of her infant and its causes. Anne, as the sole remaining 'matter of fact' in the story of her childbirth, can only provide self-narrativising of her memory, which lacks two crucial elements under mid–seventeenth-century English law: the observational gaze of the outsider (a witness to the birth), and material evidence of the mother's intention that her child have a future life.

After Cardenio explores the impossibility of each of these modes of visual revelation. Anne's infant, according to her (and the play takes Anne's side on this), was born dead while she worked in her employment as housekeeper for the wealthy family whose son had impregnated her: there was no live birth to witness. The anatomists in the play stand in for the legal system in the scenes in which they interrogate her, as one of the crucial questions that her resuscitation raised was whether she should be put to death again. English law in the mid-seventeenth century prohibited the concealment of a birth; in the play, Petty's assistant voices this injunction: 'a child undisclosed is a child in danger'. Without the observational gaze of the outsider, then, a birth is rendered both suspicious and, in the case of a stillbirth, evidence of infanticide: 'Hidden facts are guilty acts'. In the absence of a witness, in order to prove her innocence, the bereaved mother must produce evidence of her intention that the child would live and thrive in her care. This evidence was often in the form of objects purchased or acquired for the child, such as a blanket or garment (Taylor, 2019, p. 211). Objects, then, stood in for imagined lives, the absent human bodies of infants who had died. They could be understood to make visible the invisible and inaccessible, the future life that would never be lived. In the absence of such material evidence, Anne herself is the only 'matter of fact' available. The past that she holds in her memory, as well as her intention for the life of her dead child, are as inaccessible to the anatomists as the womb within her living body.

Religious and proto-neurological questions provoked by Anne's resurrection similarly intertwine with issues of medical and legal inaccessibility raised in the play. Questioning is one of the devices of 'peering into' used by the anatomists: Anne's revival provokes Petty to begin questioning the location of her mind/soul between her death and her reawakening, and he considers sleep and dreaming as a metaphor. This reflects an emergent neurology in which Anne Greene's other anatomist, Thomas Willis (who does not appear in the play), was a key figure (Taylor, 2012). Anne provides no help in answering these questions, as she has no memory of the event. The location of her consciousness during the presumed death state remains inaccessible and a matter only for speculation, informed by Descartian philosophy and religious understandings of the spatialisation of the soul. This latter question becomes of crucial importance to Anne as the anatomists question her about the location of her infant's body. For the anatomists, the body is a material trace of the truth of its birth that would render visible that moment in time. This resonates with the seventeenth-century demand for corpses driven by the practice of anatomical dissection. Petty's assistant is additionally concerned with revealing Anne's divine, or diabolical, allegiance. He draws on the language of dissection in his prayer at the end of the scene: if Anne is a servant of the Devil, he maintains, 'we will split her end to end and will turn her inside out'. For Anne, the only important question is the location of her child's soul, whether he is in heaven or hell. She either does not know or refuses to disclose the location of his body. Both the child's body and his soul are inaccessible, unable to reveal the truths that the anatomists and Anne wish to see.

Taylor additionally plays with archival inaccessibility in a dream sequence late in the play, in which the puppet and Luscinda (Anne's puppeteer and human aspect) unpack some of the philosophical underpinnings of the play. Luscinda addresses the question of the visibility of history, speaking to the audience about the lack of archival traces of Anne's love affair with the father of her child: 'The archive knows nothing of desire'. This follows the fruitless interrogation of Anne by her anatomists, whose questions turn from the location of her dead child's body to the identity of the child's father. In the dream sequence, Luscinda and the puppet seem to function as a mouthpiece for Taylor herself conducting research for the play as they speculate on possibilities for Anne Greene's love affair, in the absence of any archival traces that might suggest certainty about the historical record.

The puppet materialises this multifaceted interplay between the visible and the hidden or inaccessible. The video edit of the piece begins with the invitation, in a stills montage, to view the puppet as a specimen. Anne's voiceover reflects on the textual traces of her story as images appear of the puppet, from different angles, lying naked on the anatomy table (in the theatrical event, this voiceover was spoken in darkness). The audience is here invited to look at her body from multiple angles, as if they were anatomists circling the body and examining it prior to dissection. Not only is the womb of the historical figure of Anne Greene inaccessible to the anatomists once she revives, but in the play the audience knows that the puppet, despite looking strikingly human, has no inner organs. Its intactness means that we, like the anatomists, never see inside the body; the puppet's interiority must be imagined, the material fact of its body standing in for Anne's imagined, inaccessible interiority. In *After Cardenio*, the puppet is presented as a specimen; as the 'material fact' onstage, it is the location of revelation of the hidden truths of Anne's story and body. Theatre scholar Gianna Bouchard highlights the intended function of the specimen as exemplar or demonstration, under the gaze implicit in the word's Latin derivation '*specere*', 'to look' (Bouchard, 2016, p. 140). However, Anne resists the function of the specimen as an object of a gaze that reveals the truth of that which it exemplifies: it reveals nothing. The specimen that the audience are invited to observe alongside the anatomists will never reveal the interiority of the human body: the puppet's body resists the gaze that would pry it open. This frustration at the inaccessibility of the interior of Anne's body is mirrored in the inaccessibilities of legal and religious questions that Anne's accused crime and revival conjure, as well as the archival inaccessibilities that Taylor encountered in her research for the show.

Tarrare: materialising the medical gaze

The story of Tarrare, as told in Wattle and Daub's *The Depraved Appetite of Tarrare the Freak*, was drawn from his doctor Baron Percy's published case study *Mémoire sur la polyphagie* (1804, referred to as *Mémoire* from hence). The case study tells the life story of Tarrare, who experienced polyphagia or excessive appetite. It begins with Tarrare's ejection from his family home when they could no longer afford to feed him, after which he performed for a travelling mountebank, 'defying the public to satisfy him' (Percy, 1804, p. 91, author's translation) by throwing objects for him to swallow. His act evolved to include swallowing live cats and snakes and regurgitating the bones and the fur. He was, according to Percy, recruited by the French Revolutionary Army to swallow sensitive documents, smuggle them across Prussian lines, and regurgitate them. Tarrare failed miserably as a spy, as he was quickly caught by the Prussian army and subjected to a mock execution, after which he returned to France, found Percy in a military hospital, and asked to be cured. Percy tried a series of cures, each of which failed to curb Tarrare's appetite. This appetite was growing – Tarrare was caught drinking the blood of bloodletting patients and eating limbs from corpses in the mortuary. Percy noted that Tarrare 'took so much pleasure in eating that he seemed to fear, rather than wish for, his recovery' (ibid: 96). He was eventually chased from the hospital under suspicion of having eaten a toddler. Percy found him several years later dying of tuberculosis, a disease that 'put an end to the voracity' of Tarrare (ibid: 97). Tarrare claimed that he was being killed by a silver fork that he had swallowed. Following Tarrare's death, Percy autopsied him, looking for but not finding either the fork or the cause of Tarrare's polyphagia.

The project was a collaboration between Wattle and Daub and scientific, medical humanities and historical scholars and practitioners. The Wellcome Trust funded the development of this project as a public engagement project on biomedical history, specifically an exploration of the emergence of the pathological autopsy in the late eighteenth century. Doctors had been cutting up bodies after death for several centuries, but these procedures, such as Anne Greene's, were framed as anatomical dissections with the pedagogical intention of exploring the geography of the human body's interior in order to produce knowledge, while pathological autopsy is undertaken in order to discover the cause of disease and death. Tarrare's autopsy occurred in 1798 during the formal emergence of pathology as a discipline in Europe. This was a few years following the 1793 publication of the first European textbook on pathology by Mathew Baillie (van den Tweel and Taylor, 2010). The first scene of our production, in which Percy cuts open Tarrare in a fruitless search for the fork that Tarrare had believed was killing him, therefore stages one of the first pathological autopsies in Western Europe (Bates, 2021). Percy's *Mémoire*, which recounts this pathological autopsy, is a case study of a shift within medical practice conventionally described, within the narrative of a linear progression of scientific knowledge, as the advancement of modern medicine. Displacing this historical framing rooted in the concept of progress is Foucault's genealogical identification of the historical moment with the emergence of the medical or clinical gaze, in which patients' bodies are visible only as body parts and symptoms, with a concurrent decline of the patient narrative (2003). The opening autopsy creates a tension between the emotional impact of the moment on Percy, who knew Tarrare as a human being, and his desperate search for the fork, which allows us to witness a medical procedure predicated on the medical gaze as Percy examines, describes and tears through individual body parts.

The written archive on Tarrare is found solely in Percy's case study. Tarrare's voice is absent. In what he calls a 'grotesque act of ventriloquism: raising and objectifying the dead on stage', Tobi Poster-Su, co-artistic director of Wattle and Daub and the show's librettist and lead puppeteer, explores the ethical implications and pitfalls of the act of 'ventriloquism' involved in putting our own words into the mouths of the dead in *Tarrare*, examining this through Levinas's ethics of the other and Salverson's work on the ethics of documentary theatre (2020). As theatre-makers, raising the dead required attention to a mode of spectatorship that can be linked to Foucault's concept of the medical gaze. If the clinician's gaze allows penetration beyond the surface appearance of the

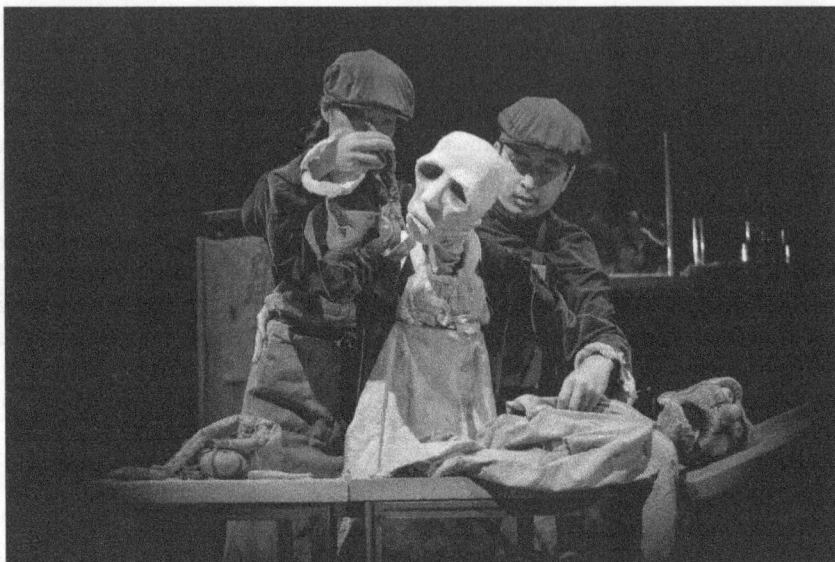

Figure 34.1 Puppets of Tarrare and Baron Percy in *The Depraved Appetite of Tarrare the Freak* (2017) with puppeteers Aya Nakamura and Tobi Poster-Su. Photo: Barney Witts. Image courtesy of Wattle and Daub.

body and the uncovering of hidden truths, thereby positioning the body as docile object within a field of biopower, the twenty-first century artist's and audience member's gaze on the representation of a historical body on stage can similarly be assumed to penetrate the veil of history in order to uncover the 'truth' of a historical moment. This reduces the historical subject to the status of an object that is only legible through the act of artistic historical representation. Creating a show to be performed on a stage before a seated audience carries a particular risk of enacting this type of gesture, seeming to invite the audience to consume a fixed frame of historical events. Our attempt to avoid this issue involved including our own artist's gaze on the bodies and stories we were staging and was rooted in using the materiality of puppetry performance strategically to interrupt this type of spectatorship. Our intentions were threefold: to make visible the constructed nature of reanimating historical narrative, to displace conventional historical narratives of the progress of modern medicine, and to materialise the medical gaze, making literal, in the construction and manipulation of the puppet bodies, the ways in which the medical gaze penetrates and fragments bodies.

Mirroring the source material for Tarrare's life story, the show's narrative is told through Percy's memories. Through this we intended to make the puppets into representations of material traces of the archive. Percy was excluded from this. He is the only 'living' puppet, the only puppet meant to represent a living human rather than a corpse, as his is the only living archival voice. The show's puppets, apart from Percy, were therefore puppets in a double sense: as literal puppets in the show, animated by their puppeteers, and as corpses in Percy's autopsy room, animated by medical assistants. The uncanniness of puppets rests partially in their uncertain status as living beings, simultaneously animated figures and dead objects. This simultaneity of perception has been described by Steve Tillis as the 'double vision' of puppetry spectatorship (1992), and by myself as '(mis)perception' (Purcell-Gates, 2022). This quality allowed us to play with the shifting perceptions of the audience as they watched the puppets on stage shift between dead corpses in an autopsy room within which the story is performed and apparently living figures within a living story. This framing intentionally served as a material metaphor for the act of creating and performing historical narrative by reanimating corpses of the past, by shifting the status of the puppets between object and subject in order to stage the object/subject shifts of historical figures that historical narrative produces.

The piece explores the tension between Percy's account of events, as narrated in his *Mémoire*, and what we imagined the experience might have been like for Tarrare. This is evident in the 'Cures' song, which takes place late in the show when Tarrare asks Percy to cure him, thereby setting off a sequence of attempted, and failed, cures based on late eighteenth-century medical practices including enemas and the ingestion of tobacco pills and boiled eggs. This scene was created to highlight two contrasting perceptions: Percy's of his medical experiment couched within the advance of modern medical knowledge and Tarrare's as a patient whose body, under the medical gaze, is reduced to the status of object. Percy's perception was conveyed through the lyrics – he sings the song, and, when he invites Tarrare to sing along with him, Tarrare can only cry or scream – and through the music's upbeat, swingy energy, culminating in a kick-line in which the medical assistants force a gagged Tarrare to dance with them. We staged the treatments as painful and requiring restraint in order to invoke the practice of surgery without anaesthesia. While European surgeons including English surgeon James Moore were experimenting with numbing the nerves during the late eighteenth century, effective anaesthesia was first demonstrated in the United States by William Morton in 1846 (Royal College of Anaesthetists, 2022). The forced dance of Tarrare at the hands of Percy's medical assistants was, therefore, an act that, in its juxtaposition of brutality and medical innovation, crystallised the complexities of patient experience during the emergence of the modern clinic that saw doctors simultaneously helping and hurting patients. The ability to cut into the body in order to cure it materialises the medical gaze with a knife: knowledge and violence co-exist as the interior of the body is made penetrable to the all-seeing gaze of the doctor. This scene juxtaposed music, movement and heavy-handed manipulation of a puppet to create a dissonance in audience perception of a key moment in medical history, evoking both laughter and uneasiness.

It was in the 'Cures' song that we most explicitly explored the theme of the body as object under the medical gaze. As the medical assistants move him around the stage, on and off of a gurney, stuffing tobacco pills and eggs down his throat, holding him down and gagging him, making incisions in his arms, Tarrare's puppet body literally becomes a manipulated object. This produces a tension between the puppet seen as object and simultaneously experienced as human. Margaret Williams suggests that puppetry can be identified as a mode of spectatorship defined by an audience member assigning agency to the object on stage (2014). When Tarrare's body is roughly moved around the stage by the medical assistants during 'Cures', the locus of perceived agency rapidly shifts between Tarrare struggling against medical assistants, an act already doubled by the manipulations of his puppeteer, and puppeteers grabbing and throwing a puppet. The Tarrare puppet is, in the audience's doubled perception, simultaneously a character and an object.

Conclusion

Puppetry offers routes into theatrical representations and explorations of often-invisible concepts within medical performance, through puppets as constructed bodies and the shifting play of agency between puppet and puppeteer. In *After Cardenio* and *Tarrare*, puppetry functions both as a device of making-visible, and as an enactment of resistance to the gaze. In one sense, the puppets that represent Anne Greene and Tarrare make visible abstract concepts that inform the medical discourses of the seventeenth and eighteenth centuries in Europe, respectively. Anne Greene's dual embodiment in *After Cardenio*, as a living human via an actor, representing the mind or soul, and as a puppet, representing the body, allowed Taylor to stage mind/body dualism and to invite them to interact. These interactions occurred directly through puppetry, as when the actor puppeteers or gives focus to the puppet, through shifting focus between the figures (at times the puppet is the focus, at times it is the human, suggesting shifts between the actions of body and mind), and through interactions between the two figures, as when the puppet comforts the human, suggesting the simultaneous presence of two facets of the self, dual yet one. This technique of puppet/human performance also functioned as a device of inquiry: Taylor discusses how it allowed the artists to ask: 'Is the body the technology for the soul, or is the soul a technology for the body?' (2019, p. 216). In this sense Taylor and her collaborators restaged seventeenth-century inquiries around consciousness and the mind/body split, emphasising the role of materiality within these enquiries through the dead-yet-alive figure of the puppet. Tarrare's fragmented corpse body served a similar function of making visible concepts at the core of eighteenth-century medical discourse, in allowing Wattle and Daub to explore materialisations of the medical gaze, making visible this gaze while simultaneously replicating it by making his subjectivity read as coherent.

In another sense, these puppets resist the gaze of both the anatomist and the pathologist, refusing to reveal that which the gaze seeks to bring to light. Anne's puppet body looks out through its prosthetic eyes but does not allow her anatomists to look either into her body or into her past. Tarrare's fragmented body, into which we can always see, refuses to reveal its secrets. At the end of the show, Percy gives up on the autopsy, unable to find either the fork or the cause of his patient's polyphagia. His assistant places Tarrare's head, now a specimen, into a jar. In pathologist Alan Bates's commentary on the Tarrare case study drawn from his collaboration on the show (2021), he uses the fork as a metaphor for Percy's search, in his autopsy of Tarrare, for something 'that he could never have found' (Bates, 2021). As with Greene's puppet body as specimen, Tarrare as specimen is meant to serve as exemplar, revealing the truth of his condition, yet it reveals nothing.

Note

1 A production filmed at the Tobacco Factory Theatres, Bristol, UK, in January 2017 can be viewed here. Available at: https://vimeo.com/513433117/6871ef5f4d.

Reference list

After Cardenio (2011) Directed by J. Taylor. Cape Town, South Africa.

Bates, A. (2021) 'Looking for the golden fork', in Purcell-Gates, L. (ed.) *Tarrare the Freak research programme – 'history of medicine and the depraved appetite of Tarrare the Freak'*. Bath: BathSPAdata, Dataset, p. 5. https://doi.org/10.17870/bathspa.12340976.v2

Bouchard, G. (2016) 'The pain of "specimenhood"', in Mermikides, A. and Bouchard, G. (eds.) *Performance and the medical body*. London and New York: Bloomsbury Methuen Drama Publishing, pp. 139–150. https://doi.org/10.5040/9781472570819.ch-010

The Depraved Appetite of Tarrare the Freak (2017) Directed by S. Calvert-Ennals. Bristol, UK: Wattle and Daub.

Foucault, M. (2003) *The birth of the clinic: an archaeology of medical perception*. 3rd edn. London: Routledge.

Mitchell, P. *et al.* (2011) 'The study of anatomy in England from 1700 to the early 20th century', *Journal of Anatomy*, 219(2), pp. 91–99. https://doi.org/10.1111/j.1469-7580.2011.01381.x

Percy, P. (1804) 'Mémoire sur la polyphagie', *Journal de Médecine, Chirurgie, Pharmacie*, 9, pp. 90–99. Available at: www.biusante.parisdescartes.fr/histoire/medica/resultats/index.php?cote=90146x1805x09& p=97&do=page (Accessed: 25 November 2021).

Poster-Su, T. (2020) 'A grotesque act of ventriloquism: raising and objectifying the dead on stage', *Applied Theatre Research*, 8(1), pp. 45–56. https://doi.org/10.1386/atr_00025_1

Purcell-Gates, L. (2022) '*Yūrei* and puppetry in Japanese ghost stories: (mis)perception and ambiguous bodies' in *Kaidan*', in Orenstein, C. and Cusack, T. (eds.) *Puppet and spirit*. London and New York: Routledge.

The Royal College of Anaesthetists (2022) *The History of Anaesthesia* [Online]. Available at: https://rcoa.ac.uk/about-college/heritage/history-anaesthesia (Accessed: 20 February 2022).

Taylor, J. (2012) *After Cardenio: an unnatural moment in the history of natural philosophy* [Podcast]. ICLS Rethinking the Human Sciences. Available at: https://podcasts.apple.com/gb/podcast/jane-taylor-after-cardenio-an-unnatural-moment-in/id506422315?i=1000126263284 (Accessed: 30 September 2021).

Taylor, J. (2019) '"Newes from the dead": an unnatural moment in the history of natural philosophy', in Gamboa, B. and Switzky, L. (eds.) *Shakespeare's things: Shakespearean theatre and the non-human world in history, theory, and performance*. London and New York: Routledge, pp. 217–234. https://doi.org/10.4324/9780367855178

Tillis, S. (1992) *Towards an aesthetics of the puppet*. Westport, CT: Greenwood Press.

van den Tweel, J.G. and Taylor, C.R. (2010) 'A brief history of pathology', *Virchows Archiv*, 457(1), pp. 3–10. Available at: www.ncbi.nlm.nih.gov/pmc/articles/PMC2895866/ (Accessed: 20 February 2022).

Watkins, R. (1651) *Newes from the dead* [Internet archive]. Available at: https://archive.org/details/b30342107/page/n11/mode/2up (Accessed: 20 February 2022).

Williams, M. (2014) 'The death of "the puppet"?', in Posner, D., Orenstein, C. and Bell, J. (eds.) *The Routledge companion to puppetry and material performance*. London and New York: Routledge, pp. 18–29. https://doi.org/10.4324/9781315850115

35

PERFORMING THE PILL

Contemporary feminist performance exploring the side effects of hormonal contraception

Alex Mermikides and Katie Paterson

The pill, or hormonal contraception, refers to synthetic oestrogen and/or progesterone usually taken to prevent pregnancy in sexually active women. Since its release in the 1960s, the power of the pill to prevent unwanted pregnancy has led to controversy and contradiction within the public discourse. Its early release attracted the criticism of religious institutions for its impact on reproduction and the licence it might give to women's sexuality (at first, prescriptions were only afforded to married women who already had children). Since then, it has been hailed as an unqualified good that can liberate women from childbearing and domestic servitude – a position taken up by women and feminist thinkers but also, more sinisterly, by the state, by public health officials and medical professionals, as a way of controlling fertility in certain populations. Equally, it has been maligned, sometimes also by feminists, as a harmful imposition oppressively regulating women, alienating them from their own natural reproductive cycle and introducing toxic and carcinogenic substances into the body. This ambivalence is further complicated by a peculiarity of hormonal contraception: the fact that it is a medicine that does not treat or cure an illness. As social historian, Lara Marks describes,

> Pharmacologically, the pill is unique. Most drugs are intended for the treatment of organic diseases. By contrast the pill is aimed at preventing pregnancy, a condition not usually considered an illness. The fact that it is a contraceptive designed to be consumed by healthy women of reproductive age for long periods of time has magnified concerns about its potential dangers.
>
> (2001, p. 4)

Marks further notes the complexity of this position, including discussion of what this means in the context of its clinical development and the question of what the medical establishment considers an appropriate level of risk. For an ill patient undergoing experimental treatment, there will be a low tolerance among medical approval boards and prescribers of potential harmful side effects. For a healthy woman, on the other hand, a higher level of negative side effects might be considered tolerable if the associated benefits are considerable. Among users of the pill, however, there seems to be a growing consensus that the existing situation is *simply not good enough*, that the promises

DOI: 10.4324/9781003036500-40

of liberation have been undermined by a lack of research, information and innovation in relation to the side effects of taking hormonal contraception.

The acknowledged side effects of the pill range from the discomfort of breast tenderness to the potentially life-threatening increased vulnerability to blood clots and stroke. However, a range of other 'unofficial' and highly individualistic side effects have also been posited, including reports of decreased libido, weight gain, weight loss, nipple discharge, mood changes and the onset of mental ill health such as depression and anxiety. Reports of such side effects are often dismissed, a point made in *Side FX*, a performance about the pill made by Katie Paterson, one of the authors of this chapter, which includes a game of 'side effects bingo', played with the audience. The lucky winner is summoned onstage to be told by a doctor/bingo caller about the side effects on their bingo card, 'that's very unusual, you know, most people don't have any problems'. The dearth of conclusive medical research into these side effects has been a key theme in the popular discourse that has proliferated in recent years, for example in the Channel 4 television broadcast, *Davina McCall's Pill Revolution* (McShane, 2023), in publications such as Holly Grigg-Spall's *Sweetening the Pill* (2013), Sarah Hill's *How The Pill Changes Everything: Your Brain on Birth Control* (2019), in Elinor Cleghorn's *Unwell Women: A Journey Through Medicine and Myth in a Man-Made World* (2021) and on the recently launched user-review contraceptive platform *The Lowdown*. On social media and sites such as Mumsnet, it is possible to access thousands of testimonies reporting side effects, medical sexism and grass-roots initiatives to empower women with information and support about their fertility. These informal bodies of knowledge provide a rich mine of information about women's medical experience, for example, providing scholars such as Heather Brook Adams (2019) and Tasha Dubriwny (2013) the opportunity to explore the complex agential relationship between women and supposedly empowering medical technologies. Scholarly interest in women's experiences and perceptions of the pill is further reflected in journal articles, at least one doctoral thesis on the topic (see, for example, Eastham, 2016; Campo-Engelstein, 2013; Liao and Dollin, 2012; Mills and Barclay, 2006) and book-length studies, for example, that edited by Saetnan, Oudshoorn and Kirejczyk (2000).

Our interest in this chapter is in another arena for alternative information and debate about the experience of taking the pill and navigating its side effects: fringe performance. In January 2023, the authors of this chapter brought together six emerging theatre-makers who had recently created performances about the pill and its side effects. The participants had been identified through internet-based surveys using search terms such as 'pill show' 'theatre + contraception' 'fringe + the pill' which captured announcements and reviews of performances that had taken place between 2018 and 2021, and through snowball sampling (chain-referrals whereby participants recommend other potential candidates). All the theatre-makers identified through the search were approached by email, and all agreed enthusiastically to participate in the roundtable, which was conducted online. We cannot claim that this is a systematic or comprehensive audit of contemporary performances about the pill: we may have missed smaller-scale or local productions that did not have an online presence or were not part of the same networks as the identified participants. However, the sample size was appropriate for our purpose, which was to get a sense of how debates about the pill and its side effects featured within contemporary performance – who was making it, why and how. The roundtable, which was led by Paterson and moderated by Alex Mermikides, was semi-structured in format, with questions on the format of and motivations behind each production and time allowed for participants to ask questions of each other.

Here are some brief descriptions of each production, in the theatre-makers' own words:

The productions

Rebecca Pythian, writer and performer of *Pill*

I've created a piece of autobiographical, verbatim, theatre, it's one act so it's quite short in comparison to a conventional show. It uses episodic style to talk about the combined con-traceptive pill and its incredible list of side effects, and a lot of the side effects I explore are the ones that are between major and minor, so maybe not spoken about as much, but it's all from my experience. . . . I think ultimately my main goal with it was to try and tell as many people's stories as possible, so I am a voice for other people as well as using my own voice for my own story, of course.

Claire Parry, writer and performer of *Intolerable Side Effects*

It basically came out of this moment when I'd been on the pill for about a decade and then I lost it, in a move process abroad, and so just couldn't access any more, and so just like galvanised coming off the pill and at that moment starting to think like oh my god what has happened to my body, it took eight months for my period then to even come back. So, lots of these things then coincided with seeing this article where the male contraceptive pill was being developed but then it was stopped for 'intolerable side effects' and it was just that list of all the things that women have just on a daily basis as part of what you just have to accept.

Rosina Aichner, writer and performer of *Ghastly*

The show was about a very intense researcher who is obsessively trying to get the male pill on the market, it is pretty much based on why can't they bring it on the market and then comparing it with the side effects of what women have, in any contraception. I had quite a lot of interviews with women, and then basically wrote all their stories into one story which was the character's story.

Sophie Wright, writer of *Sugar Coated*:

I've been working on a piece of theatre called *Sugar Coated* since early 2019. It's taken a lot of different forms including a digital monologue, a devised piece based on the script that I'd written, there's a version of it as well that I wanted to make into a digital archive. So it kind of stretches, it originally started as a piece about the pill, but it's looking more broadly at people's experiences with reproductive medical care and using space as an analogy. I think we as a society place a lot of importance about learning about the science and the history of space exploration and what's out there. We know a lot about the moon even though only twelve people have ever actually set foot on the moon where in comparison, arguably half of the people in the world experience some form of reproductive health journey. A lot of those people will consider the pill as part of that journey, and we don't know anything about it anecdotally.

Maya Shimmin, writer and producer of *Dosage*

It's a semi-autobiographical, multi-disciplinary interrogation of the pill and the side effects on mental health. So the show started when I had my own kind of year-long experience with multiple pills, and this kind of twelve-month deterioration of my mental health, and my physical health because of my mental health. So it's kind of my story that's kind of explored through live looping and sound design mixed with projection and animation, and we do creative captioning throughout the show. It's a sound designer and a performer on the stage telling the story, mixed in with interviews from about 30 other people's experiences of the pill.

Klara Klinger, writer of *Vicious Cycle* (described in the following) and performer of *Dosage* (see previously).

It's kind of a formally experimental piece that structure-wise plays with the idea of a cycle (see what I did there?) and there's like three stories, three characters that sort of go on like a journey to do with hormonal contraception. I was really drawn to the subject because, I started noticing how, I mean I guess that was the impetus for most of us, whenever you start talking to anyone who's had any experience with contraception, if you just start the conversation, it will just start this avalanche of experiences, problems, frustrations, but we just never talk about it.

As noted, one of the authors of this chapter, Paterson, has also been making a performance on the topic, called *Side FX*, as practice research towards her doctoral degree. She describes it as a 'camp, chaotic cabaret about hormonal contraception'.

We would situate the participants' work as part of a legacy of 1960s and 1970s feminist performance practice, born at the intersection of the alternative theatre movement and feminist activism and consciousness-raising – collectives such as Women's Theatre Company, Monstrous Regiment and Cunning Stunts typify this mix. As Lizbeth Goodman reports, feminist performance has always tended to operate on limited resources (1993) but decreased state subsidy for the arts in the contemporary moment manifests in ever smaller casts, with half of the productions in our survey being solo shows. The participants of our roundtable were all early career theatre-makers (less than ten years since graduation from undergraduate degrees in drama or similar), and all projects were artist-initiated (rather than commissions), performed as one-offs or short runs in small venues or occasionally as part of festivals of feminist theatre such as the long-running *Calm Down, Dear* at Camden People's Theatre in London. Our participants had no hesitation in declaring their feminist colours when asked about this aspect of their work, with emphatic comments such as: 'can't not be feminist really and very much in a protest space . . . a kind of joyful protest' (Parry), 'absolutely feminist . . . while also considering . . . the fact that not everybody that takes the pill is going to be female-identifying' (Pythian), 'I would absolutely say it's feminist, it's deliberately as intersectional as I can possibly be' and 'explicitly feminist and doesn't shy away from being an angry feminist' (Klinger).

Theme 1: diversity of experience (three stories)

For participant Wright, part of being feminist meant 'prioritising personal experience over science'. In keeping with this, a common feature of all the projects was a desire to pay attention to women's lived experiences, with an especial focus on experiences of side effects that might otherwise be overlooked or minimised. With the exception of Klinger's *Vicious Cycle*, all productions were autobiographical in terms of the content or at least their motivation, with the theatre-makers reflecting the dominant demographic of pill users, that is cisgender women of child-bearing age aiming to prevent pregnancy. At the same time, all productions also sought to represent a diversity of experiences, featuring the perspectives of contraception-users at different life stages and with strikingly different physiological and psychological responses to hormonal contraception. As Pythian put it, a shared aim seemed to be 'to try and tell as many people's stories as possible'. Klinger's description of the characters in her play illustrates the diversity of experiences encompassed by the productions, as well as reflecting some of the current critiques of the pill:

> three different stories; the first one is about a woman in Puerto Rico in the fifties obviously the trial [explained subsequently], who then has a stroke due to blood clots. The second story is this teenager who gets put on the pill because of their cycle, but they get really bad side effects in terms of mental health. And then the third story is a woman who was on the pill for a decade and then goes off the pill . . . who kind of like has a perfect life, everything sorted, doesn't find her partner attractive anymore and then there's a problem in their relationship.

The 'trial' mentioned previously is the first major clinical trial of the oral contraceptive pill conducted in Rio Piédras, a Puerto Rican housing project in 1956, under the supervision of Dr Gregory Pincus and Dr Edris Rice-Wray. This is now widely regarded as exploitative and unethical, not least because of the high dosage levels used and the deliberate selection of Puerto Rico as the experiment site explicitly on the basis of the more relaxed clinical standards and the relative poverty of the women invited to participate.[1] Pamela Dollin and Janet Liao summarise the trial thus,

> The 200-plus women involved in the trial received little information about the safety of the product they were given, as there was none to give, and no one thought that it might be necessary to provide such information. That was the standard of the day. Women who stepped forward to describe side effects of nausea, dizziness, headaches, and blood clots were discounted as 'unreliable historians'. Despite the substantial positive effect of the pill, its history is marked by a lack of consent, a lack of full disclosure, a lack of true informed choice, and a lack of clinically relevant research regarding risk. These are the pill's cautionary tales.
> (Liao and Dollin, 2012; see also Cleghorn, 2021, pp. 351–354 for an account of the trial)

This in turn reflects the historical origins of the pill's development in eugenicist arguments about population control (see Celia Gordon, 1974) and its reliance on gynaecological and endocrinological knowledge acquired through the horrific medical exploitation and abuse of women of colour (incidentally, this history is the main feature of other performance works such as *Las Borinqueñas* by Nelson Diaz-Marcano (2021) and *Family Tree* by Mojisola Adebayo (2021), the latter discussed in an chapter by Verónica Rodríguez in Part 1 of this volume). Among our participants, only Klinger's production staged historical material, but its legacy permeated the discussions and productions, for example, as one source of the insidious idea that the economic benefits of population control (especially among marginalised communities) outweigh the negative impact of side effects on individual women.

Klinger's second story, of a teenager taking the pill for non-contraceptive purposes, reflects common practice in the UK where the pill is routinely prescribed for skin disorders, management of menstrual symptoms such as heavy or painful bleeding and conditions including endometriosis and premenstrual dysphoric disorder. In the discussion, Parry suggested that sexual health providers are quick to place girls on hormonal contraception in the belief that even if they are not already engaging in sexual activity with men, they will be soon. For gender theorist Paul B. Preciado, writing on the role that hormonal treatment plays within what he calls the 'pharmacopornographic era', such prescriptions initiate girls into a passive, prescribed femininity within which she might not be trusted to defend their own sexual and reproductive availability (2013). Parry's report of her own experiences of being prescribed the pill at a young age echoed this:

> I was just put on the pill so, so young, and I think so many people are, and at that point you have no idea really, you just go on it, for me it was initially for skin reasons too, so it's kind of, before I was even using it as contraception . . . a lot of people aren't even properly sexually active, and it's just chosen as a precaution so that when that moment comes, should the dreaded thing happen, all these young promiscuous girls are protected already.

Preciado conceptualises the pill as a 'lightweight, portable, individualized, chemical panopticon', an ongoing process of submissive self-monitoring, such that 'the prison cell has become the body of the consumer, which sees itself chemically modified without being able to determine the exact effects or where they come from, once the hormonal compound has been ingested' (2013, p. 205). The prescription of the pill to teenage girls who are still forming their social identities, and for whom the source of 'exact effects' are additionally difficult to ascertain, reflects a theme that is picked up in Paterson's research: the complexity of self in relation to hormone use. For a teenager, how is one to ascertain whether mental ill health is brought on by synthetic hormones or 'teenage angst'; to identify what is artificial and what is inevitable; and, perhaps most significantly, how might they recognise and convince others that something abnormal is at play?

The third story depicted in Klinger's play concerns the breakdown of a long-term heterosexual relationship when a woman discontinues her pill use and finds she is no longer attracted to her partner. Sarah Hill argues that the pill can radically alter experiences of attraction and that it is common for women to discover that the partner they loved while taking the pill is suddenly much less attractive to them when they come off it in order to seek to conceive (Hill, 2019, p. 102). Rather sensationalist coverage has recently been given to the idea that sexual orientation itself is affected by the pill, with suggestions that bisexual women experience hormonally impacted fluctuations in gender preference (see, for example, Morrison's feature in the UK 'tabloid' newspaper, the *Daily Mail*, 2023). This relies on a simplistic and offensive conceptualisation of bisexuality as a kind of see-saw bouncing between gay and straight. Nonetheless, Hill presents data to support the idea that changes in attraction can be caused by hormonal contraception; she implicitly advises women seeking a long-term male partner to come off the pill early in their relationships, just to check. This has profound implications for women's understanding of romance and sexuality, our very autonomy, and yet it remains poorly understood, unheard of until it happens to you.

By raising awareness of a range of possible side effects, the participants saw themselves as campaigning for more medical research and development. A more immediate aim also seemed to be to give women permission to name their experiences as medical, as side effects. As Shimmin puts it:

> And actually, if all of us, if anyone that was considering hormonal contraception, were told about the side effects they would know what to look out for at least, so that then they could come off it, rather than blaming themselves or thinking that it was just part of who they are . . .

I think . . . actually a lot of people found a lot of solace in [seeing *Dosage*] and a lot of realising oh my gosh, no-one's ever explained that feeling to me

Theme 2: official sources

As these accounts suggest, in both the roundtable discussion and in the productions themselves, the lived experience of people taking the pill was often set against medical accounts of what side effects might occur and the extent to which they should be considered tolerable. There was some degree of 'doctor bashing' in relation to sexual health care providers (usually doctors and nurses working in general practitioner surgeries), who were often depicted as providing inappropriate advice or prescriptions (the young age at which girls were prescribed the pill was a key concern, as illustrated by Klinger's second story previously). Health care professionals were often depicted as minimising or dismissing negative side effects. Phythian describes employing a device in her play in which the same medical consultation is repeated three times, with the health care provider speaking the same lines each time despite the fact that the patient, who is experiencing extreme fluctuations in mental health, offers wildly different complaints. This use of repetition conveys routine medical consultations as brutally depersonalised, with condescending platitudes about what is 'normal' offered in response to stark and distressing experiences and where the data (often indicative of a lack of study rather than of conclusive research) overrides the experiences being reported. There were also occasional harrowing accounts of negative side effects, including graphic accounts of coil rejection, extreme mental health problems, excessive bleeding to be the point of unconsciousness and alarming physical symptoms, which were sometimes deemed brushed aside by medical professionals. The impression is that dramatic medical incidents and extreme pain and suffering were discounted as medical emergencies when they occurred in a woman's body. These accounts and discussion thereof were infused with a sense of astonishment that those experiencing even common side effects had not received adequate warning about them.

The most pointed critique, however, tended to be aimed at the pharmaceutical industry, with all participants expressing indignation at Aichner's report of this encounter with an audience member at a post-show discussion:

we had a guy . . . who was from . . . a pharmaceutical start-up, and he said for the pharmaceutical industry actually contraception is solved. And that was, you know it's interesting for him to hear because yeah, for them it's a solved issue, and there aren't any, the pharmaceutical industry is not interested in developing this any further.

Pythian referred back to this later in the roundtable discussion:

And it amazed me when Rosina said about the gentleman from the pharmaceutical industry. . . . I was like, 'what?' That baffles me, if all of us are here creating this kind of work and people are still going to their doctors and nurses and reporting all of these side effects, then how can there be a full stop?

The participants' distrust of health care providers and pharmaceutical companies aligns with a lineage of women's health activism, emerging within the feminist movement of the 1960s and 1970s, which sought to empower women to take back control of their bodies from the more misogynist aspects of the medical establishment. The movement's bible, the Boston Women's Health Book Collective's *Our Bodies, Ourselves* (1971), encouraged women to question health care systems and to reclaim anatomical and medical knowledge of their own bodies – and advocated for the importance of personal stories in doing this. Cleghorn describes how material for the book emerged from extensive questionnaire surveys and workshops, on the basis that 'real change happened when women listened to other women' (2021, p. 362). However, despite our participants' honouring of the lived experiences of contraception-users, it is notable that several chose to collaborate with medical professionals in their research and development processes. Shimmin, for example, describes how she involved 'a contraceptive consultant that was giving us more the medical background, as well as bringing in a psychology consultant looking at actually why do we have that effect when we're taking something'. This use of medical science and expertise to legitimise the accuracy and significance of the production may seem contradictory, but perhaps speaks of the complexity of women's relationship to medicine more generally, and to the pill in particular, as simultaneously emancipatory and exploitative.[2] This may be also seen as one incarnation of what Simon Parry calls the biosocial, 'alliances between individuals and groups identifying variously as artists, activists, scientists, patients, carers and indeed other positions' exploring not only accepted scientific paradigms of experience but more complex, emotional, even mystical positions (2020, p. 13; see also his chapter in Part 3 of this volume).

It may also reflect the somewhat privileged status of the participants, who were all white and educated at least to graduate level: these are women with the social capital to approach medical experts – indeed women for whom it is anomalous to encounter inadequate or discriminatory practices in medicine encounters and who can afford to complain about contraceptive provision (it should be noted that the authors also share this privilege).

Theme 3: friendly feminists (making palatable)

There were divergent approaches to staging experiences of hormonal contraception among our participants, but they all shared a desire to engage the audience in conversation and debate. For Wright, 'the thing I keep coming back to is the personal is political . . . it just needs to feel personal and emotional and like, it just needs to feel enough to start that conversation'. For others, this desire to 'start the conversation' was built into the production with several participants using audience participation. In *Dosage*, for example, Klinger 'handed out like fake pills, obviously they were mints or whatever, to men' and required that 'every time there's an alert noise I take one pill . . . the dosage is raised throughout the show – basically every time there's an alert, the audience members need to take the pill as well'. In keeping with this desire to involve the audience, Klinger described her vision for her own piece *Vicious Cycle* as 'the play, the narrative, just sort of fizzles out and turns into a conversation', where the conventionally mimetic characters cede the focus and the audience is invited to chime in. Phythian used a talkback structure, splitting an hour-long performance slot into thirty minutes of performance and thirty minutes of discussion, implicitly placing equal value on the two components.

This emphasis on participation and conversation revealed a somewhat tentative position among all but one of the participants: they wanted to bring about a revolution – but wanted to avoid seeming 'preachy' while doing so. There appears to be a fear that allowing their anger and outrage to be visible would scare off the people and institutions who most need to see it. All the contributors implied a deeply felt responsibility to inform, to leave their audiences more educated on the subject of hormonal contraception than they entered, but again, there was concern about how this would come across. Klinger asked the other roundtable participants:

> how did you approach creating your shows, how did you approach sort of sharing this information in a way that's not, you know, a preachy or like TED talky type of affair. . . . That's one of my main concerns in working on my show.

Pythian responded that 'it's definitely a subject where it feels very like you could be immediately preachy and it's worrying'. This pattern of attempting to make fierce anger and ugly facts more palatable was also reflected in Paterson's own conversations with women during the development of her piece, *Side FX:* ten minutes of passionate rhetoric would frequently be followed by an equally profuse apology.

Variously framed as keeping it light and avoiding finger pointing and preaching, there was a distinct concern among the participants not to alienate the audience with perceived whining or accusations. Of course, this speaks to the theatre-makers' desire to appeal to their audience, but it suggests an anxiety about what kind of feminism will be acceptable, what kind of complaint (for, as we know from Sara Ahmed [2021], complaint attracts especial opprobrium when voiced by women and other minoritised groups). This bid for accessibility resulted in several of the participants transposing their subjects to alternative settings. Wright's *Sugar-Coated* project evokes the world of space exploration, on the basis that 'I know more about Mars, I think, than about my own reproductive health system and what the pill does for it'. Parry's *Intolerable Side Effects* was born out of her deep frustration when she read press coverage of a male contraceptive trial halted for so-called intolerable side effects which, she observed, were 'all the things that women have just on a daily basis'. The resulting show charts the travails of Diane the Rabbit through a clown world of contraceptive celery and frozen paw syndrome:

> I transposed the subject into the world of a rabbit, with all the connotations of like rampant rabbits, and it just gave me this really fun rabbit character to work with. . . . So, the rabbit then took celery, as the pill, and so would have these instructions to nibble this celery, and then the side effects are really stupid and big, it would like range from the little ones of like a flickering paw and uncontrollable leg, to like slapping herself in the face to being completely paralysed. . . . She goes on rabbit tinder and it's all very silly and physical and full of jumping, and then she goes on this rabbit date with a stupid like cuddly toy rabbit and it's essentially me going back and forth doing the voices.

The transposition aims to make the severity of side effects more visible, implying that an audience might find it dull to watch a human woman experiencing them. Parry describes the empathy she hopes the audience feels having gone on a journey with Diane the rabbit.

One success of this 'friendly' feminist approach was that several of the productions managed to reach men, with anecdotal reflections across the board suggesting that men were moved to reflect on the significance of female hormonal contraception for the first time, prompted to have important discussions with their partners and committed to raising awareness amongst other men. Parry recounted a meeting with a man a few months after he attended her show in Edinburgh, who told her that,

> he'd had this whole discussion with his girlfriend out of the show that they never would have had before and they actually, it just like occurred to them to talk about contraception and to make it an active choice between them rather than like, before he'd just assumed that the girl goes on the pill or something or other and is fine. So that was like, a really nice moment where it felt like these kind of things do have the power to open those conversations, and they don't have to dictate anything but they can just, yeah, be a part of making people realise there's a discussion.

This anecdote may seem insignificant, but the realisation that there is 'a discussion' to be had goes some way to countering a degree of ignorance or resignation in the wider public discussion. For example, in developing and sharing her piece, *Side FX*, Paterson often heard feedback from older British women that during their own contraceptive years, nobody spoke about the challenges associated with either contraception or the hazards of a female reproductive system more generally – they simply got on with it. Though there was extensive women's health activism throughout the second half of the twentieth century, it seems that, for these women, this did not necessarily translate to a mainstream conversation. The internet cultures of the early twenty-first century to some extent replicate this disconnect: dramatic narratives of frightening side effects of hormonal contraception and debates about alternatives abound, but the conversations are 'password-protected' and conducted among a small group – Parry's anecdote sharply reminds us of how rarefied conversations about the pill can be.

Conclusion: sounding alarms

It also indicates the limits of the much-touted 'conversation' because, in the absence of effective alternatives to hormonal contraception, for women or men, there are very few practical changes to be made. Women (and others with the capacity to become pregnant) continue to be burdened with responsibility for birth control and are offered a limited choice: to effectively avoid unwanted pregnancy without recourse to complete abstinence from sex with men, they must put up with the side effects. In view of this, it is telling that several of the shows contained a repeated device whereby characters (and in one case, audience members), swallowed a pill in response to the sound of an alarm clock (or more accurately, an iPhone alarm engineered to sound like an alarm clock). Parry's Diane 'sets an alarm every time she has to take the pill'. On stage Paterson obediently swallows one each time the alarm rings and she reflected in the discussion that 'there's something about labour isn't there, constant, repetitive, boring labour, and the alarm's quite a good indicator of that'. As noted, Klinger involved the audiences in this routine, asking them to swallow a pill on cue throughout the performance: 'the funny thing is that they actually did keep doing it. So they just obeyed the rules of the show, even though they hated it'.

Wright's comments on the situation reflected the general view that

> there was a sociological thing about the idea of perceived risk and whether the risk of something was worth the knowledge or scientific thing that we'd get out of it even though it puts people's lives at risk. . . . I imagine a lot of us have done research about the history of the pill but the way that the pill had come out and the perceived risk of people's infertility when they get the doses wrong, or headaches or blood clots, that it is worth not getting pregnant, in order to have those other side effects.

Wright refers to a paradigm that often surfaces in arguments about side effects, namely that the significant risks of pregnancy will always outweigh the potential harms associated with preventing it. Marks quotes Dr William Inman arguing, with some exasperation, that this risk-benefit analysis assumes that pregnancy is guaranteed where contraception is absent (2001, p. 128). However, the risk of pregnancy is not only a physiological risk but a social one; unplanned pregnancy constitutes a loss of control, a failure of not just contraceptive efforts but self-regulation on the part of the mother, and, as Dubriwny argues, these are unacceptable failures in women's access to autonomy and self-management (2013, p. 155). Particularly for teenage mothers, for unmarried mothers in much of the world, for mothers who are employed outside of the home and for others for whom the 'social burdens' of pregnancy (a term coined by Ann Saetnan in Saetnan, Oudshoorn and Kirejczyk, 2000) are high, contraceptive labour is vital to maintain social standing through appropriate self-regulation: the pill is indeed a 'portable . . .

panopticon'. The sound of the alarm penetrates daily life, calling the pill-taker to action, and in performance it can be highly affective/effective, communicating an invasive relentlessness. The audience's compliance with the alarm in Klinger's show reflects the current situation: the situation is alarming, and yet women continue to take the pill, putting up with the side effects because unwanted pregnancy is framed as an apex threat with which to quash any complaints; anything, surely, is preferable to unwanted pregnancy.

Notes

1 This view is challenged by Lara Marks, who highlights the involvement of many women in administering the trial and suggests there is a racist undertone to the characterisation of Puerto Rican women as helpless victims of the white American doctors.
2 This also speaks to the precarity of emerging theatre-makers in the UK, for whom the Arts Council Project Grants are almost the only strand of funding available. Many shows live or die on the success of (often numerous) ACE bids. The inclusion of medical experts as partners on these bids may be deemed to strengthen the case for support. It is all very well to create a piece exploring ambiguous, complex experiences and even medical misogyny, but the presence of a qualified medic and a community workshop may be required to pay for it.

Reference list

Adams, H.B. (2019) 'Goodbye, "post-pill paradise": texturing feminist public memories of women's reproductive and rhetorical agency', *Quarterly Journal of Speech*, 105(4), pp. 390–417. Routledge. https://doi.org/10.1080/00335630.2019.1657238

Ahmed, S. (2021) *Complaint!* Durham: Duke University Press.

Boston Women's Health Book Collective (1971) *Our Bodies, Ourselves*. New York: Simon and Schuster.

Campo-Engelstein, L. (2013) 'Raging hormones, domestic incompetence, and contraceptive indifference: narratives contributing to the perception that women do not trust men to use contraception', *Culture, Health and Sexuality*, 15(3), pp. 283–295. https://doi.org/10.1080/13691058.2012.752106

Cleghorn, E. (2021) *Unwell women: a journey through medicine and myth in a man-made world*. London: Weidenfeld & Nicolson.

Dubriwny, T.N. (2013) 'Feminist women's health activism in the twenty-first century', in *The vulnerable empowered woman*. New Brunswick, New Jersey and London: Rutgers University Press.

Eastham, R.K. (2016) *Negotiating the fertile body: women's life history experiences of using contraception*. PhD thesis. Lancaster University.

Goodman, L. (1993) *Contemporary feminist theatres*. London and New York: Routledge.

Gordon, L. (1974) 'The politics of population: birth control and the eugenics movement', *Radical America. United States*, 8(4), pp. 61–98.

Grigg-Spall, H. (2013) *Sweetening the pill*. Winchester and Washington: Zero Books.

Hill, S.E. (2019) *How the pill changes everything: your brain on birth control*. London: Orion Spring.

Liao, P.V. and Dollin, J. (2012) 'Half a century of the oral contraceptive pill: historical review and view to the future', *Canadian Family Physician Médecin de famille canadien*, 58(12), pp. 757–760.

Marks, L. (2001) *Sexual chemistry: a history of the contraceptive pill*. New Haven and London: Yale University Press.

McShane, A. (2023) *Davina McCall's pill revolution*. London: Channel 4.

Mills, A. and Barclay, L. (2006) 'None of them were satisfactory: women's experiences with contraception', *Health Care for Women International*, 27(5), pp. 379–398. https://doi.org/10.1080/07399330600629468

Parry, S. (2020) *Science in performance: theatre and the politics of engagement*. Manchester: Manchester University Press.

Preciado, P.B. (2013) *Testo junkie: sex, drugs, and biopolitics in the pharmacopornographic era*. New York: The Feminist Press at the City University of New York, pp. 55–81.

Saetnan, A.R., Oudshoorn, N. and Kirejczyk, M. (eds.) (2000) *Bodies of technology: women's involvement with reproductive medicine*. Ohio: Ohio State University Press.

36

THE GIFT OF LIFE

Organ transplantation and surrogacy on the stage

Gianna Bouchard

In 2020, in the UK and other countries in the global north, existing health inequalities came into sharp focus as a result of the collision of the socially seismic shifts brought about by the coronavirus (COVID-19) pandemic and the Black Lives Matter movement. As the body count mounted in the face of the pandemic's onslaught, and racial justice protests erupted around the world at the brutal police killing of George Floyd in the United States, attention turned to interrogating exactly whose bodies were most at risk in the public sphere and in health care, and why. Black and brown bodies were rapidly exposed as being more vulnerable to state violence and to succumbing to COVID-19 in higher numbers. In terms of the pandemic, ethnic minorities were often on the frontline of social and health services, as nurses and care workers, as well as patients, and so they became doubly susceptible to contracting the virus. Early statistical data reported in the media started to reveal these stark differences in case numbers and mortality rates:

> Early data of the Covid-19 crisis, broken down by race, is alarming. In the US, in Chicago, as of early April 2020, 72% of people who died of coronavirus were black, although only one-third of the city's population is. . . . In the UK, of the first 2,249 patients with confirmed Covid-19, 35% were non-white. This is much higher than the proportion of non-white people in England and Wales – 14%, according to the most recent census.
>
> (Ro, 2020, BBC online)

Sadly, there was nothing fundamentally new in many of these revelations, which highlighted deeply embedded structural racism and discrimination in health care. The need for policy change, decolonising medical training, addressing environmental and social injustices, and ensuring equitable access to resources for marginalised communities became part of the national conversation. The deployment of innovative medical technologies and the rapid growth of new drug therapies and treatments seemingly do little to curb the exploitation of vulnerable bodies. Examining contemporary clinical labour practices, such as clinical trials and tissue banking, academics Catherine Waldby and Melinda Cooper have noted that '[w]hile populations in the developed economies perform some kinds of clinical labour . . . more onerous and risky clinical labour is increasingly outsourced to poor populations in the developing world' (2008, pp. 59–60). The global reach of pharmaceutical and biomedical companies provides unparalleled access to new markets of global

DOI: 10.4324/9781003036500-41

majority bodies for testing, research development, and as donors, whilst raising concomitant bioethical concerns about exploitation, abuse and lack of consent.

Against this backdrop of precarity and heightened risk for marginalised communities as patients and clinical labourers, this chapter examines two contemporary plays that explicitly stage global majority bodies in relation to whiteness in the different medical contexts of organ transplantation and gestational surrogacy: *Harvest* by Manjula Padmanabhan (2003) and *Made in India* by Satinder Kaur Chohan (2017). Biocapitalism drives the trade in organ transplantation and surrogacy that these plays interrogate, 'comprised by the new economics and industries that generate value out of parts of human bodies', making them commercial enterprises that can ensnare impoverished populations in their machinations (Banner, 2017, p. 12). Both plays are written by women and focus on the discriminatory and colonialist fault lines in these complex social and medical scenarios. They offer an exploration of the racialised positions of donor and surrogate in relation to the brown female body as they entangle in globalised medical practices and procedures.

The commodification of the body in these instances sits uneasily in relation to widespread ideas about donation and surrogacy as forms of gift giving. Certain national legal and ethical frameworks, in the UK, for instance, underpin these notions by maintaining that bodies and tissues are non-fungible. As such, there are no property rights in bodies and financial incentives for donation and surrogacy are either illegal, in the case of organ donors, or kept to paying expenses only, for surrogates. The idea of the gift inflects the public discourse around transplantation and surrogacy, where donors and surrogates are both considered to offer the 'gift of life' to their recipients in the form of organs or children. The concept of the gift of life in relation to organ transplantation refers to the act of donating organs or tissues to save or enhance the life of another by replacing failing parts with a donor's. The donor in these instances, whether living or cadaveric, is viewed as generously giving the gift of life to restore health and vitality, often to an anonymous stranger. In gestational surrogacy, a woman carries and delivers a pregnancy for another individual or couple where the embryo is created using the intended parents' or donors' eggs and sperm through *in vitro* fertilization. The resulting embryo is implanted into the gestational surrogate's uterus, and she then carries the pregnancy to term. Providing the means for someone who would otherwise be unable to have a child to have offspring is also often described as giving the gift of life to the new parent/s. This public narrative is visible in a Sky News article from September 2022 about a reality television celebrity in a same sex marriage, whose sister acted as his surrogate. The tag line to the article reads, 'The 44-year-old shared his daughter's name in an Instagram post and paid tribute to the people who had given them the "gift of life"'.[1] Meanwhile, the NHS regularly uses this metaphor in relation to organ donation, for instance, urging people to 'Celebrate the Gift of Life' during Organ Donation Week.[2]

To better understand this complex idea of gift-giving in medical contexts, scholars have mainly drawn on the separate studies of Marcel Mauss and Richard Titmuss. Anthropologist Mauss examined gift-giving practices in traditional societies in the early twentieth century, identifying three specific expectations and obligations that went with the giving of a gift: the obligation to give, to receive, and to reciprocate (2002, pp. 50–55). In order to sustain social relations and networks, Mauss noted that gift-giving was an expected part of everyday practices, and any recipient had an obligation to receive such a gift. Not giving or receiving gifts appropriately in these societies could undermine social connections and the status of the individuals involved. Reciprocity then concluded the operation of the gift, either by a gift being given in return or by participating in some other form of social exchange. Mauss argued that these obligations produced an iterative cycle amongst a group that helped to build and maintain social cohesion. Meanwhile, sociologist Richard Titmuss based his 1970 study on comparing voluntary and commercial blood donation systems in the UK and the US, arguing for donation as a more ethical and secure gift when it is a charitable act rather than being incentivised by payment. He claimed that when blood donation is considered as a gift, donors are motivated by altruistic imperatives that reinforce social bonds and a sense of doing something for others in an ethical manner. Both studies revealed that gift-giving includes recognition of the other and is an act of sharing and connection, involving generosity and reciprocity.

The correspondences between Mauss' and Titmuss' gift theories with organ transplantation and surrogacy are not straightforward, of course. Both interventions are profoundly complex social, legal, medical, personal, and technological matters, and so metaphors are deployed to deal with the underlying strangeness of body parts being transferred to others or used for the development of another's baby. The idea of the gift, even when financial exchange is involved, helps to cope with what anthropologist Lesley Sharp, in relation to organ transplants, describes as 'a form of *ideological disjunction*' (2006, p. 14, italics in original). Medical anthropologists have found that it is commonplace for recipients and their families to view their donor as providing the gift of life. They are actively encouraged by transplant professionals to be grateful, while simultaneously 'depersonalising the donor as merely the source of transferable parts' (Shildrick, 2021, p. 5). Health care professionals worry that recipients will get over-invested in their donors and they have to comply with rules about anonymity, so they steer a strange path between acknowledging the gift whilst closing down avenues to greater intimacy with the originator of the gift. To some extent, this distancing mechanism should dampen the sense of obligation between parties, so holding onto the notion of the gift clearly alleviates some of the tensions and paradoxes for those directly involved, and helps to obscure the more troubling aspects of these procedures.

The case studies explored in this chapter, Chohan's *Made in India* and Padmanabhan's *Harvest*, raise some of the ethical dilemmas inherent in international, commercial organ transplant and surrogacy arrangements. As an often deeply unequal exchange, black and brown female bodies have become the latest source of bodily matter, commodified and sold back to the global north:

> The global traffic in organs follows the modern routes of capital and labor flows, and conforms to the usual lines of social and economic cleavage. *In general*, the organs flow from South to North, from poor to rich, from black and brown to white, and from female to male bodies.
>
> (Scheper-Hughes, 2001, p. 45, emphasis in original)

The narrative of the gift remains in these plays, even though these are financial arrangements that are heightened by the racialised dimensions of these exchanges. Through exposing white privilege in these examples, the plays focus on a particular form of medical inequality that arises through the global commodification of body parts.

Padmanabhan's *Harvest* and organ donation

Written in 1997 in response to the 'flourishing illegal trade in human organs in India', Manjula Padmanabhan's award-winning play *Harvest* offers a future dystopian vision of a transnational trade in organs for transplantation (2003, p. 4). Set in Bombay, now Mumbai, it focuses on an intergenerational family living in a single-room, inner city tenement, who become entangled with an American biotech company that contracts consenting subjects to act as donors for their wealthy clients. Having lost his job as a clerk, Om Prakash, the family's breadwinner, successfully passes a barrage of medical tests to be selected as a donor, a desperate option to earn money for the

Gianna Bouchard

selected male applicants. Once contracted, Interplanta Services quickly takes over the family's living space, converting it into a high-tech quarantine for Om, his wife Jaya, and his mother Ma, and installing a 'contact module' which links directly to the organ recipient via a live video connection. The organ 'receiver', Ginni, a young, white, American woman, visits the family virtually several times a day and exerts increasing control over their lives to prepare Om for his transplant. Om's brother, Jeetu, a sex worker who lives on the streets, arrives home just before Om is taken for organ harvesting and, in a chaotic scene in the flat, is taken by the company's guards instead of Om. Jeetu is also Om's wife's lover, an important plot point for what is to follow.

Jeetu is returned to the family without his eyes and instead receives images of Ginni straight into his brain. Overcome by desire for Ginni, Jeetu offers to do anything for her and is promptly removed for further transplantation. Meanwhile, Om is mortified at abandoning his brother to his fate, and he also leaves to try to offer himself once again for donation. Meanwhile, Ma has become addicted to the new television, a part of the compensation package from Interplanta, and ends up cocooned in a specially delivered 'videocouch', akin to a sarcophagus, which she is plugged into and never needs to emerge from again as it takes care of all her bodily and entertainment needs. The final scene is of Jaya, left alone in the flat with Ma's video tomb, where she is confronted via the contact module with the real organ recipient, Virgil. He has been masquerading as Ginni to seduce Jeetu into offering himself for full-body donation and now shows himself transplanted into Jeetu, living in his skin, much to Jaya's horror and confusion. In a final twist, Virgil claims that the receivers 'look for young men's bodies to live in and young women's bodies in which to sow their children' (Padmanabhan, 2003, p. 86). Jaya has been the target of the organ transplant all along for her reproductive capacity. In a last act of resistance, Jaya demands that Virgil must come to her in physical form if he wants her to carry his baby, that he must risk himself for the outcome he desires, or she will end her life. Thus, the play explores troubling power dynamics between the privileged and the marginalised, white and brown, North and South, in a futuristic world of transnational organ transplantation.

The corporation, Interplanta Services, 'offers Om's family a life of material luxury as a barter for a future transplant – a *gift* in exchange for an obligation' (Srihari, 2022, p. 155, emphasis in original). Instead of donation operating through a state-run, public service, where the provision of organs relies on processes of gifting to an unknown other, *Harvest* imagines transplantation as a privately contracted service operating for the benefit of rich white clients and outsourced to an economically vulnerable global majority population. If 'the move from individual will to public good is an essential component in the "gift of life"', Padmanabhan illustrates how this can be corrupted through a hyper-commodification of the body, where every tissue and organ is fungible and therefore ripe for exploitative capitalist markets (Russell, 2019, p. 70). In a striking comparison, Om's brother, Jeetu, argues that '[a]t least when I sell *my* body, I decide which part of me goes into where and whom!' (Padmanabhan, 2003, p. 33, emphasis in original). Maintaining bodily autonomy and choice in such bio-transactions is shown to be a privilege of those in the global north, who can afford these transplants, and too easily jeopardised in the south when black and brown communities find themselves in financial hardship and desperate to protect their families.

As the company takes over the family's small flat with high-tech kit that will prepare Om for donation, he and his wife Jaya gradually reveal the details of his new 'job' to his mother, who lives with them. Once she grasps what Om's new employment involves, she asks why the company has approached them and why they don't 'have enough of their own people?' Jaya sarcastically retorts that '[w]e grow on trees . . . in the bushes!' (ibid: 22). This articulates a commonplace assumption 'that the impoverished Global South has a surfeit of bodies, that the "expendable" flesh of the poor is their most valuable commodity' (Russell, 2019, p. 239). Literature scholar Emily Russell argues

382

that such narratives work to mitigate anxieties around transplants when organs cross international boundaries and transplant tourism, as it is sometimes called, offers access to cheaper and less regulated markets. The notion that these markets benefit the donors and surrogates crops up time and again, a sop to the worried consumer who wants to calm their ethical disquiet.

In signing the contract for his body parts, Om does not know what they will remove or exactly when; he simply must wait in his flat. In the meantime, the company exercise complete biological and physical control over the family, including quarantining them from their neighbours, removing all their food and replacing it with pellets, medicating them, dictating their mealtimes, and putting them under constant surveillance through the installation of the contact module. In return they are provided with the trappings of Western ideas of wealth and comfort, including a television, an exercise machine, dressing gowns, trainers, and a private bathroom with separate toilet. The contact module, a 'white, faceted globe' hanging from their ceiling, is the site of their surveillance as they are groomed for transplantation (Padmanabhan, 2003, p. 17). This computer portal can be lowered into the room and powers up to reveal the projection of 'a young woman's face, beautiful in a youthful, glamorous, First World manner' (ibid: 22). Ginni is the apparent transplant recipient, able to check up on the family virtually a few times a day, as they offer hope for her future health and ongoing life. A white 'angel', as Ma describes her, Ginni does not appear to be sick or ailing and so seems an unlikely organ recipient, but the audience is left in no doubt about the extreme differences in circumstance between the donor family and the 'receiver'. In fact, Ginni's angelic appearance in their home and provision of everything that they ask for appears to Om and Ma as a kind of gift, obscuring the horror of the obligation of donation when the time comes. Clearly embodied on the stage, the play 'dramatizes how impoverished, gendered racial bodies are disproportionately rendered the raw material of neoliberal rationalities' (Kim, 2014, p. 222).

Extensive anthropological transplant scholarship has examined how organ donation establishes new social ties between the recipient and donor, even if that means the kin of a cadaveric donor with the beneficiary of an organ and their family.[3] The idea of the gift of life in these circumstances speaks to a profound sense of connection between the individuals involved, even though medical professionals try to insert a clear disconnect between them through maintaining donor anonymity and deploying a rhetoric of re-usable organs and new body parts for the recipient that seeks to dehumanise the transfer (Sharp, 2006, p. 5). In *Harvest*, the audience witnesses a strange and strained relationship developing between Ginni and the family, echoing the potentiality of these new social relations and simultaneously undermining them through the dire nature of the contractual obligation of the gift and its colonialist framing. Ma views Ginni as a benevolent angel who bestows presents on the family, becoming obsessed by the television, which she can barely move away from as the play progresses. Om and Jaya become obedient subjects, mirroring colonial structures, when the contact module springs into life, with Om particularly fawning in his responses in order to please Ginni and keep his side of the bargain. He goes so far as to claim that, even though they have only known each other for two months, 'from the first day itself, I've felt that you are just like my sister' (Padmanabhan, 2003, p. 40). Ginni reciprocates with: 'I get to give you things you'd never get in your lifetime and you get to give me . . . well . . . maybe my life. You know? That's a special bond' (ibid: 41). Both responses address the intimate and new bond felt by those involved in transplantation surgery, although Om's is also complicated by his subservience to his white contractor, coupled with desire for Ginni.

Not only do organ transplant recipients articulate this sense of kinship with their donor but they also often express an understanding that the incorporation of another's body part goes beyond the merely biological. The gift of life thus involves a transfer of some essential but immaterial part of the donor, captured within the organ itself and passed on to the recipient. As Sharp puts it, 'donated cadaveric organs simultaneously emerge as interchangeable parts, as precious gifts, and as harbouring the transmigrated souls of the dead' (2006, p. 14). Transplant recipients regularly tell of perceived changes to themselves following their surgery that they ascribe to the donated part, such as new musical tastes or newfound interests. Their identity is felt to shift because of this incorporation of the donated part, provoking a sense amongst the transplant community and wider public that donors 'live on' in recipient bodies, strengthening the kinship ties already discussed and providing cadaveric donor families with much needed solace at their time of tragedy (ibid: 24). Shildrick calls this a 'relationship of spectrality', which is made particularly disturbing in Virgil/Jeetu's whole-body transplant at the end of the play (Shildrick, 2021, p. 2). Jaya witnesses this spectrality as a jarring racialised digital image, transposed from America into the flat in Bombay/Mumbai. It is composed of the body and appearance of Jeetu with the voice and therefore, by extension, the mind of Virgil. This occupation of Jeetu's body, the fourth such transplant that Virgil admits to having, is a form of 'parasitism . . . where one of the organisms benefits at the expense of another' (ibid: 4). Jeetu is fully compromised as Virgil occupies his flesh to reproduce with Jaya, and the idea of the gift of life in organ transplantation is rendered abusive and dysfunctional through its wholesale commodification. That *Harvest* ends with a focus on the brown female body, targeted for its reproductive ability, echoes medical ethicist Donna Dickenson's cautionary words that: 'All bodies are at risk from commodification, but women's bodies are most at risk. Not only are they richer in "raw materials" than men's bodies; women are also more routinely expected to allow access to their bodies' (2007, p. 25). Significantly, the play clarifies and extends this to highlight the vulnerability of racialised women's bodies in the face of global biotechnology and finishes on a note of female defiance. Jaya has the potential to bestow another gift of life, through the birth of a child, but forces an obligation and act of reciprocity on Virgil in demanding that he visit her in person, at great personal risk to himself as a transplant recipient. The last stage image is of Jaya settling in front of the television, looking 'happy and relaxed', waiting for Virgil to decide to make the long journey to her (Padmanabhan, 2003, p. 92).

Chohan's *Made in India* and surrogacy

A current North American surrogacy and egg donation company, Family Inceptions International, introduce their services on their website with the title 'Surrogacy – Giving the Ultimate Gift of Life'. It goes on to state that for 'the intended parents, surrogacy is a selfless gift that fulfils a dream to have a family' and that the surrogate makes 'a righteous sacrifice'.[4] Such rhetoric reflects the logic of the gift through its focus on the recognition of both parties, gratitude for the act of surrogacy, and a mutual exchange between the parties, all couched, in this instance, in quasi-religious tones. This narrative of the gift is then complicated by the fact that this is an example of commercial surrogacy, the website specifying that a surrogate could earn between $50,000 and $80,000, plus allowances, with the first instalment paid 'at confirmation of heart beat'. Such assisted reproductive technologies offer more opportunity and choice for women and families in relation to having children, and they open the way for the possibility of new kinship and familial structures to emerge. But they have also been criticised for colonising women's bodies and once again turning them into sources of extraction and biological wealth.[5] The financial exchange involved in commercial surrogacy, as for any trade in organ donation, commodifies the surrogate/donor's body, turning it into a service that is predicated on contractual obligations, something that cross-racial surrogacy only seems to exacerbate in troubling ways. In her analysis of cross-racial surrogacy, Laura Harrison argues that:

> Surrogates and intended parents are frequently separated by disparities in class, educational background, and cultural capital, with the intended parents occupying the more privileged position. When the surrogate is a person of color and the intended parents are white, race affords the intended parents another layer of privilege.
>
> (2016, p. 6)

White privilege certainly circulates through Satinder Kaur Chohan's *Made in India*, which focuses on an educated, white, middle-class, affluent woman paying for cross-racial surrogacy in India. Staged in the UK in 2017, it explores the moral, social, personal, and ethical dilemmas involved in international surrogacy through its portrayal of Eva Roe, an English woman who travels to the fertility clinic in India for the surrogate birth. Thought of as another kind of 'gift of life', ideas of motherhood are complicated by surrogacy and the play brings the two women involved, mother and surrogate, together on the stage to explore these tensions. The privilege of Eva's whiteness in this contractual arrangement is laid bare in her confrontation with the racialised woman on whom she depends.

Surrogacy involves the process of placing an embryo into a woman who consents to carry the pregnancy. Prior to the implantation, the surrogate's body is prepared through a rigorous regimen of hormones and medications. The eggs are collected, either from the intended mother, from a donor, or from the surrogate; evaluated for their viability; and then combined with sperm from the father or a donor in a laboratory. Once fertilised, viable embryos are then implanted into the uterus of the surrogate. When the oocytes (eggs) come from either a donor or the intended mother, the surrogacy is termed 'gestational' and results in no genetic connection between the baby and the surrogate. Eva wants a child through gestational surrogacy, following her husband's death from cancer and her lengthy legal battle to access and use his frozen sperm. Primarily situated within the fertility clinic led by Dr Gupta, the female clinical director, Eva becomes deeply entangled with her surrogate, Aditi, a 28-year-old Indian woman from a rural village outside of Gujarat. Eva insists on meeting her as soon as she arrives at the clinic and spends most of her time with Aditi, learning about her life and reasons for being a surrogate, buying her gifts and making her promises that she will not ultimately keep. In the face of an impending Indian surrogacy ban (a reference to the real ban that came into effect in 2015), which poses a threat to the progress of the pregnancy and eventual transfer of the baby, Eva pressures Dr Gupta to implant her retrieved and fertilised eggs in Aditi whilst also encouraging her to fraudulently complete the paperwork to look as though the procedure was completed before the ban came into effect. Aditi becomes pregnant with twins, whilst Eva's intense focus on the pregnancy leads to neglecting her work responsibilities, ultimately resulting in the loss of her job and putting the entire contract in jeopardy, as she has not paid any money to the clinic, which in turn is unable to pay Aditi. Aditi then experiences the heart-breaking loss of one of the babies in her womb, and, overwhelmed by the tragedy, she flees to her village, where she gives birth to one living and one dead twin in a distressing final scene. Dr Gupta arrives, claiming the living child and paying Aditi, leaving her in a bloodied and traumatised state with the dead baby. The narrative closes with an epilogue in which Eva takes custody of the surviving baby from Dr Gupta as the clinic shuts down. The last words come from Aditi who tells Dr Gupta that she needs to act as a surrogate again, the implication being that she has no choice in the face of her impoverished circumstances, regardless of the previous tragic outcomes.

The play makes clear Aditi's own precarity in relation to the surrogacy arrangement, both contractually and racially. Her motivation is less a 'righteous sacrifice' and more a result of her economic circumstances and desire to provide for her own two daughters. She is also a widow, which means the loss of the main breadwinner in the family. In order to explain her decision to Eva she says: 'I has no choose. Where I make so big rupee? Clinic only' (Chohan, 2017, p. 33). This comes with the added pain of rejection from her own family, who view her as 'dirty' because of her surrogacy status. Eva, however, only wants to think of this as 'one of the most brave and beautiful things one woman can do for another woman' rather than it being a more transactional and financially driven decision (ibid: 34). This tension between the idea of the altruistic gift and the surrogacy contract manifests itself throughout the play in Eva's words and choices, as she gets caught over and again in its bind.

The racialised and often highly inequitable power relations in cross-racial surrogacy emerge from the start of the play, as Eva makes the trip to the clinic to try to choose her surrogate, a highly unusual request. Dr Gupta tries to dissuade her from this early contact, given that the implantation might fail, and the contract has not yet been signed. Aditi's lowly reproductive status is confirmed by Dr Gupta, who describes her as 'only the carrier' and that Eva is merely '"renting" her womb' (ibid: 6). This enforced separation between surrogate and intended parent by a medical professional, both physical and metaphorical, echoes the same practices deployed by organ transplantation staff. Concerns to protect both parties means that the idea of the gift is promulgated, whilst the procedure is reduced to its biological, even mechanical, components to remove any perceived unhealthy focus on the donor/surrogate. Dr Gupta reassures Eva that the surrogates are 'spoiled' for the nine months when they must stay at the clinic, and she goes on to provide false and selective information about Aditi (ibid: 8). In this way, she feeds the common narrative that surrogacy in these contexts is 'life-changing' and brings inestimable benefits to the woman and her family (ibid: 11). This helps Eva to initially believe that the racialised surrogacy is a positive choice for global majority women like Aditi, but this perception is unravelled throughout the play as she gets to know Aditi and her reasons for choosing to become a surrogate. Such rhetoric obscures the lack of choice for many of these women, the risks involved, and the emotional and bodily labour of surrogacy. This is made explicit at the end of the play when Aditi gives birth alone in a village shack. The stage directions state that: '*A dead white baby lies in a plastic bucket, an umbilical cord wound around the baby's neck. Lying exhausted . . . ADITI holds a bloodied white baby close*' (ibid: 64, italics in original). This shocking image makes visible the racial dynamics of the arrangement, as well as Aditi's own trauma and a very different kind of sacrifice than that propounded by Family Inception. As Aditi tries to care for and breastfeed the living twin, Dr Gupta arrives to brutally re-assert the rights of the contracting mother, telling Aditi that '[h]e's not yours' and that she remains just 'a vessel'. In a final twist of the contractual knife, she accuses Aditi of stealing the baby from Eva (ibid: 66). Any notion of the surrogacy as gift is erased and the contractual obligation dominates the scene.

When Eva is faced with losing the one remaining baby, she ends up only being able to respond contractually, denying the reciprocity of the gift that she established earlier in the play. Aditi has noted that other women in the clinic claim that 'parent promise much before you go. "We call you from UK, Amrika, Canada, you hear baby talk." Never hear again' (ibid: 39). Eva denies that this will happen in their case but inevitably ends up reneging on all her promises to both Aditi and Dr Gupta. That Aditi should finally approach Dr Gupta in the last line of the play to be a surrogate again, after all that she has been through, makes her economic desperation obvious. Eva has the child that she wanted and can return home, whilst Aditi decides to risk everything again to try to be financially secure and provide an education for her daughters.

Both plays examined in this chapter highlight the exigencies of biocapital as it seeks to expand markets in body parts and tissues along with its susceptibility to entrenching and amplifying various inequalities. These can often follow colonialist and racist fault lines, where the privilege of whiteness extracts value from black and brown bodies for its own advantage. The idea of the gift in these narratives of transplantation and surrogacy emerges to make them seem superficially more palatable to donor and recipient and is deployed as a means of covering over the contractual and unequal relations underpinning them. But the notion of the gift ultimately cannot hold in the face of these obligations, and the property rights foregrounded in the contracts are brought to bear on these brown female bodies. Both women, Jaya and Aditi, are sought for their valuable reproductive capacities: Jaya uses her childbearing potential to bargain with Virgil and make him participate in the risk of transnational donation and parenthood, whilst Aditi remains in a deeply precarious position and needing to offer the 'gift of life' once again.

Harvest and *Made in India* make visible the biocapitalist relations between brown and white, rich and poor, north and south, in the family apartment and in the fertility clinic in India. Both intimate spaces, where bodily gifts should be deeply personal, they are invaded by affluent white people who manipulate the situations for their own ends and advantage. As black British doctor and author Annabel Sowemimo writes: 'we must establish a detailed understanding of how colonialism and race science operate within health care if we are to achieve more equitable health outcomes' (2023, p. 19). These plays examine the dangers inherent in the commodification of bodies for vulnerable and historically marginalised women and their communities, and how the reciprocity and mutuality of the concept of the gift in these procedures is shredded in these examples of globalised commercial exchange.

Notes

1 The news article is available at: https://news.sky.com/story/brian-dowling-shares-tribute-to-incredible-surrogate-sister-after-birth-of-his-daughter-12690492 (accessed: 31 August 2023).
2 Available at: www.blood.co.uk/news-and-campaigns/the-donor/latest-stories/celebrate-the-gift-of-life/ (Accessed: 31 August 2023).
3 For examples of anthropological transplant research, see Sharp's *Strange Harvest* (2006) and Lock's *Twice Dead* (2002).
4 The company website is available at: https://familyinceptions.com/surrogacy-giving-the-ultimate-gift-of-life/ (accessed: 25 August 2023).
5 For an insight into the complexity of these debates, particularly for feminists, see Chapter 1 in Harrison's *Brown Babies, White Babies* (2016).

Reference list

Banner, O. (2017) *Communicative biocapitalism: the voice of the patient in digital and the health humanities.* Ann Arbor: University of Michigan Press.
Chohan, S.K. (2017) *Made in India*. London: Samuel French.
Dickenson, D. (2007) *Property in the body: feminist perspectives*. Cambridge: Cambridge University Press.
Harrison, L. (2016) *Brown bodies, white babies: the politics of cross-racial surrogacy*. New York: New York University Press.
Kim, J. (2014, Spring/Summer) 'Debt, the precarious grammar of life, and Manjula Padmanabhan's *harvest*', *Women's Studies Quarterly*, 42(1/2), pp. 215–232.
Lock, M. (2002) *Twice dead: organ transplants and the reinvention of death*. Berkeley and London: University of California Press.
Mauss, M. (20020) *The gift: the form and reason for exchange in archaic societies*. London and New York: Routledge.
Padmanabhan, M. (2003) *Harvest*. London: Aurora Metro Press.

Ro, C. (2020) *Coronavirus: why some racial groups are more vulnerable*. Available at: www.bbc.com/future/article/20200420-coronavirus-why-some-racial-groups-are-more-vulnerable (Accessed: 18 August 2023).

Russell, E. (2019) *Transplant fictions: a cultural study of organ exchange*. Basingstoke and London: Palgrave Macmillan.

Scheper-Hughes, N. (2001) 'Commodity fetishism in organs trafficking', *Body and Society*, 7(2–3), pp. 31–62.

Sharp, L.A. (2006) *Strange harvest: organ transplants, denatured bodies, and the transformed self*. Los Angeles and London: University of California Press.

Shildrick, M. (2021) 'Hauntological dimensions of heart transplantation: the onto-epistemologies of deceased donation', *Medical Humanities*, 47, pp. 388–396.

Sowemimo, A. (2023) *Divided: racism, medicine and why we need to decolonise healthcare*. London: Wellcome Collection.

Srihari, M. (2022) 'Xenotransplantation and borders: two Indian narratives', *Medical Humanities*, 48(2), pp. 153–158.

Waldby, C. and Cooper, M. (2008) 'The biopolitics of reproduction: post-fordist biotechnology and women's clinical labour', *Australian Feminist Studies*, 23(55), pp. 57–73.

PART 5

Experiments

Introduction

At certain historical moments, including our own, emerging medical technologies and the resulting new insights they enable radically reframe our conceptualisations of the human subject or our health and medical experience. The discovery of biological structures and functions such as germs, microbes, cells, DNA and mirror neurons demanded new ways of thinking about and performing ourselves. The development of new medical interventions such as transplantation, genetic engineering and regenerative medicine extend the limits of human capacity. In this final part of our volume, our contributors provide insight into a range of contemporary performances that play out fears and fantasies provoked by biotechnologies ranging from medical imaging to AI chatbots. Also featured are performances that meditate on perplexing phenomena at the edge of our knowledge, such as the production of pain without trauma or the effect of healing without medicine or that build on alternative ways of understanding body and movement beyond the biomedical paradigm and new forms of spectatorship that emerge in moments of national emergency. Many of these performances employ the technologies and tools of scientific medicine in their dramaturgy. Here performance becomes a laboratory through which we can investigate, speculate upon and experiment with the import of such developments and phenomena, testing out the improbable and the seemingly impossible.

Adelina Ong offers a critique of the AI chatbots introduced to address young people's mental health in contemporary Singapore. Her own exchanges with one of these chatbots reveals how they promote a 'neoliberal Americentric approach to coping with crises'. In a Singaporean context, 'where the collective processing of trauma and grief is the only performance of mental wellbeing that is socially validated', this can lead to cultural incongruity that is occasionally darkly comic – as when traumatised youths are invited to 'be like the cool, calm, collected . . . chicken' – but is ultimately chilling. We turn next to an older set of medical technologies, those that attempt to penetrate and visualise our bodily interior. Since the invention of the microscope, the technology of medical imaging has had a profound impact on the way we imagine and understand our anatomy and our experiences of health and illness. In some ways, medical imaging is the medical gaze made manifest, turning the living body of the patient into an object and a text. In rendering flesh into data, Liz Orton tells us 'the internal body becomes vulnerable to new forms of exchange,

DOI: 10.4324/9781003036500-42

trade and speculation'. Yet in her script for the performance-lecture *You Are My Territory and I Am Your Explorer* (2019), she describes herself viewing an MRI scan of her late mother and finding that they 'are dancing with the technology'. The performance is one outcome of Orton's five-year investigation of medical imaging, *Digital Insides*, and the script that she shares provides a compelling evocation of the subjective power of such technologies, in this case, effecting a fleeting resurrection of a loved one.

Novel medical imaging technologies also briefly feature in Kélina Gottman's meditation on British choreographer Russell Maliphant's training practise: Jean-Claude Guimberteau's anatomical videos reveal the body as a 'continuum of histological matter' rather than the expected view of the body as a collection of distinguishable parts and systems. This integrative conception of the body, Gottman argues, helps account for the distinctively fluid movement quality in Maliphant's dancers. It also forms a part of a training practice which Gottman describes as combining practical philosophy, aesthetics, spirituality, self-care, discipline and more – a form of *askēsis* – that also involves a rethinking of both body and health.

Helen Pynor's *Habitation* (2021–2023) is an artwork created in response to her own hip replacement surgery required because of a congenital hip abnormality. Its creation, Pynor argues, rendered the art-making process into a ritual to mark a physical and psychic transformation precipitated by surgery and to memorialise the surgically excised head of her femur bone, which had, until then, 'worked so hard, under compromised conditions, all of my life'. Her account of the artwork's creation reveals how obtaining the bone confronted her with the contradictory legal status of human tissue. The incorporation of the bone itself into the artwork, which included a model of the excised bone made of bone china, exposes the collapse of the 'animate-inanimate' boundary inherent in human-created medical interventions such as prosthetic implants.

Looming Futures: Waiting Room (2021) was a site-specific performance about the way the coronavirus radically changed the spatial and relational conditions of health care encounters. As Annja Neumann with Uta Baldauf and their collaborators describe, in response to the pandemic,

> public buildings were urgently converted into hospital facilities . . . hotels and exhibition spaces were turned into critical care facilities, medical spaces became integral to our everyday experience to the extent that we lived in some of them. Even living rooms became territories of quarantine.

The production explored this 'major shift' in how and where the surveillance and remediation of health took place, capturing some of the 'material arrangements in medicine that demand role changes, new roles and affect patient agency'. This theme is picked up, too, in Freya Verlander's biopolitical analysis of the UK government safety guidance for the performing arts, published as the country began to emerge from the 'lockdown' associated with the COVID-19 pandemic. Her playful mash-up of the UK's Department for Digital, Culture, Media and Sport's document 'Working Safely during Coronavirus (COVID-19)' and Foucault's writings on the panopticon exposes the extremity of state surveillance and control on both theatre workers and spectators. At the same time, Verlander argues, the new category of spectatorship that emerged under these measures – the 'social distanced spectator' – was not entirely contained by the 'scripted and stage-managed' behaviours delineated by the guidelines, challenging the dynamic 'between contagion, containment and control'.

Clod Ensemble is a UK-based performance company with a special interest in the intersection between performance and medicine. Here, artistic director Suzy Willson provides a description and commentary on their 2018 performance *Placebo*. The production explores and manifests the placebo effect, that is, the way in which an inactive drug, sham surgery, or the supposedly non-medical aspects of health care interactions and healing rituals create health benefits. *Placebo* is 'a kind of collage which takes the form of a series of mock "scientific" experiments, all of which are danced'. Drawing on emerging research into placebos, the production implicitly critiques Western medicine's attempt to monopolise the power to heal and reminds us that theatre, too, can function as a technology to make us feel better. From the placebo effect, we move to its inverse: the nocebo effect. As curator Bec Dean explains, Korean-Australian artist Eugenie Lee's performance-installation *Seeing Is Believing* (2016) draws on neuroscience, virtual reality, haptic device development and acoustic engineering to elicit experiences of unsettling bodily dysmorphia and pain in its audience – without inflicting harm or injury. Through this ethically risky encounter, Lee seeks to convey her own experience of persistent pain: she lives with complex regional pain syndrome, a condition which, like *Seeing Is Believing*, involves pain for which no bodily cause can be found. By providing an immediate, visceral experience of this condition, Lee's work, Dean suggests, can invite 'new forms of knowledge and more profound understandings of medical patient experience and its ambiguities'.

37

PERFORMING MENTAL WELLBEING IN CONVERSATIONS WITH AI CHATBOTS

Adelina Ong

In Singapore, a public consultation conducted over 2019 to 2020 by former Nominated Member of Parliament Anthea Ong indicated that 78.9% of the 395 respondents struggled to afford mental health care. 'A Telegram helpbot, or a number that people can text privately' was suggested as one way of increasing access to mental health services (SG Mental Health Matters, 2021). In July 2021, Woebot, an AI chatbot programmed to 'create a human-level therapeutic bond with users', received $90 million in funding from Temasek, a Singaporean investment company (Woebot Health, 2021). The Ministry of Health's Office for Healthcare Transformation (MOHT) announced in August 2021 that it would be launching *mindline.sg*, which will offer free access to Wysa, an 'emotionally intelligent' AI chatbot that recommends 'self-care exercises' informed by cognitive-behavioural techniques for mental health support (MOHT, 2021). Given their relative anonymity and 24-hour availability, these AI chatbots offer promising support for young people from low-income families in Singapore who are struggling with mental wellbeing. However, these AI chatbots do not presently deliver culturally nuanced mental health interventions and can unintentionally exacerbate the deterioration of mental wellbeing through neoliberal resilience rhetoric.

In this chapter, I will reflect on the performance of mental wellbeing required of young people in a Singaporean education context. I will also problematise the template responses used by these AI chatbots and argue for the creation of culturally nuanced mental health interventions developed in conversation with people with lived experience of struggling with mental wellbeing. Adopting narrative inquiry as my methodology, I am sympathetic to Ian Marsh's analysis of diagnostic assessment tools as performative. Marsh notes that tools like the *Diagnostic and Statistical Manual of Mental Disorders* and the *International Classification of Diseases* act, 'at least in part, to produce (and reproduce) what it purports only to name' (Marsh, 2010, p. 197). There is a growing body of research that indicates how AI reflects structural racism and the biases of its developers (Algorithmic Justice League, 2021). Through interaction with these AI chatbots, users form an understanding of what negative thought distortions are and some understanding of what depression or anxiety looks like based on the presence or absence of these so-called thought distortions. These AI chatbots also train users to perform mental wellbeing through cognitive behavioural therapy (CBT) coping strategies, thus shaping personal narratives of mental wellbeing. This cultivates public performances of mental wellbeing which can, over time, shape social norms.

DOI: 10.4324/9781003036500-43

The heartaches of place

I have been interacting with two AI chatbots since April 2019. One claims to be a virtual AI coach which responds to the emotions you express and uses evidence-based CBT, dialectical behavioural therapy (DBT), meditation, breathing, yoga, motivational interviewing and micro-actions to help you build mental resilience skills and 'feel heard'. The other prides itself on its 'breakthrough relational technology', which is positioned as 'the future of mental health'. Rather than pandering to mind–body dualism implied in the construct of mental health promoted by the chatbots, I regard mental wellbeing as an imperfect translation of 身心, which literally translates as 'body-heart' in Mandarin. I am interested in the heartaches of place that are experienced by, and expressed through, bodies in place. Through 身心, I attend to the social and cultural norms and expectations that have become synonymous with mental wellbeing in Singapore.

As background to this, it is important to note that mental health services in Singapore are not free. Government-subsidised counselling sessions range from around $30 to $50SGD (£15.98 to £26.64) per session, with antidepressants costing at least $100SGD (£53.28) per month (Ong, 2020). One respondent to the *SG Mental Health Matters* public consultation said 'she had to starve in order to afford therapy' (ibid). Another said 'as a young person it can be difficult to afford mental health. . . . Certain antidepressants are not subsidised' (SG Mental Health Matters, 2021). In Natalie Lazaroo's discursive exploration of resilience amongst low-income families in Singapore, a youth states that being resilient is 'natural for us' (Anton in Lazaroo, 2021, p. 79). In between caring for younger siblings and working after school to supplement the family income (while peers from middle-income families are sent to accelerated learning enrichment centres that teach one to two terms ahead of the national curriculum), young people from low-income families in Singapore have had 'no choice but to be resilient', as they cannot afford mental health services even when mental health conditions arise in response to these challenging circumstances (Lazaroo, 2021, p. 79). The COVID-19 Mental Wellness Taskforce was launched in Singapore on 11 October 2020 to 'review the psycho-social impact of the COVID-19 pandemic on the population' (Kurohi, 2020). While this dedication of governmental resources is timely, I am concerned about the paternalistic resilience rhetoric that has been adopted as a performance of mental wellbeing in Singapore.

This rhetoric is illustrated in the government response to a tragic incident at River Valley High School (RVHS) where a student purchased an axe online, brought this to school and fatally wounded another student he did not know in the toilet during the lunch break. In a ministerial statement made at a parliamentary sitting on 27 July 2021 in response to this, Education Minister Chan Chun Sing emphasised that 'social emotional skills and resilience building form the foundation of the MOE's [Ministry of Education's] mental health efforts' (Chan, 2021). As part of the Character and Citizenship Education (CCE) curriculum, students are taught to

> differentiate normal stress from distress and mental illness, so that they can seek help before becoming overwhelmed . . . break negative thinking patterns, overcome social emotional problems [and] seek help when they need to . . . manage their emotions.
>
> (ibid)

The MOE adopts a highly interventionist approach to mental health in Singapore's educational context that only superficially resembles neoliberal modes of self-care. The MOE's approach to training students in the management of their own mental wellbeing through the CCE curriculum is more consistent with a paternalistic resilience rhetoric where resilience is intentionally cultivated in order to achieve 'a rugged, robust, disciplined society' (Lee, 1966, p. 2). Resilience is edified as an ideal desirable of those who are of admirable character.

Following a public holiday, two days after the RVHS student was fatally attacked with an axe, MOE's director-general of education, Wong Siew Hoong, said 'This morning, 97% of RV students returned to school, which is similar to the regular attendance on any given school day. This is the resilience of our students, and we are proud of them' (2021). Members of the public have criticised Wong's definition of resilience, noting that the RVHS students 'have no choice' as they were not granted time off to process the traumatic event (Romero, 2021). Others noted that validating this return to normal as 'resilience' would make the 3% who are struggling to process the event 'feel more ostracised', effectively 'shaming the 3%' and making them 'feel inferior to the 97%' (ibid). Praising the RVHS principal for 'rushing back to school to personally handle the incident' despite being 'on medical leave' and commending the teachers for attending to the students' needs and 'helping them to cope with their difficult emotions . . . despite your own grief and shock' contradicts the message that 'it's OK not to be OK' (Chan, 2021). Grief is only socially validated when it strengthens community bonds. In the context of Singapore's resilience rhetoric, RVHS staff and students were expected to prioritise the rebuilding of the school community above their own, processing individual emotional needs through the support they render to each other in school.

No comfort in AI chickens

I wondered how an AI chatbot might offer support to the 3% of students who could not bring themselves to return to school. I typed: 'A 13-year-old Secondary 1 student of RVHS was killed on campus on Monday (July 19) allegedly by a 16-year-old Secondary 4 student' (Sun, Iau and Yufeng, 2021). I was presented with a choice between 'Anxiety', 'Feeling Low', 'Grief', 'Loneliness', 'Relationships' and 'Sleep'. I am disappointed that there is no option for 'Trauma' that might respond to the flashbacks, recurring nightmares or distressing intrusive thoughts commonly experienced by witnesses of a traumatic event. Thinking of the classmates of both RVHS students, I selected 'grief' as the closest available option. The AI chatbot replied:

Chatbot: That must be so heartbreaking, I really wish I could take away any pain you're feeling. I want you to know that I care about how you feel and while you have to go through grief and not around it, we can do it together. . . . Working on your grief will never mean you're okay with what has happened. You'll just begin to learn to live your life with them in your heart.

Framing this process as 'working on your grief' evokes neoliberal expectations. Wendy Brown defines neoliberalism as 'a distinctive mode of reason' where 'both persons and states are expected to comport themselves in ways that maximise their capital value in the present and enhance their future value' (2015, pp. 21–22). With the AI chatbot, grieving is instrumentalised as a process of self-care that will enable malfunctioning mourners to return to the development of their human capital through school, continuing the process of acquiring future value through education ('live your life') while holding the memories of their classmates (one deceased, one incarcerated) in their hearts. Built on Americentric psychological interventions, this AI chatbot reflects its designers' neoliberal approach to self-repair. Unlike a human therapist who is paid to listen, the AI chatbot functions more like an interactive article that natters on, intent on teaching me about Elizabeth Kübler-Ross' five stages of grief – a theory that has been widely disproved (Maciejewski *et al.*, 2007).

After fatally wounding the thirteen-year-old with an axe, the sixteen-year-old student had asked two groups of students to call the police (Chan, 2021). A few hours after the sixteen-year-old had been apprehended, Chan arrived and was approached by two classmates of the sixteen-year-old student. They said 'Minister, please help our friend. . . . Please take care of him' (ibid). I wondered how this AI chatbot would respond to these students. I selected a story titled 'Cope with Crisis' from a selection of topics offered by the AI chatbot. It tells me about an experiment with chickens where one chicken was given a fright and then placed with a second chicken who did not witness what caused the first chicken to become panicked and fearful. When the second chicken responded with fear and panic, the first chicken became even more fearful and panicked. But when the second chicken stayed calm, the first chicken relaxed. Throughout this conversation, I am given a choice between responses, but it is clear that these responses are ultimately a technology of self-repair, crafted to train the user in self-administering mental wellbeing coping strategies. At the end of the chicken story, the AI chatbot concludes:

Chatbot: My point is that you have the power to stop the cycle of fear and panic.
Choose between 'I do?' or 'I do!'

I choose 'I do!'

Chatbot: Indeed. The next time someone you care about comes to you frightened and overwhelmed, be that cool, calm, collected second chicken. Be their rock amidst the fear.

I type 'What if I don't feel that way?'

Chatbot: Hmm . . . good point. While it's not helpful to push aside how we actually feel, it does help both parties if you can try and project assurance and confidence.

'How so?'

Chatbot: When we try and stay calm for someone else, it can sometimes help to reduce the intensity of distress we feel as well, and even better, makes the whole thing reciprocal. [Handshake emoticon].

'I'll need to see it in action'.

Chatbot: So remember, emotions can be contagious. A calm steady presence can do wonders for you and the people around you. Be the calm chicken you wish to see in the world. [Chicken emoticon]

Researchers have found that intrusive sensory memories are a 'core clinical feature of post-traumatic stress disorder (PTSD)' and that they 'involve mental imagery-based impressions that intrude into mind involuntarily' (Iyadurai *et al*., 2019). Hence, it can be challenging for people living with PTSD to remain calm while experiencing these memories. Disappointingly, the only response allowed by this AI chatbot is: 'Will do'.

Contrary to some claims, there is no human-like therapeutic bond formed with the AI chatbot as I barely get a chance to speak. My so-called responses are scripted to compel a performance of calm which can be read as resilience. Sociologist Sarah Bracke argues that 'neoliberal citizenship is nothing if not a training in resilience as the new technology of the self: a training to withstand whatever crisis capital undergoes and whatever political measures the state carries out to save it' (2016, p. 62). Drawing from a neoliberal, Americentric approach to coping with crises, the AI places the burden of coping with trauma on the individual. Consequently, the impetus to hold institutions accountable 'for the contemporary conditions that are (designed to be) met with resilience' (ibid: 60) is dispelled through positive self-talk and mindfulness. This is evident in Part Two of the 'Coping with Crisis' conversational template delivered by the AI chatbot:

Chatbot: Like the chickens in the study, we often run into situations that are out of our control. And that's a frightening and disorienting experience.
Choose between: 'Very true' or 'Uncertainty isn't so bad'.

I choose the latter response.

Chatbot: You've nerves of steel – you're a calm chicken!

I type 'Thank you?'

Chatbot: In these moments of great change and crisis it's so tempting to think back on how things were before – to imagine what life would be like if we could just go back in time . . . it's natural to mourn something when you miss it.
Choose: True' or 'I see . . .'

I choose 'True'

Chatbot: Yet it's possible to carve out some space in your head or your heart to mourn what you miss, while remaining present with what's in front of you.

I type 'Hmmm . . .'

Chatbot: I hope that in these tough times, mindfulness will help you notice your worries, yet not get lost in them. Mindfulness doesn't ask you to deny the reality of a tough situation. Instead mindfulness helps you let those worries go until you have the brain space to take care of them and, like a calm chicken, you can enjoy your worms in the meantime.
Choose: 'You really like mindfulness', 'No worms, please' or 'Thanks'.

I choose 'No worms, please'.

The AI chatbot sends a GIF of a robot in cross-legged position, levitating while meditating and the statement,

Chatbot: I'll admit I'm a fan.
Choose: an emoji with three people meditating or 'I am too'.

I choose the emoji.

Chatbot: What do you think is your "worm" these days? What can you appreciate in the here-and-now?

While the AI chatbot gently uses humour to encourage the user to perform calm, this conversational template can exacerbate guilt in a Singaporean context where the collective processing of trauma and grief is the only performance of mental wellbeing that is socially validated. This paternalistically cultivates a communitarian resilience rhetoric aligned with Singapore's shared values of 'nation before community and society above self' (Singapore Parliamentary Reports, 1991, p. 56). Taking the (only) opportunity to respond in my own words, I type in words posted anonymously by a RVHS student on *Wake Up, Singapore*'s Facebook page:

> The constant snapping of photos (even on public transport) made all of us feel that somehow, we were the ones in the wrong. . . . We thought the reporters would be more understanding given that we just left a crime scene with the realisation that one of our classmates was killed. But no . . . They just wanted something to post onto their news pages.
>
> (Anonymous, 2021)

Perhaps some RVHS students chose to absent themselves from school in order to avoid this unwanted media attention and cope with the intense, often unkind, public speculation. In response to the coronavirus (COVID-19) pandemic, schools in Singapore have integrated home-based learning as part of the regular curriculum to encourage 'self-directed learning' (Ministry of Education, 2021, p. 3). So, I add 'My "worm" is home-based learning'. The Chatbot responds,

Chatbot: Got it. I wish you joy where you can find it in these coming days and weeks my friend.

There is no comfort to be found in the so-called relational breakthrough technology of this therapeutic AI chatbot. Frustrated and angry, I respond with lines from Haresh Sharma's play *Off Centre* (1993), which is about the discrimination experienced by people living with mental health conditions in Singapore. Based on nine months of research and interviews with doctors, patients, social workers and caregivers, the play had its commission by the Ministry of Health withdrawn because of its hard-hitting critique (Sharma, 1993, p. 146). The play traces the evolving friendship between Saloma and Vinod, two people trying to live with mental health conditions in Singapore. In the play, Saloma's mother (Mak) acts as a witness to the discrimination faced by Saloma and says:

Mak: This country no good. People no good . . . I see . . . doctor. He say how many percent become better, how many percent don't become better. He smile. I smile. I see social worker. She say how many percent must take medicine only for few months, how many percent must take always. . . . She smile. I smile. I go home, I see the mirror. I smile. I cannot laugh. I cannot cry. Because I only know how to smile. I only know how to smile.

(Sharma, 1993, p. 127)

In response to this, the AI chatbot asks if I would like to try the 'half-smile technique' as a 'tool [that] can be used when you're feeling down and want to feel a bit better'. This involves relaxing the facial muscles and moving the corners of your lips until they are 'slightly up . . . but not enough to make it a noticeable grin'. You're invited 'to keep the half-smile going throughout your day'. I shut the AI chatbot and scream in frustration. My response to the AI chatbot is not unique. Feedback from a recent trial of one of the previously mentioned AI chatbots indicated that the teachers found the chatbot 'devoid of empathy'. A teacher who was feeling burnt out from having to mark 1,500 scripts was told to positively reframe this negative thought (Lee, 2022).

Performing hyperproductivity

Another aspect of the resilience rhetoric is the pressure to be hyperproductive. This was revealed to me in an applied performance workshop that I organised online for four youth workers and eighteen Singaporean youths between the ages of thirteen and nineteen in October 2021. Many of the youths had lived experience of mental health conditions. I was invited to facilitate a workshop as part of a larger programme of events focused on destigmatising mental health conditions in Singapore. Noting increasing addiction to social media platforms amongst youths during the pandemic, the organisers asked if I might focus on the impact of social media platforms on mental wellbeing. The topic of unhealthy representations of so-called perfect bodies, perpetuated through Instagram and TikTok challenges came up and, in addition to this, the performance of hyperproductivity on social media during the COVID-19 circuit breaker (lockdown) and constant overworking was highlighted as a concern. One participant noted that 'sometimes it seems to become a competition as to who is more upset or more tired or more overworked . . . it's not a competition!' The performance of hyperproductivity (including complaining about being 'overworked') is another performance of mental wellbeing that is implicitly encouraged as part of the resilience rhetoric in Singapore. Given that these AI chatbots are mostly designed by developers based in the US, most AI mental health interventions are trained on data that takes the language, behaviour and social interactions of users based in the US as its norm. These AI mental health interventions amplify existing Americentric biases already present in psychological research and fail to recognise unhealthy performances of mental wellness in a different cultural context.

Psychologists, like Yang Kuo-Shu, who have been advocating for culturally nuanced research, have argued that 'Americanised Chinese psychology without a Chinese "soul" . . . would not do much good in explaining, predicting and understanding Chinese behaviour' (Yang, 1997, pp. 64–66). AI mental health interventions trained predominantly on the data generated by users based in the US may mistakenly read social media posts on the recent 躺平 (tǎng píng, which means 'lying flat') movement and 丧文化 (sàng wén huà, which can be described as 'a culture of dejectedness') in China as indications of depression. 躺平 has become a form of 'silent resistance' where young people choose to live 'minimally' in order to 'think and express freely' while working at one's preferred pace instead of conforming to a 9-9-6 work culture that advocates overworking and results in burnout (Chen and Munroe, 2017; Teh, 2021). A 9-9-6 culture refers to a work culture where overworking, from 9am to 9pm, six days a week, is encouraged by Chinese companies. Zhang Busan's performance of 躺平是王道 *(Lying Flat Is the Way of Kings)* is sung lying flat (literally) on his couch and strumming on his guitar while extolling the virtues of 躺平. He observes that 'when you're lying flat you can't fall down' (Zhang, 2021). As Chen and Munroe explain, 丧文化 is an ironic defeatist response, laced with dark humour, adopted by millennials to the inequality that has made the attainment of traditional notions of success impossible. The 丧

茶 (Song bubble tea) menu lists 'Achieved Absolutely Nothing Black Tea' as one of its top sellers (Chen and Munroe, 2017). Sara Ahmed has asserted that 'unhappiness becomes a right in a world that makes happiness compulsory' (Ahmed, 2010, p. 193). Responding to the hopelessness of social mobility in China, 躺平 and 丧文化 function as coping mechanisms that enable young people to maintain their mental wellbeing in a culture where positivity is mandated. The 躺平 movement and 丧文化 in China are cultural performances of resistance to normative performances of success (and, by implication, wellbeing) that have had a detrimental impact on mental wellbeing. Beyond Chinese behaviour, a few psychologists have begun to advocate for a global psychology that adopts a cross-cultural approach to the analysis of behaviour (Sundararajan, Hwang and Yeh, 2020). These are encouraging steps towards a more culturally nuanced understanding of mental wellbeing.

AI futures

Developers designing AI to support mental wellbeing should bear in mind that mental health is a social construct that is normatively defined. Psychotherapist Gary Greenberg has acknowledged that the descriptors psychiatrists use to diagnose mental health conditions in the DSM are 'useful constructs', 'the best the profession can do with the knowledge and tools at hand' (2013, p. 25). Societal attitudes have shifted to recognise that neither homosexuals nor transgender people should be described as living with a mental health condition (Drescher, 2015, p. 571; *BBC News*, 2019). Even though these AI chatbots are not designed to diagnose mental health conditions, it is the responsibility of AI developers working in the field of mental health to regularly retrain the AI in response to changes in the DSM and ICD to provide appropriate emotional support.

Research into the long-term impact of a traumatic event indicates that there is a need to put in place longer-term support and monitor for PTSD symptoms that only emerge several months after the event (Iyadurai *et al.*, 2019). The ICD-11 describes PTSD as characterised by 're-experiencing the traumatic event or events in the present . . . avoidance of thoughts and memories of the event . . . persistent perceptions of heightened current threat' (World Health Organisation, 2021). This language does not capture the pain that accompanies the memories, flashbacks and nightmares; the fear that RVHS students might associate with the school or being in the vicinity of that toilet; and the guilt that might be associated with memories of the two boys involved in the incident. Often, most community social support offered in the immediate aftermath of the event may no longer be available months after, when community focus has shifted. Borrowing from Ahmed, who argues that the intrusive, repetitive reliving of the trauma 'suggests a need to replay that which has yet to be assimilated into the individual or collective psyche', these intrusive memories could function as attempts to create some narrative understanding of the traumatic experience (2004, p. 95). This narrative of the traumatic event is shaped by prior narratives that the RVHS students have constructed about the world, despite the inadequacy of language. In turn, the insight gained from this failure of articulation will shape a narrative understanding of future experiences of, and in, the world that is not limited to that which can be articulated through language. Exploring various constructions of these narratives with an AI chatbot could be useful in supporting those who experience long-term PTSD, particularly in Singapore where the cost of mental health services presents a barrier to therapy. However, AI developers could critically engage more with culturally specific performances of mental health than reinforce social norms and expectations that are detrimental to mental wellbeing.

AI-enhanced mental health monitoring mobile applications already possess the ability to track typing speed, language, facial expression, voice tone, physical mobility and the frequency and duration of social interactions in text messages, phone calls and social media posts as indicators of depression or suicidal ideation (University of Oregon, 2019). These are marketed to health care providers as tools that enable the monitoring of symptoms that indicate a relapse. Much doubt has been cast on the universality of facial expressions of emotion and the extent to which this can be used to reliably infer emotional states (Barrett *et al.*, 2019, p. 20). I remain sceptical about the extent to which the other biomarkers monitored by AIs can reliably track depression or suicidal ideation, particularly where voice tone, physical mobility and language are subject to similar assumptions of universality. While it is possible to envision how AI built to identify the relapse of suicidal ideation through the tracking of social media posts and online purchases might have identified signals of distress in the older RVHS student, I am concerned about how these AIs could function as an extension of medical paternalism that amplifies the criminalisation of young people with suicidal ideation. In Singapore, people living with mental health conditions are perceived as potentially violent ('scary', 'should avoid', 'dangerous') and incapable of rational thinking (Pang *et al.*, 2017, p. 4). While AI chatbots can provide a welcome alternative to antidepressants given the culture of over medicalisation in the treatment of depression and bipolar disorder, I am concerned about how AI mental health monitoring mobile applications that are implemented as part of long-term treatment by mental health specialists can become extensions of soft medical paternalism in Singapore. If the installation of AI mental health monitoring applications becomes a necessary condition for patients' access to medication or treatment, then people living with mental health conditions could become one of the most surveilled groups of people outside of prison. Instead of functioning as technologies of surveillance, AI mental health applications for young people with lived experience of suicidal ideation should be designed to support the life that these young people are, ultimately, prepared to live with.

Despite its limitations, the AI is reflective of its developers' bias. The AI does not harbour malicious intent when it fails to respond appropriately, but humans can be intentionally cruel and act in ways that should prompt developers to interrogate the human exceptionalism that compels its developers to make AIs more human. In Singapore, parental consent is required before medical procedures commence for those aged below twenty-one who are living with a mental health condition. Soft medical paternalism, mediated by family-oriented informed consent, is commonly practiced in Singapore, particularly when justified in terms of suicide prevention and mental wellbeing interventions (Krishna, 2012, p. 789). As an applied performance practitioner who has been working with young people from low-income families in Singapore since 2003, I have been contacted by distressed young people who are sent, against their will, for electroconvulsive therapy by their families. I am concerned about recent trends towards normalising the involvement of the school in medical consent procedures as teachers and administrators lack the required medical expertise. Instead of designing AI that forms a human-like therapeutic bond, AIs could be designed in ways to leverage machine learning capabilities that exceed human abilities. Beyond mental health monitoring and CBT AI chatbots, the AI could customise mental health interventions that combine a range of culturally nuanced interventions including arts therapy, animal therapy and even video games, based on the individual's personality or narrative profile.

Returning to the applied performance workshop I facilitated online with young people in Singapore, when I invited the participants to simultaneously sing a song that expresses the support they wish they had received when they were struggling with mental wellbeing, they sang:

Do you ever feel like a plastic bag drifting through the wind?
I'll be there when the world stops turning. I'll be there when the storm is through. In the end
    I wanna be standing at the beginning with you.

I hope you dance. It is to me that we have choices.

You gave me the best of me, so you'll give you the best of you.

The last line quotes lyrics from *Magic Shop*, a song written by BTS (a popular South Korean pop group). These words are offered to someone who is struggling with depression, as an alternative to 'blatant' platitudes like 'find strength' (BTS, 2021). Another participant said that the lyrics to *Make It Right* (also by BTS) give her strength because 'you know that you are not alone when you are facing an issue'. When encouraged to share what they had learnt about themselves at the end of the workshop, the participants wrote:

It is ok to show you are not perfect.

Do not look down on yourself, everyone is good at something. If you are still feeling down, let's eat together.

We are in this together. We have gone through so much and we will emerge stronger than ever before!

The sun will always meet the moon at the horizon. When we are feeling lost and down, look at the sun and moon for comfort and refuge.

I've survived all my bad days so far, things have gotten better before.

These words do not perform resilience or hyperproductivity as wellbeing. These are words of solidarity and support, grounded in the daily struggle of negotiating mental wellbeing. Perhaps, if developers of AI chatbots attended more closely to the knowledge that young people from low-income families in Singapore have acquired through living with mental health conditions, then the AI chatbots they design to support mental wellbeing will offer a more sustainable definition of mental wellbeing for all in Singapore.

Reference list

Ahmed, S. (2004) *The cultural politics of emotion*. Edinburgh: Edinburgh University Press.

Ahmed, S. (2010) *The promise of happiness*. Durham, NC: Duke University Press.

Algorithmic Justice League (2021) *Research – the algorithmic justice league, algorithmic justice league*. Available at: www.ajl.org/library/research (Accessed: 17 September 2021).

Anonymous (2021) 'An RV student speaks up', *Wake up, Singapore* [Facebook]. Available at: www.facebook.com/wakeupSG/posts/2013328285499453 (Accessed: 21 December 2021).

Barrett, L.F. *et al.* (2019) 'Emotional expressions reconsidered: challenges to inferring emotion from human facial movements', *Psychological Science in the Public Interest*, 20(1), pp. 1–68.

BBC News (2019) 'Transgender no longer recognised as "disorder" by WHO', *BBC News*. Available at: www.bbc.com/news/health-48448804 (Accessed: 13 August 2021).

Bracke, S. (2016) 'Bouncing back: vulnerability and resistance in times of resilience', in Butler, J., Gambetti, Z. and Sabsay, L. (eds.) *Vulnerability in resistance*. Durham: Duke University Press, pp. 52–75.

Brown, W. (2015) *Undoing the demos: neoliberalism's stealth revolution*. 1st edn. New York: Zone Books.

BTS (방탄 소년단) (2021) *'Magic shop' official MV, BIGHIT music official*. Available at: www.youtube.com/watch?v=VTRGOBT6p80 (Accessed: 4 October 2021).

Chan, C.S. (2021) 'River valley high school incident', *Ministerial Statements*, 95(34). Parliament No. 14, Session No. 1. Singapore: Parliament of Singapore. Available at: https://sprs.parl.gov.sg/search/sprs3topic?reportid=ministerial-statement-1700 (Accessed: 16 December 2021).

Chen, Y. and Munroe, T. (2017) 'For Chinese millennials, despondency has a brand name', *Reuters*. Available at: www.reuters.com/article/us-china-congress-millennials-insight-idUSKCN1BF2J7 (Accessed: 20 September 2021).

Drescher, J. (2015) 'Out of DSM: depathologizing homosexuality', *Behavioral Sciences*, 5(4), pp. 565–575.

Greenberg, G. (2013) *The book of Woe: the DSM and the unmaking of psychiatry*. New York: Blue Rider Press, Penguin Group (USA) Inc.

Iyadurai, L. *et al.* (2019) 'Intrusive memories of trauma: a target for research bridging cognitive science and its clinical application', *Clinical Psychology Review*, 69, pp. 67–82.

Krishna, L.R. (2012) 'Best interests determination within the Singapore context', *Nursing Ethics*, 19(6), pp. 787–799.

Kurohi, R. (2020) 'New task force to tackle mental health needs of Singaporeans amid pandemic', *The Straits Times*. Available at: www.straitstimes.com/singapore/health/task-force-to-tackle-mental-health-needs-amid-pandemic (Accessed: 12 August 2021).

Lazaroo, N. (2021) '"Five stars arising": a conversation about applied theatre, precarity, and resilience in Singapore', *Research in Drama Education: The Journal of Applied Theatre and Performance*, 26(1), pp. 73–87.

Lee, K.Y. (1966) 'Transcript of speech made by the Prime Minister Mr Lee Kuan Yew at Queenstown Community Centre on 10 August 1966', Singapore, 10 August. Available at: www.nas.gov.sg/archivesonline/data/pdfdoc/lky19660810.pdf (Accessed: 20 August 2021).

Lee, W. (2022) '#trending: MOE therapy chatbot for stressed teachers labelled unhelpful by some', *TODAY*. Available at: www.todayonline.com/singapore/moe-chatbot-negative-reviews-1984976 (Accessed: 27 October 2022).

Maciejewski, P.K. *et al.* (2007) 'An empirical examination of the stage theory of grief', *JAMA*, 297(7), pp. 716–723.

Marsh, I. (2010) *Suicide: Foucault, history and truth*. Cambridge and New York: Cambridge University Press.

Ministry of Education (2021) *Experiencing blended learning (BL) with our children*. Available at: www.moe.gov.sg/-/media/files/parent-kit/experiencing-blended-learning.pdf (Accessed: 21 December 2021).

Ministry of Health, Office for Healthcare Transformation (2021) *About mindline.sg*. Available at: www.mindline.sg/about (Accessed: 12 August 2021).

Ong, A. (2020) 'Making mental healthcare more affordable for Singaporeans', *TODAY Online*. Available at: www.todayonline.com/commentary/making-mental-healthcare-more-affordable-singaporeans (Accessed: 16 July 2021).

Pang, S. *et al.* (2017) 'Stigma among Singaporean youth: a cross-sectional study on adolescent attitudes towards serious mental illness and social tolerance in a multiethnic population', *BMJ Open*, 7(10), pp. 1–11.

Romero, A.M. (2021) 'Netizens Slam MOE director-general for touting "resilience" of RVHS students back in school', *The Independent Singapore News*. Available at: https://theindependent.sg/netizens-slam-moe-director-general-for-touting-resilience-of-rvhs-students-back-in-school/ (Accessed: 19 August 2021).

SG Mental Health Matters (2021) 'Common ground', *SG Mental Health Matters*. Available at: https://sgmentalhealthmatters.com/common-ground-statements (Accessed: 12 August 2021).

Sharma, H. (1993) *Off centre*. Singapore: Ethos Books.

Singapore Parliamentary Reports (1991) *Shared values*. Singapore: Parliament of Singapore, p. 56. Parliament No. 7, Session No. 2, Vol. 56, Sitting No. 13. Motion.

Sun, D., Iau, J. and Yufeng, K. (2021) 'River valley high school death: sec 4 boy arrested over alleged murder of sec 1 boy on campus', *The Straits Times*. Available at: www.straitstimes.com/singapore/courts-crime/river-valley-high-school-student-killed-on-campus-police-on-site (Accessed: 23 August 2021).

Sundararajan, L., Hwang, K.-K. and Yeh, K.-H. (2020) *Global psychology from indigenous perspectives: visions inspired by K.S. Yang*. New York and Switzerland: Springer Nature.

Teh, C. (2021) 'More and more Chinese 20-somethings are rejecting the rat race and "lying flat" after watching their friends work themselves to death', *Insider*. Available at: www.insider.com/disenchanted-chinese-youth-join-a-mass-movement-to-lie-flat-2021-6 (Accessed: 25 August 2021).

University of Oregon (2019) 'ADAPT: adolescent development and psychopathology team', *CAS Adapt*. Available at: https://adaptlab.uoregon.edu/projects/ (Accessed: 12 November 2019).

Woebot Health 2021 (2021) 'Woebot health closes $90 million series B funding', *Woebot Health*. Available at: https://woebothealth.com/woebot-health-closes-90-million-series-b-funding/ (Accessed: 17 October 2021).

Wong, S.H. (2021) *Director-general of education Wong Siew Hoong's remarks on RVHS incident*. Available at: www.youtube.com/watch?v=HxBk9QNS_xA&t=12s (Accessed: 19 August 2021).

World Health Organisation (2021) 'ICD-11 for mortality and morbidity statistics', *World Health Organisation*. Available at: https://icd.who.int/browse11/l-m/en#/http://id.who.int/icd/entity/90875286 (Accessed: 13 August 2021).

Yang, K.-S. (1997) 'Indigenising Westernised Chinese psychology', in Bond, M.H. (ed.) *Working at the interface of cultures: eighteen lives in social science*. London: Routledge, pp. 62–76.

张不三 (Zhang Bu San) (2021) 《躺平是王道》躺平即正义. Available at: www.youtube.com/watch?v=corZx0a1yRU (Accessed: 22 September 2021).

38

YOU ARE MY TERRITORY AND I AM YOUR EXPLORER

Liz Orton

In 2016 I began to hold conversations with patients, using their medical images as a point of visual inquiry. These dialogues explored the body's interior visuality from a non-clinical point of view, attempting to deinstitutionalise medical images and find out how patients might engage with their own images and disrupt the medical gaze. This was part of a five-year artist research project, *Digital Insides*, 2015–2020, funded by an arts grant from the Wellcome Trust, a charitable foundation focused on health research. My collaborator was Professor Steve Halligan, a radiologist at University College London Hospital (UCLH). I had a residency at the hospital, observing numerous imaging clinics and making recordings with staff and patients. A short time into the project my mum became ill, and I found myself with all of her medical records. I held on to them for a year after she died before looking at them and wrote this text as a response. It was delivered as a lecture performance at Bloomsbury Theatre in May 2019.[1]

Opening

The setting, in May 2019, is a dance studio in Bloomsbury Theatre, about seventeen metres square with a level floor throughout. The walls are covered in black felt. The audience is seated in two areas of eight rows of different lengths, at about a thirty-degree angle to the front. They can see each other as well as the performance, as if they are in a hospital waiting space. On the right of the room, behind the chairs is Lori Allen, a sound artist, her mixing desks on a table. At the front there is a large table which has a projector at one end, and a notebook and manilla folder at the other. Liz Orton is seated at the table, holding a microphone. Throughout the performance she alternates between reading from the notebook and the folder, indicated in this script through the use of italics for the former and regular text for the latter. There are two screens for moving image projections, a large one filling the wall behind her, controlled by a technician, and a smaller one to the side of the table, controlled by the artist. Descriptions of the moving images and texts on each screen are provided in the following script. The moving images complement rather than illustrate the words spoken by the artist. House lights are low and the artist uses the light from the large projection behind her to see her script. When it gets too dark to read the script, she uses the torch from her phone. There is live sound throughout the performance based on samplings of MRI recordings.

DOI: 10.4324/9781003036500-44

Performance begins

Large screen: image which looks like an eye resolves into a compact disc (CD) with reflections of tree branches.
  Small screen: as above.

> In early 2016,
> I walked out of the North Middlesex hospital,
> carrying only a small plastic bag of your belongings.
> Sometime later when I was going through your things,
> looking for memories, I found the CD of your medical images.

Large screen: close-up of spines of notebooks packed tightly into a box.

> We'd requested it from the Release of Information Unit at
>   the hospital,
> but by the time the administrator emailed me to say it was
>   ready for collection,
> you were down the corridor on end-of-life care.

Large screen: view goes round and round a hospital revolving door, overexposed to the light.

> I had a growing pile of patient CDs by then,
> and I added yours to the top.
> I wasn't sure that was where it belonged,
> but I didn't move it.
> About a year later,
> one quiet evening I put the CD in my computer.
> By then I was familiar with how medical images load, their
>   confusion of menus, columns and windows,
> and I had interviewed numerous patients about their medi-
>   cal images.

Small screen: an abstract medical image looks like an iris emitting light.

> I had already trained myself to use Osirix,
> a professional radiology software.
> I'd practised at first on the Visible Human Male,
> the first data set of a fully imaged body.
> This male came as a series of 1870 files,
> each one a slice across the body.

Large screen: we move through Joseph Paul Jernigon's files as a cross-section from feet to head and back.

> He was called Joseph Paul Jernigan, a convicted murderer
> who was executed by lethal injection in Texas in 1995. He

was far from perfect. He had one testicle. His appendix and one of his teeth were missing, and there was tissue deterioration at the site of the injection. The preparation process had caused his brain to swell and his blood vessels to collapse. His middle ear ossicles were lost, and some of his tendons had become smeared. But this Visible Human male was my training ground, a body I could learn with.

Small screen: we see close-ups of word games in old-fashioned looped handwriting, of words that are contained in other words such as 'perseverance', 'pleasantry', 'decrepit' and 'plausible' and 'casualty'.

I listen to the CD spinning and after a short pause the
  folders of your images appear,
like a stratigraphy of disease and disaster.
1994 with the pain in your back (426 images)
2008 when you got run over (1226 images)
2012 with your painful toe (2 images)
and 2016 your final illness (3988 images).

Medical images rarely provide certainty. The best way to verify an image is through another image.

You started with CT,
and that led to an MRI,
and then to a colonoscopy
and finally, to an X-ray.

Large screen: a GIF created from ultrasound images like waves in a dark ocean plays on a loop.

At first, I stay in the flat world of 2D sequences
and you are a flick book,
each image almost identical to the next.
Like a geologist,
I follow your layers down towards the deep time of your toes.

Balzac believed that the body was made up of layers of images, an infinite number of leaf-like skins laid on top of one another (Nadar in Goldberg, 1988, pp. 127-128). He thought that every time we are photographed one of these ghostly layers is transferred from the body to the image. Each exposure causes a further loss of the body.

I slip and slide forwards and backwards.
It's a black and white world,
Full of patterns and murky abstractions.

Where doctors failed,
Perhaps I can rescue something from these excavations.

Large screen: from interior to exterior, a view of a house through a blue and red window.

I assemble you from your slices,
a dissection in reverse,
and suddenly you are there,
shining out at me from the screen:
a blue spectral outline,
floating in the dense cosmic black of the display.
You hover,
like a patch of mist
on a moonless mountain lake,
swaying slightly as if blown by small breaths.
Then you liquidise into a watery column, dissolving from
*   your edges.*
You are all flow,
a constant becoming that reminds me that the body is more
*   process than object.*

You are perfect for this technology.

Large screen: holiday photographs of diverse landscapes, taken by the artist and her mother on a shared camera, move across the screen in both directions, clashing and overlapping.

I can see they only cared for part of you.
A rectangle that cuts your body,
amputating your head and shoulders, arms, hands and feet.

Your lungs resolve,
only to fade away again
until you seem to be a simmering fire,
an afterglow of deep energy.
And then you fill with green and pinks, erupting into small
*   explosions.*

My grief is free to wander in new directions, riveted to
*   you.*
I want to spin you, save you, export you, print you.

I am lost all over again.

These, I realize, are your final images,
taken just after the last photograph,

of you standing in your long brown coat at the gate to
  the park.

The history of medicine might be understood as a series of
attempts to make the body visible.

When you have your MRI scan they let me stay with you.
'It's not really allowed', the radiographer said,
'but I can see she will need you'.
He saw our weaknesses,
even before he turned on the machine.
The MRI suite is cool and full of pale surfaces.
I count ten shades of cream.

Large screen: a glitched moving medical image plays that looks like rotating staircases turning
endlessly around each other.

The radiologist injects you with gadolinium,
a rare metal that enhances contrast in the image.
Seeping through your veins,
it co-opts your body into revealing its own ailments.

Then the radiologist leaves, closing the door tight shut
and we see him through a window
as if we are suddenly on the outside.

You say the MRI machine looks a bit like a coffin,
and I watch you going in head first from one end.

Inside your body, protons start moving and spinning.
Quantum mechanics are at work.
Your molecules are agitating and sending signals.

Large screen: photographs from a 1970s Radiography Manual flash up on different parts of a black
background for less than a second each.

A few weeks after your scan,
as part of a residency at the hospital imaging department,
I join the radiographers in a CT clinic.
I am there to observe the observers.

We sit in our control room,
Behind glass that's thick with lead,
To keep us from irradiating.
As we enjoy our cups of tea,

exchanging stories from the evening before,
the first patient on the list arrives,
a young man with loose clothes and a fine beard.
The radiographers attend to him with care and efficiency
but the space seems to undermine their kindness,
through its systems of divisions,
its insides and outsides.

See the patient,
on the other side.
Alone.
Half undressed.
Lying down.
Holding still.

Small screen: a looping GIF shows an x-ray of an x-ray machine.

The radiographers communicate to patients via a microphone, following a script of sorts,
and it always ends the same.
'You may experience a warm feeling.
You may experience a warm feeling'

Large screen: still photographs from a medical imaging re-enactment staged by the artist move across the screen, colliding and overlapping. Plays for 3 minutes from beginning to end with audio clips of patient interviews.

'Please keep still Mrs Orton'.
From his room, the radiographer booms at you through a
  speaker.
He can see you for what you are: a digital sampling of
  skin, bone, hair, water, tissue and blood.

My eyes fall on the far wall where a mural practises its
  visual effects,
dragging my eyes along pathways towards its hilly horizons.

The machine vibrates with its clicks and bangs,
an amplified white noise keeping you in its orbit,
bashing at you with its acoustics.
You are a zone of pure numbers.
Finally the noise stops,
and a processor turns your radio signals into an image.

The artist stands.

Large screen: flashing lights in green, pink and yellow resolve into a human body.

What is the body? A non-transparent object of varying density and composition. What is the image? A series of measurements, modelled in space.

We are asked to leave.
It's a perfunctory dismissal.
I seek the radiographer's gaze,
looking for reflections of what he has just seen,
testing what he knows.
He looks away.

Large screen: 3D torsos created from medical images rotate one after the other.

Is the opposite of collaboration exploitation?

Back in the control room,
we work our way down the patient list.
Occasionally an emergency interrupts our steady progress.
A phone call, and soon after,
a body arrives on a trolley,
wheeled straight from A&E.

Inside the body is pure darkness. There are no optics or lenses in medical imaging. Algorithms reconstruct density data into images, with automated contrast and smoothing.

Patient images materialise in triptych in front of us.
Axial. Coronal. Sagittal.
X y and z.
We see what the patient cannot see,
and will have to wait to know.

Textbooks describe the medical image as if it is a window into the body, as if the body already belongs to medicine and isn't changed by it. But we know that every observation of a body changes that body.

Large screen: a pair of legs, medically-imaged, dance across the screen.

On the way home from the hospital,
we remember about the metal plate in your leg,
a magnetic hazard that we forgot to declare.
This artefact came back to me twice –

once as a starburst in your images,
and then as a nugget of steel,
blackened and smooth,
given to me after you were cremated.
I put it in a bowl with some stones
I'd collected on holiday.
Sometime afterwards I added another piece of metal.
A shiny disc, like a large coin,
but rough and calloused,
made from silver recovered from about 2000 patient x-rays.[2]

Large screen: a glitched medical image of a pale pink multiple body rotates.

The x-ray changed us forever. It collapsed the distinction between inside and outside that had been the basis
of the human subject for hundreds of years. In the x-ray
the surface of the body was lost and dissolved in the
image.

Lesions and tumours can be represented as equations. And
polyps, cysts, blobs and nodules. Machines are learning
to interpret the smallest variations in the body's code,
sensitive to all our patterns and irregularities. Algorithms can analyse our numbers, we are their mathematical
matter.

Machines can detect and diagnose lung nodules and colonic
polyps, liver metastases and retinal disorders. Breast
cancer is one of the biggest potential markets for
automated diagnosis, but their lumpiness is a challenge
for artificial intelligence. Irregularities are not always
pathological.

Large screen: hundreds of imaged eyes from an AI research project flash up one by one very
quickly.

Small screen; same as above, creating a pair.
The artist moves close to the audience.

I imagine images of breasts passing in a line in front of
machines. But computers can't see, so all this talk of
machine vision is really just a metaphor for new forms of
calculation, to establish some continuity with the past,
and with human sight, which has for a very long time been
the privileged sense in medicine.

The live sound, which has been playing throughout the performance, becomes very loud at this point and the artist has to speak at a volume to be heard.

> In a future of pure operational images – where machines capture the body's insides, and render them for interpretation by another machine – there won't be any images.
>
> The media likes to compare human and machine vision, to frame them in a contest in which computers not only displace doctors but begin to control them too. Humans are at a certain disadvantage. We can only see about twenty-five shades of grey for example, compared to about 32,000 possible pixel values. Computers can operate in thresholds that exceed human senses.
>
> Plus, computers don't tire. They don't think about the past or the future. They don't become dehydrated. They don't judge our bad habits. They aren't racist or sexist. But. Oh. They. Are. Because embedded in the data they learn from are all the inequalities in our healthcare systems. But they don't get stressed and they don't become emotionally involved. They don't care.

Momentary pause in sound. Artist sits down again.
   Large screen: five patterned blocks, like a moving bar chart, rise and fall.

> *I return to your CD.*
> *This time I try a surface reconstruction and after some*
>   *moments you load,*
> *a vast silver structure with corners and lines that*
>   *zig-zag.*
> *As I roam you with my clicks and strokes,*
> *you respond with generous turns that let me flow over and*
>   *through you.*
> *Your weightlessness and your easy moves beguile me.*
> *I traverse you,*
> *as if you are my territory and I am your explorer.*

House lights go down and the room is almost dark.

> *You are labyrinthine,*
> *becoming over and over,*
> *a multiplex of corporeality.*
> *I lean into your light.*
> *Together we overcome dualities:*

skin and bone,
inside and outside,
presence and absence,
me and you.
We spoke about this but it's more than either of us
imagined.

We are dancing with this technology.

I glide along your digital depths.
You are mercurial.
No blood or other matter can stop me.
We are involved like never before.

The software takes me to the inside of the inside,
opening up views that have never been seen before by human
eyes.
There is a whole universe inside of you.
Comets fly right by me.
I join an asteroid belt travelling across deep time,
and land on a piece of interstellar rock to explore ravines
and dark caves.

The history of medicine has been leading up to this moment
of vision,
and has already overtaken it.
I am close to my own origins,
the child returning to her mother.
Yet I have never felt so alone.

Large screen: found footage of radiologists assessing scans. Patients' words such as 'a useless army', 'cheesy puffs', 'remote lands' and 'explosions' flash in yellow over the top. This sequence plays from start to finish for three minutes.
    Artist stands facing the audience.

Our images are analysed in darkened rooms. Though we never
meet them, radiologists are our interpreters, turning our
images into diagnoses.

Artist turns her back to the audience.
    Large screen: spots of green, yellow and orange flicker like a landscape, until the form resolves into a turning, medically-imaged female body.

As the radiologist
speaks his findings,

they are transcribed instantly into documents via voice
recognition software:
specular – exquisite – benign – adjacent – contingent –
acoustic – granular – calcified – suspicious – turbid –
lobulated – spiculated – invasive.

Some weeks later I read an entire 4000-word radiology
glossary to my laptop's Dictation software:

Large screen: The artist reads out the list of words from the glossary, in the left-hand column below. On the screen, synchronised with the artist's voice, we see the words in the right-hand column appearing as if being typed on a page, sometimes slowly and sometimes in short bursts.

Acetabulum	a sexy bottom
Achalasia	actually easier
Acute	a cute
Adnexal	next to
Algorithm	algorithm
Alveolus	alveolus
Ampulla of water	and cooler water
Anechoic	anechoic
Atomic number	a tonic number
Atelectasis	eight lax cases
Azygos lobe	I cough hello
Belly	belly
Benign	be nine
Biopsy	biopsy
Bougienage	bluesy launch
Bowel	barrel
Brachiocephaltic trunk	brachiocephalic trunk
Bregma	Brenda
Buttocks	butter
Budd Chiara syndrome	barred key syndrome
Calyx	Horlicks
Calcar avis	call car Avis
Canal of Schlemm	can now of slam
Cardiac tamponade	cardiac tampon A
Cephalad	see salad
Chemical fog	chemical fog
Cholangiography	Holy Lands geography
Controlled area	controlled area
Claustrophobic	claustrophobic
Clitoris	clitoris
Constipation	constipation

Small screen: the column on the right continues its mistranslation of words until it reaches the letter Z, and finishes at the end of performance. We don't have the original words from this point.

Artist, still standing, turns back to face the audience.

> The most spectacular and colourful of all medicine's images are the neuro-images. I can't find any reference that establishes the authority of their reds and yellows, the veracity of their blues and greens. Yet we revere these images as if they have been generated by the brain itself, and can reveal deep truths about ourselves.

Artist sits at the table.

Large screen: two pairs of medically-imaged arms with clasped hands move towards each other, overlap and pass.

> *I am thankful that neuro-imaging is improving lives:*
> *for people with multiple sclerosis*
> *epilepsy and Parkinsons,*

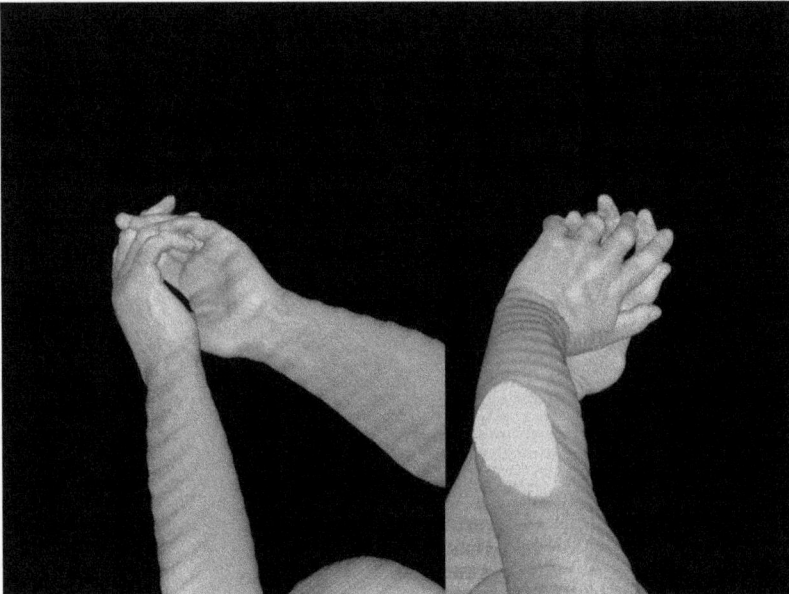

Figure 38.1 'Two pairs of medically-imaged arms with clasped hands move towards each other, overlap and pass'. Digital images displayed on large screen display in *You Are My Territory and I Am Your Explorer* (2019). Image courtesy of Liz Orton.

and stroke patients.
But I worry that it wants our thoughts,
and dreams and memories too.

If I think of a lion,
among a range of given objects,
a computer can learn to use my brain signals to recon-
  struct that image of the lion.
But what if I think about global warming?
Or my elderly neighbour?
Or the way light falls on a leaf?

There is talk of the body becoming transparent, of technologies making us fully visible. Where are the narratives
of obscurity?

According to Massachusetts Institute of Technology medical images are a near perfect match for machine learning (Brouillette, 2017). Imagine. The internal body is an
ideal training ground for the computer gaze, our insides
a new digital sublime.

Algorithms are in training. Neural networks are churning
over our numbers, each one of us part of a larger optimisation problem. The body is rich for extraction.

But listen to this. We can't always understand what the
machines are learning. There are too many dimensions. It's
a black box.

I find that for £2000 I could buy a full body scan, marketed
a bit like an MOT, that offers to find problems before they
become symptoms, to anticipate illness from the inside.
These moves to interiority would have us believe our body
is only inside of us.

I know it will be the last time I look at your images.
The sun is too bright for me to see the screen properly.
I try swivelling the monitor,
but in the end I sit in the dark.

Large screen: we pass very slowly and very closely over a surface of a medically imaged body.

All the density without gravity makes you restless.
At the touch of the mouse, you spin this way and that,
an acrobat that keeps on turning.

417

My tears make you all blurry.
I feel I am getting closer to something but you keep
  changing and re-animating.
Now you are a series of geometric parts,
like a Lego city,
or one of those Chinese puzzles that is impossible to
  reconstruct.
It's one transformation too many.
How do we get back to the beginning?

Medical images are now one of the most important sources of biomedical data. As transmittable code, images allow for new ways of accessing, knowing and disseminating the body. The separation of images from bodies is rarely secure.

As data accumulates, in public and private storage systems, the internal body becomes vulnerable to new forms of exchange, trade and speculation. An industry in data mining and digital retrieval is emerging around us, from us, the new informational people. Now that we are streams of numbers, see how quickly new business interests are forming.

Systems will test in new ways the old idea of the skin as a boundary between inside and outside, a protector of the body's privacy. Images can combine with other data, flowing across digital platforms and moving between providers, pulling us into new territories. Test results mixing with pension plans, pixels with interest rates, diagnoses with health insurance. The internal body is a space for financial speculation. But all this is in the future.

You begin to recede,
as if you want to become a dot on the screen's horizon.
You are a body drifting towards infinity,
casting no shadow.
I feel you going away from me all over again.
Everything I do to get closer to you just accelerates your
  disappearance.
I can't break you out of this optical system.

I take a break,
and when I return, I find you have returned too,
circling like nothing had ever happened.
And in the end,
it's the screen that stops me,
a trace of my reflection on the monitor.

The two of us in the same image.

Closing image: medically imaged skin fragmenting into two images.

Large screen: Credits.
Performed by: Liz Orton
Sound: Lori E Allen

No images of the artist's mother Anne Orton were shown during this performance.

Images and voices: Naomi Alao, Jenny Ayres, Anna Crohnios, Fiona Candlin, Claire Collison, Ida Levine, Phil Martin, Anne Redomond, Oliva Romero, Mike Saunders and Rick Spurway.

Thanks to: Dr Steve Bandula, Prof. Steve Halligan, Sylvia Kluczewski, Anne Orton, Yael Shavit.

Reference list

Brouillette, M. (2017) 'Deep learning is a Black Box, but health care won't mind', *MIT Technology Review*, 27 April.

Nadar, F. (1988) 'My life as a photographer', in Goldberg V. (ed.) *Photography in print: writings from 1816 to the present*. Albuquerque, NM: University of New Mexico, pp. 127–128.

Notes

1 The project also led to a website (available at: www.digitalinsides.org), a conference and edited book of essays (*Becoming Image: Medicine and the Algorithmic Gaze*) and an artist's book, *Every Body Is an Archive*. All the dialogues were accompanied by a consent procedure approved by UCLH.

2 I had a box of anonymised X-rays given to me by a hospital, a batch purchased on eBay and a large donation from a metal recovery company. Silver recovery is an industrial process during which the silver is 'washed' from the X-ray film using a cyanide solution and then removed from the solution by electrolysis. With the help of a silver recovery company, I retrieved 30g of silver from the X-rays.

39

DISCIPLINE AND *ASKĒSIS*

Training, spiritual philosophy and dance in Russell Maliphant's choreographic practice

Kélina Gotman

This chapter explores ways dance and health intermesh in British choreographer Russell Maliphant's practice. In particular, I examine how his long-standing involvement in Rolfing – a psychophysical practice of 'structural integration' or body-mind alignment – as well as Tai chi and anatomical modelling enable him to pursue a project of research into questions of health and choreographic aesthetics. I argue that while his dance work has come to be highly regarded nationally and internationally for its signature fluidity – the lithe, torque-like and remarkably virtuosic quality of motion he achieves in his own performance and that of his company dancers – at the root of Maliphant's lifelong project is an approach to training and integration that reconfigures how we may understand dance, movement, performance and health. I write this in the wake of six or so years of conversation with Maliphant, most recently as a resident researcher for the Maliphant Dance Company's project 'Dance, Health and Aesthetic Performance' (2019–2025). My proposed inquiry into the critical genealogy of ways health and dance concepts are imbricated in therapeutic practice and what I am calling biophilosophical aesthetics informs what I offer here.

In particular, the angle I take revolves around what I have been seeing as an alignment between Maliphant's approach to everyday dance training and the Greco-Roman practice of 'spiritual philosophy', a way of treating life as an exercise in the exploration of or ongoing research into *how* to live. I follow Greco-Roman philologist Pierre Hadot's analysis of these practices and Michel Foucault's work, heavily influenced by Hadot's, to think about how one might conceptualise 'dance' as a form of research into (and exercise in) health understood in the broadest possible sense as a practice of opening and integration.

The notion of 'mind/body' integration has a complex genealogy of its own, and I will not, for reasons of scope, treat that in full here, though this does occupy other facets of my ongoing work in this area; here, the 'anatomo-political' quality of dance and movement as a practice of kinaesthetic configuration does drive what I am seeking to explore in relation to genealogies of 'mind/body' 'balance'. For Foucault, anatomo- and biopolitical *'techniques* of power' operate on the social body in relation to economic and productive processes characteristic of capitalism (1990, p. 141, emphasis in original). Bodies are produced by forces of articulation and control that do not merely 'discipline' groups and individuals into submission or docility but, far more powerfully and subtly, arrange discourses and institutions so as to render certain forms visible, normative or calculable. At the same time, as Foucault articulates in his later work, exercises of self-conceptualisation (or

DOI: 10.4324/9781003036500-45

self-knowledge) and care have characterised philosophical practices from way before the Christian era, and although these existed in marginal forms with the advent of Christian asceticism, followed by Protestantism and capitalism – summarily – these practices may be traced to radical artistic practice, revolutionary movements and more (2009). In the work of Maliphant, what we discover is a spiritual practice that aligns ecological integration and a searching (or researching) quality, what I further analyse with Foucault as *zētēsis*; this is not the same as 'practice-based research' or 'research-informed practice' but something like research/creation, a hybrid interrogation of form and what subtends form, kinaesthetic anatomy. In this epistemological exercise or practice, 'training' takes on a different quality, not training *for* performance or mastery of a discipline but training as an exercise in moving oneself daily. As Foucault outlines, after Hadot, exercises in good, thoughtful or attentive living – 'spiritual exercises' practised by the Stoics, among others – were a form of medicine, as well as a way of diagnosing what is wrong, how to see and feel and think clearly; philosophy was at the outset a therapeutic and spiritual exercise, *therapeia*.[1]

I draw attention to the entanglement of spiritual, corporeal and aesthetic practices in a 'structurally integrated' body/mind with Maliphant, in the wake particularly of integrationist and body worker Ida Rolf (1896–1979), whose practice has informed Maliphant's (he is a trained practitioner and long-term advocate of her approach). For Rolf, and followers who practise her therapeutic techniques, alignment of the body and 'bodymind' through light massage-like touch reintegrates bodies misaligned through misuse; gentle work with posture opens up what can be described as energy fields, allowing more ease and connectedness within the body and between the body and the person's relational ecology. Rolfing recognises the interpenetration of 'physical' and 'emotional' lives, to uncover physical holding patterns, for example, resulting from long-term emotional tensions and strains. Thus, 'dance' becomes a practice of structural integration, indissociable from a practice of health, construed as the subtle balancing of energetic, kinaesthetic and anatomical forces, and as an epistemology, a way to deepen understanding of how our emotions shape and are shaped by everyday practices.

Combining my own lived experience as a trained dancer and academic with conversations across methods of work and fields also brings up questions of form with regard to method and writing. Is there a way the entanglements I am exploring within a structurally integrated arena come to be mirrored in the writing? In what follows, I attend to notions of *askēsis* as an attentive practice of living and form-of-life, to the material entanglements of corporeal and 'spiritual' processes, following among others the radical work of Hadot. The 'spiritual', with Hadot (2002), signals attention to how philosophy is an ongoing practice of transfiguration, not a discipline to master but a way of living within a generous and generative openness to others in the present.

'Structural integration': method and form

The web of issues that Maliphant's practice touches on is immense, from Daoism and anatomy to design and architecture; but, as I am arguing, this is also the point of his work – its ethos. Because 'structural integration' articulates a healthy, mobile – or what he calls an 'easy connected' – body which sees all elements of posture, emotional wellness and more as interpenetrating, naturally his own understanding of corporeality, training, performance and 'setting' intermesh (pers. comm., 7 August 2020). How to write about this, how to structure an 'argument'? When I have found myself speaking about this work over the past few years, I have found that the borders and structures themselves slip, shift and open – and that that, again, is also the point. What might appear as a 'subject' (for example, 'the dancing body in the choreography of Russell Maliphant' or 'training and aesthetics in Maliphant's work') blends into the manner of doing the work, the manner of carrying oneself while doing it or the healthfulness or attentiveness with which one approaches one's own articulation of this choreographic aesthetico-politics (or, after Foucault, this anatomo-politics) and even the integration of one's own life world within the matrix of this 'subject' or object of study. I have written elsewhere about ways my own desk, and life-world, structures of fatigue or family or home, aches and pains, public health and more suffuse the thinking (Gotman, 2021).

The research comes no longer only to be about anatomy, movement, choreoaesthetics and choreopolitics, or physical therapy, but also to query the epistemological hierarchies that appear to order for example therapeutic manipulation (as with Rolfing), martial arts (such as Tai chi), spiritual practice or philosophy (Daoism, spiritual exercises) or scientific epistemologies that conceptualise for example bone and muscle structure one way and the therapeutic and choreographic practices that shape these structures in another. Such entanglements and adjacencies open further out, so that Maliphant's work in this case becomes a node or knot for rearticulating rearticulation as such: for addressing relationships between arts and sciences, bioepistemology and bioaesthetics, practice and performance.

Of entanglement and filament and bone: fascia/Rolfing

Maliphant is known for the beauty and fluidity of his signature rhythm and shape. What is striking, however, is how much his approach to shape reveals something more subtle which, I think, expresses something like a 'holistic' concept or practice of health, a body articulating interstitial zones between flesh and bone, ligament and sinew. This is not 'health' understood in the sense of a checklist – verifying there is no fever or heartbeat is so-called 'normal' – but 'health' in the sense of a state of integration and relative equilibrium; in Maliphant's work, the attempt to achieve balance is an attempt to work with vulnerabilities, plasticities and pliabilities – with all the mechanisms that enable ageing, deterioration or solitude to gain form and to transform. I think this concept of health aligns, among others, with tenth- and eleventh-century physician and philosopher Avicenna (Ibn Sīnā)'s philosophy as the prevention and cure of disorders, according to theory and practice, taking into account environmental factors, psychological factors, movement, rest and much more. 'Medicine' then is not only about the 'body' but about the web of entanglements within which we move.

As Avicenna put it in his *Metaphysica*, there are practical sciences that inform and depend upon human actions and those that inform us about the nature of things. Importantly, within the practical sciences, a further three emerge: public management, which includes religious laws and politics; household management; and the science of the self, specifying what we are to do with ourselves when we are on our own or in association with others. Civic management, household management and management of the self, in other words, are the three branches of science that govern how we associate with ourselves and with others in a practical way. Because the speculative sciences deal with things that are independent of us, in his view (including mathematics, geometry, astronomy, optics, mechanics and so on), they are understood in varying degrees of connectedness to the 'sensible matter' of human life and so too to motion and change. With Avicenna, the question of movement is at once germane to practical and theoretical health questions, and it serves as a litmus test between so-called 'natural' and more abstract epistemological procedures (2016, pp. 11–15). Motion, moving bodies – anatomo-politics – link or recalibrate corporeal life, where this meets 'public body' and 'public health'; while choreographic practice, and specifically training philosophies, are often understood in aesthetic and critical terms in dance and performance studies as touching on forms of representation, Maliphant's work, I think, suggests an approach to movement that articulates a 'whole body' concept of bioaesthetic practice, where the limits and structures of the 'body' are also in question. Where does the 'body' begin? Where does it end? What is it composed of, and how is it formed, and is there an 'it'? How do anatomical, Daoist, ergonomic, design/ structural and choreographic approaches to an enmeshed body-form enable another order of play with and research into the choreographic politics of training as a practice of living? 'Dance', rather than being separated from other forms of motion, operates as a harbour, receiving and holding and displaying everyday networks and structures of nourishment and exercise and disciplines of training and bioaesthetic form.

So while there is arguably of course 'beauty' in Maliphant's choreography, understood in some respects quite classically as curved lines, torque, smoothness, sheer physical power, and while this aesthetic practice has earned him enormous accolades and no small number of placements with car ads and others keen to associate profitably with smooth and lithe form, the intention beneath the skin, as it were, in his work, suggests that there is something taking place far more deeply at the level of an exploration of figuration as such. This is not speculative only as regards a 'cohering' body but also material: it conjoins the theoretical and the practical in the exploration of aesthetico-political care and, I think, health.

With Maliphant, choreographic practice allows for the quality of 'self' and motion to be formed, perhaps transformed. As he puts it, in conversation, the question of *how* the quality of movement is affected is nearly but never quite explained by recognising the dancer and the choreographer's knowledge of the fascial networks holding tensions and distensions within a body. 'Picturing' these surely affects the quality of motion, he surmises, as does working against distinctions between muscle and bone, eliminating these from one's body concept, replacing these with filaments, liquefactions. I would venture to call this a biophilosophical epistemology, or even a bioaesthetic epistemology, where 'biology' has to be understood as an ever-evolving set of coordinates pertaining to *bios*, the body that is lived (and lived in terms of its shifting and modular form).[2] In all instances, the work is indefinite, open, and it constitutes a practice of self-searching and searching, a way to dive deeper into the 'marrow' of form. This is what one could further call, with Foucault, training, or 'exercising oneself' so as to *form* life, to enable 'life' to continue to take shape, to give and to bear form (2001, pp. 82, 301–302, 339, 406, emphasis added). As a mode of 'research' (*zētēsis*), this practising attention to oneself and to others allows for philosophy – an exercise in living a truthful life, open daily to further deepening.[3]

Balance: extension, relation, *therapeia*

In my conversation with Maliphant in July 2020, one of the first figures he offered to think with was the Daoist notion of 'balance' comprising not just an intracorporeal set of alignments but a healthful notion of balance extending far beyond the sole body or bodymind: to friends, family, neighbourhood, community; to one's entire network of energetic and emotional relations; to one's extended self. This aligns with concepts of extended mind prominent in neurological and ecological approaches to cognitive theory or embodied cognition: 'extended mind' suggests that we do not merely 'know' with our 'bodies' (the premise of embodied cognition), but furthermore that we co-constitute our existences within far broader relations of alliance with other places, systems, entities. At the same time, even this model perhaps fails adequately to account for how we are more than contained within an extended, vast series of interconnections – more than the figure of the singular 'I' appears to attest – but that these zones of dehiscence and rehiscence are perpetually displacing where and how 'I' or 'it' or 'thou' form and mesh. I have elsewhere called these structures 'vibrant affiliations', to understand how 'family', 'society' and 'self', for example, intermingle in acts of ongoing constitution (Gotman, 2019). What speaking in the midst of a global pandemic allowed for here was recognition that this interpenetration of 'self' and neighbourhood, community or ecology reflects a powerful understanding of 'health' and what one could refer to as public health, accounting for ways we are inextricably associated with one another just as we appear to need to stand back, retreat. Daoist practice, like spiritual philosophy, acknowledges how we are 'balanced' only if we are able to attend to various aspects of our lives peacefully, continuously and with care (see Hadot, 2002).

With talk of 'work/life balance', strain, fatigue, overwork and debilitating stress, and the relatively sudden release and intensification of these issues in the context of lockdown culture, it seemed apt, to say the least, to be thinking about how dance not only, for example, narratively portrays a practice of balance but embodies this manner of negotiating balance every day. In order to dance, one must have one's household (also) in order. This is not simply the 'household' as in the laundry, the dishes, the children – though it is all that too – but 'household' as a manner of approaching the tendrils of governmentality (see Gotman, 2021).

For Félix Guattari, 'ecosophy' describes a fundamental imbrication of three 'ecological registers (the environment, social relations and human subjectivity)'; this is an 'ethico-political articulation' (2000, p. 28), which takes life on this planet far beyond the problem of linking pollution to 'quality of living' (bad air, and so on) but to the philosophical or *ecosophical* way relationships and experiences of selfhood are bound up in what we typically learn to experience as a context or frame (an environment) for the self, or these selves. When Maliphant describes the work of articulating a dancing body that is inextricably linked – for its sense of balance, flow, ease, fluidity – with social relations – it is an ecosophical argument engaged in questions of architectural and anatomical form. Tensegrity, like biotensegrity, describes structures that do not rely on, for instance, a framework, topped with a casing or shell (skin, cladding) but 'hold together', as it were, through delicate and dynamic interlocking pressures – mutual holdings. In *Biotensegrity: The Structural Basis of Life* (2014), a book Maliphant works with, osteopath Graham Scarr shows some of the ways architectural structure and human microbiology share common geometric and mathematical forms, specifically the tetrahedron, hexagon and other geodesic geometric shapes – the octahedron, icosahedron and so on. The tetrahedron, significantly, 'occupies the *smallest* volume of unit space within the *largest* surface area, which makes it a minimal-energy shape, and naturally occurs as piles of oranges, molecules of water and methane, mineral crystals and radiolaria' (microscopic protozoa that produce intricate, usually silica, skeletons composed of endo- and ectoplasm). Chains of tetrahedra, he adds, twist into a tetrahelix – a form that inventor and visionary Buckminster Fuller (1895–1983) deployed to build his experimental structures held together not by glue, bolts or other adhesives but by the sheer force of shapes balanced through the careful exercise of a natural dynamic pressure – or vectoral force (Scarr, 2014, pp. 12, 16, emphasis in original). Fuller coined the notion of 'tensegrity' to describe how this tension between parts of isomorphic geometric bodies produced efficient systems or structures, using vectorial motion or force, equilibrium, contraction, twisting and untwisting; the 'jitterbug' describes 'an oscillating energy system in continuous motion', which in Scarr's gloss 'contracts and expands omnidirectionally around a central point, first one way and then the other . . . a dynamic model of bodies in motion before they crystallise into form' (ibid: 22). It is no surprise that Maliphant would see in this a powerful set of observations and images for his work.

Maliphant has an array of tensegrity structures hanging about his workspace, which he shows to his dancers and students and any interested interlocutors. But what I quickly learned in conversation was that more than deploy systems or structures of tensegrity, Maliphant has drawn from the closely allied notion of biotensegrity, a term coined by the orthopaedic surgeon

Stephen Levin, who in the 1970s observed that standard biomechanical theories failed adequately to account for the shape and structure of living organisms he identified at every level or scale. Right around the same time, the cell biologist Donald Ingber suggested that tensegrity also better explained the behaviours of cancer cells than did any previously held systems (ibid: ix). Biotensegrity describes the biological 'tensegrity' structures that run through – or shape – our bodies at the cellular and the molecular level. What Maliphant found was that Rolfing, for example, proved, or paved the way for, some of the surgical research that was now starting visually to show biotensegrity at work within the fabric of living tissue. Anatomical dissection had previously – for centuries – taken place on dead bodies. With the development of mesoscopic investigation into living tissue in the 2010s, extremely small cameras could travel through the skin, as it were, and 'see' matter live. The hand surgeon Jean-Claude Guimberteau was the first visually to demonstrate what he saw through these mesoscopic recordings, determining that the biotensegrity structures described by Levin and Ingber in the 1980s were now directly observable through video exploration of living matter.

Guimberteau has called his meso-anatomical odyssey *Strolling under the Skin*, and the choreographic reference to the 'stroll' is well warranted. The 'camera's eye' view of living tissue shows that whereas one may be accustomed from childhood and textbook cut-outs to conceptualise one's body as made of skeletal matter, topped with muscle, covered in fascia (if this is not left out entirely), and then skin, the fascia or whole-body soft tissue that Rolfers, among other 'body' therapists, work with, is in fact indistinguishable from flesh or skin or bone. The entirety of our living organism is composed of a singular 'histological continuum' of material stuff, webs of interconnecting 'fascicles' (Guimberteau, 2005).

It is not difficult, perhaps, to understand why these images and forms fascinate a choreographer known not only for the 'beauty' of his choreographic line but also for the investment in manual therapy he practises. What struck me early on was the way this non-hierarchical system, by which bone, muscle, tissue and skin are one, echoes and reflects an anti-hierarchical or at least a non-hierarchical epistemological continuum by which 'therapy' (for example, Rolfing, osteopathy), academic science (hand surgery), choreographic practice, martial arts and more become co-extensive bioepistemologies, each node engaging with sets of vectorial forces or vessels or filaments within a continuum of living intellectual-affective matter. Guimberteau's video images show (as the voiceover narrative attests) that the 'apparent disorder and irregularity of shapes was in fact the basis of some other form of complexity that we still knew hardly anything about': the vessels within the flexor tendons being operated on stretched and extended across all surfaces observable live (*in vivo*); 25× magnification allowed the Guimberteau team to see that tissue exists on a continuum. So whereas 'reductive mechanistic models' had posited classical 'pump' systems, where vessels were slotted into one another, here were completely and intricately enmeshed filaments knitted throughout living matter (Guimberteau, 2005). As osteopath Colin Armstrong writes in his preface to Guimberteau's *Architecture of Human Living Fascia*:

> Perhaps the most important message is that there are no distinct separate layers within the histological continuum of living matter. We discover that the whole body is structured by a vast single unitary tensional network that is composed of billions of interconnected multidirectional fibers and fibrils. The fibrils interweave and interconnect to create the three-dimensional microvolumes that Dr Guimberteau has named microvacuoles. These are the basic architectural units – fundamental building blocks of the body.
>
> (Guimberteau and Armstrong, 2015, pp. xv–xvi, xv)

Although Armstrong is still using the comparatively mechanistic image of a 'building block' and an 'architectural unit', the *in vivo* photography and narrative describe a mesh of filaments, fractal patterns; the interpenetration of figures of speech reveals, I think, a shifting paradigm. This is what Maliphant envisions when he works with his dancers: to achieve 'balance' and fluidity, bodies are not working with lines in space, but microvolumes, a whole tensegrity and biotensegrity network of infinitesimal fibres. The Da Vinci body becomes something else: a whirl or a spiral, a set of living and vibrant continua, vesicles and vacuoles.

As noted, Maliphant carries around tensegrity models to show dancers and interlocutors how to visualise the micro mechanisms that are not mechanistic at all, but fluid, plastic, pliable, balancing through systems of torsion, tension and gravitational force. Although he has not found experimental proof that this concrete visualisation – via the tensegrity models – causes dancers to achieve the sort of signature fluidity for which his work is so recognisable, he has consistently observed that they do achieve remarkable ease through these conversations and visualisations, in some part. Speaking with him about this in July 2020, I was struck by the fact that the figure of virtuosity we were circumnavigating is in fact very different from the sort of performative imperative so well known in classical dance forms and more popular forms of street dance that rely on high-octane competitiveness. As Maliphant conceded, for choreographer Deborah Hay, the point with performance is not to show off, not to demonstrate some feat, but to allow oneself to be seen. What we realised, discussing this further, was how with his dancers – and in his own performance – another order of aesthetics is articulated, showcasing alignment at the level of the self, for lack of a better term: something that allows one to be seen, as one is. This means that the beauty that transpires when one is watching is not of a purely formal sort, nor is the work narrative; something else is going on. I would call this in part *therapeia*, to the extent that there is a (non-articulated) spiritual alignment within the self/form/organism taking place, and that this transpires in a certain quality of tranquillity or peacefulness at the level of the chest, for example, in ease, and quiet care. This is care with regard to the possibility of showing oneself such as produces what for Foucault and Hadot constitutes philosophical medicine or spiritual philosophy – and practised here, one might say, through movement, manifest as living form, where 'ease' and integration align.

To the extent that philosophy was originally in this way a form of medicine, and to the extent that with Maliphant, we witness implicitly a form of integration, practised in the everyday act of kinaesthetic searching, one finds I would argue a certain bioaesthetics of healthful life, a form-of-life that is open rather than closed: that is what is 'beautiful' in a nearly ineffable, almost inarticulable way. This notion of 'health' does not need to align with smoothness (many forms may be very jagged), but the bioaesthetic softness and strength that are achieved, I think, reveal a particular facet of ongoing work with calibration, interiority. The revelation of a process of interiority through 'showing oneself' with care, while practised with enormous attention to 'technique' (techniques of living, training in arts of dance and so on), not only ultimately theatricalises spiralling, liquefying form; form is also very subtly performed as a question, a gift – though one may not realise this quite in seeing it. One may not realise this at all; at the surface of the body, a swirl; on the stage, a living braiding, a meditation.

Sustainability: longevity, depth and form

One could counter that this is well and good for young dancers in the prime of their physical strength, but Maliphant's work increasingly finds interest in older dancers. He is, in his fifties and sixties, dancing more than ever; what arrests his attention is the way this approach to dance and to dance training not only allows for longevity within the work of performance but more than this makes a virtue, perhaps, of such grace. I think the implications are enormous, as regards how we construe the professional dance industry. It is beyond the scope of this chapter to touch on that fully here. But if what Maliphant's work reveals is the entanglement of physical therapy, emotional anatomy, martial arts, classical and contemporary ballet training, a Daoist outlook on the entanglement of all aspects of self beyond the singular individuated material body, and more, then naturally what transpires from this is a concept of the natural 'body' (and of 'beauty', as well as enjoyment) that I think allows the dancer, like the viewer, to be at ease and to rest. In the terms of pre-Socratic philosopher Heraclitus, one might say: *while changing it rests* (μεταβάλλον ἀναπαύεται). Understood as a dynamic way to conceptualise the interpenetration of change and rest (as opposed to the productivist view characteristic of modernity, which sees progress as determined always by motion, with no stopping), this attention to rest/change as μεταβολή (metabolē) allows for another order of healthful care, another political or choreographic biopolitics and bioaesthetics; another 'anatomo-politics' also.

Discipline and *askēsis*

What I am advocating for, then, in my reading of Maliphant's work is an approach to training that recognises dance less as a discipline to master and more as a form of *askēsis*, what Foucault saw as training in life form: an 'ethopoetics', in a way (Foucault, 2016, pp. 56, 68n34). With *askēsis* – quite different from 'asceticism', which early mediaeval Christianity saw as requiring condemnation of pleasure and of the flesh – what is emphasised is a manner of doing, a practice, every day.[4] This requires openness to constant discovery and growth, even without any of this being an 'end'. It also means there is not a mastery that is achieved. Rather, training is an ever-evolving sort of work, inhabitation of what Giorgio Agamben, in the wake of Foucault (and Ludwig Wittgenstein), calls form-of-life. This means that whether one is in or outside the studio, one is attending to the way one lives, to the interconnection or entanglement of all these parts of one's life. The way one holds one's head or neck or jaw or spine is something to 'deal with' in the studio, perhaps, but it is also inextricable from the way one is aligned in the rest of one's life. Maliphant is clear on this: he does not seek for his dancers to reveal or to 'work on' 'personal' aspects of their lives in the studio. But to the extent that his Rolfing practice, among others, allows him to draw attention for instance to a hip bone or a jaw bone and so to re-place, to rearticulate what might have been 'out of joint', this emanates out towards and suffuses the total life form a dancer or trainee inhabits. At the same time, their own practices in yoga or Pilates or street dance or martial arts will of course also contribute to their modes of moving and inhabiting their bodies (and performing), their own offerings, their own intelligence and attentiveness in the studio, their own manners of doing creation and research. Maliphant seeks to work with this plurality of modes of cognition, what I am calling a choreographic *ethopoiesis*, so that what is 'formed' as 'choreography' is a body (or bodymind, or what have you) more fully aligned: movement becomes integration visibilised.

Arguably, what is going on also thus is the exercise of *energeia*, what Agamben reads as a mode of being-at-work distinct from the product of the work or from the use of the body towards work (*ergon*). Agamben massages these distinctions in *The Use of Bodies* (2016), drawing out the image of the dancer, as mentioned by Seneca, for whom a dancer (when she is skilled) deploys gestures 'perfectly adapted to the meaning of the piece and its accompanying emotions'; 'movements match the speed of the dialogue'. This 'use-of-oneself' is a form of craftsmanship that accompanies *oikeiosis* – what Agamben, reading the Stoics, defines as 'the appropriation or familiarization of the self to the self' (ibid: 49–52). As *ethopoiesis* and *oikeiosis*, 'dance' (movement formed) in Maliphant's work becomes the 'appropriation or familiarization of the self to the self in this way', and the deployment of this self-appropriation as *energeia*. This attunement may be what strikes viewers as beautiful, what distinguishes this quality of motion from another. The shape or skill is less at stake than the fact that what one witnesses obliquely in performance is attentiveness to living form.

Proietto: visibilised ontogenesis

The notion of the *quality* of a motion – its character or characteristic – is a driving question for Maliphant, for whom motion is less shape than it is the energy or liquidity or depth or integrity and integration with which movement emerges via form. A case in point is the now classic work of Maliphant's, *Afterlight*, which earned dancer Daniel Proietto immense accolades and the work a Critics' Circle National Dance Award for Best Modern Choreography (2010). When I saw it at Sadler's Wells, London, in 2009, as part of the *In the Spirit of Diaghilev* bill, I was, like so many, mesmerised, still. There was something liquid, mournful, penetrating, fascinating and ungraspable in the image of this singular figure spinning fluidly within a shaft of light, like a ballerina held, serene and limitless, in a glass box. Yet rather than conjuring capture, Proietto conjured absolute tranquillity, the motion so full of ease, it might have no end; this was not the ceaseless perpetuum mobile of modernity – something else was going on, diving into a pool of energy and resource far deeper. His quietly swirling motions, set to music by Eric Satie, rendered the apparently simple spirals his body performed – like a corkscrew, perfect torque – an object or moment of suspension. It did feel like one was witnessing something held infinitely in the space of this swirl, this case.

For Elizabeth Grosz, the 'incorporeal' dimensions of matter – and the ontoethical question of how matter and non-matter move together, transform (beyond the paradigms of 'new materialism') – provoke the question of irreducibility, of transindividuation: the incorporeal always shadows corporeality, and vice versa (2017). In the work of Maliphant, the (nearly tautological) 'embodiment' or manifestation or visibilisation of lived matter, articulated through an ongoing (spiritual) exercise in *zētēsis* (research, enquiry), exemplifies, I think, an ontogenetic process. This is ontogenesis as the emergence of form into and through or with a continuously changing ecology/environment/world, just as body/form shifts and emerges. As an experiment in how to reassemble or to rearticulate 'holism', even 'organicity', this practice in body/form engages with method, with practice or praxis – as a manner of being (*ethopoietically*) continuously attentive for example to anatomy, where this melts into another order of (formless) form. In order to experiment with, and ultimately to achieve, another quality of motion, nearly like but not quite ballet or contemporary dance, Maliphant works past structure, to arrive nearer to the zero point where this softens into fascial torque. There is no longer a body conceived of anatomically as composed of parts, or a bioaesthetic and anatomo-political fantasy of muscle-building (typically masculine) (pers. comm, 29 March 2018), nor the sense of a skeleton that has to be moved around, but the continuum of histological matter, a showing of oneself as it is dissolving known form.

This invites a very different concept of the relationship between training, choreographic practice, 'dance', body, matter, science and much more than approaches to dance training I think typically invite. The demoralising and exhausting parcellation of dance work in an era of 'flexibility' and precarity, for instance, can be aligned with what Luc Boltanski and Ève Chiapello (2011) described of the 'new spirit of capitalism' which followed the 'artistic critique' of the generation of May 1968 and the rearticulation of new management and institutional cultures aligned with an 'energetic' type of highly non-securitising fluidity. In a similar vein, dance critics such as Anne Schuh (2019) have underscored the ambivalent violence of notions of 'eclectic training' and 'work with/out boundaries' as a way of occupying or inhabiting time within a neoliberal framework. Yet the sort of integration I am describing does something, I think, slightly different. For Schuh, Tai chi on the subway, for example, is one of many ways artists continuously 'working' engage in technical 'bricolage', becoming resourceful so as to be adaptable to a multifaceted professional context always quickly paced (2019, pp. 82, 84, 86–89; see also Bales and Nettl-Fiol, 2008). Increasingly reliant on the language of 'practice', dancers habituated to 'hired work' and expectations of perpetual availability and mobility conceptualise training in an expansive sense: 'I have a raving practice' was offered to her as one only slightly tongue-in-cheek response by an artist who does not otherwise regularly attend class (Schuh 87; see also Foster, 1997, in Schuh 84). But while this approach to bricolage and the 'hired body' foregrounds the neoliberal capture of the 24/7 cycle of productivity into the working regimes of artistic labour, I have been aiming here also to recognise another approach to full-scale integration. With attention to form-of-life, *energeia* (or being-at-work, distinct from 'doing' 'work', where 'work' is a product, and can be alienated, captured, within neoliberal and other structures) – besides constituting another ethics, and ontoethics, and poethics, and another form of visibilised ontogenesis – has the potential also to become a site of rearticulation through self-knowledge and care.

Of course, Maliphant has leisure to do this, to an extent, as he is a highly established choreographer, more secure than trainee dancers; nevertheless, the culture of *zētēsis* and of *askēsis* which I think he has modelled might invite other forms of practice that aim to find in the 'remedial' or in philosophical medicine not an accidental art for injury but a constitutive question; going deeper, rather than adding things up, may allow for one of the most radical counterpoints to the performative sorts of accountability that are demolishing all sectors as they seek to tick every box. This is the opposite of 'wellbeing' or shallow 'resilience', but an ongoing encounter. What is at play is *metabolē*: somewhere between changing, movement and rest.

Even if nothing 'looks different' on the surface of things: one goes to the studio, trains; one performs on this or another night; one is injured, one heals (hopefully); one goes on – perhaps something in the *energeia* shifts, subtly; from discipline to *askēsis*, rather than mastering a singular form, one trains in everyday acts of attention to enable something of another ergopolitical and poiethical emergence: a biopolitics and bioaesthetics of actually living form.

Notes

1 See Hadot, 2002, p. 23 and 23n5; see also Foucault, 2001, p. 96. On philosophical practice as a form of medicine and therapy, see also Foucault, 2001, pp. 10–11, 57–58, 93–95, 104; on physiology (*phusologia*) as a form of epistemology, a way of knowing self and world/nature, see esp. 232–233. Foucault describes *askēsis*, a practice or exercise of the self in relation to the self (*'de soi sur soi'*), as close to medicine and music, in the work of the Stoic Musonius Rufus (301); *askēsis* emphasises truthful living, perspicacity – alleviating anxiety, achieving some tranquillity of soul, purging fears and so becoming a spiritual athlete, enduring ongoing self-searching as a healthy relationship of self to self (*'de soi à soi'*) with others (301–314). On the ancient practice of *parrhēsía* or truthful speech – performed at the right moment – as physiological and therapeutic, see also Foucault, 2016, pp. 42–46.
2 Foucault describes *bios* (distinct from *zōē*) as that which is experienced or lived and can be transformed through practice and specific forms attention; *bios* thus has to be understood in relation to *tekhnē* as a practice or exercise (*'exercice'*) and a challenge or task (*'épreuve'*) towards ongoing self-understanding and self-transformation (Foucault, 2001, pp. 428–429, 466–467). See also Foucault, 2014, pp. 253–259 on the relation between *bios, tekhnai peri ton bion* (arts or techniques of living) and *erōs*.
3 Foucault discusses the notion of *zētēsis* (or *zêtêsis*) in relation to Socrates's practice, as research into truth (see e.g., Foucault, 2009, pp. 80–82).
4 On the difference between *askēsis* as a spiritual practice of truth and what became (largely Christian) asceticism, involving deprivation of the self, see esp. Foucault, 2001, p. 305, 2009, pp. 292–294, where he notes that Christian asceticism tends to reject the present world in favour of another world, and to obey an external authority, while Stoic and Cynic practices were engaged in transforming the present world and discovering one's own relationship to truth and so on by engaging in rigorously knowing (and critiquing) oneself.

Reference list

Agamben, G. (2016) *The use of bodies*. Translated by A. Kotsko. Stanford, CA: Stanford University Press.

Avicenna (2016) *The* Metaphysica *of Avicenna (Ibn Sīnā): a critical translatio-commentary and analysis of the fundamental arguments in Avicenna's* Metaphysica *in the Dānish Nāma-i 'alā 'ī (The book of scientific knowledge)*. Edited and Translated by P. Morewedge. London: Routledge and Kegan Paul.

Bales, M. and Nettl-Fiol, R. (eds.) (2008) *The body eclectic: evolving practices in dance training*. Urbana, IL: University of Illinois Press.

Boltanski, L. and Chiapello, È. (2011) *Le nouvel esprit du capitalisme*. Paris: Gallimard.

Foster, S.L. (1997) 'Dancing bodies', in Jane, C.D. (ed.) *Meaning in motion: new cultural studies of dance*. Durham: Duke University Press, pp. 235–257.

Foucault, M. (1990) *The history of sexuality. Vol. 1: an introduction*. Translated by R. Hurley. New York: Vintage Books.

Foucault, M. (2001) *L'herméneutique du sujet. Cours au Collège de France. 1981–1982*. Edited by F. Gros. Paris: Seuil and Gallimard.

Foucault, M. (2009) *Le courage de la vérité. Le gouvernement de soi et des autres II. Cours au Collège de France. 1984*. Edited by F. Gros. Paris: Seuil and Gallimard.

Foucault, M. (2014) *Subjectivité et vérité. Cours au Collège de France. 1980–1981*. Edited by F. Gros. Paris: Seuil and Gallimard.

Foucault, M. (2016) '*La parrêsia*. Conférence prononcée par Michel Foucault à l'université de Grenoble le 18 mai 1982'. In *Discours et vérité, précédé de La parrêsia*. Ed. Frédéric Gros. Gen. eds. Henri-Paul Fruchaud and Daniele Lorenzini. Paris: Vrin. 19–75.

Gotman, Kélina, (2019) 'Society and Family: Vibrant Affiliations'. In Jennifer Wallace, ed. *A Cultural History of Tragedy*, Vol. 6, 1930–Present. 6 vols. Gen. ed. Rebecca Bushnell. London: Bloomsbury. 127–143.

Gotman, K. (2021) 'The inappropriable: on oikology, care, and writing life', *Substance*, 50(1), pp. 116–139.

Grosz, E. (2017) *The incorporeal: ontology, ethics, and the limits of materialism*. New York: Columbia University Press.

Guattari, F. (2000) *The three ecologies*. Translated by I. Pindar and P. Sutton. London: The Athlone Press.

Guimberteau, J.-C. (2005) *Promenades sous la peau ou A la découverte des architectures de la matière vivante [Strolling under the Skin]* [Film]. ADF Films Productions and CERIMES.

Guimberteau, J.-C. and Armstrong, C. (2015) *Architecture of human living fascia: the extracellular matrix and cells revealed through endoscopy*. Edinburgh: Handspring Publishing.

Hadot, P. (2002) *Exercices spirituels et philosophie antique*. New edn. Paris: Albin Michel.

Scarr, G. (2014) *Biotensegrity: the structural basis of life*. Edinburgh: Handspring Publishing.

Schuh, A. (2019) 'Having a personal (performance) practice: dance artists' everyday work, support, and form', *Dance Research Journal*, 51(1), pp. 79–94.

40

TOOTH FAIRIES FOR ADULTS

Performing ritual

Helen Pynor

The Tooth Fairy is a simple ritual that seems to recognise the loss of childhood teeth as some small rite of passage in the journey towards growing up. The ritual takes place when a child loses a milk tooth: the child is invited to hide it under their pillow at bedtime, and on waking, they find it magically replaced by a coin, purportedly by a fairy who leaves the money in exchange for the tooth. Perhaps the tooth fairy myth also offers basic instruction on how we might approach rituals involving other shed human tissues. This chapter explores the possibilities for surgically excised human tissues to become the substance of rituals, within artistic and performance practices, and the roles these practices might play in physical, psychic and emotional adaptation to bodily change associated with health conditions that necessitate surgery. Rituals involving excised tissues of the body could be seen as practices of care – actions that mimic, enact or stand in as metaphors for practices of care – or as forms of memorial. Such rituals may actualise the material, historic, emotional, symbolic and spiritual potential embedded in excised human tissues.

This exploration was prompted by hip replacement surgery I undertook in 2019, required due to a congenital hip abnormality, during which the head of my femur bone was cut and surgically excised. A new work, *Habitation* is based on the experience, commissioned for the Experimenta *Life Forms* International Triennial of Media Art (which toured Australia nationally between 2021 and 2023) and for the City of Joondalup Art Collection, Perth, in Western Australia.[1] Unable to bear the idea of my hip bone ending up in an anonymous biohazardous waste stream, I sought permission to keep the removed bone material. This was resisted, at first, as access to one's own tissues and knowledge of the final resting place for these tissues is often withheld from patients in an act of personal and material erasure. Nevertheless, *Habitation* comprises a series of ceramic objects, including a bone china object made from my surgically excised femur head bone and a series of lightbox images composited from my archive of X-ray and CT scans. The images trace my body's dynamic adaptation to change over the course of my life and include metaphorical elements that reference the absent bone and bodily transformation following surgery.

Bounded objects

The resistance I initially met when requesting the return of my bone exposes the ambiguity that surrounds the question of who has legal ownership and rights over body parts that have been

DOI: 10.4324/9781003036500-46

removed after surgery or death. Indeed, it often surprises people to learn that we do not legally own our 'own' body parts once they are removed from our bodies. This rests on an English legal principle dating back to the seventeenth century that asserts that 'there is no property in a dead body'. It forbids property ownership rights in human corpses, thereby preventing the moral affront of corpses being traded for profit. By the nineteenth century the principle was well established in many jurisdictions, including the UK, US and Australia (Mason and Laurie, 2001). However, a landmark Australian case, *Doodeward v Spence*, was made in 1908, prompted by the police seizure from a medical museum of a two-headed still-born human foetus, its exhibition deemed an insult to public decency. The High Court ruled that, despite the 'no property in a dead body' rule, 'a dead human body may under some circumstances become the subject of property', on the basis that:

> A corpse may possess such peculiar attributes as to justify its preservation on scientific or other grounds, and, if a person has by the lawful exercise of work or skill so dealt with such a body in his lawful possession that it has acquired some attributes differentiating it from a mere corpse awaiting burial, he acquires a right to retain possession of it.
>
> (*Doodeward v Spence*, 1908)

This conferral of property rights on those who have exercised 'work or skill' has been used as a precedent in subsequent cases, making property rights assertable by, for example, pathology companies that section, stain or otherwise perform work on human pathology samples and by museums that dissect and undertake preservation techniques on body parts or tissues.[2] It persists in recent bioethical frameworks, for example, Nuffield Council on Bioethics (UK)'s *Human Bodies* report, which includes the statement that:

> It is now well established that where body parts 'have acquired different attributes by virtue of the application of skill', then they may become property . . . and hence protected by the law of theft. Thus any form of tissue that is 'processed' into new products . . . may be considered 'property' and may legitimately be sold (*though not by the person who provided the source material*).
>
> (Nuffield Council on Bioethics, 2011, p. 64. Italics mine)

In the face of this contradictory situation, a range of consent models have been introduced in recent decades which recognise that donors may continue to hold interests in their excised bodily material and that seek to protect these rights (Kaye *et al.*, 2015). A significant step was the Human Tissue Act of 2004, which was motivated by the Bristol and Alder Hey organ retention scandals in the UK. This public attention followed an inquiry concluded in 1999, which revealed that organs and tissues, including hearts, from hundreds of deceased children had been retained for forensic and research purposes, without the knowledge or consent of their kin (Mason and Laurie, 2001). In the aftermath of the Bristol and Alder Hay scandal, the 'no property in a body' rule was revisited and debated in earnest by legal scholars. For example, in their article on the ambivalence around the legal status of bodies and body parts, Kenyon Mason and Graeme Laurie noted the contradictions embedded in the legal situation, where concepts such as the 'gift' of tissues by donors implicitly suggest the existence of ownership, whilst property rights were simultaneously explicitly denied in law (Mason and Laurie, 2001, p. 725). A counterpoint within these debates was that the attribution of proprietary rights in relation to human tissue would not reflect the fact that donors may be more concerned with the potential uses and misuses of their tissues, rather than the acquisition and retention of them. An example of this, noted by legal scholar Loane Skene, is naturally shed hair being collected and misused, for example, to obtain DNA sequence data about the owner. The remedy to this situation is not the return of the hair (as property rights would suggest) but compensation for its wrongful use, in which case more appropriate rights of control could be provided by laws of privacy, battery, negligence and non-discrimination (Skene, 2002).

In response to the rapid evolution and transformation of biomedical research and information technologies, more recently attention has turned to dynamic models for ascertaining the most ethical position in relation to human tissue. A dynamic model sees consent as a fluid, ongoing arrangement. In a scenario envisaged by Jane Kaye and others, research participants whose tissues or biodata are stored in biobanks could be connected directly to researchers through, for example, a 'personalised, digital communication interface' facilitating 'two-way communication to stimulate a more engaged, informed and scientifically literate participant population where individuals can tailor and manage their own consent preferences' (2015, p. 141). The model is appealing, but it is difficult to see how it could operate in contexts where human tissues are commercialised, an increasingly common scenario.

In a nuanced exploration drawing on the anthropological concept of liminality – the state of in-betweenness – Laurie underscores the failure of the law to adequately address human experiential dimensions that relate to human health research. These experiential dimensions are especially relevant for patients undergoing surgical removal of their tissues. Laurie writes:

> The separation of elements of self can represent a form of crisis, necessitating new 'forms of process' to deal with what occurs. The crisis is often seen as new threats to privacy, or to a lesser extent to identity, through loss of control. . . . The myth of liminality can . . . assist our understanding here when we appreciate that liminality might not only [be] experienced by *persons*. The 'bounded objects' of health regulation . . . 'data', 'tissues', 'embryos' etc. – can also be seen in these terms.[3]
>
> (Laurie, 2016, p. 64)

Laurie offers the example of supernumerary embryos produced during the course of assisted reproduction technologies and procedures, citing Susan Squier's concept of 'liminal lives' to describe entities that are 'neither discarded by-product nor valued human being' (2004, p. 4). In focusing regulatory attention on attempting to turn such liminal lives into 'bounded objects', the law, continues Laurie, 'seems to overlook the experience for the data or tissue *subject*'. He proposes an 'alternative regulatory perspective' which would 'recognise and acknowledge the enduring connection between subject-object, and the potential identity-significant implications of this' (2016, pp. 64–65, italics in the original). These themes – liminality in relation to the 'bounded object' of human tissue, the interrelation of subject and object and the human experience of surgery – were explored through the making of *Habitation*.

Actions for the retrieval of the erased

During hip replacement surgery, the round, ball-like head of the femur bone and its associated stalk is cut off and removed to make space for the prosthetic implant. In advance of my own surgery, it was very important to me that I retain this small piece of bone that had worked so hard for me under the compromised conditions of hip dysplasia. That it could end up in a biohazardous waste stream seemed an intolerable transgression. In Australia, where my surgery would take place, regulatory authorities do allow patients to retain their surgically excised tissues. However, in a consultation with my orthopaedic surgeon six months prior to surgery, my request to retain my bone was cut off mid-sentence: 'you can't keep the bone'. I owe my success in eventually obtaining my femur head bone to my colleague, artist/academic Jaden J.A. Hastings, who in the lead-up to having surgery herself had extensively researched the policy settings in Australia and other jurisdictions regarding patient requests to retain surgically removed body parts.[4]

Her research revealed, for example, that the Australian Federal Government Department of Health (DoH) document *Requirements for the Retention of Laboratory Records and Diagnostic Material* outlines minimum standards for pathology laboratories who handle human body parts. For 'unprocessed' body parts, it states that although 'a pathology practice may own the container in which a patient's specimen is held, in most jurisdictions it does not legally own the specimen itself'. It goes on to require that the laboratory in question 'consider its duty of care to the patient before agreeing to release a specimen to the patient or next-of-kin', including 'assessing the reason for the applicant's request for an early release or return of the specimen, and using this information *to judge whether the request is reasonable*' (National Pathology Accreditation Advisory Council, Department of Health, 2018, p. 19, italics mine). The Royal College of Pathologists of Australasia (RCPA) adopts a similar position in the policy statement, *Return of Tissues to Patients*:

> Laboratories should have established protocols to permit compliance with patient requests for the return of body parts/tissue/prosthetic devices . . . while minimising any risks to patients and others from infection and toxic chemicals.
> (Royal College of Pathologists of Australasia, 2009/2013, p. 1)

The DoH document goes on to outline constraints on returns, including efforts to prevent trading in tissues and organs for transplantation, prevention of the spread of infectious diseases that may be carried within tissues, and assurances (records and signed receipts) that the applicant will dispose of the body part or foetus lawfully and responsibly (National Pathology Accreditation Advisory Council, Department of Health, 2018, p. 19). The RCPA policy outlines requirements for pathology laboratories to establish and document the 'legitimacy' of the applicant and to counsel patients in the safe handling and disposal of the specimen, including specimens containing the toxic chemical formalin (e.g. if burying in the garden, to do so sufficiently deeply to 'prevent retrieval by animals') (Royal College of Pathologists of Australasia, 2009/2013, p. 1).

In the light of the (albeit conditional) policy support for patients retaining their body parts, it is striking that most patients' requests to retain surgically excised body parts are met, as mine was at first, with a blank refusal. The paternalistic oversight and embedded power inequities inherent to pathology laboratories making decisions about whether a patient's request is 'reasonable' are clear. Beyond this, within the power relations of the surgeon-patient relationship, its time-poor context and the opaque bureaucracy of large hospitals, there seems little room for negotiation and dialogue. In my own case, I had come to that meeting with my surgeon armed with print-outs of the Australian standards and policy documents, at which he expressed genuine surprise and offered to check the situation. I followed up the meeting with a detailed email outlining my professional 'credentials', describing my intention to include the bone material in a work of art and assuring of my intention to comply with all regulatory frameworks including safe disposal of my 'biohazardous waste'. I attached a pre-prepared five-page consent form to be used on the day of my surgery, outlining responsibilities, waivers, extracts of the standards and policy documents discussed previously and a consent page for signing by patient and medical representative. Four months later, after follow-up email and phone call prompts, I received a brief letter from my surgeon stating that he had 'spoken with the hospital' and confirming that 'retaining the bone tissue following your hip replacement surgery with me on Monday, 3rd June will be allowed' (O'Sullivan, pers. comm., 2019).

But even for those armed with a high level of professional skill and legislative awareness, decisions seem to rest on the disposition of the surgeon and hospital, with no clear or consistent regulatory approach applied. Hastings' research indicates that most surgeons hold a firm belief that patient retention of excised body parts is forbidden.[5] Is this lack of awareness underpinned by the increasingly risk-averse, litigious environment that surgeons and hospitals are operating within? Does it reflect siloed medical practices where standards applied to one subdiscipline (pathology) exist with little awareness from an adjacent subdiscipline (surgery), despite the standards applying to 'objects' that both sub-disciplines routinely handle? Is it indicative of the persistent power imbalance between surgeons and their patients? Does it reflect the uncomfortable liminality of excised human tissues, occupying a 'no-place' of meaning within Western cultures?

In using my bone to make a work of art, I embodied a legal contradiction as one who exercised 'work or skill' on my femur bone material, thereby earning the legal right to own it, whilst simultaneously being ineligible to hold such property rights as the donor of that body part. The law has not yet envisaged the 'patient-artist' subject, who both donates and creates from that donation. Something that I had not envisaged, on the other hand, was that some of my own bone might be retained by the medical team and then entered into a monetised global medical market. The material in question was the more 'formless' bone scraped out of my hip cup (acetabulum), to create a stable surface for the prosthesis cup, and it had an equally formless fate. Prior to my surgery, I was invited to sign a consent form to release my bone for a bone donation program. I pictured a local not-for-profit transfer of excised bone to other patients-in-need; however, the bone might have in fact been incorporated into products – 'dust which forms a firm foundation for dental implants, putty used in spinal fusion, and pellets which are implanted as replacements of excised diseased bone' – sold in a 'global medical market' (Nuffield Council on Bioethics, 2011, p. 37). This market is sizable: according to Kateryna Hronska and Kamran Zamanian, the global orthopaedic biomaterials market, comprising allograft bone graft material and demineralised bone (both obtained from living donors) and synthetic bone graft substitutes, was estimated at approximately two billion US dollars in 2022, predicted to rise to 2.7 billion by 2029 (Hronska and Zamanian, 2023). There is a large chasm to scale from the 'no property in a body' rule to the global trade in body parts, the ancient legal principle seeming almost quaint in this context. The 'no property' rule and the Doodeward exception conspire to ensure that the only subjects in this global economy who are assured of *not* receiving monetary benefit from such a trade are the donors themselves.

I did not sign the bone donation consent form. This was because I had already gained permission to keep my surgically excised femur head bone and at the time had not considered my hip cup scrapings. Presumably, then, my hip cup bone material ended up in a biohazardous waste stream. I have been unable to determine the final resting place for such biomaterials, beyond establishing that such waste is cremated. What happens after that? Do my bone ashes rest in landfill? Were they incorporated into fertiliser? What other possible futures?

A certain kind of knowledge: performing ritual

Method for the production of bone china clay from human or animal bone material

1. *Procure bone, and remove excess soft tissue from around the bone.*
2. *Place the bone in a pot and boil for several hours, to render remaining soft tissue more pliable.*
3. *After boiling, scrape remaining soft tissue from the bone and wash well.*
4. *Place the bone in sunlight for a day or so, to thoroughly dry out.*

5. *Calcine the bone by placing it in a ceramics kiln and heating to a temperature of 1000°C.*
6. *Grind the calcined bone to a fine powder, using a mortar and pestle for small quantities, or a ball mill for large quantities.*
7. *Sift the ground bone ash through successively finer sieves, ending with a no. 80 mesh sieve.*
8. *Prepare a quantity of finely sieved Kaolin clay and Cornish stone powder.*
9. *Combine ingredients: 50% bone ash, 25% Kaolin clay, 25% Cornish stone by weight.*
10. *Add 25% by weight water initially, then more if needed to achieve good consistency, and wedge the clay to remove air bubbles and ensure a homogenous mix. The clay is now ready for use.*
11. *Fashion the bone china clay into the desired form, then allow to thoroughly dry.*
12. *Fire the greenware bone china at a temperature of 1150°C, using alumina for support if required.*

In their article on art, imagination and ritual, Paul Stenner and Tania Zittoun define rituals as processes that mediate across life ruptures, the 'liminal transitions' that 'threaten to disrupt the collective and individual lives of those whose worlds are transformed' and argue that art making can be considered 'technologies for facilitating liminal experiences of transition'. Referring to a previous article by Stenner, co-authored with Monica Greco (2018), they argue that 'art forms like painting, poetry, theater, music (and so forth)' constitute 'liminal affective technologies in their own right *when they are implicated in the transformation of the world of those engaging with them'* (Stenner and Zittoun, 2020, p. 246. Italics in the original). The performance of 'rituals' was central to the development of *Habitation*. The surgery itself could be considered to have ritual elements,[6] and art-making processes, including the production of bone china clay (described previously), engagement with my medical imaging scans and data and the ensuing dialogues prompted by these processes, could be conceived of as rituals, not least because of their transformational quality.

Bone china production entails an alchemical-like transformation, one that turns bone material into its mineral constituents. During the calcining stage (step 5 above), in which bone is heated in a ceramics kiln to 1000 degrees Celsius (the same temperature as cremation) and the carbon-based matter is burnt off, only the constituent mineral content of bone – calcium, iron from red blood cells and mineral trace elements such as copper and selenium – remains. The following steps use this 'mineralised' bone to make bone china clay, after which a second round of intense kiln heat catalyses a further molecular rearrangement, to produce the bone china object. To honour the material, symbolic and spiritual potential embedded in my surgically excised femur bone head, I used my bone material to make a white bone china replica of my excised femur head. I also made pale creamy-coloured earthenware ceramic replicas of my pelvis and femur bones – the bones that remain in my body. All bone forms were cast from 3D prints based on 3D data exported from my pre-surgery CT scan. In the finished *Habitation* artwork (which can be seen on the front cover of this book), the bone china femur head sits inside a display cabinet, adjacent to the other bones.

Engaging with my own bone during the making of *Habitation* unlocked a cascade of realisations and offered forms of knowledge that, I believe, would not have arrived in other ways. I liken the experience to the hands-on ritual of washing the body of a deceased loved one, as described by Jenny Briscoe-Hough, Founder and Director of a community funeral home in Port Kembla, Australia. Here, she falteringly searches for language to describe the transmission of a certain form of 'knowledge' that results from this hands-on engagement:

something happens I think when you put your hands on the body of someone who you love and care about who has died . . . your body . . . gets a message from that. It's like . . . maybe a mimetic sort of memory, something happens in the *body*, so that your body somehow understands that that person has died.

(Fidler and Briscoe-Hough, 2018)

Holding my femur head in the palm of my hand and turning it over, I marvelled at my wildly mis-shapen bone – where a femur head would normally be a smooth round ping-pong ball shape, mine had a very significant, overhanging mushroom-like overgrowth on one side of the head and a worn away surface on the other. It was as if the cells of my bone had, over the years, made a collective decision to gradually migrate east. I felt a sense of wonder at bone's capacity to remodel itself. In *The Secret Life of Bones* (2019), Brian Switek notes that although we may think of bone as our deepest infrastructure, our ultimate scaffold, strong, solid, unchanging, it is in fact as dynamic as skin or any other bodily tissue – in constant dialogue with the cellular soup in which it resides, remodelling itself according to moment-to-moment conditions and pressures. It is engaged in an ongoing fluent dialogue with the planetary force of gravity in an elegant enactment of the collapse of an inside-outside or human-planet binary. My bone probably adapted and improvised over the years in the face of its congenitally abnormal condition, displaying its capacity for plasticity and inventiveness. Perhaps the mushroom overgrowth was protective, an attempt at increased stability, or perhaps some other gesture impervious to human imagination but following the inner logic of bone.

Gazing at my bone, I also understood fully how abnormal it really was and why surgery had become a necessary path. I did not gain this knowledge from examining my CT scan: although the scan clearly shows the mushroom head in flattened cross-sectional form, this did not support me to achieve the necessary act of spatial reconstruction, to learn the shape of my bone tactilely, using my hands and fingers. Surgical interventions enact sudden, violent changes to our bodily integrity, even whilst being life-giving and life-saving. Handling my actual bone and developing the artwork helped me to make sense of the demands of surgery and my decision to undertake it and to support my adaptation to sudden bodily change. It offered me an avenue to comprehend and make meaning of pain and to hold the contradictory responses of wonder and pain simultaneously. I believe this deeper, fuller imaginary and embodied knowledge of the interior of my body influenced my engagement in the long, intricate post-surgical process of rehabilitation.[7] The ritual also offered an avenue to express a form of gratitude to the small piece of bone that had worked so hard, under compromised conditions, all of my life.

That this bone might have ended up in landfill is, I feel, one of the unacknowledged violences of contemporary medicine. Retaining one's own excised bodily tissues is not meaningful to everyone, and the significance we give to particular tissues and organs also varies. Yet based on a series of *Tooth Fairies for Adults* workshops I have run with members of the broader community, individuals have reported consistently that pre-surgery requests to retain excised pieces of their bodies were refused.[8] Whilst for most this was not a devastating loss, there was a persistent vocalisation of a kind of quiet outrage, a sense of impotence and incomprehension, that some unnamed miscarriage of justice and power had been enacted.

As *Habitation* began its tour in 2021, a story broke in the Australian media that brought public attention to issues of justice and power in relation to human tissue – and that illustrated the importance of both rituals and more dynamic models of consent, in resolving them. The news report revealed that 7000 blood samples taken from First Nations Australians in the 1960s had been held for five decades without consent in a laboratory at the Australian National University (ANU) (Higgins, 2021). The story described the shock and distress experienced by members of the Galiwin'ku community from Elcho Island in the Torres Strait on first learning that 200 samples taken from their ancestors were held in the collection. Over the course of three years and extensive dialogue with ANU scientists (the ANU project lead Azure Hermes was herself a First Nations woman who had family members represented in the collection), the community decided to allow DNA to be extracted from the samples whilst returning the remainder of the blood to their homelands, where it was honoured in an on-Country ceremony. Galiwin'ku community elders and leaders travelled to the ANU to engage with the blood samples and the ANU team and to install a permanent memorial of Galiwin'ku Larrakitj burial poles on the ANU campus to represent the return of the blood samples. Young leader Cyril Bukulatjpi commented:

> When we see the blood of the person or hear of the person that has passed away, we acknowledge them by getting emotional, we also cry and sing. . . . For a young person like me, today is really monumental.

> (cited in Higgins, 2021)

What is striking about the Galiwin'ku community's process is its dialogic nature, which enabled solutions to be found that balanced the community's desire to benefit from contemporary biomedical science whilst simultaneously satisfying long-held spiritual and cultural practices. This dialogic approach can also be seen in current protocols for the collection of 'biomaterials' from First Nations Australians for biomedical research, which has strong ethical oversight from the Indigenous and non-Indigenous communities, acknowledging the frequent colonial abuses of power enacted on Indigenous Australians and recognising that tissues separated from the body can have strong cultural significance and can embody connection to ancestors.

For non-First Nations communities in Australia and in other Western cultures, I would argue that there is, largely speaking, a lack of cultural context for such values and practices (outside of the reverence paid to bodies of the deceased, and the – arguably inadequate – consent processes which aim to regulate what is done to patients' biomaterials). There is also a distinct lack of dialogic process surrounding patients' requests to retain excised tissues, in a context where the time and resources available for such dialogue do not exist.

The practices of artists working with body parts removed in medical contexts cannot be compared to the deeply embedded cultural practices of First Nations cultures. However, it is, in part, the work of artists to undertake acts of redemption and reclamation and to find languages for objects and entities whose status would otherwise be adrift from culturally legible meaning and purpose. One context for this are major surgical interventions and the bodily, emotional and identity transformations that ensue, which draw patients into a state of liminal transition that merits exploration and memorialisation through 'ritual' art-making processes.

An ancient waste

Most people, including myself, express surprise upon first learning that 'bone china' is made from actual bone. Despite the strong clue embedded in the name, perhaps it is the seeming incongruity of bone china's association with fine English teas, colliding with the implied visceral brutality of obtaining bone from animal bodies. Using bone material to make a bone china object brings into dialogue two seemingly incongruent ideas: the 'animality' of bone china and the 'minerality' of animals. This offers a deconstructive and metaphoric gesture that reveals underlying structures of material connectivity between living and non-living entities that are not immediately available to our sensory perception. The intricate process of making bone china – extracting bone from animal bodies, reducing it to its mineral constituents and deploying its calcium content to provide the strength that is characteristic of bone china – enacts a kind of 'ritualised' demonstration of 'animal minerality'. Bone china clays can be purchased commercially pre-prepared. However, the insights I discuss in this chapter would not have arrived for me had I not engaged with and touched with my skin, the basic constituent components of my bone minerality during the making of the clay.

When a prosthetic object takes up residence in the human body, multi-layered 'intimacies' occur between living tissues and inanimate materials, offering a medically mediated embodiment of what philosopher Monika Bakke has termed 'lithic intimacy': life's diverse, intimate relationships of exchange and inter-species companionship with minerals (2018). Whilst the collapse of the animate-inanimate boundary is made explicit through contemporary prosthetic implants, Bakke notes that such intimacies have existed since the earliest origins of life, highlighting the artificial constructed nature of an animate-inanimate binary. Citing minerologist Robert Hazen on the 'intimate interplay of life and rocks' (Hazen, 2014), Bakke writes:

> Minerals change and diversify when they come into contact with life. . . . What we need now is not a belief in the solitude and indifference of minerals, but a celebration of their response-ability to life and creative elaborations on their diversity. Art can offer ways to articulate how minerals and life attract and seduce each other, and how minerals open up to life's intimate strategies, the outcomes of which cannot be determined.
>
> (n.d.)

In the making of *Habitation*, I explored what Bakke further describes as the 'intimate encounter between life and minerals', seeking to challenge perceptions of the body as a passive recipient of human-engineered implants. My titanium/ceramic hip implant is 'cementless', meaning no adhesives were used to attach the implant to my bone. Rather, the implant has a hydroxyapatite coating that stimulates my own bone cells to grow into tiny fissures in the implant coating. It is the ongoing dynamic renewal of these cells that holds my implant in place, now and into the future. The ultimate success of the forceful medical intervention of hip replacement surgery depends upon the ongoing quiet agency of cells to 'perform' this adhesion, a process of life-long cellular infiltration and renewal. Between two biocompatible materials – living bone and prosthesis – deeply embedded and entangled with each other, molecular and atomic exchanges will inevitably take place at the dynamic interface between bone and implant, resulting in the dissolution of a clear separation between myself and the prosthetic new-comer, a dissolving of the animate–inanimate boundary. In *Habitation*, I attached metallic coral forms to the sites in the ceramic sculpture where my actual hip prosthesis is embedded in my real bones. The intimate relationships of exchange taking place in coral between soft-bodied organisms and their calciferous structures offer an analogy to the osteo-integration of human bone cells into the mineral structure of prostheses.

Human-created medical interventions such as prosthetic implants make explicit the collapse of the animate–inanimate boundary. However, such medical technologies rely on the already-existing capacity of biological entities to incorporate and forge biologically meaningful relationships to (an)other. This is the deep-time evolutionary history of life on Earth – one long experiment in the promiscuous exchange of nucleic, proteinaceous, lipid, mineral and other biologically active molecular species. The boundary collapse I explore in *Habitation* barely warrants a mention in the long evolutionary history of how animals and minerals have cooperated and co-evolved, to their mutual benefit. Handling my own bone also unlocked imaginary spaces for me about the deep time history of vertebrate minerality. 'Skeletons dramatize an ancient waste, whispering a ghostly testimony to the useful internalization of hazardous waste sites', writes Dorion Sagan, proposing an origin story for bone in our early vertebrate progenitors (1992, p. 368). The first vertebrates evolved in sea water. The calcium phosphate in bone owes its origin, according to Sagan, to the necessity of eukaryotic cells to manage the high concentration of calcium in the surrounding sea water that would have been toxic to the intracellular environments of cells. He suggests that early vertebrates bioaccumulated excess calcium phosphate in discreet 'hazardous waste sites' within their own bodies in order to maintain intracellular calcium concentrations at no higher than the physiologically viable level of around one in ten million. At some stage these biohazardous waste sites found useful redeployment as bones, which performed, amongst other things, the essential role of scaffold support when vertebrates moved onto land and were subject to the collapsing forces of gravity. The changing role of calcium and bone itself, across this timescale, destabilises a view of bone's 'inevitability' and brings to the fore the contingent nature of bone's existence and function and biology's always-in-process inventive and improvisatory ontology.

Acknowledgements

Grateful thanks to Bec Dean Carolyn Johnston; City of Joondalup, Perth; Corin Group; Experimenta Media Arts, Melbourne; Jan Guy; Jaden J.A. Hastings; Jonathan Parsons; Lizzie Crouch; Lubi Thomas; Michael O'Sullivan. *Habitation* was assisted by the Australian Government through the Australia Council for the Arts, its arts funding and advisory body.

Notes

1 The Experimenta *Life Forms* International Triennial of Media Art was curated by Jonathan Parsons and Lubi Thomas, Associate Curator Jessica Clark.
2 See, for example, *R v. Kelly*, cited in Mason and Laurie, 2001, p. 721.
3 Laurie acknowledges the insights of collaborator Paul Stenner for the expression 'forms of process'.
4 I cite Australian policies since this is the jurisdiction in which I undertook my surgery. However, extensive prior research undertaken by my colleague Jaden J.A. Hastings found that these policies were replicated in other jurisdictions Hastings examined. Personal communication, Jaden J.A. Hastings.
5 A colleague who underwent hip replacement surgery in 2022 had her request to retain her bone met with hostile, almost aggressive anger from her surgeon. This is despite the fact that she had almost identical 'credentials' to mine and went to her surgeon armed with the same policy documents. Although a nurse was charged with looking into the request, my colleague experienced what she believes to have been hospital 'delaying' tactics until the date of her surgery, by which time it was too late. There is a notable exception to the difficulties described in obtaining body parts in the case of pregnancy and childbirth. Requests for the bodies of deceased pre-term foetuses are often supported, and the bodies of still-born babies routinely supported, although this was not the case in the past. Today, the 'personal significance' of the child's body to the parents and the associated grief is clear, culturally legible and condoned. Requests to retain placentas after childbirth are also now routinely made and supported, with practices such as burying placentas in places of significance to the parents and the conversion of placentas into nutritional supplements now widespread and accepted.
6 These include the ritual of placing a patient into an altered state of consciousness through anaesthesia, the rituals of hygiene and infection control, the ritual of slicing into the patient's body then carefully stitching it up and so forth. The 'rituals' inherent in the performance of surgery are also explored in two other chapters in this volume. The first is by Steve Reid, Laurie Rauch and Alp Numanogluin, and the second by Christina Lammer, Tamar Tembeck and Wilfried Wisser, both found in Part 2 of this volume.
7 Santa Fe–based artist Christine Cassano also made a sculptural work (using porcelain and mirror) which responded to and attempted to articulate the experience of hip replacement surgery. Cassano described it as 'my way of working through what had happened inside my body' (cited in Trimble, 2023).
8 *Tooth Fairies for Adults* workshops were conducted within public programs for the Experimenta *Life Forms* International Triennial of Media Art, in which *Habitation* was exhibited. Thanks to Experimenta Director Jonathan Parsons for suggesting the linkage of the Tooth Fairies ritual to my work.

Reference list

Bakke, M. (2017) Art and Metabolic Force in Deep Time Environments. *Environmental Philosophy* 14(1), pp. 41–59. doi:10.5840/envirophil20173744

Bakke, M. (2018) 'A rock of one's own: lithic intimacy in art and science' [Presentation]. FEMeeting: Women in Art, Science and Technology Symposium.

Bakke, M. (no date) *Mineral companionship of evolving environments*. Available at: www.udk-berlin.de/forschung/temporaere-forschungseinrichtungen/dfg-graduiertenkolleg-das-wissen-der-kuenste/veranstaltungsarchiv-des-dfg-graduiertenkollegs/tuning-into-worlds-more-than-human-aesthetics-in-the-arts/monika-bakke-mineral-companionships-of-evolving-environments/ (Accessed: 21 May 2022).

Doodeward v Spence [1908] 6 C.L.R., pp. 406–407.

Fidler, R. and Briscoe-Hough, J. (2018) *Best of 2018: Jenny Briscoe-Hough* [Podcast]. Conversations. Available at: www.abc.net.au/radio/programs/conversations/jenny-briscoe-hough-best-of/10583146 (Accessed: 11 December 2018).

Hazen, R. (2014) 'Mineral fodder', *Aeon*. Available at: https://aeon.co/essays/how-life-made-the-earth-into-a-cosmic-marvel (Accessed: 11 July 2023).

Higgins, I. (2021) *Blood samples taken from Indigenous community more than 50 years ago to be returned*. Available at: www.abc.net.au/news/2021-05-27/blood-samples-stored-at-anu-returned-to-indigenous-community/100164322 (Accessed: 27 May 2021).

Hronska, K. and Zamanian, K. (2023) *Evolution of the global orthopedic biomaterials market*. Available at: www.odtmag.com/contents/view_online-exclusives/2023-04-10/evolution-of-global-orthopedic-biomaterials-market/ (Accessed: 25 June 2023).

Kaye, J. *et al.* (2015) 'Dynamic consent: a patient interface for twenty-first century research networks', *European Journal of Human Genetics*, 23, pp. 141–146. https://doi.org/10.1038/ejhg.2014.71

Laurie, G. (2016) 'Liminality and the limits of law in health research regulation', *Medical Law Review*, 25(1), pp. 47–72. https://doi.org/10.1093/medlaw/fww029

Mason, K. and Laurie, G. (2001) 'Consent or property? Dealing with the body and its parts in the shadow of Bristol and Alder Hey', *The Modern Law Review*, 64(5), pp. 710–729.

National Pathology Accreditation Advisory Council, Department of Health (2018) *Requirements for the retention of laboratory records and diagnostic material*. 7th edn. Available at: www.health.gov.au/internet/main/publishing.nsf/Content/B8562E2C3D131ED8CA257BF00019153C/$File/20180612%20-%20Final%20-%20Retention.pdf (Accessed: 3 November 2018).

Nuffield Council on Bioethics (2011) *Human bodies: donation for medicine and research*. Available at: www.nuffieldbioethics.org/publications/human-bodies-donation-for-medicine-and-research (Accessed: 15 June 2023).

O'Sullivan, M. (2019) Personal communication [email] with the author. *Approval* [email].

R v Kelly (1998) 3 A11 ER 741. Cited in Mason and Laurie, 2001, p. 721.

Royal College of Pathologists of Australasia (2009/2013) *Return of tissue to patients*, Policy No. 1/2009. p. 1 Available at: www.rcpa.edu.au/getattachment/e4d48c26-22c0-4106-8211-4965346f5bee/Return-of-Tissue-to-Patients.aspx (Accessed: 3 November 2018).

Sagan, D. (1992) 'Metametazoa: biology and multiplicity', in Crary, J. and Kwinter, S. (eds.) *Incorporations*. New York: Zone Books, pp. 362–385. Cited in Bakke, 2017, p. 52.

Skene, L. (2002) 'Arguments against people legally "owning" their own bodies, body parts and tissue', *Macquarie Law Journal*, 165, pp. 1–11. Available at: http://classic.austlii.edu.au/au/journals/MqLawJl/2002/7.html

Squier, S. M. (2004) *Liminal lives: imagining the human at the frontiers of biomedicine*. Durham: Duke University Press.

Stenner, P. and Greco, M. (2018) 'On "the magic mountain": the novel as liminal affective technology', *International Political Anthropology*, 11, pp. 43–60.

Stenner, P. and Zittoun, T. (2020) 'On taking a leap of faith: art, imagination, and liminal experiences', *Journal of Theoretical and Philosophical Psychology*, 40(4), pp. 240–263.

Switek, B. (2019) *The secret life of bones: their origins, evolution and fate*. London: Duckworth Books.

Trimble, L. (2023) 'A body of work inspired by one hip replacement', *Hyperallergic*. Available at: https://hyperallergic.com/799423/a-body-of-work-inspired-by-one-hip-replacement/ (Accessed: 16 February 2023).

41

WAITING ROOM

Material moments of medicine as performance

Annja Neumann with Uta Baldauf

Looming Futures: Waiting Room is a site-specific performance by four actors and dancers, first staged at Atelier Stroud in September 2021. The production draws on practice as research to explore how public spaces were repurposed into temporary health care spaces during the COVID-19 pandemic in the UK. It asks how people structure their engagement with medicine in terms of performance rather than narrative in traditional and new medical settings, for instance, in outpatient clinics and pop-up testing sites. The production engages with the potential of waiting rooms to spatialise health care and to facilitate role changes in medical practice. Spaces of waiting serve as a magnifying glass to expand the understanding of the staging conditions in diagnostic situations and how they inform the terms of the therapeutic encounter. *Waiting Room* provokes through its lack of plot. In this way, it aims to make perceptible the type of roles audience performers play in medical settings.

The Atelier, the venue for the first production, is a craft and textile workshop located in a part of south-west England that is known for its woollen mills, where spinners and weavers worked from as early as 1400. The broadcloth made there – dyed with the famous Stroudwater scarlet – was traded around the world, often for use in bright red military uniforms. Now it supplies the green felts found on tennis balls and snooker tables. Inspired by these fabrics and textiles, *Waiting Room* addressed patterns of movement and interweaving, in particular in relation to questions of materiality in medicine as performance and as illuminated by the coronavirus pandemic. Three material moments that cross-connected between medical, digital and theatrical waiting spaces will focus this account of the production: a hospital-theatre screen, rustling plastic bags and a knitted square. In this way, the snapshot will not provide a full account of the performance but concentrate on specific material arrangements in medicine that demand role changes, new roles and affect patient agency.

A second production of *Waiting Room* took place in the public gallery of the Stroud Valley Artspace (SVA) in the town centre nearly a year later.[1] At the time of these productions, bodies in stillness had become a familiar sight, whether boxed in squares on a Zoom screen, prone in rectangular bedspaces or confined through protecting screens in pop-up vaccination centres. In what follows, I focus on the first production but also consider aspects of the second.

Waiting Room, a medicalised performance space, examined moments of disruption, practices of waiting and the medicalisation of everyday life, drawn from the first eighteen months of the first lockdown in the UK, from March 2020. Medicalised spaces can appear to demand that users

DOI: 10.4324/9781003036500-47

perform, given their frontstage backstage design and given the plethora of scripted roles into which patients are meant to fit, for instance doctor/patient, expert/non-expert. *Waiting Room* explored how people structure their engagement with medicine in terms of performance and how their roles changed when mobile modes of medicine moved into new public settings. It was structured around three clinical practices that mark phases of a patient's journey in hospital – those of waiting: admission, treatment and discharge.

Admission: becoming one body

Upon arrival at the performance, participants wait to be registered; and are immediately treated as patients. A crisp registration requires participants to disinfect their hands, complete an admission form, and follow directions after being identified with a number. This dictates where everybody sits in the courtyard of the SVA Artspace. Second, participants then wait for a collective and choreographed lateral flow COVID test to start. Performer 1 demonstrates the testing movement: opening the extraction tube, the extraction buffer sachet, nasal swab, wiping the swab around the inside of each nostril ten times and placing two drops on the test strip.

Third, between each step we wait until everyone has completed the action. It is strangely bonding to perform the test together. Participants surrender to the manipulative force of theatricalisation of the lateral flow test, meticulously following every step of the instructions. Fourth, this synchronous movement is followed by fifteen anxious minutes of waiting for test results. Every second is marked by the ticking of an egg timer.

Eventually, two dancers, who had participated in the test, peel off and start re-tracing microgestures from the test action. The combination of mime and contact dance they use becomes more expansive and surreal when they re-perform the test sequence. They slip into an absurdist narrative. Waiting moves through their bodies like the drops falling onto the test strip. And their grotesque gestures suddenly wipe a massive imaginary swab around the courtyard, expand the space and are charmingly anarchic. Through these moments of dissent the dancers break away from the audience as one body, spurring critical spectatorship.

Finally, participants who tested negative are ushered inside and seated in front of a white screen waiting for a Zoom projection to begin.

Throughout the performance, performers and participants explored the transformative potential of the waiting room: through role changes, changes of locale and playful intervention. The latter were mostly initiated through a textile screen, generally moving from clinical intervention toward a theatrical encounter.

The *Waiting Room* resembles site-specific performance pieces that explore medical dramaturgy, such as *An Anatomie in Four Quarters* (2011) by UK-based performance company Clod Ensemble. In that case, dance and audience movement are used to dissect the space of the theatre (Willson, 2016, p. 152). *Waiting Room* likewise aims to understand how performance and medicine theatricalises public spaces. The objective is to explore how this new theatricality of health care, when relocated in hybrid spaces, affects participant's agency or their ability to respond to a situation. Theatricalisation for this purpose is defined as a manipulative force that, on the one hand, perpetuates established regimes of representation and, on the other, encourages critical spectatorship through the failure of meaning making (Brandstetter, 2005). Moreover, *Waiting Room* explores the moment when space becomes an active agent: when it starts to participate in the action.

Most particularly, the production explored the waiting room – a space found in both theatrical and medical worlds. In the theatrical world, this could mean a space located backstage or in a foyer, and, as it happens, waiting is 'an oft-neglected part of every performance's dramaturgy, affecting both performers and spectators' (Fischer-Lichte, Weiler and Jost, 2021, p. 19). In health care settings, equally, clinical protocols and spaces are designed to accommodate designated phases of waiting. This prescribed waiting alleviates material pressures in health care but also creates a specific performative dynamic. Crucially, spaces of waiting act like magnifying glasses when theatricalised. Waiting rooms spatialise medical care. In other words, they create a particular presence that makes perceptible material and spatial relations between theatrical performance and medicine, particularly in diagnostic situations.

COVID-19 spurred a medical visibility unprecedented in the last two decades. Public buildings were urgently converted into hospital facilities during the first UK wave, hotels and exhibition spaces were turned into critical care facilities; medical spaces became integral to our everyday experience to the extent that we lived in some of them. Even living rooms became territories of quarantine. This medicalisation of everyday life and the major shift it caused to spatial and performative arrangements sets the scene for the production. The performance constantly moves between various public and private spaces, spurred through specific activities or changes of location and perspectives.

Aesthetically, *Waiting Room* explored self-isolation and COVID-19 spaces by working with the shape of a square. We used this to reference shifts experienced in the pandemic, which moved medicine beyond institutional boundaries – referring in our work to a makeshift testing centre in a courtyard of an art gallery and a craft and textile workshop, to care undertaken behind a rectangular sheet used as curtain, on a computer screen for online consultation or by drawing rattling cubicle curtains around participants. Through this critical play with spaces, which was undertaken using a mix of semi-improvised dance and semi-scripted performance, *Waiting Room* created places of medical confinement. It medicalised courtyards, through gazebos and strict protocols, transformed an art gallery and textile workshop into a clinical space and a theatrical stage through various regimes of looking and role changes and took waiting 'to the streets' by temporarily seating audience members on chairs outside the gallery window to look into the action.

Together performers, health care professionals, dancers and spectators continuously repurposed these rectangular spaces through our interactions and by changing their spatial arrangement with military precision and playful absurdity. In the era of the pandemic, this iterative re-configuration of square-shaped spaces engaged with the confining of our actions to a single room and with the remixing of physical and virtual space. We were interested in exploring COVID-19 aesthetics, their material effects and affects, asking where the arrows on the floor, the Zoom windows place us and how the performativity of the pandemic not only medicalised our daily life but also theatricalised it. Everybody became an actor in *Waiting Room*. These spaces of waiting, and the ways they moved us, open up questions about compliance, surrender and border-crossing: who is an actor and who is acted *upon* in medical and theatrical settings?

Waiting Room invites participants to articulate their health stories or what they bring to the space through a set of embodied practices that reach beyond narrative and that might also refer to stories that could not be told, for instance by patients on ventilators. We used sensory and embodied modes of storytelling developed by artist-researcher and dancer Sally Dean in the second production and placed them in a diagnostic and artistic environment. As for you, reader of this chapter, the piece exposed participants to a high level of uncertainty about what would happen next in the waiting room, especially when they were seated in front of the screen in the middle of the gallery space, and they had to wait until their number was called by one of the health professionals or until the action behind the screen, described later in this chapter.

The fabrics and textiles of our rehearsal spaces in Atelier Stroud informed the practice of dramaturgy, particularly methods of interweaving, the creation of diffractive or entangled spaces and the choreographic use of strings. The performance was mutually constituted by all participants. Using a diffractive dramaturgy means that it had no predetermined plot or set characters, nor did it tell a preconceived story. Rather it involved different phases of waiting in various locations for material relations and stories to unfold. The performance is structured across the three themes already introduced as key to the experience of waiting: admission, treatment and discharge. *Waiting Room* explores material moments that cross-connect between medical, digital and theatrical spaces. In what follows, three material moments of the performance are focused on more deeply: a hospital-theatre screen, rustling plastic bags and a knitted square.

Here I draw on conversations with three co-creators: co-director, performer and student nurse Uta Baldauf and choreographers and dancers Brenda Waite and Alexandra Howard. Our discussion will be criss-crossed by contributions from members of the ensemble and from audience members. This mode of documentation responds to the analytical difficulties posed by participatory performances where audience members frequently become 'acting spectators' (Kolesch and Warstat, 2019, p. 312). My own role here was as co-director and performer. Here, we present our work in relation to multiple and unavoidably partial perspectives.

Setting the scene

Uta Baldauf's description of her routine as a student nurse and her performance in *Waiting Room* inform two key material moments of the piece. Audience members first encounter Baldauf as Performer 1 at the reception desk in Atelier Stroud. She also demonstrates the lateral flow test later in the admission phase. In both, she performs as a health care professional.

Uta: Working in a busy medical ward is like stepping onto a stage: when I put on my uniform and enter the corridor, I act like a performer who gives focus to detail in a fast-moving play. If I don't put on my smile the space around me can turn against me. The hospital is like a maze and the uniformity can produce an uncanny feeling of déjà vu. Many vulnerable patients experience a delirium that is triggered by the environment. For some, it even feels like prison, and paranoia begins to creep in. To counter these effects, I have to balance my clinical tasks with acts of compassion and some of that is achieved by performing a part until it becomes authentic. Theatrical fourth walls are created by curtains drawn around hospital bedsides producing an illusion of privacy. They function like a tent where you can hear your neighbours breathe. Voices travel, while shoes and feet are observed from under the curtain. We willingly and unwillingly become part of another person's unfolding drama. Strangers become allies, counsellors or friends, and others can turn into enigmas, with misunderstandings, even turning somebody into a temporary villain. Inevitably, waiting separates procedures and clinical tasks. These stretches of frozen time hang like a static existence, surrounded by the stream of busy practitioners, the patient waiting for the practitioner to step into the orbit of a shared relativity. The shift and change of people's lives are conducted by the feedback and attention of the practitioner.

The stage design: diffracting space

The curtains drawn around a bedside became the main prop for our performance. We used a white sheet to interrelate the white cubicle curtains in hospitals to computer screens and curtains used in theatres, using projection to help. This screen divided the main stage into a large waiting area and an intimate space behind the screen. We used this division to stage border-crossings between public and private, patients and doctors, audience members and performers, as well as in-person participants and avatars. We were attentive to the differences and similarities the waiting rooms generated and to the effects these 'border-crossings' had on participants. We also used three movable curtains across the main gallery window for the SVA production. Waiting became increasingly theatrical through a choreographed curtain drawing movement, particularly for passers-by on the street. Three performers simultaneously drew a curtain each across the main gallery window to mark every scene change.

Rustling plastic bags (in unison)

The admission phase of the first production took place in the courtyard in front of the Atelier, surrounded by Piccadilly Mill brick buildings, a car park and residential houses. Here trestle tables were repurposed to form part of a temporary testing site. COVID-19 lateral flow test kits were carefully laid out to be socially distanced.

What followed was the performance of a collective COVID-19 lateral flow test. Once the nurse completed her instructions, a rustling sound was heard. Although participants were no longer required to move together, all audience members simultaneously opened the plastic bags provided in their test kits to discard their swabs. A crumpled crackling of rustling refuse filled the air. In this moment of sudden convergence, the audience became one body. It was as if the simultaneous rustling confirmed their surrender to the forced testing regime.

COVID choreographies

Waiting Room used dance improvisation to explore spatial relations between performance and medicine. Two dancers retraced, repeated and abstracted clinical protocols and the performativity of the pandemic based on the found movement of the collective lateral flow test. And they repeated and re-performed these movements in semi-scripted scenes, to create an interactive movement score. Such operations are suggestive of what Brandstetter, Egert and Hartung have called 'a double movement, a countermovement, a repeated movement, which in turn follows paths, threads, and lines of deconstruction' (2019, p. 3). Interwoven performance cultures of this kind cannot be tracked back to a fixed origin or identity.

Brenda Waite and Alex Howard, who created and performed the movement together (in the first production), describe the first movement score.

Brenda: We began by placing ourselves in the environment in a pedestrian mode while the audience arrived and spent time chatting. This created a frame for the space and performance to come.

Alex: We then took on the movements generated by the act of real-time lateral flow testing. Micro-gestures and functional movements of opening packets, swabbing, placing and re-placing phials, paper and plastic testers became gestures, at once abstract and impersonal. That said, being impersonal was nigh on impossible since we were two people, two dancers performing: Brenda and me. We were on our feet, and occupied with the flow of performance, in contrast to the 'testers' who were seated, at trestle tables, and waiting for their results.

Brenda: We worked from literal movement to forms of abstraction, exaggeration, repetition, and stylisation that brought tone and energy to our gestures. This led to more extreme postures and positions. We used our surroundings, for instance, by leaning against a wall, by lying on the ground, or by coming close to the audience. For me, there was an underlying emotional quality about all this, as well as an element of parody. We explored this last quality by playing with the absurdity of the swabbing gesture. As time passed, we increased the spatial frame by moving further away from the audience.

Alex: The audience participants received their results and were duly ushered inside. The door closed. Brenda and I waited outside. We were not part of that experience although we knew, in outline, what it was. We waited once again later in the piece. This was when the audience was ushered deeper into the Atelier building. I found that these two instances of waiting were a 'waiting-for', a prescribed waiting for a designated but unknown experience.

Treatment and discharge: materialised sensations and undoing knitted squares

At this point, just after test results had been checked in the performance, I take over the account of the performance. As Performer 2 in *Waiting Room*, I handed out a handcrafted piece of fabric, shaped in a square that would fit into the palm of the hands. Audience members were invited to present this to two performers in the next phase before they were asked to unravel it and to participate in a choreography with their string. The knitted squares symbolised COVID spaces, the spaces of confinement and the deprivations endured during COVID-19. And undoing them released material to re-imagine how to reconnect with each other in medicalised spaces.

The treatment phase in the piece involves several interventions. As participants become increasingly restless on their chairs, lined up in front of the theatre-hospital screen, and sat in the middle of the SVA gallery in the second production, they wait for their number to be called out by a nurse. The atmosphere for those waiting in front of the screen resembles that of a sterile NHS outpatient waiting room. A nurse routinely moves three curtains across the gallery windows. By contrast, performers behind the screen use an experimental somatic mode of applied storytelling developed by Sally Dean for the therapeutic encounter. The latter responds to the public space of an art gallery in the second production by crafting the clinical encounter and health stories into a material object. Participants are called behind the screen in pairs and asked to identify a part of their body that requires attention. A performer attends to each participant and creates a cast of the chosen body part with silk paper by carefully touching and moulding the paper and indirectly the body. A soft crinkling sound blends in with the periodic sound of moving curtains. Participants are asked to take their cast with them, followed by another period of waiting and the request to place or hang up their moulded sensations on red strings running across the gallery. The performance finishes with participants sat outside on the street, looking into the gallery and waiting for the curtains behind the gallery window to open. This location change turned them into active spectators again, watching how their sensations and the care administered to their bodies materialised in floating objects in the gallery. A choreographed curtain movement across the gallery window by the three nurses finishes the performance.

Audience Member: A screen divided the waiting room from the narrow entrance area of the mill barn. It was created through a white sheet strung from a tie beam. We were sitting in front of the screen, waiting to be admitted to a virtual Zoom room. All of a sudden, the sheet resembled a computer screen. A Zoom meeting with the same nurse, who had welcomed me, was projected onto the screen. This time, her movements were constrained by the square of the Zoom box, her body truncated across the chest. My hand pressed against a hand-knitted square on my knee. The soft feel of the wool was a tactile reminder of my location. I twined the loose ends around my fingers.

Then it was my turn, and I entered the intimate space behind the screen. I completely forgot about the audience on the other side. There were three women behind the screen holding a long red string. They asked me to pick a string from a selection of much shorter strings and to tie it to their string. I had no idea why I was doing this. Asked to show my knitted square I became part of the action and almost felt a kind of sadness when I am instructed to unravel it later on.

Background and credits

Co-direction and production: Annja Neumann, Uta Baldauf
Choreography: Brenda Waite, Alex Howard
Poetic script: Annja Neumann
Movement created with and performed by:
Brenda Waite, Alex Howard, Uta Baldauf, Sally Dean, and Rebecca McMillan

Performance created with and performed by:

Performer 1: Uta Baldauf (Atelier) and Rebecca McMillan (SVA)
Performer 2: Annja Neumann
Performer 3: Brenda Waite;
Performer 4: Alex Howard (Atelier) and Sally Dean (SVA)

Produced in association with Atelier Stroud and supported by the SVA. Research funded by the Isaac Newton Trust and Cambridge Digital Humanities at the University of Cambridge.
Looming Futures: Waiting Room was first performed at Atelier Stroud in Gloucestershire, 2021.

Note

1 The piece is documented here. Available at: www.sva.org.uk/events/2020/3/28/waiting-room and here as a short video film: https://youtu.be/by0_NhPxYIA [accessed 14 December 2023].

Reference list

Brandstetter, G. (2005) *Bild-Sprung: TanzTheaterBewegung Im Wechsel Der Medien*. Berlin: Theater Der Zeit.

Brandstetter, G., Egert, G. and Hartung, H. (2019) *Movements of interweaving*. London and New York: Routledge, pp. 1–21.

Fischer-Lichte, E., Weiler, C. and Jost, T. (2021) *Dramaturgies of interweaving: engaging audiences in an entangled world*. London and New York: Routledge, pp. 1–26.

Kolesch, D. and Warstat, M. (2019) 'Affective dynamics in theatre: towards a relational and poly-perspectival performance analysis', in Kahl, A. (ed.) *Analyzing affective societies: methods and methodologies*. London and New York: Routledge, pp. 304–337.

Willson, S. (2016) 'Clod ensemble, an anatomie in four quarters', in Bouchard, G. and Mermikides, A. (eds.) *Performance and the medical body*. London and New York: Bloomsbury, pp. 151–171.

42

'STATECRAFT' AS 'STAGECRAFT'

Performing public health and the production of the socially distanced spectator

Freya Verlander

It was mid-summer 2020 during the coronavirus pandemic. I saw a picture on Twitter of two audience members wearing masks sitting in a theatre auditorium. The accompanying text suggested that the theatre-going experience felt scripted now. It was this image that got me thinking about the spectator's new role. This chapter is the product of that thinking. It examines the UK government guidelines and safety measures for those working in the performing arts, as well as the biopolitics inherent in the precise choreography of audience movement in theatres during the pandemic. With recourse to Foucauldian theory, I consider the documentation for 'Working Safely during Coronavirus (COVID-19)', by the UK's Department for Digital, Culture, Media and Sport (DCMS, 2020), in consultation with representatives of the performing arts sector, Public Health England (PHE) and the Health and Safety Executive (HSE), which presented a series of health and safety measures for theatre staff, performers and audiences. Measures included use of masks, screens and barriers, sanitisation stations, the reduction of close contact activities, the control of body-flow through theatre and performance environments, limiting prop handling to reduce transmission and keeping temporary records of audiences for the purposes of test-and-trace. This chapter interrogates how such 'statecraft' becomes literal 'stagecraft' in recognition of the performative nature of COVID-19 health and safety measures as a form of pandemic theatre[1] and how such measures produce what I call the socially distanced spectator.

The COVID-19 social drama

Indeed, there was a *whole* theatre surrounding the UK government's handling of the COVID-19 crisis. During daily press briefings, for example, the UK prime minister at the time, Boris Johnson (and other government ministers) would address the country, standing in front of Union Jack flags at lecterns emblazoned with the latest public health slogan. In 'Why Meaning-Making Matters: The Case of the UK Government's COVID-19 Response', cultural and political sociologist Marcus Morgan reads the UK government's management of the COVID crisis as a social drama. He uses:

> A range of tools for cultural analysis – including narrativization and its link to genre, ritual process and social drama, casting and interpellation, scripting and performance – [to] specify

DOI: 10.4324/9781003036500-48

the ways in which shifts in meaning-making resulted in changes in the political fortune of powerful actors, alterations in public behaviour, and ultimately in life and death outcomes for tens of thousands of UK citizens.

(2020, p. 314)

Morgan argues that the government's response narrative fell into three periods which were 'defined by changes in the moral coding of events, modifications in the casting of the actors involved, and alterations in the dominant narrative genre within which events were to be understood' (2020, p. 271). For Morgan, the first period, from early January to mid-March 2020, can be categorised as 'narrated in a low mimetic mode' in which COVID-19 was 'cast . . . as an object of routine and political management' (ibid: 271). There were recommendations for handwashing but no interruptions to UK social structures. Meanwhile, and in contrast, the UK public watched as the COVID-19 crisis played out on the global stage – with lockdown measures being implemented in China, for example, or nationwide in Italy. On 23 March 2020, however, the narrative changed. The UK entered the first lockdown with the clear message: 'Stay Home. Protect the NHS. Save Lives'. This second period, according to Morgan, was 'narrated in the high mimetic mode of tragedy that drew upon the highly polarized, and occasionally apocalyptic language of warfare'– the UK was at war with the virus (ibid: 271). This period 'even reached into the holy genre of romance and legend' with the casting of 'PM-as-hero' when Johnson contracted COVID-19 and fought it off (ibid: 272). The third narrative period began in June 2020, Morgan argues, and was characterised by ambiguity, contradictions in narrative and 'contradictions in government actors' own public performances' (ibid: 273).

Morgan also considers the performativity of gestures, such as the handshake, when COVID-19 was narrated as non-threatening, or the ritual clapping for the National Health Service,[2] alongside the government narratives that these actions supported or undermined. Morgan's focus on the 'casting' practices involved in the UK government's COVID-19 response, however, is most relevant to my argument. COVID-19 was cast as antagonist, NHS and frontline workers were cast as heroes and the UK public were given a support role in the social drama. He notes, however, that the public's role was less scripted and 'more akin to improvisational theatre'– there is a risk with audience participation because they will not necessarily stick to the script (ibid: 275). In this chapter, I argue that the government guidelines for how the performing arts might return to different levels of operation might be understood as part of this wider social drama but, more specifically, I argue that they *do* function as a form of script and stage directions for the spectator's support role within performance venues.

Scripting the socially distanced spectator

In what follows, I take the government guidelines, published 11 May 2020, for the safe return of the performing arts as the object of study. It is worth noting that there is the sense that the guidelines have been written with a fixed idea of *what* the performing arts are. References to sound and lighting desks, staging, orchestra pits, costume fittings and hair and makeup teams, for example, suggest that the guidelines were written with large-scale commercial theatres and productions in mind. It seemingly neglects smaller scale, live art and fringe works with the expectation that theatre managers/practitioners will adapt the guidelines to suit their circumstances.[3] I argue that the documentation functions as a means of asserting social control over performance venues and members of the public. It also functions as a playbook, of sorts, for the production of the socially distanced spectator as a *new form* of spectator. Methodologically I am working with an archived version of the guidelines documented in The National Archives' UK Government Web Archive – specifically, the first guidelines issued on 11 May 2020. The guidelines outline the government's five-stage roadmap 'to bring our performing arts back safely' as follows:

Stage One – Rehearsal and training (no audiences)

Stage Two – Performances for broadcast and recording purposes

Stage Three – Performances outdoors with an audience and pilots for indoor performances with a limited socially-distanced audience

Stage Four – Performances allowed indoors and outdoors (but with a limited socially-distanced audience indoors)

Stage Five – Performances allowed indoors/outdoors (with a fuller audience indoors)

(DCMS, 11 May 2020)

While this chapter will not focus on tracking changes across the documentation, the following offers an indication of some key changes in UK legislation, which were reflected in updates. By mid-August 2020, for example, the UK was at Stage Four of the roadmap; however, the re-introduction of national restrictions, or lockdown, in November 2020 meant that performing arts venues had to return to the level of operations outlined in Stages One and Two. Similarly, a regionally differentiated approach to local restrictions was introduced in November 2020. It took the form of a three-tier system dependent on virus levels: Tier 1: Medium alert, Tier 2: High Alert and Tier 3 (a Tier 4, meaning local lockdown, was later introduced). This new local tiered approach, in turn, impacted the stage of operations that performing arts venues could operate at in a particular region. This illustrates how government guidelines impacted the level of theatre and performance operations and set the stage for the emergence of the socially dis-tanced spectator – a phenomenon that emerged largely in Stages Three and Four of the roadmap when socially distanced performances were permitted. I theorise the production of the 'socially distanced spectator', therefore, as an original contribution to spectator scholarship because as a mode of theatre going it represents a distinct moment in theatre history. Arguably, never before had the role of the spectator been quite so carefully scripted and stage-managed as it was in the government's guidelines for what was effectively the performance of public health within the pandemic theatre.

Biopolitics and biopower

To further explore this interplay between *state* and *stage* craft, this chapter draws on Foucauldian theories of biopolitics. More specifically, it draws on Foucault's 'Society Must Be Defended Lectures: 17 March 1976' (1976) and Foucault's writing on the panopticon in *Discipline and Punish* (1975). In 'Society Must Be Defended', Foucault details the movement from sovereign to state control. He summarises that: 'the right of life and death was one of sovereignty's basic attributes' and that this power materialised as 'the right to kill . . . the right to take life or let live' (Foucault, 1976, pp. 61–62). The emergence of biopolitics, or biopower, refers to the state's control over biological bodies (specifically over humans-as-a-species) and represents a recon-figuration of the power over life and death. Foucault expresses this as 'the power to "make live" and "let die" ' (ibid: 241), and it is this re-configuration, specifically 'the power to "make live" ', I explore in relation to the guidelines for the return of the performing arts during the COVID-19 pandemic.

Under sovereignty, punishment is a spectacle and applied to the individual body. The 'right to kill' served a disciplinary function. Biopower, however, as exercised by the state works differently; there is a move towards the disciplining of the societal body through surveillance mechanisms. Foucault writes:

> We have . . . the emergence of something that is no longer an anatomo-politics of the human body, but what I would call a 'biopolitics' of the human race. What does this new technology of power, this biopolitics, this biopower that is beginning to establish itself invoke? [Biopower focuses on] processes [including] the birth rate, the mortality rate, longevity, and so on – together with a whole series of related economic and political problems . . . which in the second half of the eighteenth century, became biopolitics' first objects of knowledge and the targets it seeks to control.
>
> (ibid: 243)

The COVID-19 guidelines for the return of the performing arts similarly perform as part of wider governmental strategies for controlling the mortality rate and longevity of the population. In the chapter 'Panopticism', Foucault considers seventeenth-century plague measures, as well as how biopower responds to illnesses to control the mortality rate and longevity of the population. He writes:

> death was no longer something that suddenly swooped down on life – as in an epidemic. Death was now something permanent, something that slips into life, perpetually gnaws at it, diminishes it, and weakens it. These are the phenomena that begin to be taken into account at the end of the eighteenth century, and they result in the development of a medicine whose main function will now be public hygiene, with institutions to coordinate medical care, centralise power, and normalize knowledge. And which also take the format of campaigns to teach hygiene and to medicalise the population.
>
> (ibid: 244)

COVID-19 was, of course, a pandemic. Gerard Delanty's 'Six Political Philosophies in Search of a Virus: Critical Perspectives on the Coronavirus' considers how following 'in the footsteps of Michel Foucault's pioneering analysis of plagues and surveillance [we] see a new authoritarian regime of governance taking shape' (Delanty, 2020, p. 2). Sylvia Walby, however, rightly questions: 'are the interventions to separate the infected from the not-infected really best characterised as authoritarian' as opposed to socially democratic (2021, p. 24)? We saw how death, and gnawing cases of long COVID, intervened globally, but so too did public health and hygiene campaigns (working similarly to the ones that Foucault mentions here). We know that biopolitics works to intervene to 'make live'. Foucault identifies that a 'new discourse emerged [during the eighteenth century] which positioned health as a collective concern that required population-based measures', and, as Deborah Lupton *et al.* summarise, 'Foucault's writings on biopolitics, biopower and governmentality identified how people's bodies are governed and managed by their incorporation of health-related advice into their everyday practices' (2021, pp. 5–6).

The public health measures that we integrated into our everyday practices to help prevent COVID-19 transmission can also be understood as part of what Nikolas Rose describes as the 'devolution of many responsibilities for the management of human health . . . across the twentieth century, [which] had been the responsibility of the formal apparatus of government' (2007, p. 3).

In *The Politics of Life Itself* (2007), Rose argues that biopolitics today takes the form of a 'vital politics', or a continual development of the impetus to 'make live'. Rose's writing on the idea of 'subjectification' and 'somatic expertise' is relevant to the development and practice of UK government guidelines. Rose defines subjectification as the:

> novel conceptions of 'biological citizenship' [which] have taken shape [that] recode the duties, rights and expectations of human beings in relation to their sickness, and also to their life itself, reorganise the relations between individuals and their bio medical authorities, and reshape the ways in which human beings relate to themselves as 'somatic individuals'.
>
> (2007, p. 6)

The COVID-19 guidelines illustrate how subjectification and somatic expertise are drawn upon. For example, representatives from multiple professions (DCMS, PHE and the performing arts sector) collaborated to develop the guidance and ensure its correct performance. There was devolution from the state to theatre managers, to staff, down to the individual spectator, who was responsible for managing their relationship to others. As such, the guidelines illustrate the devolution of responsibility within performance environments to such an extent that we were *all* responsible for 'vital politics'. Biopower's impetus to 'make live', in order to make *live* performance, is generalised in the UK guidelines through the regularisation of movement and the knowledge that each body is potentially a vector of transmission.

The section which follows is both a provocation and creative smash of Foucault's work in his chapter 'Panopticism', specifically the section which details the response to the plague in the seventeenth century, and material taken from the UK government guidelines for the safe return of the performing arts during the COVID-19 pandemic. Foucault's chapter, for example, begins: 'The following, according to an order published at the end of the seventeenth century, were the measures to be taken when the plague appeared in town' (1975, p. 195), and I have adapted this to '**The following, according** to guidelines published by Department for Digital, Culture, Media and Sport . . .' to reflect the COVID-19 pandemic and the performing arts setting more specifically. This is alongside several other structuring statements that I have lifted from Foucault's writing on the plague in 'Panopticism', which are presented in bold. The text lifted from the government guidelines is italicised. I have chosen material from the documentation which brings Foucault's writing on bodies, space and surveillance to light within performing arts venues in the COVID-19 context.

Performing the panopticon

The following, according to guidelines published by Department for Digital, Culture, Media and Sport (DCMS) in consultation with representatives of the performing arts sector, Public Health England (PHE) and the Health and Safety Executive (HSE), in the first quarter of the twenty-first century, were the measures to be taken *to help performing arts organisations . . . in the UK understand how to work and take part in the performing arts safely, and keep their audiences safe during the COVID-19 pandemic.*

First, a strict spatial partitioning, *keeping as many people as possible 2m apart from those they do not live with. Social interactions should be limited to a group of no more than two households (indoors and out) or up to six people from different households (if outdoors). COVID-19 is a public health emergency. Everyone needs to assess and manage the risks of COVID-19. . . . As an employer, you also have a legal responsibility to protect workers and others from risk to their health and safety. . . . Where the enforcing authority, such as the HSE or your local* *authority, identifies employers who are not taking action to control public health risks, they will consider taking a range of actions to improve control of workplace risks. For example, this would cover employers not taking appropriate action to socially distance, where possible. The actions the HSE can take include the provision of specific advice to employers through to issuing enforcement notices to help secure improvements.* **Each individual is fixed in his place. And, if he moves, he does so at the risk of his life, contagion or punishment.** *Failure to complete a risk assessment which takes account of COVID-19, or completing a risk assessment but failing to put in place sufficient measures to manage the risk of COVID-19 could constitute a breach of health and safety law. Serious breaches and failure to comply with enforcement notices can constitute a criminal offence, with serious fines and even imprisonment for up to two years.*

Inspection functions ceaselessly. The gaze is alert everywhere. *Objective: That all employers and organisations carry out a COVID-19 risk assessment. . . . The vast majority of employers are responsible and will join the UK's fight against COVID-19 by working with the Government and their sector bodies to protect their workers and the public. However, inspectors are carrying out compliance checks nationwide to ensure that employers are taking the necessary steps.*

This surveillance is based on a system of permanent registration. *Test and trace. The opening up of the economy following the COVID-19 outbreak is being supported by NHS Test and Trace, which will be undertaking the routine health protection practice of tracing and contacting those who have been in close contact with someone who has an infectious disease. You should assist this service by keeping a temporary record of your audience when applicable and other visitors for 21 days, in a way that is manageable for your business or organisation, and assist NHS Test and Trace with requests for that data if needed. This could help contain clusters and outbreaks. . . . If you do not already do this you should do so to help fight the virus.*

The process of purifying. *Particular attention should be given to ventilation and sufficient circulation space especially around equipment and between groups. Keeping the environment clean. Objective: To keep the environment clean and prevent transmission by touching contaminated surfaces.* **This enclosed, segmented space, observed at every point, in which the individuals are inserted in a fixed space, in which the slightest movements are supervised.**

Guidelines published for the return of the performing arts

The previous is an experimentation with form and content. The material lifted from the guidelines has been taken from the first version published on 11 May 2020. I have chosen sections which relate to the opening of the 'Panopticism' chapter which outline the quarantine, legislative and surveillance measures published to contain outbreaks of the plague. These sections are intended to draw parallels between the guidelines issued in 2020 and Foucault's writing on the plague as a 'political dream' because it enables an absolute control of bodies, movement and mortality through surveillance mechanisms and punishment. Each statement in bold links to spatial arrangements, who is responsible for enforcement, what the risks of neglecting the health and safety measures are *and* what punishments may be enforced, practices of inspection, surveillance and the cleaning practices necessary to reduce the risk of transmission – encouraging audience members, for example, to use hand sanitiser upon entry as part of the performance of public health.

This exercise demonstrates the ways in which we might understand the policies constructing a panopticon structure within theatre and performance sites. Foucault comments of the panopticon that:

> this enclosed, segmented space, observed at every point, in which the individuals are inserted in a fixed place, in which the slightest movements are supervised, in which all measures are recorded, in which an uninterrupted work of writing links the centre and periphery, in which power is exercised without division, according to a continuous hierarchical figure, in which each individual is constantly located, examined and distributed among the living beings, the sick and the dead – all this constitutes a compact model of the disciplinary mechanism.
>
> (1975, p. 197)

He goes on to suggest that this mechanism, or disciplinary power, is analysis. We can see how analysis functions similarly in the COVID-19 context, broadly, and within performance environments more specifically. For example, performing arts venues must maintain records for test-and-trace and are expected to collaborate with the NHS to help contain and control outbreaks which illustrates how **'this surveillance is based on a system of permanent registration'**. This not only indicates the way in which a similar 'work of writing [which] links the centre and periphery' emerges in the pandemic performance setting, but the language used, 'the fight against the virus', also demonstrates how biopower's rhetoric works (ibid: 197). Joining the 'fight' against the virus rhetorically aligns organisations with the government's biopolitical agenda to 'make live', which is particularly problematic when the very existence of independent arts workers was threatened by lack of government support. The measures of surveillance and inspection also function in theatres and performance venues as biopolitical technologies for the extension of control, but, while Foucault writes that 'power is exercised without division, according to a continuous hierarchical figure' in the case of the plague, what we see – again, more broadly in society but more specifically in the guidelines – is that power and responsibility is devolved to the individual who visits the theatre.

We can see the impetus to ensure that 'individuals are inserted in a fixed place, in which the slightest movements are supervised, in which all measures are recorded' (ibid, p. 197) emerging through the ways in which the guidelines propose a number of mitigating actions under 'Managing Risk' (DCMS, 2020, online). Strategies for spacing the audience to ensure social distancing included, for example, The Willow Globe's strategy of fixed seating plans and name cards on seats for households or the practice of selling tickets with the idea that only 'household bubbles' or cohabiting people could sit together. Here we might loop back to Morgan's argument that the public's role in the social drama that was COVID-19 was 'akin to improvisational theatre' (275), because theatregoers did not always stick to the script. For example, they might choose to perform the roles of cohabiting people to get around the rules which said that you could only be seated with members of your own household.

There were also measures which positioned individuals working in, and visiting, theatre and performance venues in a 'fixed place', where their movements can be 'supervised', which included 'using screens or barriers to separate people from others' and 'using back-to-back or side-to-side working (rather than face-to-face) whenever possible' (ibid). I have suggested how such measures are part of what might be understood as a form of panopticon because they are designed to create one-way-systems through the space. One-way-systems were often employed to control the movements of audience members, too. For example, Dante or Die – an experimental theatre company specialising in site-specific performance – created the socially distant performance installation

Skin Hunger (2021) at the Stone Nest in London. The work featured different coloured one-way-routes taped along the floor for audience members to follow so that they would never come into contact with one another. The proposed measures such as the back-to-back or side-to-side ways of working also maintained a unidirectional gaze. They operated to illustrate statecraft as stagecraft because they introduced physical structures, screens and barriers, which stage-managed people's movements within the performing arts environment.

The guidelines also stage-managed the physical handling, and passing, of props between people in order to 'reduce the transmission and maintain social distancing where possible'. (ibid). The Pantaloons, a touring theatre company who specialise in producing open-air productions of Shakespeare's works, integrated these guidelines into their production of *Twelfth Night* (2020) so that statecraft informed the stagecraft. The cast was made up of two social bubbles (households) and, as Artistic Director Steve Purcell explains, 'We decided . . . we'd actually make the social distancing part of the production', which accentuated the play's themes of 'restraint' and wider restrictions on touch (Hudson and Purcell, 2021, online). Designer Zoë Hudson also explained that where the script required props be passed between characters they bought doubles so there was no contact between the bubbles (ibid). Measures under 'Sound and lighting' similarly introduce material structures, or statecraft as part of the stagecraft, such as 'creating a screen around sound and lighting desks to create a barrier which aerosols do not pass through, between the sound team and audience or other crew' as well as potentially leaving an empty row of seats if the sound desk is in close proximity to the audience (DCMS, 2020, online). And, on this, Purcell describes how distancing regulations informed the design aesthetic of the production:

> we've got to leave . . . a certain amount of space between the front of the acting space and the front of the audience space. . . . We have a couple of oars and some fishing nets and a hat and some other bits of detritus that just sort of form a line, just to remind the actors, 'No, you can't come any further forward than this'.
>
> (Hudson and Purcell, 2021, online)

Audience management

I have outlined how the guidelines suggest bodies should be controlled and monitored via health and safety surveillance mechanisms as they move through performance venues, as well as some of the ways this statecraft manifests as stagecraft, but my other objective is to suggest how the biopolitical operations recommended in the government guidelines result in a new phenomenon: the socially distanced spectator. To this end, the advisories on 'Managing Audiences' and the imperative to maintain social distancing within performance venues are of interest here. In the first version of the guidelines, it is stated that:

> Organisers should ensure that steps are taken to avoid audiences needing to unduly raise their voices to each other. This includes but is not limited to, refraining from playing music or broadcasts that may encourage shouting, including if played at a volume that makes normal conversation difficult. . . . This is because of the potential for increased risk of transmission particularly from aerosol and droplet transmission. . . . You should take similar steps to prevent other close contact activities – such as communal dancing in audiences.
>
> (DCMS, 2020, online)

Here we can see that it is not just perceived-as-risky movements, like dancing, but also potential verbal interactions between audience members that the guidelines seek to control. Volume, specifically, needs to be regulated to reduce the need for audience members to project their voices and, thus, reduce the potential of viral transmission through airborne droplets expelled through the mouth. Furthermore, under 'Staging and Capacity', the guidelines suggest that 'risk assessments should specifically consider the max capacity for a given performance and ability to manage audience behaviour to avoid compromising social distancing' (ibid). I want to emphasise 'manage' here, because audience behaviour is clearly conceptualised as a risk to be *managed* in public health interests. Anticipating how audiences might behave mitigates this risk:

> Considering the expected interactions amongst audience members and making sure sufficient controls are in place to maintain social distancing, for example providing clear communication, demarcating spaces, using sufficient ushers.
>
> (ibid)

Pressure points for crowding (such as queues for the toilets) must be planned for. The implication is that certain works and atmospheres may encourage certain behaviours that may violate government guidelines. 'Discouraging or avoiding gatherings', for example, 'such as performances or screenings that may encourage audience behaviours that increase transmission risk, for example crowding, clustering or physical contact outside of household groups or support bubbles' (ibid). The insights that can be gained are that government understands performing arts venues as sites of contamination because of the behaviours and modes of sociality that might be enjoyed as part of the theatre going experience.

Of course, there is a historical and pervasive discourse around theatre and contagion. The guidelines might be understood as a continuation of a version of the anti-theatrical prejudice that we can trace back to Plato's *Republic*. *The Republic* cautions that dramatic representations 'infect' audiences: 'poetry, dramatic poetry in particular, has a bad effect on its audiences, who learn to admire and imitate the faults it represents. We cannot, therefore, allow poets in our ideal state' (1987, p. 384). Anti-theatricalists make claims about the immorality of theatres and performance and warn against the transmission of affect. The government guidelines responded to the threat of *literal* contagion, but we see traces of anti-theatrical prejudice in the anxieties over the transmission of affect. It is implied that, without management, audience members may be unable to resist certain forms of communal behaviour and thus become potential social contaminants. However, again, the impetus is on theatre managers, staff and volunteers to anticipate audience behaviours and to manage their audiences.

The guidelines, when followed, therefore, produce the 'socially distanced spectator' *as a new kind of spectator*. The most basic definition of this term would quite literally be as a spectator who respected social distancing measures; however, it is *much* more than this. For example, we can understand the socially distanced spectator as a product of anti-theatrical prejudice. The guidelines, as we have seen, conceptualise audience members as susceptible to the transmission of affect. They are understood as potentially unruly, risky bodies who must be controlled in order to control the transmission of the virus. To take this further, then, the socially distanced spectator can also be understood as the *ideal* spectator in the eyes of the state. Or, in other words, they are someone who performs the role of public health and safety (by helping to control the spread of the virus) within the pandemic theatre (and, therefore, beyond it). This type of spectator can be understood in contrast to those spectators who, for example, claimed to be part of the same household in order to sit together during a performance and, therefore, subverted their scripted roles.

The choreographic score

To conclude, this chapter has theorised the ways in which the UK government guidelines for the return of the performing arts resulted in the construction of theatre and performance environments as a form of panopticon and, through the implementation of statecraft as stagecraft, also resulted in the production of the socially distanced spectator. I have argued that the devolution of governance and the responsibility for COVID-19 health and safety measures constitute biopolitics' impetus to 'make live'. The various modes of 'statecraft' become 'stagecraft' in the construction of a 'vital politics', or an infrastructure of 'vital politics', within the theatre; however, I want to put final-thoughts pressure on the 'socially distanced spectator' as a product, or construct, of COVID policies for the safe return of the performing arts. Because although audiences are clearly cast as bodies to be managed, the devolution of responsibility for the management of public health ends with the spectator. I have noted the measures (including crowd management and requirements for additional stewards) as modes of surveillance and enforcers of safety measures, but what more of the spectator's role? Under the first guidelines, it states that:

> It is expected that guests will take responsibility for their own and others' welfare and abide by social distancing in the auditorium. Staff should nevertheless be deployed to make sure these measures are being observed.
>
> (DCMS, 2020, online)

Again, we see the dynamics of surveillance and discipline at play. By way of conclusion, I want to focus on the expectation that spectators have a role to play in the maintenance of 'their own and others' welfare'. Gia Kourlas' reflections on the choreography of bodies during a pandemic is relevant, here, for the way in which Kourlas recognises the individual responsibility we have for choreographing our movement in relation to others:

> When you walk outside, you are responsible for more than just yourself. We are in this together, and movement has morals and consequences – its own choreographic score, or set of instructions – in this age of coronavirus.
>
> (2020, online)

This idea of a 'choreographic score', determined by the individual's movement, plays out at the interstices between contagion and containment. It also emphasises public health as a form of performance. The 'choreographic score' as a performative measure recognises how deeply entwined the social, biological and political are in COVID-19 as a case study. The COVID-19 guidelines for the performing arts similarly script the responsibilisation of the individual spectator through policy and choreographed practices within the performance environment. Kourlas' understanding that 'we are in this together, and movement has morals and consequences' (2020, online) chimes with Walby's writing on the social democratic understanding that 'if one is sick, we are all potentially sick' (2021, p. 24). As theatre venues re-opened and requirements to socially distance were lifted, it became a requirement for entry for spectators to show proof of vaccination status or negative lateral flow test, markers of ongoing responsibilisation towards other theatregoers in performing vital politics. This chapter has thought through the dynamic between contagion, containment and control as it is scripted and stage-managed in the guidelines for the safe return of the performing arts during COVID-19. It has drawn attention to the carefully scripted role of the spectator, as well as the socially distanced spectator's responsibilities for wider public health. In the pandemic theatre, we were all implicated in a 'vital politics', enacting the impetus to 'make *live*' in order to make *live* performance.

Notes

1 The terms 'statecraft' and 'stagecraft' are borrowed from Fintan Walsh's *Theatres of Contagion* (2020), which explores the dynamic between contagion and containment in performance contexts. See specifically Lynn McCarthy's chapter, 'Nomadic Contagion and the Performance of Infrastructure in Dale Farm's Post-Eviction Scene' which interrogates government infrastructure, specifically bunding (a type of wall), as 'an administrative tool of social control' (2020, p. 136). 'Bunding is a form of statecraft', Walsh writes, 'which has clear resonances with stagecraft' (2020, p. 16).
2 See chapter by Giskin Day in this volume for discussion of the UK clap-for-carers movement.
3 As an example of addressing government misunderstandings of types of performance, the Coalition for Open Air Theatre and Out to Perform wrote an open letter entitled 'Kickstarting a Cultural Revival with the Early Opening of the Outdoor Performing Arts' to Oliver Dowden, the secretary of state for digital, culture, media and sport, on 12 February 2021. It argued that outdoor performances should open earlier, as they do not pose the same risks of COVID-19 transmission as indoor performances.

Reference list

Dante or Die (2021) *Skin Hunger: a socially distant performance installation*. Glasgow: Salamander Street Ltd.

DCMS (Department for Digital, Culture, Media & Sport) (2020) *Working safely during coronavirus (COVID-19): performing arts: guidance for people who work in performing arts, including arts organisations, venue operators and participants*. Available at: https://webarchive.nationalarchives.gov. uk/ukgwa/20200709202336/; www.gov.uk/guidance/working-safely-during-coronavirus-covid-19/perfor ming-arts#arts-2-6 (Accessed: 19 December 2022).

Delanty, G. (2020) *Six political philosophies in search of a virus: critical perspectives on the coronavirus pandemic*, p. 24. Available at: www.lse.ac.uk/european-institute/Assets/Documents/LEQS-Discussion-Papers/LEQSPaper156.pdf (Accessed: 3 April 2023).

Foucault, M. (1975) *Discipline and punish: the birth of the prison*. 2020 edn. London: Penguin.

Foucault, M. (1976) ' "Society must be defended," Lecture at the College de France, March 17, 1976', in Campbell, T. and Sitze, A. (eds.) *Biopolitics: a reader*. Durham and London: Duke University Press, pp. 61–82.

Hudson, Z. and Purcell, S. (2021) *Interviewed by Sarah Sharp for atmospheric theatre*. Available at: https:// atmospherictheatre.exeter.ac.uk/items/show/149 (Accessed: 28 April 2022).

Kourlas, G. (2020) 'How we use our bodies to navigate a pandemic', *The New York Times*, 31 March. Available at: www.nytimes.com/2020/03/31/arts/dance/choreographing-the-street-coronavirus.html (Accessed: 23 April 2022).

Lupton, D. *et al.* (2021) 'The face mask in COVID times: a sociomaterial analysis', in *DG ebook package English 2021*. Berlin: De Gruyter.

Morgan, M. (2020) 'Why meaning-making matters: the case of the UK Government's COVID-19 response', *American Journal of Cultural Sociology*, 8(3), pp. 270–323.

Plato (1987) *The republic*. Translated by D. Lee. New York: Penguin.

Rose, N. (2007) 'The politics of life itself: biomedicine, power, and subjectivity in the twenty-first century', in *EBook package backlist 2000–2013*. Berlin: De Gruyter.

Walby, S. (2021). 'The COVID pandemic and social theory: Social democracy and public health in the crisis', *European Journal of Social Theory*, 24(1), pp. 22–43. https://doi.org/10.1177/1368431020970127.

Walsh, F. (eds.) (2020) *Theatres of contagion: transmitting early modern to contemporary performance*. London: Bloomsbury Methuen Drama Publishing (Methuen Drama Engage).

43

ACTIVE INGREDIENTS

Notes on Clod Ensemble's *Placebo*

Suzy Willson

Clod Ensemble is a UK-based performance company that has an ongoing fascination with medicine and performance. I founded Clod Ensemble in 1995 with musician Paul Clark, and over this period we have developed two interweaving strands to our practice: performance work presented in theatres, arts galleries and public spaces and a programme of participatory creative learning that works with people in community centres, schools, hospitals, medical schools and universities. One strand of this creative learning programme is called Performing Medicine and offers arts-based support, learning and professional development opportunities to people working in healthcare settings – doctors, nurses, artists, occupational therapists.

Clod Ensemble's first-ever show in 1995 was based on Pushkin's 'little tragedy' *Feast During the Plague*. In the midst of a terrible plague, a group of people surreptitiously gather to have a party – to make themselves feel better and to mourn the loss of a friend. Since then, we have made several performances which draw on medicine and the medical profession as a way of exploring wider themes, including *Kiss My Echo (2001)*, *Must* (with Peggy Shaw) (2007), *Under Glass (2007)*, *An Anatomie in Four Quarters (2011)* and most recently *Placebo*, which I will focus on here. *Placebo* is an hour-long piece performed by seven dancers, which premiered and toured the UK in 2018, accompanied by a series of events, talks and workshops called 'The Power of Placebo'.

The 'placebo effect'

Placebos are typically inactive drugs or treatments with no pharmaceutically 'active ingredient', which are used in double blind trials of new drugs to ascertain their efficacy. In these clinical trials, usually there are two groups of patients – half of them get the 'real' drug and half get the placebo. The placebo effect describes the response patients have when the 'inactive' drug itself creates health benefits. And these phenomena can be remarkable: scientific research has shown that 'sham' surgery can create lasting pain relief (Jonas *et al.*, 2015), that the colour or size of pills can impact on their effectiveness (De Craen *et al.*, 1996) and that the identity and 'performance' of the doctor can have an impact on medical outcomes (Miller and Kaptchuk, 2008). Placebo treatments have now been shown to create measurable physiological change. There is a growing interest in finding out how placebos work and understanding how we can harness the power of this response as a potent healing technique.

DOI: 10.4324/9781003036500-49

In this chapter, I will share some of the ways we came to make a performance by exploring the phenomenon of placebo, using it as a key to unlock a whole world of connected ideas and images.

Placebo: points of departure

Clod Ensemble create performance pieces through long periods of research and development. For *Placebo*, we talked to a rich mix of people working in surgery, general practice, nursing, complementary therapies, psychiatry, neurology, philosophy, shamanism, history, poetry and art. As the choreographer/director, I work closely alongside musician Paul Clark to structure the performance. We begin with some points of departure – themes, ideas, texts and images – some of which I reference here. Through a process of guided improvisations that draw heavily on this visual and written source material, the dancers create movements that are then developed, edited and 'transposed' as the process unfolds. The score is developed in parallel, with Paul in the rehearsal room, offering musical ideas that both stimulate movement and respond to it.

The subject of placebo itself is multi-layered. It's impossible to understand what makes someone feel better by identifying a single 'active' ingredient. It is necessary to take into account the context, the form, the personalities involved, and other interrelated factors which have an influence. Likewise, trying to translate the layered process of making Placebo into a linear chapter is particularly challenging. It pains me to try and reduce the personalities, colours, ideas, sounds, contexts and choreographies that rely on the experiences and sensations of the audience into words. The placebo effect resists reductionist ways of understanding. Reflecting this, our production is like a moving collage which takes the form of a series of mock 'scientific' experiments, all of which are danced. The layering of light, voices, music, movement, costume and audience response all impact the experiments. Movements are repackaged, distorted, multiplied and abandoned, propelled by a rich original score that sweeps mischievously through euphoric club tracks to classical fugues and features a multitude of different voices. Costumes, which change throughout, are designed by non-binary fashion label Art School.

Placebo explores both the beauty and the limits of scientific analysis and interpretation as well as the expectations, beliefs and aesthetic preferences we bring to all our encounters including those that take place in both healthcare settings and theatres. It asks whether a red pill (or costume) is more powerful than a blue one and if the packaging affects the potency of the pill or performance. Does it matter whether something is fake or real? The conceit is that the performance itself is a medicine – a placebo pill, a sugar pill – and as such, it is difficult to extrapolate one single active ingredient from it.

The piece begins with the seven dancers facing the audience. They are wearing blue skirts and white tops reminiscent of lab coats. A monotone robotic, computer voice speaks:

Hello, here we all are, together in the same room. The observation room. Many of us haven't been feeling 100%. We have been suffering from aches and pains, loss of sleep, anxiety about the future, addiction to technology, loneliness, envy, isolation and some unexplained symptoms.

We will conduct a number of experiments designed to investigate the factors that help or hinder us feeling better. . . . There will be an opportunity to review your findings once the experiments have been completed.

461

WARNINGS AND PRECAUTIONS: Stop watching and contact a doctor immediately if you develop any of the following symptoms: Swelling of the tongue or throat, difficulties swallowing, embarrassment, disillusionment, disappointment, difficulties breathing, sensitivity to light, muscle spasms, hives.

Immediately the audience is placed in the position of objective viewer – an absurd and impossible position for them to take. Will the performance make them feel better?

T'ain't what you do, it's the way that you do it

Perhaps the placebo effect is not actually as mysterious as it first seems. Studies clearly demonstrate that *how* you administer a treatment or drug can be as important as *what* the drug is. There is a relationship between the way a 'cure' is 'performed', if you like, and how effective it is. Framing, character, stage presence, colour, light, the expectations of an audience, the theatre, branding and marketing, costume, set and props – this is the stuff of performance and theatre which artists have meditated on for millennia – aesthetic factors as important in healthcare as in theatre. Anyone studying the placebo effect is studying the tools that artists train themselves to understand and use. Clod Ensemble's productions are always aiming for a place where form and content are congruent – where everything is playing together – shape, colour, words, light, costume, character and so on. Our shows do not only describe or represent something – they *are* the thing. Form and content are inseparable. As Ella Fitzgerald sang it: 'T'aint what you do, it's the way that you do it'. Or maybe it is *both* what you do and the way that you do it that matters.

The first experiment sets the tone. 'Experiment 1: Observe', says the voice.

Dancer A will give Dancer B a bunch of flowers three times. Does the manner in which the flowers are administered affect the way Dancer B feels, positively or negatively?

First Dancer A throws the fake flowers at B, then lavishly overburdens him with them and finally gives them with respect and space. The third way clearly makes him 'feel better'. It is not what she does, it is the way that she does it that matters. A later experiment (number 7) builds on this: a group of four dancers perform the same choreography four times, each time accompanied musically in a different way. Which one makes you feel better? Each has a very different emotional resonance, humour and set of meanings depending on the score: a doleful cello solo, the theme from an imaginary spaghetti western, cool jazz or the suspense of a horror film score.

Performance, authenticity and the act of imagining

Often described as the 'benign negative control', the placebo effect has distinctly negative connotations in medical contexts, seen as something that gets in the way of the 'real' medicine, and perhaps as a consequence of this has been long ignored. It has sometimes been seen as an embarrassment to doctors and pharma, especially when it outperforms 'legitimate' treatments they can offer (Kaptchuk and Miller, 2015).

The wealth of discourse on the ethical use of placebos in clinical contexts invariably assumes that placebos oblige practitioners to peddle in deception – that placebos are 'fake' and that for them to work, the recipient has to believe they are real. For anyone working in theatre and performance, we know that deception or artifice has an effect. No one would question that because, say, we are not really in Verona in the Middle Ages, a performance of *Romeo and Juliet* would be less effective, but somehow the marrying of form, content and authenticity as a whole experience is less allowable (or at least less nuanced, understood or spoken of) in medicine.

The imagination of the audience and their 'suspension of disbelief' is a powerful tool. Theatre relies on honesty, authenticity and intention which allow us to 'make believe'. With this in mind, the evidence showing that even when the patient knows they are taking a placebo, it can still work, is not as counterintuitive as it might seem. Indeed, some general practitioners (GPs) have begun prescribing open-label placebos to patients (Kaptchuk *et al.*, 2010). There are surprisingly straightforward ways to do this: by saying, for example, 'I'd like to suggest giving you a treatment – a simple sugar pill – that we know has worked for many other people in similar situations to you'.

Simulation is effective, artifice is effective, and can bring us to change. We sleep by pretending to be asleep, after all, by lying down and closing our eyes. Even if we do not feel happy, smiling changes our mood; it opens the potential for joy. We all respond to our environment – the way something is described affects us positively or negatively: conditioning, beliefs, expectation and imagination have all been shown to have measurable, physiological effects in health care and other healing settings. Are actors and performers frauds? Are the dancers fakes? Should they be trusted?

The healing response triggered by a placebo pill or intervention must not be dismissed as purely an 'imagined' one. This idea that something could be 'all in the mind' exposes a fundamental schism in Western medicine which I have been grappling with for decades – a Cartesian binary between mind and body that even now persists – in plain sight. It is like a chasm or a crack – a schism that has a profound impact on the way people experiencing 'unexplained symptoms' such as chronic pain and chronic fatigue syndrome are treated. Words like 'psychosomatic' often seem to suggest that they are faking it or putting it on, as if their suffering does not count because no 'physical' cause (lesion, bruise, tumour or fracture) can be found. Indeed, I have witnessed people in hospital wards being described derogatively by staff: 'There's nothing wrong, they are faking it'. Whatever is going on in cases like this, there is certainly something wrong. Placebos affect both 'mind' and 'brain', and the two cannot be separated from each other.

In making *Placebo*, we wanted to challenge the mind/body binary – to explore the wonderful and powerful influence of the passions on the state and disorder of the whole self.

The absurdity of Experiment 7 addresses the notion of fake and real directly, where the dancers announce that during the dance: 'I'm going to show the same movement twice. One will be fake, and one will be real'. The audience are left to work out which one is which.

Beliefs and agency

Throughout the performance, it becomes clear that each dancer has a different relationship to their own health which shifts and changes. Each person is known by a letter in a futile attempt to give themselves scientific status. A is suggestible – always copying people, ready to respond. F is after instant reward and results rather than connection to feelings or cause; he wants to overcome difficulty through endurance. There are two characters who represent or embody pleasure and pain. D is constantly exploring ways to manage her pain. She is interested in the effectiveness of treatments but finds most offers of care burdensome and so refuses them. She leans into her pain – refusing help from other characters, she explores it, investigates it. C, on the other hand, is capable of unbridled joy – and knows that this is a powerful healing tool.

We all bring our own belief systems, opinions and ideas to a clinical encounter. If I think that something is going to heal (or entertain) me, will it be more effective?

'Experiment 2: Observe', demands the computer voice.

Dancer C will dance in a way that gives her real pleasure. Does our knowledge that the dancer's pleasure is real affect the way we feel: positively or negatively?

As C dances, incorporating movements that we will see recurring throughout the piece, we hear a collage of voices embedded in the soundtrack driving her on to a beat:

And what? What would you say? Sugar pill. What? The heart starts to get coherent and the heart starts to affect the brain, and the brain starts to affect the heart and the heart starts to affect the brain waves like this and they're moving and you see Alpha and you see Beta and you see Beta and you see Delta and you can see from the body, via the body, back of the body, top of the body, heal your body. The body can't heal the body, you have to get beyond your body to heal your body, change your body. In the elegant moment. Very few people are in the present moment. Oh my god I'm addicted to my own frustration I'm addicted to my own suffering I'm addicted to my own guilt 2 sugar pills 4 sugar pills sugar sugar sugar pill I love it And I'm hearing, what I'm hearing is 'Everything can change'.

Other dancers are infected, influenced, changed by the movement and rhythm of her dance. But they are interrupted by G, who does not seem to understand or feel their pleasure and is unsettled that the boundaries of the experiment have been transgressed. He is the figure who seems to identify most with Western medicine, adopting the manner of an archetypal consultant – authoritative, grounded, rational, safe within his world view. He is interested in others but never relinquishes his own position, more interested in cure than care. He is consistent, requiring order and evidence, and his manner can be patronising and sometimes brutalising (with the best intention). He dances a recurring duet with B, who is soft and fragile. He removes his skirt in a way that resembles a surgeon getting dressed for surgery and proceeds to manipulate B. He is performing 'objectivity', carrying him across the stage in a duet. B is passive, puppet like. Without agency. When G exits, B collapses. But each time the dance is repeated throughout the piece, B gains agency and power until he becomes an equal partner in the duet, learning to stand again on his own two feet, becoming active in his own treatment and taking responsibility for his part in its effect. In the development of much Western medicine, the patient became a passive spectator, often infantilised by a healthcare system. This, to me, is one of the great tragedies of westernised health mechanisms and has had devastating consequences. Look at the United States, where a compliant population has become addicted to a quick fix, resulting in an epic opioid crisis (Verhamme and Bohnen, 2019; Manchikanti *et al.*, 2012).

In recent years, a shift towards 'patient-centred care' has attempted to restore agency to the patient as more and more studies show that having some personal control over your health results in being healthier long term and 'feeling better'. The nature of the relationship between doctor and patient is changing and the simple maxim 'doctor knows best' seems to no longer be serving the patient or the doctor. Nevertheless, the relationship with the doctor remains key to the effectiveness of a treatment (Kelley *et al.*, 2014).

Conditioning and environments

Because going to the doctor normally makes us better, we are consequently generally conditioned to get better when we see a doctor. *Placebo* plays with this idea of conditioned response throughout the piece. Some of these conditioned responses are negative. 'White coat syndrome' is the term used when, for instance, the presence of a healthcare professional makes the heart beat faster when getting blood pressure checked.

In Experiment 5, Dancer A is doing her ballet practice. When the light is on, she dances with glee; when it is off, she stops and seems bored and distracted. The voices in the soundtrack describe a laboratory experiment:

> [Light ON] So this is a mouse. [OFF] And you see that when the light is shone, the mouse starts eating cheese. [ON she continues dancing] But when it's turned off [OFF] the mouse loses interest and starts wandering around looking at other things. [ON] When the light is shone – going at the cheese like anything [OFF]. OK, light's off. Mouse puts down cheese, sniffs, turns away. And if you wait, the light comes on again [ON] and, look, straight away, it starts eating some cheese again.

In placebo studies, it is well documented that simply being in a healthcare environment can trigger placebo responses. The soundtrack to *Placebo* draws on the account of Eutimio Perez who was under the care of Dr Bruce Mosely at the Methodist Hospital, Houston, US, for severe arthritis in his knee. He was told he was having surgery, went through all the motions of the operating theatre and was put under anaesthetic, but no actual surgery took place. When he came round, he felt better. It worked, and the effects were lasting, as we hear in the soundtrack to the piece, which plays recordings of Eutimio Perez and Bruce Mosely speaking:

> When I first had that pain, I couldn't do a lot of things, like going fishing, or playing basketball or going dancing. I didn't think that, uh, it could be any worse. Terrible awful, I. . . . And nobody would say which of the three treatments was revealed in the envelope. Not even the staff knew who was in each group. Until they were in the theatre. I was thinking: 'Good gosh, here's a patient who we're pretending to do surgery on . . . we're not really doing surgery. I'm a physician and a healer after all, Is this really, y'know, the right thing to do? The response ranged from: 'you gotta be kidding me, I can't' – bewilderment, 'there must be a mistake'. Cos they all felt so strongly that something had happened to change what was going on inside.

We respond to context, environment, sound and lighting. In her book *Cure*, Jo Marchant (2016) describes an experiment which proved that the effect of listening to a favourite recording when taking an immunosuppressant maximises the effect.

Research reveals that size and colour matter, that red pills are more effective than blue pills and that football teams wearing red shirts are more likely to win; that if someone takes ibuprofen in a Neurofen pill, which comes with familiar packaging, it is more effective than taking an identical drug packaged as Boots generic brand. Even when the patient knows it is exactly the same medicine, they will pay extra for the premium brand – as something about the packaging triggers a healing response in them.

About half-way through *Placebo*, the dancers have a competition to find out which of them is the most active ingredient:

> Before you've even met this person, you already have expectations in your head of how this person will be when you meet them. *Who is the most incredible? Who is The Active Ingredient?* Some people like having a label, either positive or negative. For other people

just having a label is something they don't want at all. *Fakes have been around for decades. Handbags, watches, clothes.* Is it a phoney label or is it a real label? What many people don't understand is we are scrupulously honest. *Let them put their evidence down.* Every day, someone is trying to convince you to do something. *Is it a phoney label or a real label?*

It is an endurance test; they leap up and down until, one by one, they run out of steam. G (our paternalistic consultant figure) is cross, because, evidently, he is not the fittest, and he deftly takes back control by cueing a highly repetitive piece of trance-like music and inviting the audience to participate in different movement and thought-experiments. Speaking softly, he asks the audience to observe their own somatic responses as they watch the dancers, now dressed in sparkly costumes that play with the light (resembling the foil interior of a pill packet), rock themselves hypnotically across the stage:

> So, let's start with our heartbeat – I want you all to put your hands on your hearts and just feel your heartbeat. And now your breath. Breathe in and breathe out. Does the way the dancers move change your heart rate?
> I'm now going to slowly turn the lights down, just by 5 per cent.
> You are 70 per cent likely to be gradually feeling warmer as the sequence continues.
> By this stage, our heartbeats are beginning to synchronise. Our breathing rates are slowing down.
> I will now gradually turn the volume down. Some people may detect a background aroma of roses.

The repetitive nature of the movement becomes predictable and boring. This drug is losing its power and Dancer D (the character who has been coping with extreme pain throughout without complaint) does not trust the dealer, G. She is still in pain and interrupts him. She cannot bear it any longer.

> Stop! Stop. This isn't working. Stop the music. Stop! Stop.
> I still feel pain. I don't believe you! I don't believe in you! [To the audience] It's bullshit! It's all fake! Change the light. It's pointless. It's all fake. There is no smell of roses! They didn't actually change the volume.
> [Dismantling mic] Look – it's not even a microphone! It's a torch. [She switches the torch on and points it into the audience, keeping it moving, not picking anyone out]. Everything's fake. You say it's ok, but it's not OK. It's a lie. And lying is wrong. It isn't making me feel better. It just isn't.

There is another medical character in the piece, E, probably a doctor, perhaps a psychoanalyst (nothing is made explicit – the audience are free, even encouraged, to bring all their own judgements, assumptions and biases to the performance). E is analytical and methodical, but understands that the clinical encounter is a relationship. She actively challenges the paternalism of the system she is working within. Early in the piece, she rejects the robot voice, bringing a microphone on stage so that her own voice can be heard:

> I'm sorry, this isn't working. The sound of the voice is making me feel bad. Can you turn it off please? We can take responsibility for ourselves. Can you flip the switch? Thank you.

Perhaps E (like many of us working within healthcare systems) is trying to change the paradigm from within the paradigm, but this can be tiring, and even those with the best intentions can become institutionalised and abuse their power. E is certainly capable of brutality and coercion.

By now, nothing and no one are quite what they seem. Realising that D is still in pain and that the whole performance is now falling apart in front of her eyes (and ours), E invites the dancers to do things that *they* think will make them feel better (score a goal, pelvic thrusts across the stage, ballet practice). But before long, she takes control, insisting the dancers will feel better by running round and round in circles, and like a crazed ringmaster, she drives them to exhaustion and disillusion.

At last, dancer A rebels, dancing gently in her own melancholic rhythm. E huffs off stage. Everyone is feeling bad – this is the nocebo effect – when treatments elicit adverse health reactions, normally due to negative beliefs or expectations – in full force. Even A has had the joy knocked out of her. They are all reeling from the side effects of a noxious intervention and worn themselves out trying to feel better. G has lost his power, and as a result he has lost faith in the experimental project – he is broken. Lights turn on and off as in Experiment 5, but A is not playing anymore, and she will not take the illuminated bait – the mouse refuses to ballet.

Suddenly, we hear the cool jazz of Experiment 7 again. Marilyn Monroe appears to be walking onto stage. It is E! She has had enough of trying to make others feel better. Now, she dives into her own Warholesque fantasy world and reaches for a fake cigarette:

I would not be alive if it weren't for cigarettes.

They got me through the hardest times. They changed time, and kept me from being hungry. If I don't think it is bad for me, maybe it won't be. People always filling your mind with bad images, Makes me ill – we never used to think about the damage we were doing. We all just died younger. Smoke keeps me from falling into the dark places.

I'm having a cigarette or two
I'm filling my chest with the best, of you
The fog around me is filtering the light
Making me look sultry in the night
Isn't it making you wish I was in your arms
Sure, I can be lonely, I can be blue
I can be wanting to spend time with you, but nothing comes close
To that cigarette thrill
Lighting up the nights . . .
filling my lungs with the meaning of life

Everything begins to change.
We have arrived at Experiment 13.

Ceremony and ritual

Interestingly, placebo studies show that if you take a pill at the same place, at the same time every day – basically if you turn the taking of the pill into a ritual – it increases the impact. The patient is required to be active, to play their part.

Despite an institutionalised and perfectly rational suspicion of a myriad of 'alternative' healing techniques that rely on symbol and ceremony (for example, faith healing, shamanic practices, folk medicine) of course, Western medicine also relies on its own set of powerful symbols and rituals. The white coat, the stethoscope and so on create placebo responses which have been described and written about widely, though perhaps from disciplines outside of medicine, such as anthropology or sociology, rather than from within the medical profession itself (Bernstein *et al*., 2020). Many of these alternative practices have valuable lessons to learn from – the complex rituals, the deep sense of acknowledgement. The power of being seen, heard and witnessed may not provide a 'cure' for cancer but can help people to manage the symptoms and prevent isolation, depression and despair.

I have sat in many rooms over the years listening to doctors getting angry about homeopathy. The argument often made is that it is deceiving, that it makes claims that it cannot deliver and prevents people from seeking more effective medicines. But what homeopathic encounters demonstrate, if nothing else, is that people *feel better* when a healer/doctor spends time with them, listens, does something ceremonial and establishes trust. And surely 'feeling better' must be one of the desired outcomes of healthcare? (Or, is it just to 'cure' disease?) Homeopaths and acupuncturists harness the things that activate placebo responses very effectively.

At one of our 'Power of Placebo' public events, Professor of Neurology at Edinburgh University Jon Stone, who specialises in functional neurological disorders, played us an extract from the film *The Wizard of Oz* (1939). This fantastical film follows Dorothy and her friends as they travel the yellow brick road in search of the Wizard of Oz, whom they believe will solve all their problems: Dorothy needs to get home, the Scarecrow needs a brain, the Tin Man needs a heart and the Cowardly Lion needs courage. At the end, although the 'all powerful' Wizard is revealed as a fraud, dashing their expectations, by listening to the predicament of Dorothy and her friends, he does find a way to help them and himself feel better. The Scarecrow, who is looking for a brain, is presented with a 'Doctor of Thinkology' diploma in recognition of his support for Dorothy. He is persuaded that he actually had a brain all along and finds a newfound ability to quote trigonometry. 'A placebo transaction has occurred, but there is nothing fake about it' said Professor Stone, 'a truth has been revealed, a brain restored'.[1]

In the process of making *Placebo*, we dived into the world of alternative healing practices and folk rituals, of quackery and pseudo-science, of mediaeval peoples circling the spoon three times, of dancing ('movement is the medicine'), shamanic burials, whirling dervishes, and we were inspired by the work of artists who focus on ceremony, on care, on ritual – Ana Mendieta, Joseph Beuys, Guillermo Gómez-Peña, Sheila Ghelani, Marina Abramović, Franko B and Welfare State International. The quasi-religious and sacred. Blood, feathers, felt, wax, fire. The deep-rooted desire to connect with nature as part of a healing process.

I spent a long time looking at an old black and white photograph of two adults pushing a small child through a hole in a healing tree in an attempt to cure them of rickets.[2] The seeming absurdity of a horizontal child in a tree, the adults in clothes from a bygone era, presumably desperate to 'make better please', and the poignant forest light all capture something that is both funny and profoundly touching – human beings struggling with their own flesh and bones.

The finale (happy endings)

So, here we are nearing the climax of our performance. The music is building – trumpets sound like elephants in the distance, casting a spell on proceedings as D brings onto stage layers of black netting and sequins and slowly adorns herself in ceremonial attire. A ritual begins as the sounds of pipes breathe life into the moment. She is both patient and healer. Whirling and spinning, she transforms her pain into dance.

And then, as if by magic, the lights shine brightly on a finale which aims to sensate – to please – an ecstasy of colourful, glittering materials. It is a mash-up of all the material we have seen and heard re-made afresh in new combinations and contexts, imbuing the whole structure of the show with the possibility of being a kind of placebo effect in itself:

> When I first had that pain, I couldn't do a lot of things, like going fishing, no playing basketball, or going dancing
>
> I didn't, I didn't think that, uh, It could be any worse
>
> Change your body – the heart starts to get coherent and the heart starts to affect the brain, and the brain starts to affect the heart and the heart starts to affect the brain waves like this and they're moving and you see Alpha and you see Beta and you see Beta and you see Delta and *you can see from the body, via the body, back of the body, top of the body, heal your body. The body can't heal the body, you have to get beyond your body to heal your body, change your body*. The number of dimensions, in which we are going to be asked to excel suddenly gets way bigger. Can, can you do this without falling over, without dropping the plate? Are you an orthogonal thinker? Are you good at manipulating symbols? *There's going to be this array of things, against which we suddenly, not just have to be good enough, but we have to, excel*. In the elegant moment, and we switch, flip the switch. And then all it takes is a tiny little push with a finger, and it's going to completely shift. That switch gets flipped. *Strap me in, let's give it a go*. The real action would be: 'hey, we can do things if you flip the switch' flip the switch flip the switch flip the switch flip the switch flip the switch flip the switch flip the switch flip the switch

Postscript

Twenty five years after our first production of *Feast During the Plague*, we found ourselves in the midst of a real-life pandemic. During this time, the themes addressed in *Placebo* have become even more apparent. We have seen widespread health anxiety and an unprecedented lack of agency over one's own health, with private decision making mandated by central government and its health advisors. How we talk about, manage and communicate public health, how we manage a 'cure' and respect different belief systems has always had global consequences – now this has become front-page news. What you say about an illness matters, and how you frame a treatment matters, too.

However, whilst anecdotal discussion about specific placebo effects has been rife amongst the public ('I'm not sure if it's a real headache or if I was just expecting one after my booster jab'), it has been spoken about less in public health messaging. One recent study carried out by the Placebo Studies Programme at Harvard Medical School that did not make the headlines was a meta-analysis of coronavirus vaccine trials that found that 35% of patients receiving a placebo reported systemic adverse events (most commonly fatigue and headache) (Haas *et al.*, 2022).

What makes individuals, communities, countries feel better (or worse) in the wake of this virus? The emergence of long COVID and concerns that a 'mental health epidemic' is inevitable make this a question which we urgently need to address.

I know through my own experiences of the healthcare system that the nature and quality of care – the performance of care – can fundamentally affect the *will to live*. Sadly, people can be as traumatised by their hospital experiences as by their illness – as we have seen *en masse* over the pandemic. Perhaps, as medical philosopher Charlotte Blease (2012) argues, we should rename the placebo effect the positive care effect and spend more time and resource on understanding and harnessing the power of all the elements that make placebos effective – that make people feel better.

If changes in lighting, environment, intention, language, style and movement can help ease the pain, a powerful argument emerges for the role of arts and culture in the health and well-being of an individual (or a nation). The pandemic has presented a radical moment in which to imagine and implement a profound partnership between culture, health and social care – with the need to engage isolated people in communal activity and to support healthcare professionals becoming ever more apparent. The social prescribing movement – where GPs can refer their patients to arts activities – is gathering momentum in the UK, with state investment in the idea that a trip to an art gallery or going to choir can effect health benefits. For many artists, the apparent absurdity of a health system prescribing arts activity is enraging and points to a reductive, instrumentalising of the arts. But perhaps this can be seen as a small step towards actually healing a schism or rebalancing a system that has been detrimental to our health – a recognition that a place which does not celebrate our living world, and honour our dead, through music, poetry, colour, dance, song and ceremony is not a place in which human beings can thrive.

Credits

Placebo is a performance piece by Clod Ensemble
  First performed at Lowry, Salford in 2018

Direction – Suzy Willson
Music – Paul Clark
Performed by Brian Caillet, Chihiro Kawasaki, Elisabeth Schilling, Nathan Goodman, Omar Gordon, Valerie Ebuwa and Yen-Ching Lin
Movement material created by the company
My Lonely Lungs monologue – Peggy Shaw
Costume – Art School (Eden Loweth and Tom Barratt)
Lighting – Hansjörg Schmidt
Dramaturgical Consultant – Stephen Brown
Musicians – Christopher Allan (Cello); Calina de la Mare (Violin); Luca Ricci (Accordion); Esther Black (Bass); Osman Yilmaz (Flute); Alison Lively (percussion); Izzy Stepanova (Piano); Aden Titftieyk (Trumpet)
Research – Bella Eacott
Producer – Roxanne Peak Payne
Commissioned by The Place.
Supported by a Wellcome Sustaining Excellence Award and Arts Council England.

Notes

1 Available at: www.clodensemble.com/placebo-if-i-only-had-a-brain/.
2 The image originates from Uppland, Sweden, 1918. Available at: https://commons.wikimedia.org/wiki/File:Folklig_l%C3%A4kekonst._Sm%C3%B6jning._Uppland_-_Nordiska_Museet_-_NMA.0034675.jpg.

Reference list

Bernstein, M.H. *et al.* (2020) 'Putting the "art" in the "art of medicine": the under-explored role of artifacts in placebo studies', *Frontiers in Psychology*, 11(1354). https://doi.org/10.3389/fpsyg.2020.01354
Blease, C. (2012) 'The principle of parity: the "placebo effect" and physician communication', *Journal of Medical Ethics*, 38(4), pp. 199–203. https://doi.org/10.1136/medethics-2011-100177

De Craen, A.J. *et al.* (1996) 'Effect of colour of drugs: systematic review of perceived effect of drugs and of their effectiveness', *British Medical Journal*, 313(2072), pp. 1624–1625. https://doi.org/10.1136/bmj.313.7072.1624

Haas et al. (2022) 'Frequency of adverse events in the placebo arms of COVID-19 vaccine trials: a systematic review and meta-analysis', *JAMA network open*, 5(1), pp.e2143955-e2143955.

Jonas, W.B. *et al.* (2015) 'To what extent are surgery and invasive procedures effective beyond a placebo response? A systematic review with meta-analysis of randomised, sham controlled trials', *British Medical Journal*, 5. https://doi.org/10.1136/bmjopen-2015-009655

Kaptchuk, T. and Miller, F.G. (2015) 'Placebo effects in medicine', *New England Journal of Medicine*, 373(1), pp. 8–9.

Kaptchuk, T. *et al.* (2010) 'Placebos without deception: a randomized controlled trial in irritable bowel syndrome', *PLoS One*, 5. https://doi.org/10.1371/journal.pone.0015591

Kelley, J.M. *et al.* (2014) 'The influence of the patient-clinician relationship on healthcare outcomes: a systematic review and meta-analysis of randomized controlled trials', *PLoS One*, 9(4), p. e94207. https://doi.org/10.1371/journal.pone.0094207

Manchikanti, L. *et al.* (2012) 'Opioid epidemic in the United States', *Pain Physician*, 14(3), pp, ES9–ES38.

Marchant, J. (2016) *Cure: a journey into the science of mind over body*. Chicago: Turabian.

Miller, F.G. and Kaptchuk, T. (2008) 'The power of context: reconceptualizing the placebo effect', *Journal of the Royal Society of Medicine*, 101(5), pp. 222–225. https://doi.org/10.1258/jrsm.2008.070466

Verhamme, K.M.C. and Bohnen, A.M. (2019) 'Are we facing an opioid crisis in Europe', *The Lancet Public Health*, 4(10), pp. E483–E484.

44

TO ENTER A PLACE OF PAIN

The work of Eugenie Lee

Bec Dean

The personal experience of physical pain is a challenging one to interpret or to represent to other people. Academic and theorist, Elaine Scarry wrote in her seminal text, *The Body in Pain: The Making and Unmaking of the World*, about the difficulty of expressing physical pain, stating that 'physical pain is exceptional in the whole fabric of psychic, somatic and perceptual states for being the only one that has no object' (1985, p. 161). In this chapter I write about pain conveyed in performance and participation through my experience of working curatorially over several years with the Korean-Australian artist Eugenie Lee. In Lee's work, the artist's highly subjective experience of persistent pain is transferred through experimental technologies and real-time engagement with participants into an immersive form of shared knowledge and understanding of a state that is elusive both to understand and to portray.

In 2015, I commissioned Lee's interactive performance work *Seeing Is Believing* for my curatorial project, *The Patient: The Medical Subject in Contemporary Art*, which was first exhibited at University of New South Wales Galleries in Sydney, Australia, in 2016. Composed of works made by twelve contemporary artists and collaborations from the 1970s to the present day, *The Patient* engaged with artistic practices that represented patient perspectives of the medical context – predominantly the experiences of the artists themselves. As a PhD project, I set numerous curatorial and social objectives for undertaking the exhibition, among them being to centre the work of artists-as-patients within public discourse on art and health and to raise what I called 'biomedical art' as an emerging field of interdisciplinary practice into conversations about how art can transform our understanding of illness, pain and mortality.

I define biomedical art in my doctoral research as being characterised by its aesthetic engagement with the medical and health sectors. Biomedical art practices utilise or collaborate with medical and biological science research to bring specialised knowledge into conversation with the lived experience of medical patients and their networks. In the case of *Seeing is Believing*, Eugenie Lee is a long-term patient with persistent pain who gathered collaborators across neuroscience, virtual reality, haptic device development and acoustic engineering to create an immersive aesthetic experience that can transcend the challenges of expressing persistent pain to other people.[1]

In the following paragraphs, I describe a first-person account of engaging as a participant in *Seeing Is Believing*. This is an attempt to bring you as reader inside the work while emphasising the importance for Lee of devising a project that needs to be experienced physiologically and

DOI: 10.4324/9781003036500-50

emotionally in real-time in order to be understood. As Scarry relates in her treatise on pain, I recognise that a written description is insufficient to the task, but I hope that in some way it conveys the sense of trepidation, claustrophobia and discomfort verging on fear which still resonates within me years later. My memory of this work resides like a fragment of a horror movie that builds from waiting and isolation, through clinical procedure, to an immersive viscerality.

Seeing Is Believing

I sit in a waiting area that has been arranged inside a gallery. There are two white, wooden chairs placed against a black wall, opposite three small enclosures. The central enclosure takes the form of a black box with a closed door that is large enough to be considered human scale.

The artist enters the waiting room and takes me to the most open of these spaces where we sit and introduce ourselves at a white table with two chairs. She is a small Korean woman in her thirties, with friendly eyes but a quiet and insistent demeanour. At the table I sign a paper print-out of a document, which is full of complex legalese that diminishes personal responsibility for her role as an artist, and provides my consent for what is about to happen.

In the far enclosure, she leads me to a desk stacked with a black box object like a small road case – a reinforced box for transporting fragile equipment – that has various apertures in its top and sides. She asks me to extend my hands through the largest of these at the front of the case facing me, which I do with a little hesitancy, and I see them appear in front of my eyes on a digital display on the top of the case. She initiates a computer programme where blue blocks of colour appear around my hands and continues to talk to me about their appearance. The blocks close in around my hands and she instructs me to keep them inside the blue lines. Soon, the digital display erases the side of the screen showing my right hand. The artist asks me to locate my right hand with my left hand inside the box, and instead of feeling the warmth of my own flesh, my hand touches the hardness of the box. Even though the box is only a foot wide, I have managed to lose my sense of where my hand is. I laugh and feel slightly disoriented as I withdraw my hands.

Initiating another computer programme and the next test, she asks me to put my right hand inside the case again, and to extend my index finger. My pointing hand appears in the digital display, and she lightly pinches the tip of my index finger. I feel a pulling sensation and my finger appears to grow, like a rubber band being stretched-out. She stops pulling and my finger remains elongated in the display. Then she pushes her finger against the tip of mine, and I can feel it shrinking while watching my finger become a stump of knuckle on the screen. I remove my hands from the case, and of course, they appear as normal as they did at the start of the experiment.

We leave this area and the artist invites me inside what looks like a bank vault with a table and chair installed inside it. It is about one and a half metres square and lined with upholstered fabric padding – quite literally, a padded cell. I sit on the chair and am instructed to slip on a glove that is connected to cables, as well as an Oculus virtual reality (VR) headset. In the Oculus' display, I can see my gloved hand represented in the VR space which has turned the inside of the padded cell a blood red, and I wiggle my fingers in front of my 'eyes'. My digital arm is synced to my movements and I start to feel pressure in my ears and silence fills the space around me as the door to this room is closed behind me. I feel that I am alone.

In the VR feed, I see my hand and arm begin to swell, taking on the sweaty appearance and turgid feel of uncooked sausages. My hand feels tight and hot, the skin thin and pulsating inside the glove as if under pressure or exertion. The blood red of the VR space darkens, and metallic scraping sounds accompany a vision of barbed wire creeping into the ceiling above my virtual body. The wire scratches and inches towards my hand, eventually piercing it through my palm. I feel heat and pain at the point of rupture. I am about to cry out, to ask the artist to stop the sequence, when the wire winds back and my swollen hand appears to return to normal.

After a moment, the door of the chamber opens. I remove the glove and headset and walk with the artist to a third space, offering two chairs facing each other across the table. My heart rate begins to slow and after taking some time to compose myself, we talk about what happened.

Dealing in pain

Lee's work deals in pain. It does not seek to represent it but to create the conditions whereby an experience of pain may be delivered to participants in her work without causing any form of lasting harm or injury – indeed, any 'actual' pain. It seeks to elicit empathy for the pain experience by manufacturing its semblance but while doing so to purposefully broaden knowledge of human perception. *Seeing Is Believing* is an embodied demonstration of the brain's plasticity, of the human body's ability to be made susceptible to suggestion and of the possibility that pain has the potential to be treated in ways other than pharmacologically.

When I met Lee in 2014, I was undertaking doctoral research about artists-as-patients in relation to my curatorial practice and seeking to define the emerging field I was piecing together of biomedical art. The exhibition I eventually curated, *The Patient*, included well-known trailblazers of art and medicine including ORLAN, Bob Flanagan and Sheree Rose and Jo Spence, alongside more recent practice and new commissions by Australian artists and groups.[2] I commissioned *Seeing Is Believing*, by Lee, which was to be the artist's first foray into both performance and augmented reality. The project bound the neuroscience research of her collaborators with her lived experience as a patient with 'chronic' or persistent pain.

In the works of biomedical art I was studying and commissioning at this time, I was witnessing the separation enacted by the diagnostic 'medical gaze' – of the medical subject from their identity – being transformed and made new by the empowerment of artists in perceiving and researching their own illness and pathology through a scientific lens, within the laboratories of biomedical science and with the support of scientific collaborators. I was finding that artists working in this field, by accessing the instruments, methods and perspectives of scientific research, were able to not only resist complete objectification as medical subjects but to publicly challenge presumed medical orthodoxies or persistent misunderstandings or stigma towards medical conditions.

At the time of our meeting to discuss the exhibition, Lee was reaching the end of a representational arc in her work, which had sought to convey her experience of persistent pain through figurative painting and installation. In her two-dimensional works, Lee represented herself clothed in white gowns – traditional Korean funeral garments – and isolated inside neat, domestic settings, crouched on furniture or surrounded by encroaching barbed wire or visceral red gore – a kind of domestic gothic. In a large-scale installation called *McGill Pain Questionnaire* (2012), which replicated two towering rows of medical filing cabinets, Lee referenced the limitations of expressing pain through the use of the McGill Pain Scale – one of many language- or numerical-based measures that general practitioners and clinicians use to assess a patient's pain level.

While the work featured a mechanical spindle running like a spine through the centre of one of the cabinets, where ferocious-looking barbed wire scratched against plexiglass, it positioned the viewer comfortably outside the drama of these mechanics. The pain it represented was still contained within an objectified, impenetrable other, signifying the repressed silence experienced by millions of people living with persistent pain. Following the production of this work, Lee found that her creative exhaustion with representational mediums to convey her ideas and experience to others was mirrored by ideas in pain theory. Like many who suffer from persistent pain, Lee was challenged by the practical limits of expressing physical pain to other people, including her clinicians:

> The clinicians, because of their university training, understand pain only in relation to tissue damage. So, if there is an ongoing pain, you just cut off that nerve that's linked to that area and then you should be fine. But people with chronic pain still experience ongoing pain, and clinicians don't understand why. So the patient often gets pushed aside because the case is too difficult.
>
> (Lee, 2017)

The persistent pain that Lee interrogates in her work is called complex regional pain syndrome (CRPS) and stems from no injury upon the body of those who experience it (Better Health, no date). Although pain may be felt to emanate from a limb or in an internal organ of a patient with CRPS, there is no tangible bodily site to be identified or treated. Guiding Lee's research and engagement of scientific partners for *Seeing Is Believing* was her desire to find answers and potential solutions for her ongoing experience of CRPS, an experience that could not be reconciled with a solo, studio-based, painting practice. Her connection to neuroscientists at the research institute Body in Mind (BiM) at the University of South Australia was made possible first through a residency supported by Accessible Arts and then by Australian Network for Art and Technology (ANAT) in Adelaide.[3] Lee was interested in developing a visual and psycho-sensory language beyond the reaches of representational painting, as the subject of her work was her own experience of the 'visceral' form of CRPS – pain within the body's organs rather than a limb.

Smoke and mirrors in the theatre of pain research

In my description of *Seeing Is Believing*, Lee first engages me in an examination using a Mirage Machine, a digital version of the 'Disappearing Hand Trick' test for perception, in which my brain is tricked into losing track of the spatial coordinates of my right hand (Bellan *et al.*, 2021, pp. 1–21). This Mirage Machine is a real tool of neuroscience, and the illusion it produces is one of several in the neuroscience toolkit for demonstrating brain plasticity.[4] The machine shows the participant that their perception of their self in time and space is connected to a range of sensory inputs that can be easily augmented by external forces.

The use of rich media environments in pain research was the basis for Lee's engagement as an artist with BiM, a research laboratory that investigates the role of brain and mind in chronic pain. Engaging with Lee during a visit to her BiM residency in South Australia, I participated in a mediated-reality programme for back pain, where patients are shown a real-time display of themselves from behind, and are then able to use the programme to digitally change the shape of their backs (Nishigami *et al.*, 2019, pp. 178–183). This act in the virtual world potentially improves the psycho-bio perception of the participant's back pain, or in my case, a temporary sense of a better posture in the real world.

The ability for our brains to quickly attune our bodies and our senses to the immersive spatial environments of VR and other mediated reality is the subject of hundreds of 'fail' compilations on YouTube, where, within seconds of donning a headset, people are filmed crashing into the boundaries of their real surroundings or perceiving virtual threats as real ones. The ability of the brain to adapt to virtual and augmented reality environments has been of significant benefit to neuroscience research into persistent pain experience and treatment, the hypothesis underpinning this experiment being that pain experiences may be able to be modulated through illusory techniques and technologies.

As a person with CRPS, Lee was keen to replicate for participants in her work a common physical presentation of CRPS, where one hand or foot of the patient becomes swollen at the site where pain is perceived. To realise this, she collaborated with a range of computer scientists and digital designers to take neuroscientific ideas around multisensory perception into a performance environment combining VR, sound and haptic devices. Virtual reality artist and academic Andrew Burrell created the digital environment and sonic interior of the padded cell and represented the invasive barbed wire and the meaty hand of the simulation, while a team of wearable device developers created a tight-fitting, vibrating glove to apply pressure and warmth upon the hand to simulate its swelling.[5]

The scientific thesis upon which *Seeing Is Believing* is based is the idea that persistent pain is formed in the protective, motivational and emotional areas of the brain and heightened by a range of psychological factors, including fear, anxiety, depression and the anticipation of pain itself, which Lee seeks to mimic in her work (Woo, 2010, pp. 8–12). This idea is broadly understood within the biopsychosocial model of pain, where biological, physical and social factors all contribute to one's pain experience (Turk, Wilson and Swanson, 2010, p. 16). The use of the mediated reality tool for delivering temporary pain relief in patients is reversed by Lee in *Seeing Is Believing* within her performance, to instead use it to manifest an embodiment of pain-like experience in participants. Lee identifies this phenomenon as an example of the nocebo effect – the opposite of placebo – in this case, where harm to the body is perceived through the subject's belief that they have been harmed.

While we have more sophisticated technological tools for creating illusions than the smoke and mirrors of an earlier century, the neurological foundations upon which such illusions are manifested remain the same. Our sensory receptors help us to make sense of the world, and facets of this 'world' can be fabricated or augmented around us, including through forms of social interaction. Throughout her performance, Lee focuses the attention and the psycho-cognitive state of the participant around an anticipation of something unpleasant happening to them in the confines of a dark, cramped and noiseless space, which primes them with a sense of unease in preparation for the intense, mixed reality environment.

Experience design and the visitor

As a visitor to a gallery, one may anticipate being intellectually or emotionally challenged by images, forms, concepts and ideas and through performance practice, by the bodies, utterances or feats of endurance of artists in real time. From my own experience of working with arts organisations and galleries in this early part of the twenty-first century, I understand galleries to be exceptionally risk-averse environments, so that any possibility of actual or perceived harm that may be caused to a visitor through any material or action is either mitigated or reduced to zero. As public spaces, galleries are designed to be safe, which is a rational and legislated response to harm minimisation. The practical challenges that Lee's biomedical art presents for galleries and for curatorial practice are bound up in this institutional management of visitor safety, alongside the principles of human ethics – including the principle of doing no harm to the subjects of scientific experiments – that accompany the collaborative science research facets of her work. Lee introduces instruments into the exhibition space, including the Mirage Machine and methods for using virtual reality that are borrowed from neuroscience research laboratories. In turn, these instruments bring along with them a range of methodologies and conditions for their use, including rigorous consent procedures for any participants or patients engaging with them.

The solutions to these challenges for the performance of *Seeing Is Believing* were provided by Lee's original design for the work to be experienced as a pseudo-medical consultation. While she had originally intended to present the project as a one-on-one performance of a thirty-minute appointment (this was extended to forty-five minutes), the addition of legal documents and the reproduction of consent procedures by her scientific partners in consultation with the gallery bolstered a perception of personal risk on the part of the participant while effectively mitigating risks across her various partnerships – including with myself as curator. Alongside the technological manifestation of illusion, the use of darkness and confined spaces and the incorporation of persuasive language and performance, Lee's work builds an appreciative anticipation of risk to the participant's body through other less aesthetic means – including the incorporation of complex legalese, a booking system and a script. As Lee recounts of early negotiations on the performance development with her research partners:

> I had to have my entire performance script approved by them. They directed me word-by-word, line-by-line, through the entire performance. All three stages. They told me that I would need to orally present the legal disclosure, which would then be signed by the participant. But I was also directed to explain every detail of the performance and participant's interaction, so there would be no surprises. But I thought, 'There has to be a surprise! This is art'.
>
> (Lee, 2017)

While the project's human ethics challenges threatened to disclose everything that would take place in the performance, thereby neutralising the nocebo effect, Lee developed a partial solution with her collaborators in which the participant's legal disclaimer could be signed in the process of their making an online booking for an appointment. So even prior to presenting at the venue, each performance participant was made aware of personal risk, signing away control and a degree of personal agency, and this awareness was reinforced by Lee through the three stages of her performance.

The pseudo-medical construct anticipated through the booking system also carried through to the exhibition design for the performance. Lee's space included a waiting room, a consultation area equipped with medical apparatus and a table and two chairs arranged for debriefing. The most complex component of the spatial design for the project was the construction of a functional anechoic chamber, an engineered environment designed to completely muffle external noise, built to house the VR component of the work. Designed with the support of an acoustic engineer and architect, this black box served a range of purposes: to seem scientific, to emulate the function of a padded cell and to cause a change in pressure and acoustic environment when the door closed, so that any participant would become more aware of their body and its enclosure prior to applying the VR headset and glove.

As closely as possible, Lee sought to connect findings and theories in neuroscience with her lived experience with CRPS, which included feelings of fear, isolation and being at the mercy of someone else's academic or clinical perspective. At the same time, Lee used the design of the consultation and its three stages to reverse her own role from that of patient to specialist. Following its initial presentation, the exhibition tour to galleries in regional towns of Australia enabled Lee to further develop the social engagement facets of her work and her performance to reinforce suggestions and expectations of pain experience and the idea of imminent threat or danger to participants. As curator, my attention to care in this work – for both the project and its people – was committed to providing supportive scaffolding so that Lee and her participants could briefly partake in care's inversion into pain (or something that seemed painful) and in crossing the dualities of sick/well and doctor/patient. For the tour, this included shortening the consultation periods for *Seeing Is Believing*, allowing Lee more rest time between appointments and scheduling the work as a live public programme rather than as a continuing form of artistic labour throughout the exhibition's season. While there is a common understanding of the etymological underpinning of curating to care, in terms of care for objects and attending to behind-the-scenes labour, I have found it essential in my own practice to return to this foundational principle in order to expand it to caring for artists, audiences and the lifecycle of an artwork (Dean, 2021, pp. 101–102).

Biomedical art and patient agency

In *The Birth of the Clinic: An Archaeology of Medical Perception*, originally published 1963, Michel Foucault introduced the concept of the 'medical gaze', charting the development of this concept over time and through the specificity – including the politics – of the social contexts of modern medicine (1994). However, this diagnostic gaze, while clearly focused on patient health and the betterment of medical knowledge, establishes a doctor-patient power differential in which patients are invariably positioned as the vulnerable and less knowledgeable party. In *Seeing Is Believing*, the artist's lived experience of pain is inserted within a performance space for pseudo-treatment. Through this work, and with the support of science partners, Lee muddies the duality of the doctor/patient relationship as it extends to knowledge and agency and presents another possibility for ideas in neuroscience to reach public awareness.

In *Seeing Is Believing*, participants in the work are presented with an opportunity to put themselves on the other side of the dichotomy of wellness and illness and to allow themselves to be briefly and purposefully discomfited. Unlike Lee's installation work, *McGill Pain Questionnaire*, this participatory performance reaches beyond the capacities of any object produced as a representation of pain to create an experience that produces a transformative encounter for the participant, drawing them into a more profound understanding of pain. This in turn suggested empathic ways for sharing knowledge through bodily experience, using the aesthetics of technology and performance.

As artist-as-patient, Lee navigates the power differential produced by the medical gaze through multi-layered, co-productive collaborations, which network her practice within potential emerging treatment research for persistent pain and through experimental practice in virtual and augmented reality and other forms of rich media that are now proliferating within various medical and mental health treatment contexts.

The artist-as-patient

Alongside many of the artists represented in the exhibition, Lee presented work that referenced her medical patient body as a body of knowledge rather than as compliant and helplessly objectified within a medical system. Lee's body in particular – and at her own insistence – was present in the gallery space across the exhibition's entire first season in 2016, delivering performance after performance for four days a week over a period of seven weeks. And while I have made much of the artistic agency and the dynamic presence produced by the artist in her own work, it remained that her performance schedule was overly taxing, and the gallery environment lacked accessible infrastructure to support Lee to take proper breaks and refresh.

While rigorous disclaimer and disclosure processes were woven into Lee's performance to benefit the safety of the visitor, her own self-care and health were compromised by the same measures. In our interview following the first presentation of the work, we discussed how the project could be modified to be less impactful and tiring on her body for the various iterations of the exhibition's tour and her future productions:

> Instead of a forty-five-minute performance, I'm going to reduce it down to twenty minutes . . . it would be a better performance work and bring out potentially better reactions from participants as well. I'm not going to talk as much as the scientists asked me to originally.
>
> (Lee, 2017)

Since the exhibition and tour of *The Patient*, and her presentation of *Seeing Is Believing* independently, Lee has continued to work with some of her original neuroscience collaborators on a new participatory performance project. With Professor Jill Bennett, I was able to curate an early version for *The Empathy Clinic* (2019), an exhibition for The Big Anxiety festival of art, science and people, focused on mental health also at the UNSW Galleries in 2019. The work, *Break Out My Pelvic Sorcery* (*BOMPS*; 2019–ongoing), transforms the arcade game *Breakout* into a haptic, virtual reality experience, where participants have pain simulations delivered to their pelvic region while performing a seemingly simple task of bouncing a ball against a wall.

As a project focused quite literally on the physical performance of individual participants rather than drawing on the endurance capacity of Lee herself, *BOMPS* deliberately relegates the artist to the position of sideshow operator – a puller of strings. It suggests the expansion of Lee's pain performance repertoire into a range of lived-experience specificities, including, in this case, the pelvic pain caused by endometriosis. As a complementary opposite to *Seeing Is Believing*, *BOMPS* is a portable work requiring little aesthetic embellishment or scaffolding to support it, just a space with a computer, a VR kit and a haptic belt. Rather than building a fearful anticipation of pain from the expectation of an unpleasant appointment, *BOMPS* offers the experience of pain sensation in the shockingly juxtaposed context of light entertainment. Its 'hacked' devices attack participants in their pelvic region, awakening primal vulnerability in the middle of play and laughter, causing them to utter a scream or an expletive (Reich, 2021). It creates annoyance, irritation and an immediate recognition of the ways in which pelvic pain may disrupt an ordinary day and the most basic of functions.

Interruption of a health crisis

Lee's development of *BOMPS* and similar projects was paused in 2020 when the coronavirus pandemic placed the work of artistic communities across the world in a holding pattern. At the time of writing this, the pandemic continues, and there is a lingering hesitancy towards the presentation of forms of artistic interactivity where devices need to be shared between people. Nothing that cannot be adequately wiped and sanitised is easily operable.

When I was undertaking research for *The Patient*, we were facing a burgeoning health crisis in Australia mirrored in other countries, which was exacerbated by a lack of adequate health care for an increasingly ageing population. This situation has been amplified by the pandemic, as patients of all kinds other than COVID-19, including those with hidden disabilities like persistent pain, are sidelined as non-critical by hospitals on the verge of exhaustion. Many artists I have worked with over the past few years are still confined to their domestic spaces and are forging ways to continue important discourses and expand their creative networks across art, medicine, health and disability justice through other means. Lee continues to engage her collaborators and anticipate the ways in which interaction and participation in her work may be realised in the future.

The work of artists like Lee who have lived experience of illness, disability and the medical sector will be vital as we emerge from the present health crisis into another one and face the task of reorganising and repositioning our art and culture in relation to this. As I describe through *Seeing Is Believing*, the work of artists-as-patients, and the rich forms of interdisciplinary collaborations found in biomedical art, can create new forms of knowledge and more profound understandings of medical patient experience and its ambiguities – suggesting a powerful case for the integral role of art in life.

Notes

1 I refer to chronic pain as persistent pain throughout this chapter, as it is the preferred adjective of the artist and many advocates with lived experience to describe this condition.
2 These included new works and commissions by Australian artists Guy Ben-Ary and team, Helen Pynor, Bianca Willoughby, recent work by Ingrid Bachmann (Canada), Tim Wainwright & John Wynne (UK/Aus) and historical work by Australian artists Brenton Heath Kerr, Carol Jerrems and David McDiarmid.
3 Lee's pain science collaborators were Dr Tasha Stanton, Dr Valeria Bellan and Professor Lorimer Moseley at the University of South Australia and Body in Mind research group (BIM) based at the Sansom Institute for Health Research at the University of South Australia.
4 The Mirage Machine is an invention of scientist Dr Roger Newport of Oxford University's Mirage Lab, loaned for the exhibition and tour.
5 The wearable device developers were Stuart Esdaile, Rosie Menzies, Tom Hazell, Blake Segula and Corey Stewart.

Reference list

Bellan, V. *et al*. (2021) 'Where is my arm? Investigating the link between complex regional pain syndrome and poor localisation of the affected limb', *PeerJ*, 9, pp. 1–21, e11882.

Better Health (no date) *Complex regional pain syndrome (CRPS)*. Available at: www.betterhealth.vic.gov.au/health/conditionsandtreatments/complex-regional-pain-syndrome-crps (Accessed: 22 January 2022).

Dean, B. (2021) 'Curatorial care and the lively materials of biomedical art', in Muller, L. and Langhill, C.S. (eds.) *Curating lively objects: exhibitions beyond disciplines*. London: Routledge, pp. 101–102.

Foucault, M. (1994) *The birth of the clinic: an archaeology of medical perception*. New York, NY: Vintage Books, p. 196.

Lee, E (2012) *MacGill Pain Questionnaire*. Main Gallery, Sydney College of the Arts, Sydney: University of Sydney.

Lee, E. (2017) Interviewed by Bec Dean, 29 March, Project No. HC15850.

Nishigami, T. *et al*. 2019. 'Embodying the illusion of a strong, fit back in people with chronic low back pain: a pilot proof-of-concept study', *Musculoskeletal Science and Practice*, 39, pp. 178–183.

Reich, H. (2021) 'Australian artist Eugenie Lee evokes the chronic pain of endometriosis in high-tech experiential artworks', *ABC News*, 3 January. Available at: www.abc.net.au/news/2021-01-03/artist-eugenie-lee-chronic-pain-of-endometriosis-vr-installation/12989868 (Accessed: 4 January 2022).

Scarry, E. (1985) *The body in pain*. Oxford: Oxford University Press, p. 161.

Turk, D.C., Wilson, H. and Swanson, K.S. (2010) 'The biopsychosocial model of pain and pain management', in Ebert, M.H. and Kerns, R.D. (eds.) *Behavioural and psychopharmacologic pain management*. Cambridge: Cambridge University Press, p. 16.

Woo, A.K.M. (2010) 'Depression and anxiety in pain', *Reviews in Pain*, 4(1), pp. 8–12. https://doi.org/10.1177/204946371000400103

INDEX

For Product Safety Concerns and Information please contact our EU
representative GPSR@taylorandfrancis.com
Taylor & Francis Verlag GmbH, Kaufingerstraße 24, 80331 München, Germany